D0857251

ATLAS OF THE HEART

Editor-in-Chief

J. Willis Hurst, MD

Candler Professor of Medicine (Cardiology)
Emory University School of Medicine
Chief of Cardiology
Emory University Hospital and Emory Clinic
Atlanta, Georgia

Associate Editors

Robert H. Anderson, MD

Director and Joseph Levy Professor of
　Paediatric Cardiac Morphology
The Cardiothoracic Institute, University of London
Honorary Consultant, Brompton Hospital
London, UK

Anton E. Becker, MD

Professor of Pathology
University of Amsterdam
Academic Medical Center
Amsterdam, The Netherlands

Benson R. Wilcox, MD

Professor of Surgery
Chief, Division of Cardiothoracic Surgery
University of North Carolina
School of Medicine
Chapel Hill, North Carolina

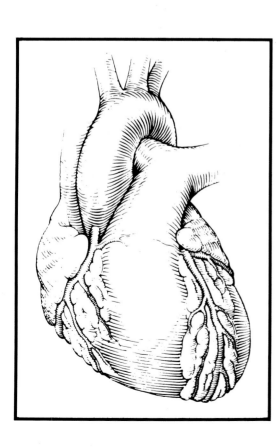

McGRAW-HILL BOOK COMPANY

New York St. Louis San Francisco Colorado Springs Oklahoma City
Auckland Bogotá Caracas Hamburg Lisbon London Madrid Mexico Milan
Montreal New Delhi Panama Paris San Juan São Paulo Singapore Sydney
Tokyo Toronto

GOWER MEDICAL PUBLISHING
New York London

ATLAS OF THE HEART

Copyright © 1988 by Gower Medical Publishing,
a division of J.B. Lippincott Company.
101 Fifth Avenue, New York, NY 10003

All rights reserved. No part of this publication may be reproduced, stored in a retrieval system, or transmitted in any form or by any means electronic, mechanical, photocopying, recording, or otherwise, without prior permission of the publisher.

Library of Congress Cataloging-in-Publication Data

Atlas of the heart.

   Includes bibliographies and index.
   1. Heart—Diseases—Atlases.   I. Hurst, J. Willis
(John Willis), 1920–   [DNLM: 1. Heart Diseases—
atlases.   WG 17 A8844]
RC682.A82   1988   616.1′2′00222   87-37839

ISBN 0-07-031501-9 (McGraw-Hill)

NOTICE
Medicine is an ever-changing science. As new research and clinical experience broaden our knowledge, changes in treatment and drug therapy are required. The editors and publisher of this work have made every effort to ensure that the drug dosage schedules herein are accurate and in accord with the standards accepted at the time of publication. Readers are advised, however, to check the product information sheet included in the package of each drug they plan to administer to be certain that changes have not been made in the recommended dose or in the contraindications for administration. This recommendation is of particular importance in regard to new or infrequently used drugs.

Cover illustration reproduced with permission from King SB, Douglas JS: *Coronary Arteriography and Angioplasty.* Copyright © 1985, McGraw-Hill, NY. Illustration by Michael Budowick, Medical Artist, Emory University School of Medicine, Office of Medical Illustration.

      Editor: William J. Gabello
   Designer: Carol Drozdyk
  Illustrators: Laura Pardi, Sue Ann Fung
Art Director: Jill Feltham

10 9 8 7 6 5 4 3 2 1

Printed in Hong Kong by Imago Productions (FE) PTE Ltd.

To patients with heart disease
and to those dedicated to helping them

PREFACE

Abe Krieger of Gower Medical Publishing and Dereck Jeffers of the Health Professions Division of McGraw-Hill Book Company visited me in my office at Emory University Hospital in the early part of 1986. They were there to determine my interest in the creation of an atlas based on *The Heart,* for which I have been editor-in-chief for six editions.

I was interested in their proposal for two reasons. First, *The Heart* is a comprehensive text on the heart and blood vessels. Because of this, it is necessary to limit the size of such a book in every conceivable way; otherwise, it would be a yard thick. Accordingly, as author and editor, it has been necessary for me to limit the number of illustrations in *The Heart.* The solution to this problem, I thought, would be an atlas based on *The Heart,* in which color illustrations of pathology and surgery would be emphasized. I was informed that Dr. Robert H. Anderson of London, Dr. Anton E. Becker of Amsterdam, and Dr. Benson R. Wilcox of Chapel Hill, North Carolina, were prepared to supply the color illustrations. I was elated because I was familiar with Becker and Anderson's *Cardiac Pathology* and Wilcox and Anderson's *Surgical Anatomy of the Heart.* Both books are viewed by cardiologists as being informative and beautiful.

Secondly, as one who has struggled to teach, I have always appreciated the value of carefully designed illustrations in the art of communication. Visual stimuli are more likely to communicate than auditory stimuli. This is why reading is more valuable than listening to lectures. Accordingly, I have always favored the use of illustrations in communication.

So, I enthusiastically accepted the offer of Gower and McGraw-Hill. I then set about organizing an *Atlas of the Heart* that would complement *The Heart.* The first chapter of the *Atlas* on normal cardiac anatomy would be written by Drs. Anderson, Wilcox and Becker, and the second chapter on cardiac remodeling by Dr. Becker. For the most part, the remaining 16 chapters would be based on a selection of chapters from among the 138 chapters in *The Heart* and enhanced by the addition of new color photographs of pathology and surgery. The goal was to decrease the amount of text, retain a sufficient number of figures to illustrate clinical information, and increase the number of illustrations depicting pathology and surgery. Permission from the authors of *The Heart* was obtained, and they were asked to review and contribute to my synopsis of their chapters. Accordingly, their names have been added as authors of the chapters in the *Atlas.* In the case of Chapter 3, "Congenital Heart Disease," Dr. Anderson's name was also added as an author because of the amount of work he did on the text of this chapter.

We thank McGraw-Hill for permission to abstract selected chapters from *The Heart* and to reproduce illustrations published for the first time in any of the six editions of *The Heart* or other McGraw-Hill publications of which I was an author, such as *Atlas of Electrocardiography* (formerly published by Blakiston), *Introduction to Electrocardiography,* and *Electrocardiographic Interpretation.* For the use of other illustrations from *The Heart* that were previously published elsewhere, we obtained permission from the original source. Some of the illustrations used in *Atlas of the Heart* have been published by Gower in *Cardiac Pathology* and *Surgical Anatomy of The Heart.* In all cases, appropriate credit has been noted in the legend of the illustration and cited in full in the Figure Credits at the end of each chapter.

I have edited several books and authored a number of articles, but I must confess that this task was, without a doubt, the most difficult I have ever tackled. I persevered because of my belief that the final product would be valuable and because of the opportunity to work with Robert Anderson, Anton Becker, and Benson Wilcox who, I believe, are masters of their work. I thank them for their contributions to the text of each chapter and the beautiful illustrations. Their work is priceless. It is a joy to work with them. I again thank the authors and editors of the sixth edition of *The Heart* for permitting me to abstract the 16 chapters that were used to create the chapters in *Atlas of the Heart.*

I thank Gower and McGraw-Hill for giving me the opportunity to develop this *Atlas.* The task assigned was not easy, but I sensed it was worthwhile. Gower and its illustrators are first rate; I especially thank Laura Pardi for her magnificent artwork. I thank Abe Krieger of Gower and Dereck Jeffers of McGraw-Hill for their administrative ability in seeing this book to fruition. Bill Gabello of Gower deserves special thanks for his superb editing ability and administrative talent.

As I lean exhausted against the ropes, I wish to thank Carol Miller. Without her skill in organizing and typing, this book would not be.

I thank my wife Nelie. No Nelie, no book.

Now for a little rest—at least over the weekend.

J. Willis Hurst, MD

CONTENTS

I Anatomy of the Normal Heart and Its Response to Disease

II Diseases of the Heart

III   The Heart and Other Conditions

CONTRIBUTORS

Walter H. Abelmann, MD
Professor of Medicine, Harvard Medical School;
Physician, Beth Israel Hospital, Boston, Massachusetts

James K. Alexander, MD
Professor of Medicine, Baylor College of Medicine;
Chief of Cardiology, Veterans Administration Hospital,
Houston, Texas

Joseph S. Alpert, MD
Professor of Medicine; Director, Division of Cardiovascular
Medicine, University of Massachusetts Medical School,
Worcester, Massachusetts

James E. Dalen, MD
Professor and Chairman, Department of Medicine, University of
Massachusetts Medical School; Physician-in-Chief, University of
Massachusetts Hospital, Worcester, Massachusetts

David T. Durack, MB, DPhil
Professor of Medicine, Microbiology and Immunology;
Chief, Division of Infectious Diseases, Duke University
Medical Center, Durham, North Carolina

Harriet P. Dustan, MD
Professor of Medicine; Director, Cardiovascular Research
and Training Center, University of Alabama in Birmingham,
School of Medicine, Birmingham, Alabama

Gary Gerstenblith, MD
Associate Professor of Medicine, Johns Hopkins University
School of Medicine, Baltimore, Maryland

John F. Goodwin, MD
Emeritus Professor of Clinical Cardiology, Honorary Consulting
Physician, Royal Postgraduate Medical School,
Hammersmith Hospital, London, UK

Robert J. Hall, MD
Clinical Professor of Medicine, Baylor College of Medicine
and the University of Texas Medical School at Houston; Medical
Director, Texas Heart Institute; Director, Division of
Cardiology, St. Luke's Episcopal Hospital, Houston, Texas

W. Dallas Hall, MD
Professor of Medicine (Hypertension); Director, Division of
Hypertension, Emory University School of Medicine,
Atlanta, Georgia

Bernadine P. Healy, MD
Chairman of the Research Institute,
The Cleveland Clinic, Foundation Cleveland, Ohio

J. O'Neal Humphries, MD
O.B. Mayer Sr. and Jr. Professor of Medicine; Dean, School of
Medicine, University of South Carolina, Columbia, South Carolina

Hiroshi Kuida, MD
Professor of Internal Medicine and Physiology; Associate Dean,
Student Programs, University of Utah School of Medicine,
Salt Lake City, Utah

John H. Newman, MD
Associate Professor of Medicine, Elsa S. Hanigan Chair in
Pulmonary Medicine, Vanderbilt University School of Medicine and
St. Thomas Hospital, Nashville, Tennessee

Elizabeth W. Nugent, MD
Associate Professor of Pediatrics, Cardiology Division,
Emory University School of Medicine, Atlanta, Georgia

Scott J. Pollak, MD
Cardiac Fellow, Department of Medicine, Emory University School
of Medicine; Chief Resident in Medicine, Emory University Hospital
(1984–1987), Atlanta, Georgia

Edward L.C. Pritchett, MD
Associate Professor of Medicine, Division of Cardiology,
Duke University Medical Center, Durham, North Carolina

Charles E. Rackley, MD
Anton and Margaret Fuisz Professor of Medicine; Chairman,
Department of Medicine, Georgetown University Medical Center,
Washington, DC

Timothy J. Regan, MD
Professor of Medicine; Director, Division of Cardiovascular
Diseases, University of Medicine and Dentistry of New Jersey,
New Jersey Medical School, Newark, New Jersey

Joseph C. Ross, MD
Associate Vice-Chancellor for Health Affairs, Vanderbilt
University Medical Center, Nashville, Tennessee

Robert C. Schlant, MD
Professor of Medicine (Cardiology); Director,
Division of Cardiology, Emory University School of Medicine;
Chief of Cardiology, Grady Memorial Hospital,
Atlanta, Georgia

Ralph Shabetai, MD
Professor of Medicine, University of California San Diego; Chief
of Cardiology, San Diego Veterans Administration Medical Center,
San Diego, California

Panagiotis N. Symbas, MD
Professor of Surgery, Thoracic and Cardiovascular Surgery
Division, Emory University School of Medicine,
Atlanta, Georgia

Elbert P. Tuttle, Jr., MD
Professor of Medicine (Nephrology), Emory University School of
Medicine, Atlanta, Georgia

Andrew G. Wallace, MD
Kempner Professor of Medicine and Vice-Chancellor for
Health Affairs, Duke University Medical Center, Durham,
North Carolina

Myron L. Weisfeldt, MD
Professor of Medicine; Director, Cardiology Division,
The Johns Hopkins Hospital, Baltimore, Maryland

Nanette Kass Wenger, MD
Professor of Medicine (Cardiology), Emory University School of
Medicine; Director, Cardiac Clinics, Grady Memorial Hospital,
Atlanta, Georgia

Gary L. Wollam, MD
Formerly Associate Professor of Medicine (Hypertension),
Emory University School of Medicine, Atlanta, Georgia

I

ANATOMY OF THE NORMAL HEART AND ITS RESPONSE TO DISEASE

1
ANATOMY OF THE NORMAL HEART

Robert H. Anderson, MD
Benson R. Wilcox, MD
Anton E. Becker, MD

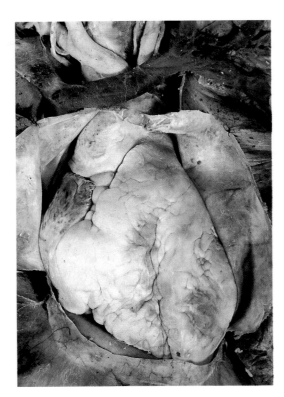

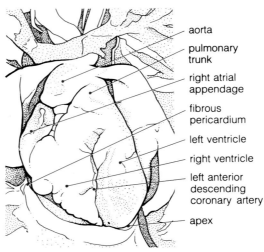

aorta
pulmonary trunk
right atrial appendage
fibrous pericardium
left ventricle
right ventricle
left anterior descending coronary artery
apex

FIG. 1.1 *The heart is seen within its pericardial cavity with the anterior thoracic wall removed and the fibrous pericardium incised. Note that the pericardial cavity is between the fibrous layer and the epicardium (see Fig. 1.2). Note also that the pulmonary trunk is anterior and to the left of the aorta.*

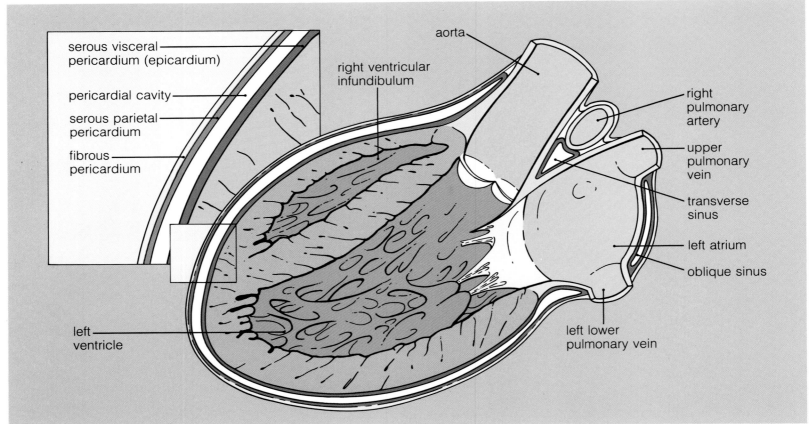

serous visceral pericardium (epicardium)

pericardial cavity

serous parietal pericardium

fibrous pericardium

right ventricular infundibulum

aorta

right pulmonary artery

upper pulmonary vein

transverse sinus

left atrium

oblique sinus

left ventricle

left lower pulmonary vein

FIG. 1.2 *A diagram of the long axis of the heart at right angles to the outlets shows the arrangement of the pericardium. The outer fibrous sack is firmly attached to the great arteries and veins at the base. The heart itself invaginates a second sack, the serous pericardium. The two layers of this serous membrane, however, are densely adherent to other structures. The inner layer (visceral) is attached to the surface of the myocardium as the epicardium. The outer layer (parietal) is attached to the fibrous* *pericardium. Effectively the pericardial cavity is located between the tough fibrous layer and the surface of the heart. Within this cavity are two recesses: transverse and oblique sinuses. As shown in the diagram, the transverse sinus is in the inner heart curvature while the oblique sinus is behind the diaphragmatic aspect of the left atrium, limited by the attachments of the pulmonary veins (see Fig. 1.19).*

To understand the normal action of the heart and to diagnose its abnormalities, particularly those due to congenital malformation, it is necessary to have complete and full knowledge of the usual arrangement of cardiac structure.

This knowledge starts with a consideration of the *position of the heart* within the chest. A mediastinal structure, the heart lies within its pericardial sack such that one third of its bulk is to the right of the midline (Fig. 1.1). The long axis of the heart is oblique, with the base in right-sided superior location and the apex extending well to the left. The right atrial appendage is a key landmark on the right border of the silhouette, while the pulmonary trunk occupies the left superior border, lying anteriorly and to the left of the aorta. The arrangement of the covering pericardial sack ensures smooth action of cardiac contraction. The pericardium has a firm fibrous layer which encloses and fuses with the outer membrane of a double serous layer. The inner layer of the serous sack fuses with the surface of the heart itself to form the epicardium. The pericardial cavity therefore is between the epicardium and the outer layer of serous pericardium, itself fused with the tough fibrous pericardium. Within the overall cavity thus formed are two distinct recesses, the oblique and transverse sinuses of the pericardium (Fig. 1.2).

The *arrangement of the cardiac chambers* themselves can be understood on the basis of the structure of the short axis. Figure 1.3 shows the structure of the atrioventricular valves relative to the aortic root. The latter structure is wedged deeply between the mitral and tricuspid orifices; the atrioventricular junctions then are encircled by major branches of the coronary arteries.

Further dissection (Fig. 1.4) shows the firm fibrous continuity existing between the sinuses of the aortic valve and the annulus of the mitral valve; this is the *cardiac skeleton,* which is much less well formed around the leaflets of the tricuspid valve. There is a very well formed block of fibrous and collagenous tissue where the support structures of the mitral, tricuspid, and aortic valves are all continuous. This is the central fibrous body, shown from its atrial aspect in Figure

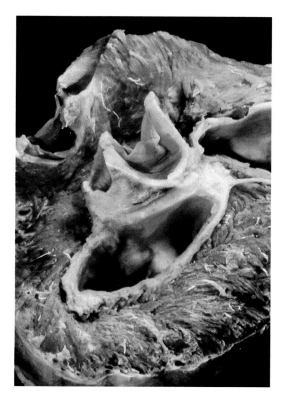

FIG. 1.3 *The superior aspect of the base of the heart is shown after removal of the atrial chambers. This view reveals the interrelationships of the aortic, tricuspid, and mitral valves, which underscores the arrangement of the fibrous skeleton (see Figs. 1.4–1.6). The aorta is deeply wedged between the two atrioventricular orifices. The coronary arteries emerge from the two* aortic sinuses closest to the pulmonary trunk and run round in the atrioventricular grooves. The leaflet arrangements of the atrioventricular valves are well seen, with mural and aortic (anterior) leaflets guarding the mitral orifice, and septal, anterosuperior, and inferior (mural) leaflets in the tricuspid orifice.

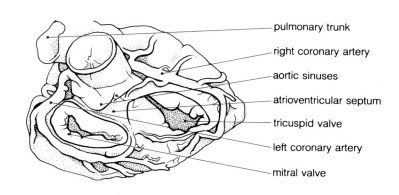

— pulmonary trunk
— right coronary artery
— aortic sinuses
— atrioventricular septum
— tricuspid valve
— left coronary artery
— mitral valve

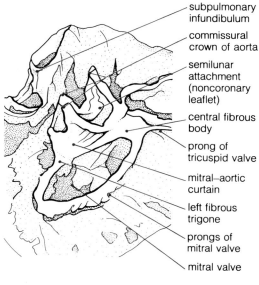

— subpulmonary infundibulum
— commissural crown of aorta
— semilunar attachment (noncoronary leaflet)
— central fibrous body
— prong of tricuspid valve
— mitral–aortic curtain
— left fibrous trigone
— prongs of mitral valve
— mitral valve

FIG. 1.4 *The fibrous skeleton has been dissected in this heart specimen, which appears in the same orientation as the specimen in Figure 1.3. The atrioventricular junction is bared down to the annulus of the mitral valve, while the aortic valve leaflets are removed to the level of their semilunar attachments. (Figure 1.5 shows these attachments from the ventricular aspect.) The fibrous skeleton is made up of the aortic–mitral unit together with much weaker extensions around the tricuspid orifice. The keystone of the skeleton is the central fibrous body, formed from fusion of the aortic, mitral, and tricuspid orifices. The dissection also shows well the extensive area of fibrous continuity between the aortic and mitral valves. This is thickened at each end to form the right and left fibrous trigones. The right trigone is then incorporated into the central fibrous body. The atrioventricular conduction axis penetrates through this body to reach the subaortic outflow tract (see Fig. 1.30). (Reproduced with permission of the authors and publisher; see Figure Credits)*

1.4 and from the ventricular aspect after removal of the skeleton from the ventricular mass in Figure 1.5. The leaflets of the aortic and mitral valves are then continuous, forming the roof of the subaortic outlet; they also form a block of fibrocollagenous tissue within the left margin of the outflow tract. This thickening strengthens the left margin of fibrous continuity and is called the left fibrous trigone. It complements the right trigone, which is incorporated into the central fibrous body. The remainder of the fibrous body is the membranous septum, which separates the subaortic outlet from the right atrium and ventricle, respectively (see below).

The function of the fibrous skeleton is to support the leaflets of the various valves and bind them to the myocardial masses. As can be seen from Figure 1.5, the skeleton is less well formed around the tricuspid valve orifice. In this position the leaflets spring from the fibro-fatty atrioventricular groove and are directly apposed to the right ventricular muscle mass. By and large it is the substance of the atrioventricular grooves which serves to isolate the atrial from ventricular musculature at all points save the site of the atrioventricular conduction axis (bundle of His). This insulates the atrial and ventricular segments of myocardium except at the point of normal conduction

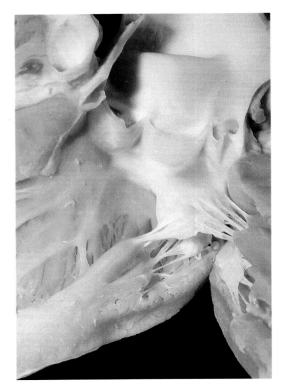

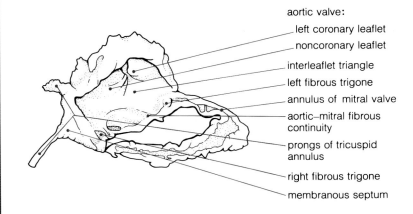

FIG. 1.5 *The fibrous skeleton shown in Figure 1.4 has been removed from the heart and photographed from beneath. It shows the firm annulus of the mitral valve, the limited extensions around the tricuspid valve, and the subvalvar fibrous skirt of the aortic valve (see Fig. 1.6). The central fibrous body is made up of the fusion of the right fibrous trigone with the membra-*

nous part of the septum. Examination of this figure together with Figure 1.4 shows that the fibrous skeleton has no relationship to the pulmonary valve. As demonstrated in Figure 1.13, the leaflets of the pulmonary valve arise directly from the musculature of the right ventricular outlet component and have no fibrous support.

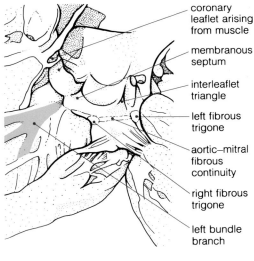

FIG. 1.6 *This dissection illustrates the subaortic outflow tract. It shows that the aortic root is a partly fibrous and partly muscular structure sculpted by the semilunar attachments of the leaflets of the aortic valve. There is no annulus as such supporting these leaflets. Anteriorly they arise directly from the musculature of the ventricular septum. Posteriorly they arise from the membranous septum, the fibrous trigones, and the area of aortic–mitral fibrous continuity. Fibrous sheets fill the interleaflet triangles in these areas and contribute to the fibrous skeleton. It is a mistake to conceptualize the skeleton itself as ascending in the form of tricorn cords to support the attachments of the valve leaflets.*

(see below). The fibrous elements of the skeleton are well represented in the aortic root, where they form its roof and border with the right-sided heart chambers (Fig. 1.6).

The overall arrangement of the *cardiac valves* in short axis is shown in Figure 1.7, while the ventricular short-axis equivalent is seen in Figure 1.8. The key feature is the deeply wedged position of the aortic valve between the tricuspid and mitral valves. The expression of this within the ventricles is that the subaortic outlet lifts the leaflets of the mitral valve away from the septum such that a crevice of the outlet reaches to the diaphragmatic surface of the heart. In contrast the inlets and outlets of the right ventricle are widely separated by the muscular roof of the right ventricle (the supraventricular crest); the outlet extends out to the left border of the heart, and the septum, seen in short axis, has a considerable curvature.

Taken in isolation, each of the *cardiac chambers* possesses intrinsic features which permit its unequivocal recognition. In the case of the atrial chambers each possesses a venous component, an appendage, and an atrioventricular vestibule. It is the appendage which constantly retains its structure in congenitally malformed hearts and therefore is most reliable for identification. The morphologically right ap-

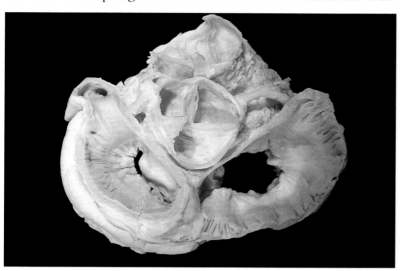

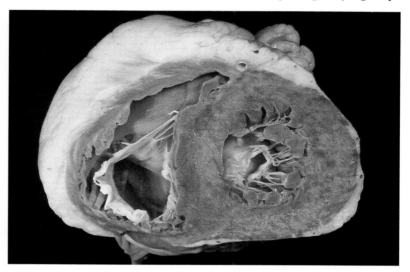

FIG. 1.7   *This dissection of the heart reveals the atrial aspect of the short axis when both atrial chambers and both arterial trunks have been removed (compare with Fig. 1.3). The deeply wedged position of the aortic valve between the atrioventricular valves is readily apparent, as is its central position within the outline of the heart. Note the different appearance of the mural and aortic leaflets of the mitral valve, the mural leaflet occupying two thirds of the annular circumference. Note also that two of the commissures of the arterial valves face each other, permitting two of the leaflets of each valve accurately to be described as the facing leaflets while the third leaflet in each case is the nonfacing leaflet. The dissection shows that the coronary arteries arise from the sinuses supporting the facing leaflets of the aortic valve. Because of this it is customary in the aortic valve to identify the leaflets and sinuses as right coronary, left coronary, and noncoronary, respectively.*

FIG. 1.8   *This photograph shows a short-axis section of the heart viewed from beneath and replicates the view obtained by the echocardiographer. The section is through the ventricular mass just above the junction of inlet and apical trabecular components (see Figs. 1.12, 1.20). The section shows how the mural (inferior) leaflet of the tricuspid valve hugs the diaphragmatic wall of the right ventricle. The septal leaflet, in contrast, is firmly adherent to the ventricular septum. The third anterosuperior leaflet hangs as a curtain between the inlet and outlet components of the ventricle. In the left ventricle the section shows how the wedged position of the subaortic outflow tract lifts the mitral valve away from the septum and gives it an oblique orientation. Its leaflets are described most accurately as being aortic and mural in location. The valve commissures are attached to the paired anterolateral and posteromedial papillary muscles. The mitral valve never has cordal attachments to the ventricular septum. Note the extensive swing of the septum itself; the inlet part is virtually in the sagittal plane while the outlet component is in the coronal plane. Note also the characteristic medial papillary muscle (of Lancisi) in the right ventricle and the extensive supraventricular crest separating the tricuspid and pulmonary valves (see Fig. 1.14).*

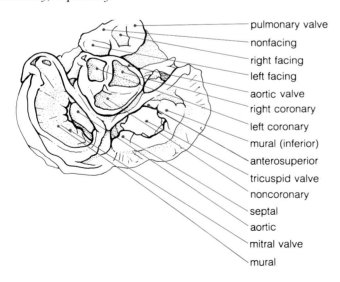

pulmonary valve
nonfacing
right facing
left facing
aortic valve
right coronary
left coronary
mural (inferior)
anterosuperior
tricuspid valve
noncoronary
septal
aortic
mitral valve
mural

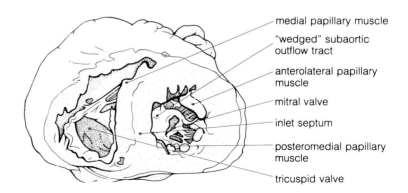

medial papillary muscle
"wedged" subaortic outflow tract
anterolateral papillary muscle
mitral valve
inlet septum
posteromedial papillary muscle
tricuspid valve

pendage (Fig. 1.9) is a triangular structure having a broad base with the venous component marked externally by the terminal groove and internally by the terminal crest. The crest is the junction of the trabeculated appendage with the smooth-walled venous component, which receives the superior and inferior caval veins together with the coronary sinus (Fig. 1.10).

The venous orifices surround the septal surface of the right atrium, this being the oval fossa characterized by its broad rim and smooth floor. The oval fossa is of vital significance during fetal life, when it is patent. Then its proximity to the inferior caval vein permits the richly oxygenated blood coming from the placenta (reaching the inferior caval vein through the venous duct) to pass directly into the left atrium and thence to the left ventricle, aorta, and brain. In contrast the deoxygenated blood returning from the brain through the superior caval vein is deflected away from the fossa by its extensive rim, being directed instead towards the right ventricle, pulmonary trunk, and the arterial duct. The vestibule of the right atrium contains and supports the tricuspid valve with leaflets in septal, anterosuperior, and inferior (or mural) location; the valve orifice is encircled by the right coronary artery (see Fig. 1.3).

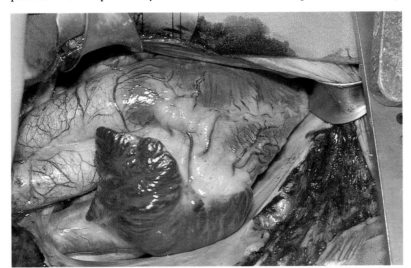

FIG. 1.9 *An operative view taken through a median sternotomy shows the triangular shape of the right atrial appendage, illustrating the extent of its junction with the venous component of the right atrium. Note the upper end of the terminal groove marking this junction.*

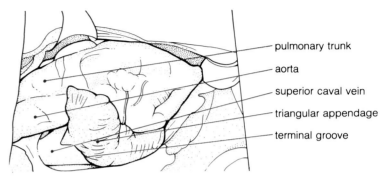

- pulmonary trunk
- aorta
- superior caval vein
- triangular appendage
- terminal groove

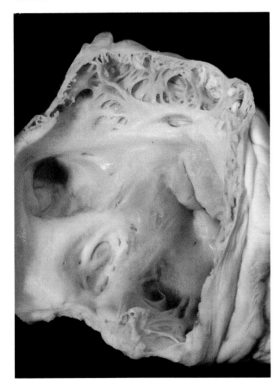

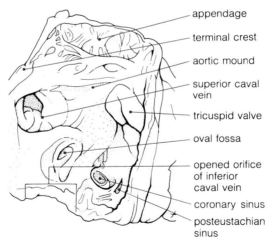

- appendage
- terminal crest
- aortic mound
- superior caval vein
- tricuspid valve
- oval fossa
- opened orifice of inferior caval vein
- coronary sinus
- posteustachian sinus

FIG. 1.10 *This photograph shows the internal appearance of the morphologically right atrium. It is taken obliquely from behind the heart after opening the atrium through the orifice of the inferior caval vein. The broad opening of the superior caval vein is sandwiched between the terminal crest (the muscle bundle marking internally the site of the terminal groove; see Fig. 1.9) and the superior infolding of the atrial roof which makes up the upper rim of the oval fossa. The oval fossa itself is the site of the atrial septum. This is far less extensive than often thought, the septum itself being confined to the floor of the fossa and its immediate surrounds. The fossa is separated by the sinus septum from the orifice of the coronary sinus. More anterosuperiorly both these structures abut on the atrioventricular septum (see Figs. 1.12, 1.13), which separates both from the vestibule of the tricuspid valve. The internal aspect of the triangular appendage is distinguished by its prominent trabeculations in contrast to the smooth lining of the venous sinus and the vestibule. In the morphologically right atrium these pectinate muscles extend around the atrioventricular junction to its posterior aspect (compare with Fig. 1.17).*

The major distinguishing feature of the right ventricle is the coarse nature of its apical trabeculations, together with the fact that the septal leaflet of the tricuspid valve has extensive attachments distally to the ventricular septum, a feature lacking for the mitral valve (Fig. 1.11). This is well seen in the simulated four-chamber cut of the heart, which, when taken posteriorly (Fig. 1.12), demonstrates also the offsetting of the proximal attachments of the atrioventricular valves. Because of this offsetting there is overlapping of the atrial and ventricular septal structures producing a muscular atrioventricular septum between right atrium and left ventricle. The extent of this muscular septum, however,

is limited because of the posterior extension of the subaortic outlet. For their larger part, therefore, four-chamber sections reveal the subaortic outflow tract interposed between the mitral valve and the septum. These sections also well demonstrate that part of the central fibrous body which is interposed between the subaortic outlet and the right-sided heart chamber. As described above, this component of the cardiac skeleton is called the membranous septum. It is crossed on its right ventricular aspect by the attachment of the septal leaflet of the tricuspid valve, thus dividing it into interventricular and atrioventricular components (Fig. 1.13).

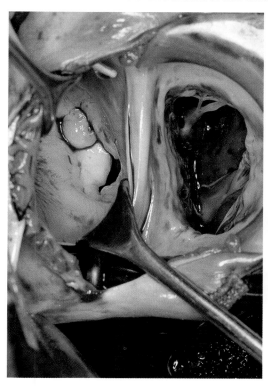

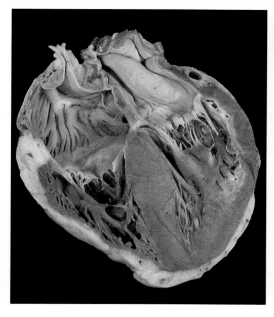

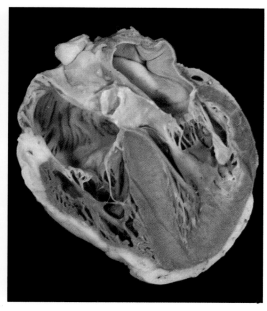

FIG. 1.12 *This long-axis section through the heart is taken at right angles to the inlet part of the ventricular septum. It produces the so-called four-chamber view of the echocardiographer since it displays the four basic cardiac chambers. The significant point in this posterior cut is the offsetting of the attachments of the mitral and tricuspid valve leaflets at the atrioventricular junction. The leaflet of the tricuspid valve is attached more toward the ventricular apex. Because of this, part of the atrial septum overlaps the muscular ventricular septum with a sloping junction between them. This part of the septum therefore is neither atrial nor ventricular but is the muscular atrioventricular septum.*

FIG. 1.13 *This section is immediately anterior to the section of the heart shown in Figure 1.12. It shows the limited extent of the muscular atrioventricular septum since, in this cut, the subaortic outflow tract has intervened between the mitral valve and the septum, lifting the leaflet of the mitral valve away from the septum. The place of the muscular atrioventricular septum is now occupied by another atrioventricular septal structure, since the septum immediately below the aortic valve continues to separate the left ventricle from the right atrium. This part of the septum, however, is made up of fibrous tissue and is part of the central fibrous body (see Figs. 1.4–1.6). Specifically it is the atrioventricular component of the membranous septum.*

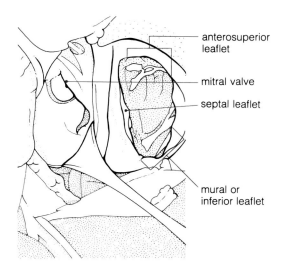

FIG. 1.11 *A surgical view oriented in anatomic fashion shows the arrangement of the leaflets of the atrioventricular valves. The tricuspid valve has septal, anterosuperior, and mural (or inferior) leaflets while the mitral valve has aortic and mural leaflets.*

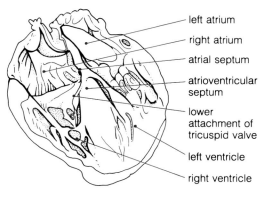

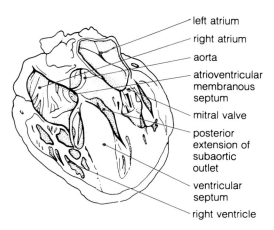

Although a ventricle is traditionally considered as having only inlet (or sinus) and outlet (or conus) components, we find it advantageous to recognize also the extensive apical trabecular component (Fig. 1.14), thus describing the ventricle in tripartite fashion. There are no discrete boundaries between the components, but the overall arrangement of inlet, apical trabecular, and outlet portions is readily appreciated. The

outlet component is extensive in the right ventricle, the leaflets of the pulmonary valve being exclusively attached to the ventricular musculature and having no connection with the cardiac skeleton. Because of this, the larger part of the subpulmonary infundibulum can be completely removed from the heart without disturbing any left ventricular structures (Fig. 1.15). It follows also that the pulmonary valve

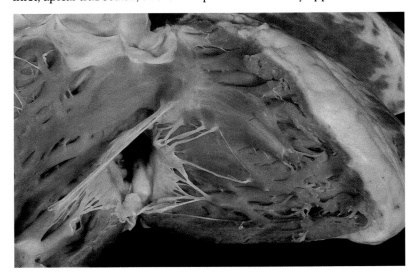

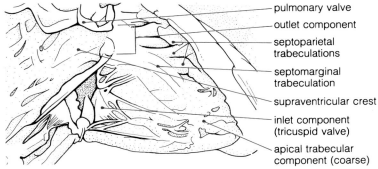

- pulmonary valve
- outlet component
- septoparietal trabeculations
- septomarginal trabeculation
- supraventricular crest
- inlet component (tricuspid valve)
- apical trabecular component (coarse)

FIG. 1.14 *The vestibule of the tricuspid valve connects in the normal heart with the morphologically right ventricle. As shown in this picture, the right ventricle can readily be analyzed in terms of three components: the inlet, apical trabecular, and outlet portions. The inlet part contains the tricuspid valve and extends from the atrioventricular junction to the attachments of the valvar tension apparatus. The outlet component is the smooth sleeve of muscle supporting the semilunar attachments of the pulmonary valve leaflets. The apical trabecular component merges with these other components and has more obvious boundaries at the inlet than the outlet. Nonetheless it is recognized because of its heavy and coarse trabeculations. The nature of these trabeculations also serves to distinguish it from the morphologically left ventricle (see Fig. 1.20). One muscular trabeculation is much more obvious in the morphologically right ventricle. It is a straplike structure that extends down from the area of the membranous septum, having two limbs at this site which extend into the inlet and outlet components, respectively. The body of this strap then runs down towards the ventricular apex where it*

gives rise to the prominent anterior papillary muscle of the tricuspid valve. This structure is the septomarginal trabeculation (or septal band). From its anterior surface a further series of trabeculations originates and runs to the parietal wall of the ventricle; these are the septoparietal trabeculations. One of these is usually prominent and is described as the moderator band. This section shows also the characteristic arrangement of the tricuspid valve and its papillary muscles. The septal leaflet has extensive cordal attachments directly to the inlet part of the muscular septum. It is limited by the medial papillary muscle (of Lancisi) anteriorly and by the prominent inferior papillary muscle posteriorly. The anterosuperior valve leaflet extends across like a curtain between ventricular inlet and outlet to the more prominent anterior papillary muscle. The inferior leaflet is then seen also to be mural, running along the diaphragmatic surface of the inlet. Note the extensive muscle shelf that separates the tricuspid and pulmonary valves. This is made up of the inner curve of the heart wall and is called the supraventricular crest.

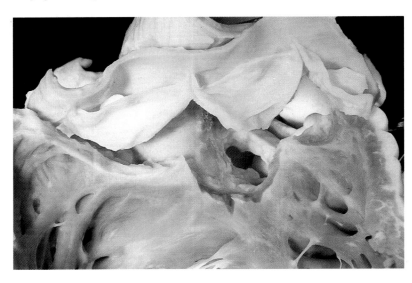

- pulmonary leaflet
- aorta
- muscular outlet component

FIG. 1.15 *This dissection illustrates the anatomy of the outlet component of the morphologically right ventricle. It shows the three semilunar attachments of the leaflets of the pulmonary valve. These are exclusively connected to the sleeve of outlet musculature. There is no annulus supporting these leaflets in the sense that the fibrous skeleton forms a ring around the mitral valve (see Fig. 1.5). The dissection also shows that the area often*

considered to be septum in the region below the two facing leaflets of the valve is in reality the inner wall of the heart. There is a space in this position between the right ventricular infundibulum and the aorta. The origin of the coronary arteries from the aorta can be seen through the incision which liberated the leaflets from the ventricular outlet (see also Fig. 1.32).

has no annulus in terms of a discrete fibrous ring. Instead, the leaflets are simply supported in semilunar fashion by the infundibular musculature.

The left atrium, like the right, has an appendage, a venous component, and a vestibule. The appendage is long and tubular, usually crenellated, and has a narrow junction with the venous component (Fig. 1.16). The junction is not marked, either internally or externally, by a terminal crest or groove such as seen on the right side (Fig. 1.17). The venous component receives the four pulmonary veins at its corners (Fig. 1.18). The septal surface of the atrium is roughened and shows no rim as in the right atrium (Fig. 1.17). Dissection shows that the greater part of the rim of the oval fossa is simply a deep groove

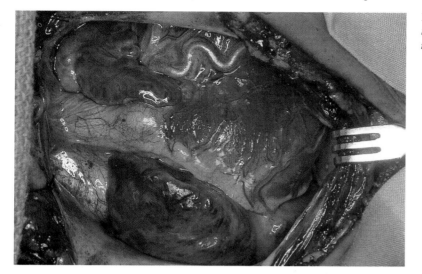

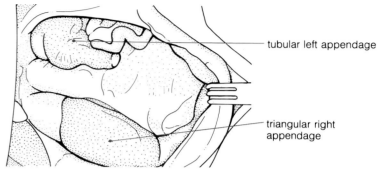

FIG. 1.16 *A surgical view through a median sternotomy contrasts the long tubular shape of the left atrial appendage with the broad and triangular right appendage.*

— tubular left appendage

— triangular right appendage

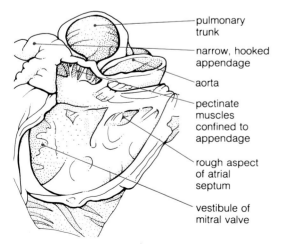

FIG. 1.17 *This dissection depicts the narrow junction of the appendage with the vestibule of the mitral valve and also illustrates how the pectinate muscles are confined within the appendage. There is no prominent terminal crest in the left atrium (compare with Fig. 1.10). The four pulmonary veins enter the corners of the smooth-walled venous component (see Fig. 1.18). Note that the left atrial aspect of the septum is roughened and shows no rim to the oval fossa such as is found in the right atrium (see Fig. 1.10).*

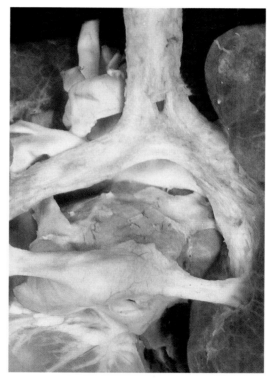

FIG. 1.18 *The pulmonary veins enter the four corners of the diaphragmatic surface of the left atrium, as shown in this dissection of the posterior aspect of the heart. The four venous connections limit the oblique sinus of the pericardium (see Fig. 1.2). This dissection also shows the site of the descending aorta (left aortic arch) and the typical pattern of the normal tracheal bifurcation. The left bronchus is twice as long as the right bronchus and is crossed by the lower lobe pulmonary artery before bifurcation.*

— pulmonary trunk

— narrow, hooked appendage

— aorta

— pectinate muscles confined to appendage

— rough aspect of atrial septum

— vestibule of mitral valve

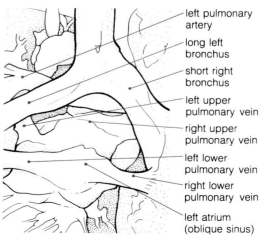

— left pulmonary artery

— long left bronchus

— short right bronchus

— left upper pulmonary vein

— right upper pulmonary vein

— left lower pulmonary vein

— right lower pulmonary vein

— left atrium (oblique sinus)

between the venous components of the two atria (Fig. 1.19). Termed Waterston's groove, this crevice is important since it can be dissected during surgery to provide one means of access into the left atrium.

Although not as obviously differentiated as the right ventricle, the left ventricle can also conveniently be described in terms of inlet, apical trabecular, and outlet components (Fig. 1.20). This tripartite approach highlights the fine apical trabeculations which are the most characteristic and constant feature of the left ventricle in congenitally malformed hearts (see Chapter 3). In the normal heart, however, both the inlet and outlet components of the left ventricle have their own distinctive characteristics. The major distinguishing feature of the inlet is that the leaflets of the mitral valve have no distal attachment to the septum. The two leaflets themselves are supported by paired papillary muscles and are located such that one is in direct fibrous continuity with the aortic valve while the other springs from the parietal part of the left atrioventricular junction (see Fig. 1.13). For this reason the leaflets are best described as being aortic and mural. They have grossly dissimilar circumferential extent, the aortic leaflet guarding one third and the mural leaflet two thirds of the junction (see Fig. 1.3). Because the aortic leaflet is much deeper, they have similar areas (Fig. 1.21). Usually the mural leaflet is divided into three components called scallops, but this arrangement is variable.

The feature of the left ventricular outlet is its abbreviated nature due to the aortic wedge position and its interposition between the inlet and the septum (Fig. 1.22). Unlike the pulmonary valve, the leaflets of the aortic valve are intimately related to the fibrous skeleton such that the overall circumference of the valve orifice is half fibrous support. Despite this the leaflets of the aortic valve do not have an

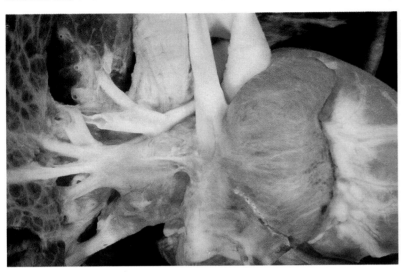

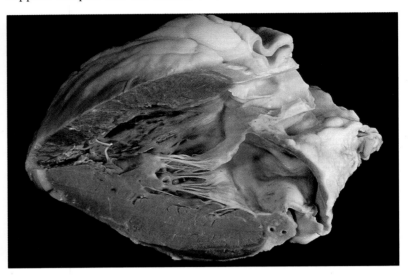

FIG. 1.19 *This dissection illustrates the important relationships between the right pulmonary veins and the venous sinus of the right atrium. There is a deep furrow, termed Waterston's groove, between the pulmonary veins and the caval veins which forms the upper margin of the oval fossa. In this position it is often taken to be a septal structure instead of the infolding of the atrial roof. Note also that the site of the terminal groove is lateral to the venous sinus of the right atrium separating it from the appendage. This groove marks the site of the terminal crest and contains the sinus node (see Fig. 1.27).*

FIG. 1.20 *This photograph shows the morphologically left ventricle opened through an incision in its parietal wall. Like the right ventricle, it can readily be described in terms of inlet, apical trabecular, and outlet components (see Fig. 1.14). The inlet component contains the mitral valve with its two leaflets supported by prominent paired papillary muscles. As shown in this dissection, the anterior or aortic leaflet is separated by the subaortic outflow tract from the ventricular septum. The mitral valve, unlike the tricuspid valve, never has direct attachments to the ventricular septum. The apical trabecular component in the left ventricle is characteristically fine and has no septomarginal trabeculation reinforcing its smooth septal surface. The outlet component is abbreviated in comparison with that of the right ventricle, since there is fibrous continuity between the mitral and aortic valves. Thus there is no muscular supraventricular crest within the left ventricle. There is, however, a marked posterior extension of the outflow tract that separates the mitral valve from the septum. (Reproduced with permission of the authors and publisher; see Figure Credits)*

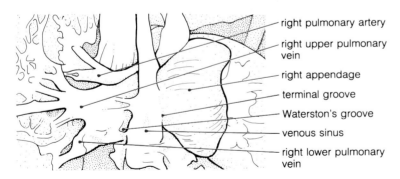

- right pulmonary artery
- right upper pulmonary vein
- right appendage
- terminal groove
- Waterston's groove
- venous sinus
- right lower pulmonary vein

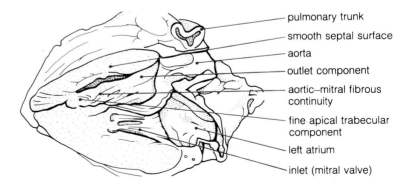

- pulmonary trunk
- smooth septal surface
- aorta
- outlet component
- aortic–mitral fibrous continuity
- fine apical trabecular component
- left atrium
- inlet (mitral valve)

annulus in the sense of a complete ring such as exists in the mitral valve. The leaflet support is again conditioned by the semilunar attachments, the zenith of the commissures being appreciably higher than the nadir of the leaflet troughs. The leaflets of both arterial valves are unsupported by tension apparatus so that they close simply due to the hydrostatic pressure of the column of blood they support during ventricular diastole (Fig. 1.23).

The *arterial trunks* in the normal heart ascend into the mediastinum in a particular fashion called "normal relations." Because of the wedge location of its root (see Fig. 1.3), the aorta springs from the cardiac

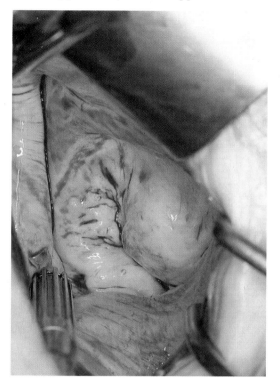

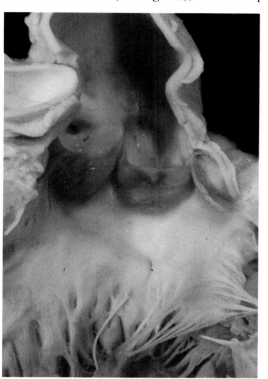

FIG. 1.21 *A surgical view of the leaflets of the mitral valve is oriented in anatomic fashion. Note that the annular attachment of the two leaflets is markedly different, the aortic leaflet taking up only one third of the overall circumference. This leaflet, however, is much deeper than the mural leaflet so that the overall area of the two is comparable.*

FIG. 1.22 *This dissection shows the outlet component of the left ventricle. The anatomy is determined by the semilunar attachments of the leaflets of the aortic valve. Unlike the pulmonary valve, which has exclusively muscular attachments, the leaflets of the aortic valve are attached in part to the muscular walls of the ventricle and in part to the fibrous skeleton (see Figs. 1.4–1.6). Note also the extensive posterior extension of the subaortic outflow tract, which is bordered to one side by the mitral valve and to the other by the atrioventricular septal structures (see Figs. 1.12, 1.13).*

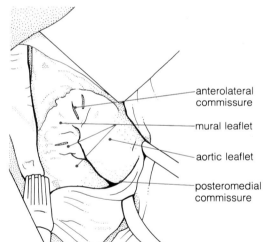

anterolateral commissure

mural leaflet

aortic leaflet

posteromedial commissure

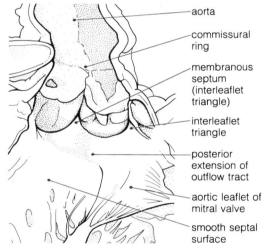

aorta

commissural ring

membranous septum (interleaflet triangle)

interleaflet triangle

posterior extension of outflow tract

aortic leaflet of mitral valve

smooth septal surface

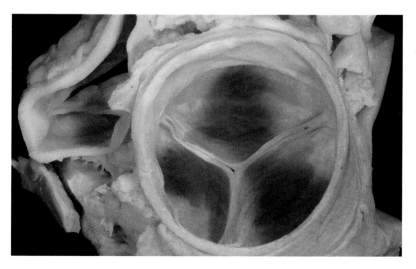

FIG. 1.23 *The aortic valve is viewed from above, illustrating the simple closing mechanism of an arterial valve. The three leaflets are forced together by the hydrostatic pressure of the column of blood they support during ventricular diastole. The function of the valves, however, depends on the normal formation of the subvalvar supporting tissues, the integrity of the leaflets, the normal arrangement of the commissural ring, and the normal configuration of the sinuses of Valsalva.*

base posteriorly and to the right of the pulmonary trunk (Fig. 1.24). The trunks then spiral around one another as they pass to supply the systemic and pulmonary circulations respectively. The arch of the aorta gives off brachiocephalic (innominate), left common carotid, and left subclavian arteries from its superior aspect while the pulmonary trunk divides into right and left branches (Fig. 1.25). During fetal life an important channel connects the arterial trunks so that deoxygenated

blood returning through the right side of the heart from the head can be shunted into the descending aorta, to be returned to the placenta for reoxygenation. This channel is the arterial duct which runs from the left pulmonary artery to the aorta, marking the origin of the descending component of the aorta. The segment of the aortic arch between the left subclavian artery and the junction of the duct with the descending aorta is itself called the isthmus (see Fig. 1.25). The

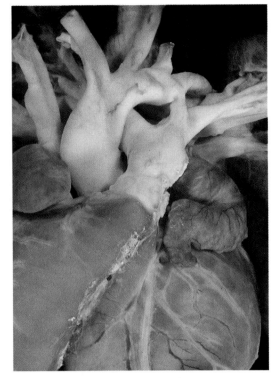
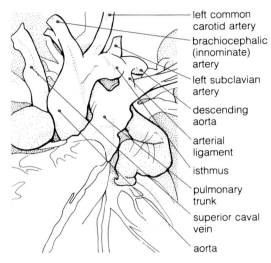

left common carotid artery
brachiocephalic (innominate) artery
left subclavian artery
descending aorta
arterial ligament
isthmus
pulmonary trunk
superior caval vein
aorta

FIG. 1.24 *This infant heart illustrates the normal relationships of the great arteries as they leave the base of the heart. The pulmonary trunk is to the left and anterior relative to the centrally positioned aorta. The trunk having bifurcated, the right pulmonary artery swings beneath the aortic arch. The arch gives rise superiorly to the brachiocephalic (innominate), left common carotid, and left subclavian arteries. It then continues as the isthmus until it becomes the descending aorta at the site of the arterial ligament. This structure arising from the left pulmonary artery is the remnant of the arterial duct which in fetal life conveys the right ventricular output to the placenta. In this specimen the duct has already closed and is in the process of conversion to a fibrous cord.*

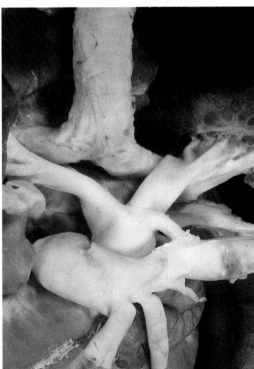
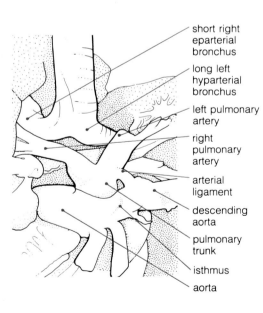

short right eparterial bronchus
long left hyparterial bronchus
left pulmonary artery
right pulmonary artery
arterial ligament
descending aorta
pulmonary trunk
isthmus
aorta

FIG. 1.25 *In this superior view of the arterial trunks shown in Figure 1.24 the aorta is deflected forward. The smooth bifurcation of the pulmonary trunk is seen along with the site of the arterial duct. It demonstrates further the anatomy of the tracheal bifurcation shown from behind in Figure 1.18. This view shows how the lower lobe artery of the left lung crosses over the long left bronchus before it has given rise to any branches. The short right bronchus gives rise to its eparterial branch prior to being crossed by the lower lobe pulmonary artery.*

arterial duct stays patent only during fetal life, normally becoming constricted and closed in the first days after birth. Within the next six weeks it then becomes converted into the arterial ligament and, by adult life, is simply a fibrous cord.

Normal action of the heart demands the synchronous activity of the *cardiac subsystems,* namely the conduction system, the arteries and veins, and the nervous and lymphatic systems. The conduction system generates and dissipates the cardiac impulse (Fig. 1.26). A vital part

of this system is the fibro-fatty atrioventricular tissue plane which insulates the atrial from the ventricular muscle masses at all points except the penetration of the specialized conduction axis. When speaking of the conduction tissues, however, we usually refer only to the nodes and their ramifications. The impulse is generated by the sinus node, a small, cigar-shaped structure lying within the terminal groove, usually laterally relative to that part of the sinuatrial junction marked by the crest of the right atrial appendage (Fig. 1.27). The node is

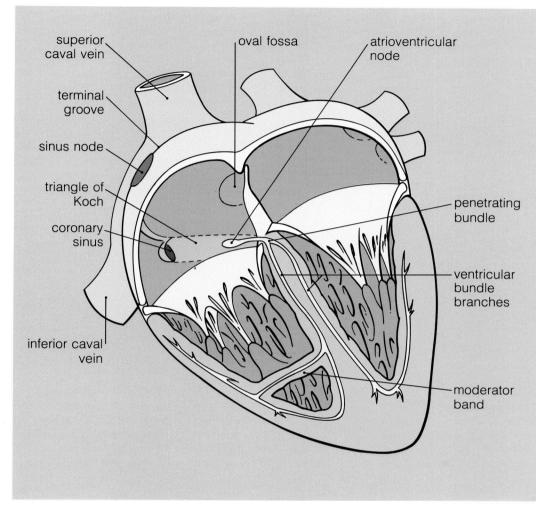

FIG. 1.26 *This diagram demonstrates the arrangement of the conduction system in the normal heart. The sinus node sits laterally in the terminal groove (see Fig. 1.27). It gives rise to the cardiac impulse, which is then carried through the atrial myocardium toward the ventricles, at the same time activating the myocardium. Conduction through the atrial chambers occurs through the working atrial myocardium, the geometric arrangement of the muscle bundles in the septum, and the terminal crest, being responsible for any preferential spread that does exist. There is no evidence to support the concept of histologically discrete tracts of specialized conduction tissue extending between the sinus and atrioventricular nodes. The atrioventricular node, which produces the greater part of atrioventricular delay, is located within the triangle of Koch (see Fig. 1.29). The atrioventricular conduction axis continues from the node into the ventricles with penetrating and branching components before becoming the ventricular bundle branches. These branches are insulated from the septum in their proximal portions, activating the myocardium of the trabecular components through the so-called Purkinje cell network. The Purkinje cells in the human heart have small dimensions and do not resemble the large and clear cells found in the hearts of cattle and related mammals.*

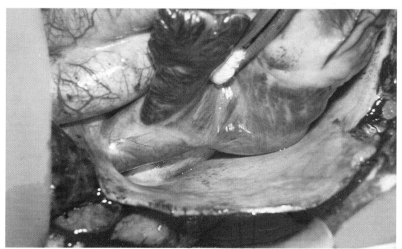

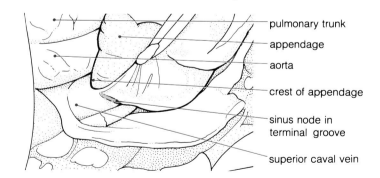

FIG. 1.27 *This photograph, taken in surgical orientation in the operating room, shows the location of the normal cigar-shaped sinus node within the lateral extent of the terminal groove at the superior cavoatrial junction.*

discrete histologically, is immediately subepicardial, and is generally arranged around a prominent nodal artery (Fig. 1.28). Although several textbooks now illustrate "specialized tracts" emanating from the sinus node in triradiate fashion, there is no convincing evidence, either anatomic or electrophysiologic, to support the existence of these purported structures. Instead, preferential conduction through the atrial musculature is governed by the geometric arrangement of the ordinary atrial muscle cells. The atrial impulse is gathered together, delayed, and distributed to the ventricular myocardium by the specialized atrioventricular conduction axis. The atrial component is the atrioventricular node, which produces the greater part of atrioventricular delay. It is located within the triangle of Koch, a most useful surgical landmark (Fig. 1.29). The node penetrates through the central fibrous body at the apex of the triangle, being no more than the size of a strand of cotton as it penetrates (the bundle of His) (Fig. 1.30). Having penetrated, it reaches the subaortic outflow tract and branches into right

and left bundle branches. The left branch spreads out in fanlike fashion (Fig. 1.31), while the right branch is a thin cordlike structure. Both branches, however, pass out to the ventricular apices before arborizing into the myocardial masses as the so-called Purkinje networks.

Equally important as the conduction system is the arrangement of *coronary arteries* supplying the heart. The two major arteries, right and left, arise from the sinuses of the aortic root (Fig. 1.32). Since there are usually three sinuses but only two arteries, and since each artery usually arises from a separate aortic sinus, one sinus does not give rise to an artery. Always, irrespective of the relationship of the arterial trunks in congenitally malformed hearts, the sinus lacking an artery is the one most distant from the pulmonary trunk (see Fig. 1.3). This sinus is therefore conveniently designated as the nonfacing sinus while in the normal heart the other sinuses are designated right coronary and left coronary, respectively. The two mainstem coronary arteries then extend and branch so as to irrigate the atrioventricular

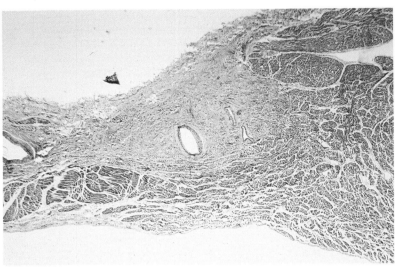

FIG. 1.28. *This histologic section, stained by the trichrome technique so that muscle appears red and fibrous tissue blue, is taken at right angles to the cigar-shaped sinus node. It shows how, in short axis, the node is a wedge-shaped structure set in the angle between the wall of the superior caval vein and the terminal crest. Note the discrete boundaries between node and muscle and the arrangment of the node around a prominent artery.*

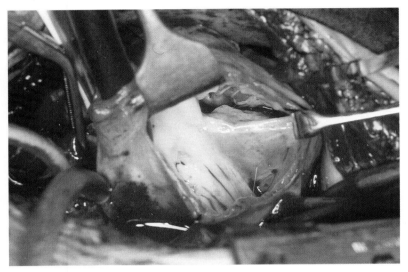

FIG. 1.29 *This view, taken in surgical orientation in the operating room, shows the landmarks of the triangle of Koch. The triangle itself is clearly visible, limited distally by the septal attachment of the tricuspid valve and proximally by the sinus septum. If the surgeon scrupulously avoids this area, there is no way that the atrioventricular conduction axis can be damaged. (Reproduced with permission of the authors and publisher; see Figure Credits.)*

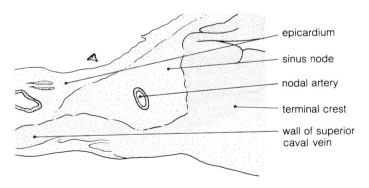

- epicardium
- sinus node
- nodal artery
- terminal crest
- wall of superior caval vein

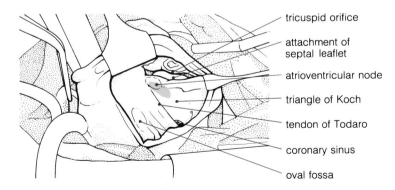

- tricuspid orifice
- attachment of septal leaflet
- atrioventricular node
- triangle of Koch
- tendon of Todaro
- coronary sinus
- oval fossa

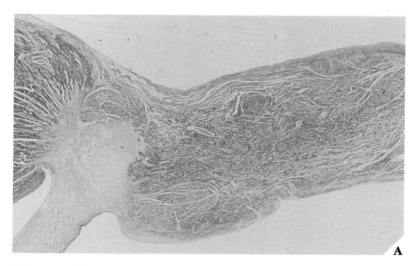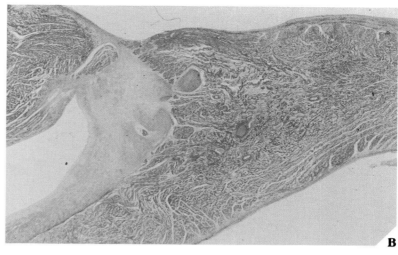

FIG. 1.30 *These sections, stained with the trichrome technique, show the position of the atrioventricular node within the triangle of Koch (A) and*

the penetrating atrioventricular bundle (of His) within the central fibrous body (B).

- triangle of Koch
- tendon of Todaro
- atrial septum
- atrioventricular node

- penetrating atrioventricular bundle
- atrial septum
- tendon of Todaro

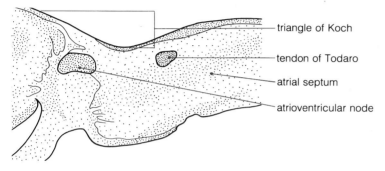

FIG. 1.31 *This diagram is taken from the monograph of Tawara (1906), which established and elucidated the significance of the atrioventricular conduction axis. It shows the fanlike arrangement of the left bundle branch. The clinical value of the so-called concept of hemiblocks should not be extended to presume that the left bundle branch is arranged anatomically in bifascicular fashion. As shown here, it is arranged as a fan and, if it divides at all, it forms three rather than two divisions. (Reproduced; see Figure Credits)*

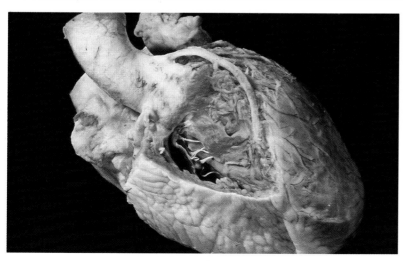

FIG. 1.32 *This dissection shows the origin of the coronary arteries from the aortic root. As shown in Figure 1.3, these arteries emerge from the two aortic sinuses which face the pulmonary trunk. The left coronary artery immediately divides into anterior interventricular and circumflex branches. The interventricular artery is well seen in this dissection along with its septal perforating branches. The circumflex and right coronary arteries encircle the orifices of the atrioventricular valves as shown in Figure 1.3. (Reproduced with permission of the authors and publisher; see Figure Credits)*

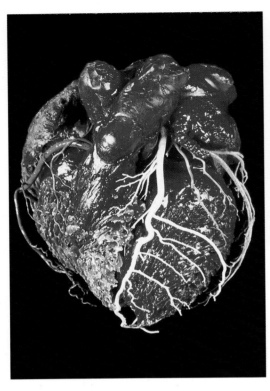

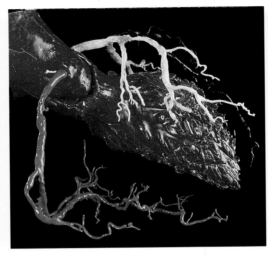

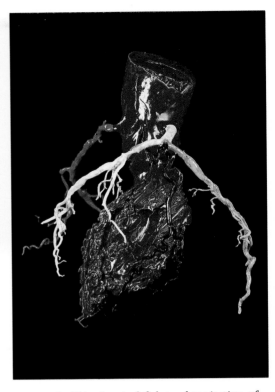

FIG. 1.33 *The anterior view of this cast of the coronary arteries and ventricles shows the position of the anterior interventricular branch of the left coronary artery in white together with its infundibular and diagonal branches. The circumflex branch of the left coronary artery together with its obtuse marginal branches are shown in yellow. The right coronary artery and its acute marginal branch are depicted in green. (Cast prepared by and photograph courtesy of Sally Allwork, PhD, London, England)*

FIG. 1.34 *This cast illustrates the anatomy of the coronary arterial tree as demonstrated in the right anterior oblique angiographic projection. The extent of the right coronary artery is well seen along with its posterior interventricular artery. As in this cast, the posterior artery is a branch of the right artery in nine tenths of individuals, an arrangement termed right dominance. In one tenth of cases, as shown in Figure 1.3, it is the circumflex artery which gives rise to the posterior descending artery—left dominance. (Cast prepared by and photograph courtesy of Sally Allwork, PhD, London, England. Reproduced with permission of the authors and publisher; see Figure Credits)*

FIG. 1.35 *This view in left lateral projection of the same heart as shown in Figure 1.34 shows the left mainstem artery and its anterior interventricular and circumflex branches. Also present in this heart is a so-called intermediate artery (colored black). It is usual now to consider such arteries as diagonal branches of the anterior interventricular artery. (Cast prepared by and photograph courtesy of Sally Allwork, PhD, London, England. Reproduced with permission of the authors and publisher; see Figure Credits)*

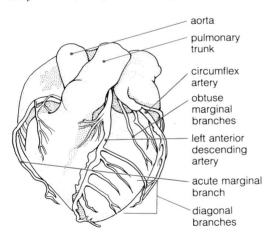

aorta
pulmonary trunk
circumflex artery
obtuse marginal branches
left anterior descending artery
acute marginal branch
diagonal branches

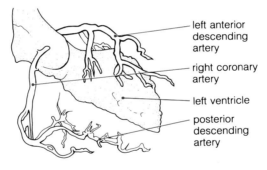

left anterior descending artery
right coronary artery
left ventricle
posterior descending artery

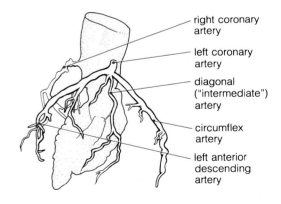

right coronary artery
left coronary artery
diagonal ("intermediate") artery
circumflex artery
left anterior descending artery

and interventricular grooves (Fig. 1.33). In most hearts this is accomplished by the right coronary artery continuing as a solitary channel encircling the right atrioventricular junction (Fig. 1.34; see also Fig. 1.3) and descending within the posterior interventricular groove. In contrast the left artery runs a very short course prior to its bifurcation into anterior interventricular and circumflex branches (Fig. 1.35). The interventricular branch then occupies the anterior interventricular groove while the circumflex branch extends to varying points around the left atrioventricular junction. In a minority of individuals (perhaps one tenth), it is the circumflex artery which reaches the crux and runs down into the posterior interventricular groove (see Fig. 1.3). The *coronary veins* also occupy the atrioventricular and interventricular grooves, returning blood into the coronary sinus, which itself runs

along the left atrioventricular groove and opens into the right atrium (Fig. 1.36).

In terms of *nerves,* the heart is supplied from both sympathetic and parasympathetic sources. Although it was at first thought that the nerves may conduct the cardiac impulse, this impression had been shown to be spurious by the start of the twentieth century. The nerves monitor the function of the heart, being intimately related to the conduction system, and are also widely distributed along the coronary arteries. The supply to the musculature of the heart itself is relatively limited compared with these richly supplied areas. The parasympathetic nerves come from the vagus and are relayed via ganglion cells confined to the atrial tissues. Indeed there are few if any vagal fibers within the ventricles of the human heart. In contrast the sympathetic fibers, de-

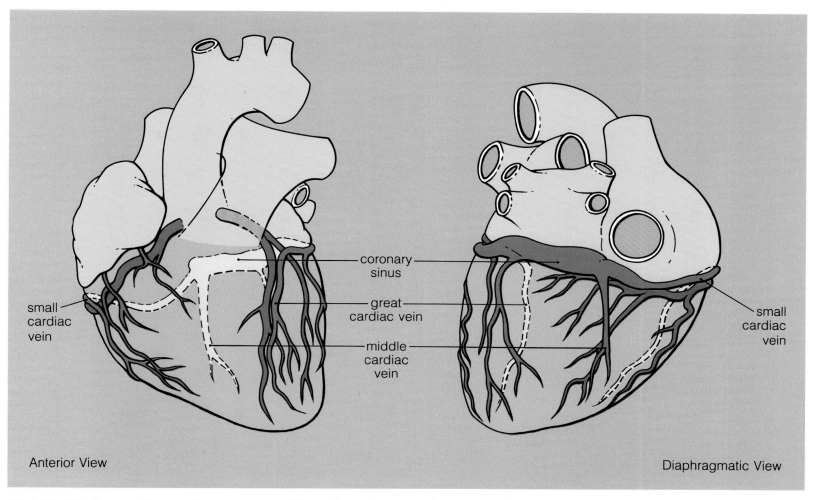

small cardiac vein

coronary sinus

great cardiac vein

middle cardiac vein

small cardiac vein

Anterior View

Diaphragmatic View

FIG. 1.36 *This diagram illustrates the arrangement of the cardiac veins, from the anterior aspect (left) and the diaphragmatic aspect (right). The veins follow the great arteries, running in the interventricular* and atrioventricular grooves. They terminate in the coronary sinus, which drains to the right atrium. In addition to these larger veins, smaller veins, called thebesian veins, drain directly to the right atrium.

rived from the cervical and upper thoracic ganglia of the sympathetic chains, are distributed more widely within the atria and ventricles, running primarily in concert with the branches of the coronary arteries (Fig. 1.37).

Histologically the heart is made up of masses of *myocardial fibers* which are intermediate in their structure between voluntary (striated) and involuntary (smooth) muscle. Although the cardiac muscle is involuntary, it has marked cross-striations, which are readily visible using the light microscope. Examination with the electron microscope shows that, as with skeletal muscle, the striations are due to the interdigitation of actin and myosin fibrils (Fig. 1.38). Thought at one time to be syncytial in nature, the cardiac cells are now known to be multiple

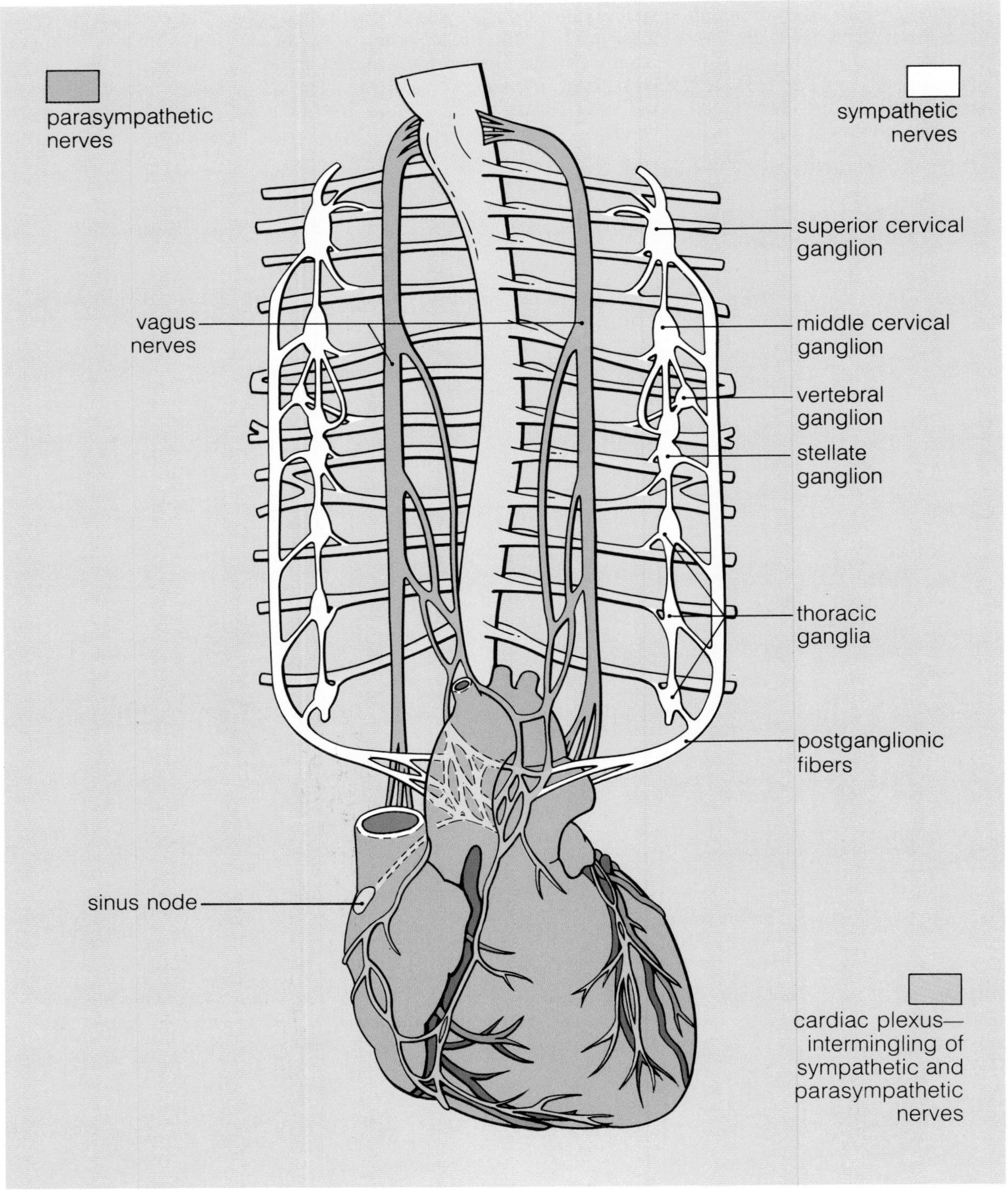

parasympathetic
nerves

sympathetic
nerves

vagus
nerves

superior cervical
ganglion

middle cervical
ganglion

vertebral
ganglion

stellate
ganglion

thoracic
ganglia

postganglionic
fibers

sinus node

cardiac plexus—
intermingling of
sympathetic and
parasympathetic
nerves

FIG. 1.37 *This diagram shows the extent and origin of the cardiac nerves. The sympathetic nerves supply both ventricles and atria, while the parasympathetic supply is largely confined to the atrial chambers. (Redrawn; reproduced with permission of the authors and publisher; see Figure Credits)*

individual units joined by intercalated disks (Fig. 1.39). Each cell therefore takes origin from and inserts into its neighbors. The cardiac skeleton is in no way analogous to the appendicular skeleton in terms of giving origin and insertion to the muscles. Instead the cardiac skeleton supports most of the leaflets of the atrioventricular valves and helps in the insulation of the atrial and ventricular muscle masses (Fig. 1.40). The specialized conduction system of the heart is less obviously cross-striated than the ordinary "working" myocardium, although the precise arrangement differs within the different components of the system.

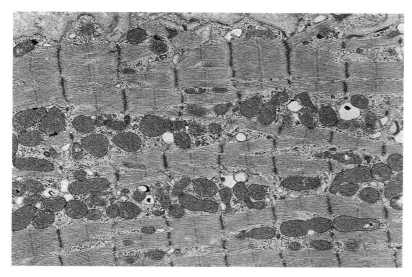

FIG. 1.38   *An electron micrograph shows the typical striated arrangement of normal cardiac muscle. The cross striations are due to the interdigitation of actin and myosin fibrils.*

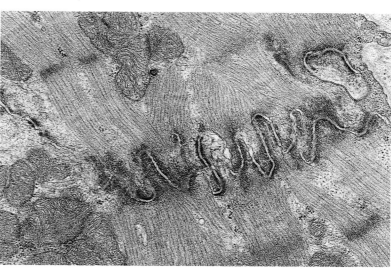

FIG. 1.39   *An electron micrograph shows the structure of an intercalated disk.*

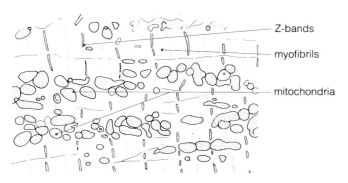

- Z-bands
- myofibrils
- mitochondria

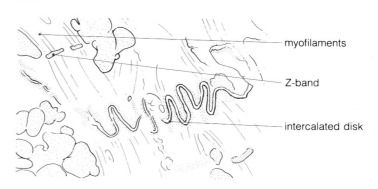

- myofilaments
- Z-band
- intercalated disk

FIG. 1.40   *A histologic section demonstrates the structure of the left atrioventricular junction. Note that the fibrous skeleton supports the leaflet of the mitral valve and insulates the atrial from the ventricular muscle masses.*

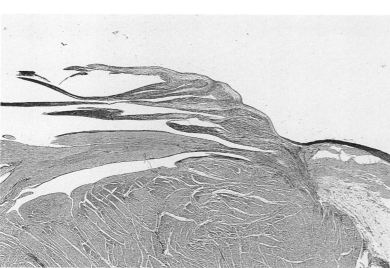

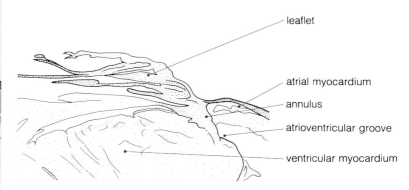

- leaflet
- atrial myocardium
- annulus
- atrioventricular groove
- ventricular myocardium

The coronary arteries are arranged as typical arteries with intima, muscular media, and adventitia (Fig. 1.41). The arterial trunks are characterized by the presence within their walls of multiple elastic lamellae while the arterial duct, during fetal life, is a muscular artery (Fig. 1.42).

FIGURE CREDITS

FIG. 1.4 From Anderson RH, Becker AE: *Cardiac Anatomy.* Edinburgh, Churchill Livingstone, 1980, p 5.4.

FIG. 1.20 From Anderson RH, Becker AE: *Cardiac Anatomy.* Edinburgh, Churchill Livingstone, 1980, p 4.3.

FIG. 1.29 From Wilcox BR, Anderson RH: *Surgical Anatomy of the Heart.* New York, Raven Press, 1985, p 2.8.

FIG. 1.31 From Tawara S: *Das Reizleitungssystem des Saugetierherzens.* Jena, Gustav Fisher, 1906.

FIG. 1.32 From Anderson RH, Becker AE: *Cardiac Anatomy.* Edinburgh, Churchill Livingstone, 1980, p 6.2.

FIG. 1.34 From Anderson RH, Becker AE: *Cardiac Anatomy.* Edinburgh, Churchill Livingstone, 1980, p 7.13

FIG. 1.35 From Anderson RH, Becker AE: *Cardiac Anatomy.* Edinburgh, Churchill Livingstone, 1980, p 7.15

FIG. 1.37 Adapted from Anderson RH, Becker AE: *Cardiac Anatomy.* Edinburgh, Churchill Livingstone, 1980, pp 6.30, 6.31; Schlant RC, Silverman ME: Anatomy of the heart, in Hurst JW (ed): *The Heart,* 6th ed. New York, McGraw-Hill, 1986, p 24.

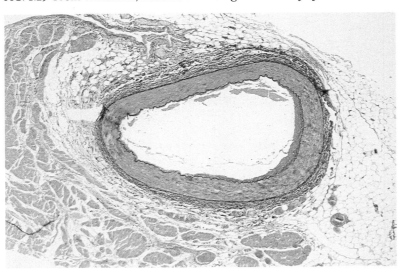

FIG. 1.41 *A cross-section of a coronary artery shows the typical arterial arrangement with intima, muscular media, and adventitia.*

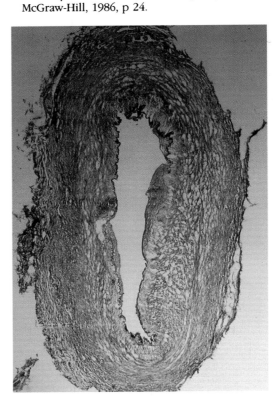

FIG. 1.42 *A cross-section of the arterial duct shows that this has the typical muscular arterial arrangement.*

2

MYOCARDIAL REMODELING AND ITS COMPLICATIONS

Anton E. Becker, MD

Based on Becker AE, Anderson RH: Cardiac adaptation and its sequelae, Chapter 1, pp 1.1–1.8 in *Cardiac Pathology*. Edinburgh, Churchill Livingstone, 1983; Anversa P et al: Quantitative structural analysis of the myocardium during physiologic growth and induced cardiac hypertrophy: a review. *J Am Coll Cardiol* 7:1140–1149, 1986; Maron BJ, Epstein SE (eds): Symposium on the athlete heart. *J Am Coll Cardiol* 7:189–243, 1986. Figures reproduced in this chapter from *Cardiac Pathology* are also reprinted with permission of the authors and publisher.

The morphologic mechanisms that underlie remodeling of the heart as an adaptive phenomenon are limited. The cardiac chambers may dilate, often due to an increased volume load, or the myocardial wall may hypertrophy as an expression of increased work load.

Several factors are important when considering the pathophysiologic effects of remodeling. The time available for adaptation plays an important role. For example adaptation in response to a sudden change in left ventricular volume load, as in a patient with ruptured cords of the mitral valve, differs from adaptation in a patient who develops a gradually progressive mitral insufficiency on the basis of rheumatic heart disease. Heavy chain isozymes of myosin may differ among various forms of remodeling. The adjustment of the capillary network may not necessarily keep pace with myocardial hypertrophy. Moreover, little is known about the role of the fine fibrillar connective tissue meshwork that wraps around individual heart muscle cells, forming a tensile element that resists stretch and provides a restoring force that may cause individual muscle cells to return to their original length after contraction.

Myocardial remodeling therefore is a process that involves many of the elements that normally constitute the heart as a whole, both at the cellular and subcellular levels. Although basically reversible in nature, the adaptive changes may in themselves introduce secondary alterations that render the heart prone to injury.

PHYSIOLOGIC GROWTH

During intrauterine life the heart supports the fetal circulation. The myocardium initially develops mainly by cellular multiplication. Functional organization of the myocytes occurs very early during development. At this early stage cellular enlargement, e.g., increased myocyte diameter and length, becomes an important mechanism contributing to the augmentation of the myocardial mass. Myocardial cellular enlargement is accompanied by growth of capillaries.

In this context two important aspects merit further consideration. During intrauterine development the growing myocardium adapts to the presence of cardiac malformations to guarantee the optimal functional capacity of the heart. Secondly, fetal myocytes also have the capacity to adapt to abnormal circumstances by hypertrophy. This implies not only that myocytes increase their dimension but also that they expand their cellular organelles responsible for oxygen consumption and adenosine triphosphate synthesis and utilization. Subsystems such as the vascular network and the fine fibrillar connective tissue support should also adapt to these changes.

Little is known at present regarding intrauterine remodeling and its functional implications. Nevertheless the considerations discussed above imply that the myocardium in a case of congenital malformation may function at a different level from that of a normal heart. This aspect may be important when considering myocardial vulnerability in the postnatal state, such as myocardial susceptibility to hypoxia.

The transition in postnatal myocardial growth from the fetal to the adult circulatory system is accompanied by a progressive increase in volume load affecting both sides of the heart. There is marked increase in pressure load on the left ventricle. The main morphologic counterpart of these functional changes is further enlargement of myocytes, producing a left ventricle that rapidly outgrows the right (Fig. 2.1). At the cellular level the myocyte organelle composition changes rapidly after birth. There is a significant increase in the volume fractions of mitochondria and myofibrils, which reach adult levels shortly after birth, together with a proportional increase in the capacity of the vascular bed.

The normal maturation of myocardium is a well balanced compensatory response in which the myocytes, including their cellular organelles, and the capillary microvasculature grow in proportion to the requested work load. As a side effect the compensatory response may render vulnerable the myocardium of hearts with congenital heart malformations.

HYPERTROPHY

Hypertrophy is defined as increased myocardial muscle mass due to enlargement of myocytes (Fig. 2.2). Ultrastructurally the hypertrophied myocyte is characterized mainly by an increase in mitochondria (Fig. 2.3), which are responsible for oxygen consumption and adenosine triphosphate synthesis and an increase in contractile proteins assembled in the myofibrils and responsible for adenosine triphosphate utilization. Basically myocardial cell hypertrophy is accompanied by dilation of the main coronary arteries (Fig. 2.4) and expansion of the capillary network in order to maintain adequate oxygen supply. This produces a rise in the total myocardial oxygen consumption demand, which may become highly significant in the clinical setting (see later discussion).

Myocardial hypertrophy often is categorized morphologically as concentric or eccentric. In concentric ventricular hypertrophy the wall thickness is increased without chamber enlargement. Such a response is encountered in patients with compensated pressure load hypertrophy of the left ventricle (Fig. 2.5). Eccentric ventricular hypertrophy

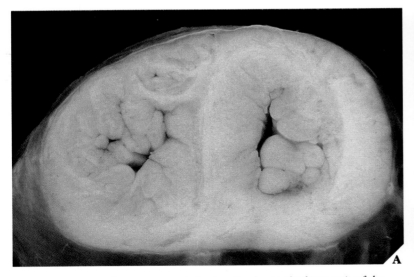

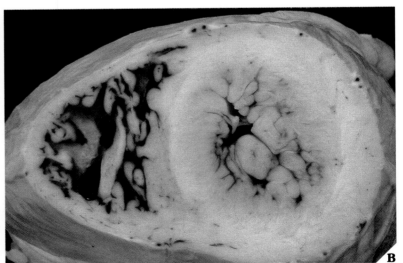

FIG. 2.1 *Cross-sections were made perpendicular to the long axis of the heart in specimens from a newborn baby (A) and a one-year-old child (B). In the newborn the right and left ventricular wall thickness is about equal,* *and the interventricular septum is almost straight. In the older infant the left ventricular wall thickness has increased over that of the right ventricle, and the septum now is convex towards the right ventricular cavity.*

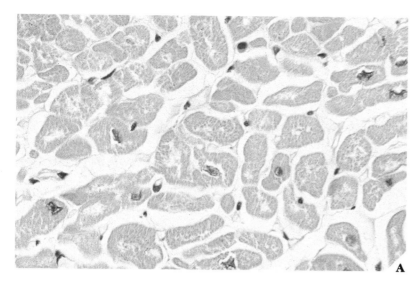

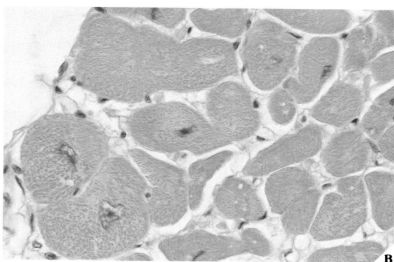

FIG. 2.2   (A) *Histologic section of normal myocardium is compared with hypertrophic myocardium* (B). *The myocardial cells are shown in cross-section at the same magnification. Hypertrophied myocytes show a*

considerable increase in size over their normal counterparts. (Fig. 1.6, Cardiac Pathology, *p 1.4)*

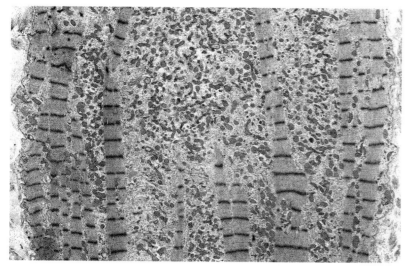

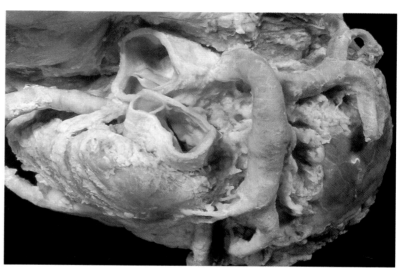

FIG. 2.3   *Electron micrograph of an hypertrophied myocyte shows a marked increase in mitochondria. This accommodates for increased demands in oxygen consumption and adenosine triphosphate synthesis. (Fig. 1.7,* Cardiac Pathology, *p 1.4)*

FIG. 2.4   *Superior view of the heart shows the aorta and main coronary arteries. The latter are markedly dilated as an adaptive phenomenon related to myocardial cell hypertrophy.*

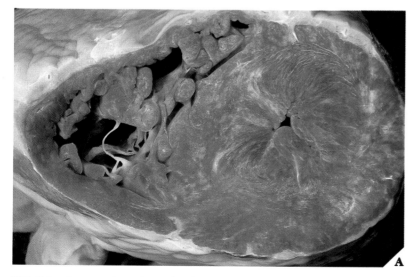

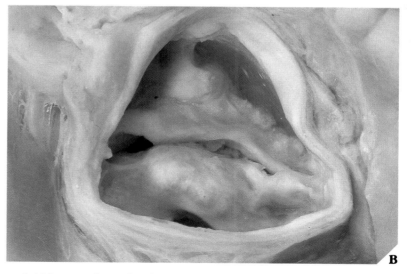

FIG. 2.5   *Cross-sections through a heart with isolated aortic stenosis show* (A) *concentric ventricular hypertrophy characterized by an increase in*

wall thickness without chamber enlargement, and (B) *a calcified and stenotic congenitally bicuspid aortic valve.*

is marked by a hypertrophic wall associated with an enlarged chamber volume, although the ratio between ventricular volume and wall thickness remains unaltered (Fig. 2.6). This arrangement is often encountered in compensated volume load hypertrophy of the left ventricle.

PRESSURE LOAD HYPERTROPHY

The classic conditions producing pressure load hypertrophy of the left ventricle include systemic hypertension, aortic coarctation, and aortic valve stenosis (see Fig. 2.5B). Right ventricular pressure load may be due to pulmonary valve stenosis, disease of the left side of the heart (with heart failure), or primary pulmonary disease. Pulmonary vascular resistance is increased in the latter two examples.

An increase in pressure load induces concentric ventricular hypertrophy as previously defined. The degree of myocyte hypertrophy differs in the various layers of the myocardium, although the overall effect is an increase in wall thickness. The increased wall thickness counteracts the elevated systolic pressures and the potentially high peak systolic wall stress according to Laplace's law (Fig. 2.7).

Growth adaptation is accompanied by hyperplasia of myofibrillar units and initially exceeds myofibrillar growth. Eventually there is a reduction of the mitochondrial-to-myofibrillar volume ratio. A critical perimitochondrial radius, which is necessary in order to supply adenosine triphosphate to the contractile proteins, may become a limiting factor in myocardial adaptation. This ultimately may impair the energy supply and compromise myocardial function. The capillary bed then increases concomitant with the increase in dimension of myocytes. In these instances the perfusion of heart muscle increases in proportion to the mass of muscle and the work it must perform. Lack of microvascular adaptation may severely impair myocardial function.

VOLUME LOAD HYPERTROPHY

Adaptation to exercise, particularly in dynamic forms of conditioning as seen in endurance athletics (running or swimming), may be accompanied by an elevated preload and eccentric hypertrophy as a compensatory mechanism. Examples of pathologic conditions that cause volume load hypertrophy of the left ventricle are aortic and mitral valve regurgitation (see Fig. 2.6B).

Structurally volume load hypertrophy consists of chamber enlargement and accompanying myocardial hypertrophy expressed mainly as increased myocyte length. The latter counteracts the increased end-diastolic wall stress by accommodating the enlarged chamber volume that otherwise may lead to spatial rearrangement and lateral slippage of the myocytes (see Fig. 2.7). The volume fractions of mitochondria and myofibrils remain almost constant. This may constitute the morphologic counterpart for the normal or improved contractile and relaxation properties of the myocardium.

Moderate exercise hypertrophy is associated with expansion of the capillary network in proportion to the increased muscle mass. In contrast there is evidence that strenuous exercise may be accompanied by inadequate capillary compensation, thus jeopardizing oxygen supply to the myocardium. Hence excessive volume load hypertrophy may lead to a state in which the myocardium is more susceptible to ischemia than expected from hypertrophy alone.

REACTIVE HYPERTROPHY

The classic examples of this form of myocardial remodeling are ischemic cardiomyopathy and myocardial infarction (Fig. 2.8). Under these circumstances muscle cells are lost, either diffusely or focally, and replaced by scar tissue. Compensatory hypertrophy of viable myocytes occurs, probably proportionally to the amount of myocardial cell loss. Under the given circumstances the ability to hypertrophy is largely determined by the underlying vascular obstructive disease. In general myocytes will increase in mean diameter while the mitochondrial-to-myofibrillar volume ratio remains constant in proportion to cell growth. Depending on the extent of myocardial cell loss, however, the ventricle may suffer chronic volume overload and subsequent lengthening of myocytes may occur. Moreover, the capillary vascular response to infarction lags behind the adaptive growth of the myocytes. Hence the hypertrophied infarcted ventricle is more vulnerable to subsequent ischemic episodes.

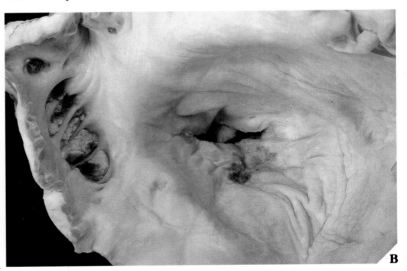

FIG. 2.6 (**A**) *Cross-section through a heart with eccentric ventricular hypertrophy shows increased wall thickness in the presence of an enlarged chamber volume. The ratio between ventricular volume and wall thickness remains unaltered.* (**B**) *Left atrial view of the regurgitant mitral valve is shown in this specimen.*

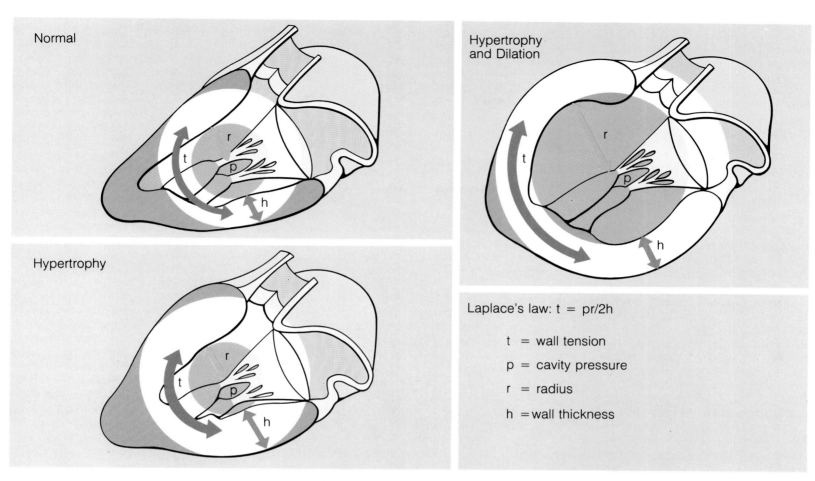

Normal

Hypertrophy

Hypertrophy
and Dilation

Laplace's law: t = pr/2h

   t = wall tension

   p = cavity pressure

   r = radius

   h = wall thickness

FIG. 2.7 *As represented in this schematic diagram, Laplace's law predicts that the load on the myocytes (wall tension = t) is determined by the product of pressure (p) and radius (r), divided by twice the wall thickness (h). (Redrawn; Fig. 1.10,* Cardiac Pathology, *p 1.6)*

FIG. 2.8 *Cross-section shows a heart with a left ventricular inferior wall aneurysm filled with thrombus due to previous myocardial infarction. There is marked reactive hypertrophy of the remaining viable left ventricular myocardium.*

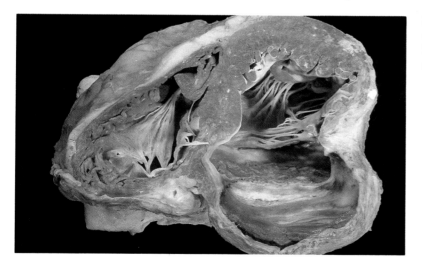

DILATION

Dilation is defined as an increase in the volume of the cardiac chamber. Sudden changes in volume load affecting a chamber usually lead to instant dilation. Chronic dilation may be related to compensated volume load hypertrophy (see above) or heart failure (Fig. 2.9). Depending on the cause dilation may resolve or persist, either as a compensated adjustment or as part of chronic volume overload with impaired hemodynamics.

COMPLICATIONS OF MYOCARDIAL REMODELING

Hypertrophy of myocardium and dilation of cardiac chambers induced as compensatory mechanisms may ultimately set the scene for secondary complications.

Dilation of a ventricular chamber, whether acute or chronic, may initiate papillary muscle dysfunction and, hence, mitral regurgitation (see Fig. 2.9) The latter condition itself causes further remodeling of the left ventricle as evidenced by enlargement of the ventricular chamber due to augmented volume load.

Hypertrophy, whether concentric or eccentric, may affect ventricular geometry. This becomes particularly pronounced in cases of marked right ventricular hypertrophy with chamber dilation. In this circumstance, the interventricular septum assumes an almost straight configuration (Fig. 2.10); it is not yet known whether this has functional implications. The reverse situation, an extreme left ventricular wall hypertrophy with a bulging septum transforming the geometry of the right ventricle, is known as Bernstein's disease, which may be a cause of right ventricular impairment.

The most important consequences of the aforementioned compensatory mechanisms relate to impaired myocardial perfusion. Marked volume load of the left ventricle with distinct chamber dilation in the setting of eccentric hypertrophy may affect the transmural perfusion pressure and may lead to impaired oxygenation of the subendocardial myocardial layers. This phenomenon is particularly prone to occur when volume load and dilation coexist with obstructive coronary artery disease (Fig. 2.11). Hence compensated chronic volume load hypertrophy may ultimately transform into a diseased state consequent to myocardial ischemia. Once induced, this process will further aggravate the impairment of myocardial perfusion by further dilation of the ventricular chamber; this allows increased end-diastolic left ventricular volume and concomitant increased pressure (Fig. 2.12). The consideration that volume load hypertrophy due to strenuous exercise may not necessarily be compensated by adequate adaptation of the microvasculature makes this sequence of events more likely.

ATHLETE'S HEART

The term athlete's heart is used to describe the cardiac effects of long-term conditioning as it occurs in highly trained competitive athletes. Enlargement of the heart is the most important feature from a morphologic viewpoint. The enlargement is due to hypertrophy of the myocardial wall, particularly in the left ventricle, and enlargement of the ventricular cavities. These features are easily demonstrated with cross-sectional echocardiography. Particularly in endurance athletes, such as marathon runners, cavity dimension is increased almost constantly. The hypertrophy of the left ventricular wall under such conditions is symmetric and the compensatory conditioning may well be summarized as eccentric hypertrophy. Occasionally an asymmetric pattern of left ventricular hypertrophy may ensue. Usually the absolute thickening of the septum is minimal and the echocardiographic septal/free wall ratio remains below 1:3. This suggests disproportionate septal thickening rather than asymmetric septal hypertrophy as part of hypertrophic cardiomyopathy (see Chapter 5). Nevertheless, once noticed, this particular aspect should always be carefully evaluated.

It remains speculative whether the type of exercise is important with respect to the changes in cardiac structure. It has been demonstrated that athletes participating in dynamic endurance sports are exposed primarily to conditions producing a volume load and thus develop eccentric hypertrophy. On the other hand, athletes involved in sports that are primarily static, such as weightlifting, are conditioned to produce primarily a pressure load hypertrophy. In view of these considerations, one may expect that endurance athletes will be more prone to secondary myocardial complications, at least when additional pathologic circumstances such as obstructive coronary artery disease are present. Indeed sudden death in competitive athletes is almost always caused by additional cardiovascular abnormalities, which may have passed unnoticed clinically. Nevertheless one may occasionally encounter instances of sudden death in athletes where no additional abnormalities can be detected other than chamber enlargement and myocardial hypertrophy without obstructive coronary disease. In some of these instances the heart shows extensive fibrosis and, occasionally, definite scars, indicating previous infarction clinically unrecognized (Fig. 2.13). In other cases, however, there is no detectable abnormality and the mechanisms underlying sudden death remain unclear.

AGING HEART

The increased longevity in the western world has led to an increased interest in geriatric cardiology. The myocardium of the elderly may be expected to show atrophy unless other circumstances prevail to

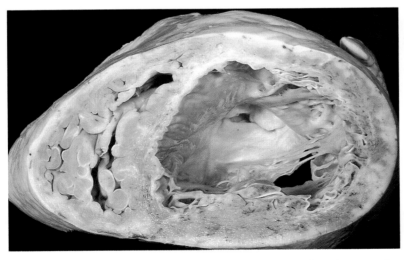

FIG. 2.9 *Heart cross-section shows a marked increase in the left ventricular chamber volume as an expression of chronic ischemia leading to a failing heart. Chronic dilation under these circumstances may lead to papillary muscle dysfunction and mitral regurgitation. The latter in itself may further jeopardize myocardial perfusion, which may aggravate left heart failure already present. (Fig. 1.3, Cardiac Pathology, p 1.2)*

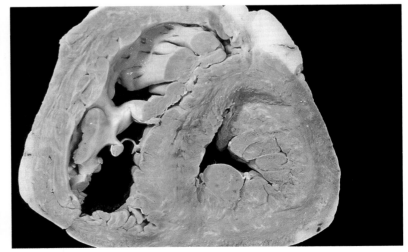

FIG. 2.10 *Cross-section through a heart with marked right ventricular hypertrophy and right ventricular chamber dilation reveals an almost straight configuration of the interventricular septum, thereby affecting left ventricular geometry.*

induce compensatory changes. As such, systemic hypertension is a frequent disorder, and a substantial number of elderly patients have myocardial hypertrophy on that basis. With increasing age, moreover, major abnormalities can occur in the fibrous tissues that constitute the cardiac skeleton, including the cardiac valves. In elderly patients therefore morphologic abnormalities of the valves, particularly of the aortic and mitral valves, are the rule rather than the exception.

In a significant proportion of patients these alterations are functionally important although not necessarily clinically manifest. It is not infrequent to detect severe isolated calcific aortic stenosis at autopsy with colossal myocardial hypertrophy. This can underscore sudden death in an elderly patient in whom the valve abnormality was never apparent clinically. Likewise a calcified mitral ring may induce mitral valve regurgitation and volume load hypertrophy of the left ventricle that, in the presence of obstructive coronary artery disease, may easily lead to myocardial ischemia, infarction, and death.

At a cellular level it is still uncertain whether the adaptive phenomena are equal to those that occur in children or adults. Such features may nonetheless prove to be important in the future for better understanding of the pathophysiology in this category of patients.

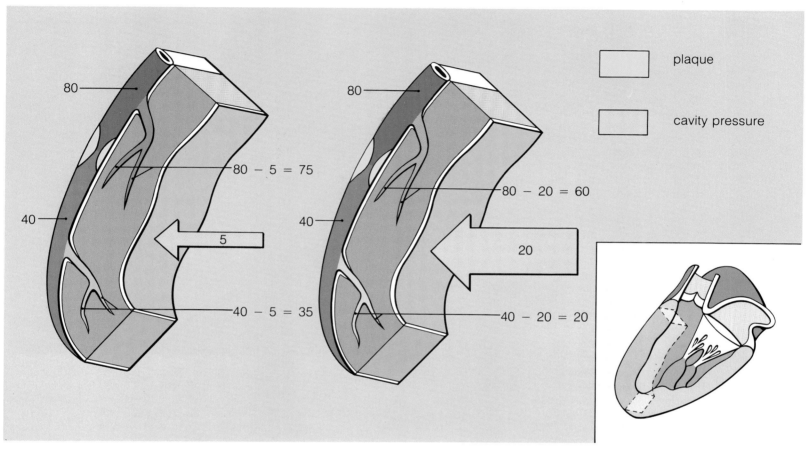

FIG. 2.11 *Schematic representation shows the interaction between myocardial perfusion and intracavitary and diastolic pressures in the presence of an obstructive coronary artery lesion. Elevated end-diastolic pressure may lead to impaired subendocardial perfusion of the left ventricular myocardium; ischemia and infarction thus may result. (Redrawn; Fig. 1.14,* Cardiac Pathology, *p 1.8)*

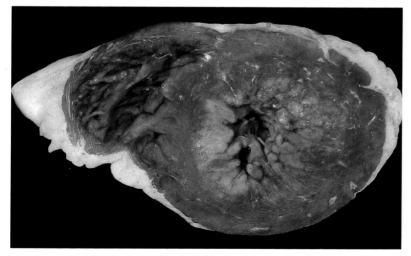

FIG. 2.12 *Cross-section through a heart reveals impairment of left ventricular subendocardial perfusion and circumferential infarction due to increased end-diastolic left ventricular pressure with chamber dilation in the setting of critical obstructive coronary artery lesions.*

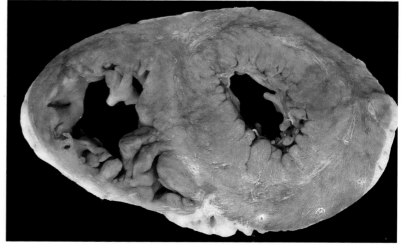

FIG. 2.13 *Cross-section through the heart of an endurance athlete shows left ventricular chamber dilation and hypertrophy of the left ventricular wall. There is extensive, almost circular and bandlike scarring of the left ventricular myocardium without evidence of obstructive coronary artery disease.*

MYOCARDIAL REMODELING AND ITS COMPLICATIONS

II

DISEASES OF THE HEART

3
CONGENITAL HEART DISEASE

J. Willis Hurst, MD
Elizabeth W. Nugent, MD
Robert H. Anderson, MD
Benson R. Wilcox, MD

CLINICAL ILLUSTRATIONS SUPPLIED BY

Elizabeth W. Nugent, MD
Scott J. Pollak, MD

Abstracted with permission of the authors and publisher from Nugent EW, Plauth WH Jr, Edwards JE, Schlant RC, Williams WH: Congenital heart disease, Chapter 36, pp 580–728, in Hurst JW (ed): *The Heart,* 6th ed. New York, McGraw-Hill, 1986. Figures, tables, or extracts of text reproduced from the above chapter, other chapters in *The Heart,* or other sources are also reprinted with permission of the authors and publishers. For the full bibliographic citations of the sources of figures or tables other than the above chapter, see Figure Credits at the end of this chapter. The greater majority of the illustrations of cardiac morphology shown in this chapter are of hearts in the Cardiopathological Museum of Children's Hospital of Pittsburgh. The photographs were taken with the permission and extensive collaboration of J.R. Zuber-buhler, MD. His considerable help is gratefully acknowledged.

Congenital cardiac defects are caused by environmental factors and chromosomal abnormalities, such as trisomy, deletion, and mosaicism. The rubella virus may cause patency of the arterial duct and is associated with peripheral pulmonary arterial stenoses.

The overall incidence of congenital heart disease is 8 per 1000 live births; the prevalence of specific lesions is shown in Table 3.1.

The complications of congenital heart disease are death, congestive heart failure, arterial oxygen unsaturation with consequent cyanosis and cerebral thrombus, bacterial endocarditis, pulmonary arterial hypertension and pulmonary vascular obstructive disease, retardation of growth and development, and exertional intolerance and restrictions. Many patients with congenital heart disease have no complications for many years.

The following discussion includes only the most common types of congenital heart disease, since the list of all types of malformations is virtually unlimited.

Table 3.1 Prevalence of Specific Lesions of Congenital Heart Disease

LESION	CASES OF CONGENITAL HEART DISEASE (%)				
	KEITH (1978)	NÀDAS (1972)	MITCHELL (1971)	HOFFMAN (1978)	FYLER (1980)
Ventricular septal defect	28.3	19.4	29.5	31.3	16.6
Pulmonary stenosis	9.9	7.5	8.6	13.5	3.5
Patent arterial duct	9.8	15.5	8.3	5.5	6.5
Atrial septal defect, secundum	7.0	4.5	7.4	6.1	3.1
Ventricular septal defect with pulmonary stenosis*	9.7	10.5	6.4	3.7	9.4
Aortic stenosis	7.1	5.7	3.8	3.7	2.0
Aortic atresia	1.5	NL	3.1	0.6	7.9
Atrioventricular septal defect†	3.4	2.7	3.6	3.7	5.3
Coarctation of aorta	5.1	8.1	2.6	5.5	8.0
Peripheral pulmonary stenosis	NL	1.0	3.6	NL	NL
Endocardial fibroelastosis	0.9	NL	2.4	NL	NL
Complete transposition	4.9	4.0	2.6	3.7	10.5
Common arterial trunk	0.7	0.8	1.7	2.5	1.5
Total anomalous pulmonary venous connection	1.4	1.3	NL	0.6	2.8
Tricuspid atresia	1.2	1.0	1.2	NL	2.7
Double-outlet right ventricle	0.5	0.2	1.0	0.6	1.6
Pulmonary atresia without ventricular septal defect	0.7	0.3	0.01	0.6	3.3
Number of patients	15,104	10,624	56,109	19,502	2,251

(Table 36-1, *The Heart*, 6th ed, p 582)
*Includes tetralogy of Fallot.
†Includes partial and complete.
NL, not listed

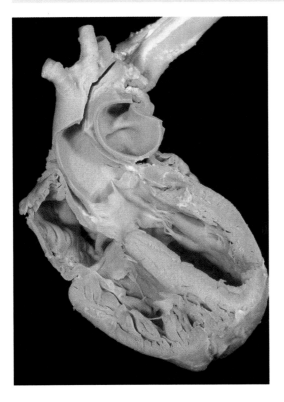

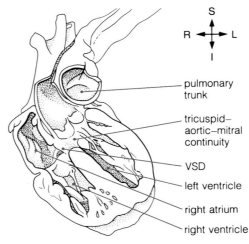

S

R ◄──┼──► L

I

pulmonary trunk

tricuspid–aortic–mitral continuity

VSD

left ventricle

right atrium

right ventricle

FIG. 3.1 *This simulated four-chamber long-axis section of a heart with a perimembranous inlet VSD shows the essential feature of the defect: Its posteroinferior border is made up of an extensive area of fibrous continuity between the mitral, aortic, and tricuspid valves. The aortic valve is located in the roof of the defect.*

VENTRICULAR SEPTAL DEFECT
DEFINITION AND PATHOLOGY

A ventricular septal defect (VSD) is defined as an opening in the ventricular septum that separates the left and the right ventricles. Seventy-five percent of these are perimembranous (Fig. 3.1); they may open into the inlet (Fig. 3.2A) or outlet (Fig. 3.2B) components of the right ventricle, or they may become confluent. Defects in the septum may also be located within the muscular septum; these are termed muscular defects (Fig. 3.3). Defects located in the outflow tract roofed by the conjoint leaflets of the aortic and the pulmonary valves

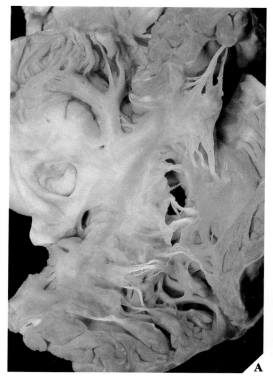

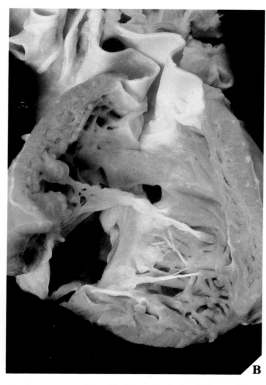

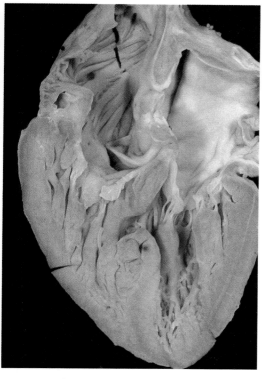

FIG. 3.2 *Perimembranous VSDs, photographed here from the right ventricular aspect, may ex-*

*tend to open primarily into the inlet (**A**) or the outlet (**B**) components of the right ventricle.*

FIG. 3.3 *This simulated four-chamber long-axis section shows a muscular inlet defect embedded within the musculature of the septum. This can be differentiated from a perimembranous defect opening to the inlet of the right ventricle by a muscle bar that forms the roof of the defect, separating it from the septal attachments of the tricuspid and mitral valves (see Fig. 3.1).*

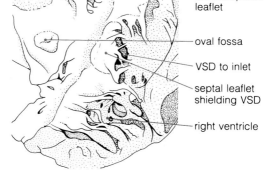

S
P ← → A
I

- anterosuperior leaflet
- oval fossa
- VSD to inlet
- septal leaflet shielding VSD
- right ventricle

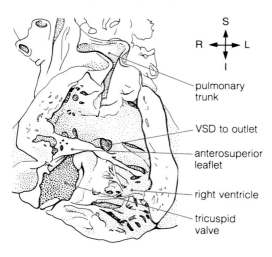

S
R ← → L
I

- pulmonary trunk
- VSD to outlet
- anterosuperior leaflet
- right ventricle
- tricuspid valve

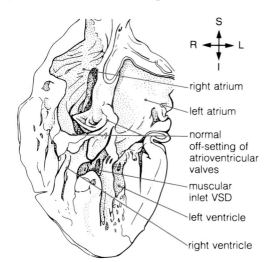

S
R ← → L
I

- right atrium
- left atrium
- normal off-setting of atrioventricular valves
- muscular inlet VSD
- left ventricle
- right ventricle

are termed doubly committed juxta-arterial defects (Fig. 3.4). A ventricular septal defect that is located immediately beneath the leaflets of the aortic valve may result in aortic regurgitation (Fig. 3.5).

ABNORMAL PHYSIOLOGY

Patients with VSDs can be divided into three groups according to the associated altered physiology. This depends upon the size of the defect and the reaction of the pulmonary arterioles. The first group is composed of patients with a small defect (less than 0.5 cm²/m²), no elevation of the pulmonary arterial pressure, and a small left-to-right shunt. The patient is at little risk except for endocarditis. In the second group the defect is of medium size (0.5–1.0 cm²/m²); the pulmonary arterial and the right ventricular systolic pressures may become elevated to about 80% of the left ventricular systolic pressure. A moderate-sized left-to-right shunt is present, and volume overload of the left atrium and the left ventricle occurs. In the third group the hole is 1.0 cm²/m² or larger. It is as large as the aortic valve orifice, so that the systolic pressure is equal in the aorta, the left ventricle, the right ventricle, and the pulmonary arteries. The amount of blood delivered to the lungs and the periphery is determined by the pulmonary and peripheral vascular resistance.

There may be very little left-to-right shunting at birth, because the pulmonary vascular resistance is high. After birth the pulmonary vascular resistance decreases and the left-to-right shunt increases, which may lead to left ventricular failure. This is usually detected clinically at 3–12 weeks of age; however, in premature infants it may occur earlier.

The large pulmonary blood flow can lead to pulmonary arteriolar disease and a high systolic pressure in the right ventricle and the pulmonary arteries. When the pulmonary arterial resistance exceeds the systemic arterial resistance, a right-to-left shunt and arterial oxygen unsaturation are found; this is termed Eisenmenger's syndrome. The pulmonary vasculature is abnormal in such cases.

CLINICAL MANIFESTATIONS

A ventricular septal defect may occur as an isolated defect or in combination with other anomalies. The incidence is the same in males and females.

SYMPTOMS

Infants, children, and adults with small defects have no symptoms. Infants with moderately large defects develop heart failure at 3–12

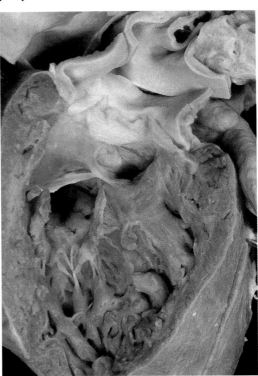

FIG. 3.4 *This outlet defect has a muscular posteroinferior rim separating the margin from the area of the membranous septum. A fibrous roof is formed by the continuity between the leaflets of the aortic and the pulmonary valves. Such a defect is well described as being doubly committed and juxta-arterial, although some may recognize it as supracristal.*

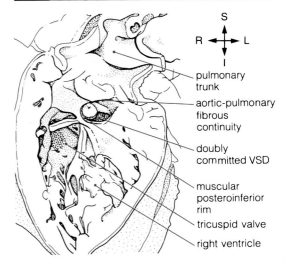

pulmonary trunk

aortic-pulmonary fibrous continuity

doubly committed VSD

muscular posteroinferior rim

tricuspid valve

right ventricle

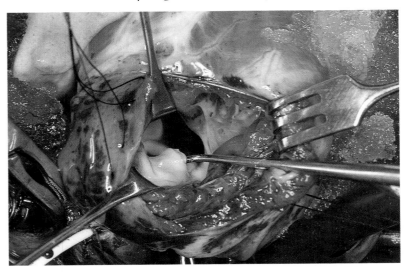

FIG. 3.5 *Operative view shows an aortic valve leaflet prolapsed into the roof of a perimembranous VSD. The aortic valve itself was regurgitant because of the prolapse.*

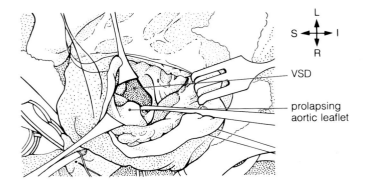

VSD

prolapsing aortic leaflet

weeks of age; parents notice breathing difficulty and fatigue during feeding. Patients with severe pulmonary hypertension and arterial oxygen unsaturation develop heart failure, hemoptysis, and cerebral thromboses.

PHYSICAL EXAMINATION

When the defect is small, a loud, usually holosystolic murmur is heard with maximal intensity at the mid- to lower left sternal border. It may be midsystolic or decrescendo, suggesting that the defect is located in the muscular septum. A thrill may be present. The pulmonary component of the second sound is normal, and the right and the left ventricles produce normal precordial pulsations.

Infants with large defects who have large left-to-right shunts together with pulmonary arterial hypertension exhibit different features. A thrill may be felt to the left of the mid- to lower sternum. A loud holosystolic murmur is heard in the same area with a low-pitched, diastolic rumble at the apex. The latter signifies a pulmonary-to-systemic blood flow ratio of 2:1 or more. The second sound is normally split, and the pulmonary closure sound is abnormally loud. The right and the left ventricular precordial pulsations are hyperactive. Respiratory distress, liver enlargement, or rales may be detected. With time the shunt may diminish as the defect becomes smaller, right ventricular outflow tract obstruction develops, or pulmonary arteriolar disease increases. When the defect becomes smaller, the murmur and second heart sound are altered in a predictable way; the murmur becomes less loud with increasing pulmonary hypertension, and the intensity of the pulmonary component of the second sound increases.

Eisenmenger's syndrome, seen in older children and adults, also has typical features. Cyanosis is apparent and a prominent a wave is detected in the internal jugular veins. A left anterior precordial lift signifies right ventricular hypertrophy. Pulmonary valve closure and pulsation of the pulmonary trunk may be palpable in the second left intercostal space. The murmur generated by the VSD is located in early systole and may be faint. The second sound is loud due to an increased intensity of closure of the pulmonary valve. The murmur of pulmonary valve regurgitation, called a Graham–Steell murmur, may be heard along the left sternal border. The systolic murmur of tricuspid regurgitation may also be heard. With time, signs of heart failure may be detected. Any patient with a defect located immediately beneath the aortic valve may have aortic regurgitation due to prolapse of an aortic valve cusp.

LABORATORY STUDIES

CHEST RADIOGRAPHY.   The chest film is normal in patients with a small VSD. The chest radiograph of a patient with a moderate-sized VSD shows a slightly enlarged heart with prominent pulmonary arteries (Fig. 3.6). The chest film of a patient with Eisenmenger's syndrome demonstrates an enlarged heart with large pulmonary arteries

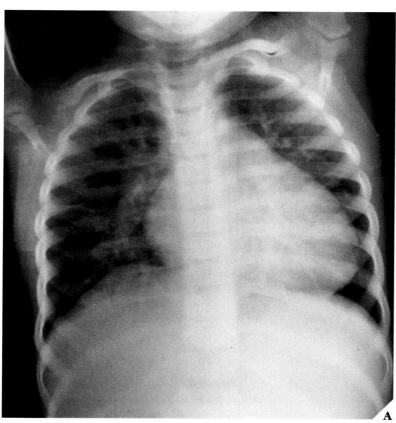

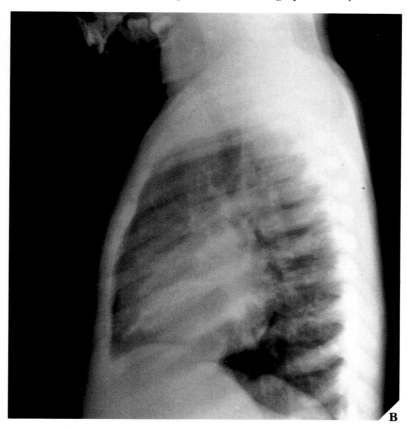

A

B

FIG. 3.6   (A) *Posteroanterior chest radiograph of a three-year-old child with a moderate-sized VSD shows moderate generalized cardiac enlargement and increased pulmonary blood flow. The right pulmonary artery is* increased in size. (B) *Lateral view shows generalized cardiac enlargement, particularly of the left atrium. (Courtesy of the X-Ray Department, Henrietta Egleston Hospital for Children, Atlanta, Georgia)*

(Fig. 3.7). The tapering of the right branch of the pulmonary artery suggests pulmonary hypertension.

ELECTROCARDIOGRAPHY. The electrocardiogram (ECG) may be normal in patients with a small interventricular septal defect. In the ECG of a patient with a moderate-sized defect the increased QRS voltage suggests left ventricular hypertrophy (Fig. 3.8). The presence of right ventricular hypertrophy is evident in the ECG of a patient with Eisenmenger's syndrome (Fig. 3.9).

ECHOCARDIOGRAPHY. Echocardiography has become increasingly useful in the diagnosis of congenital heart disease. The cross-sectional echocardiogram may be used to identify the type of VSD (Capelli et al, 1983). Perimembranous defects are juxta-aortic, being directly related to the central fibrous skeleton supporting the aortic valve. The muscular defects are surrounded by muscle, while the doubly committed juxta-arterial defects are roofed by aortic and pulmonary valves in fibrous continuity (Fig. 3.10). A Doppler recording of a patient with an isolated interventricular septal defect is shown in Figure 3.11.

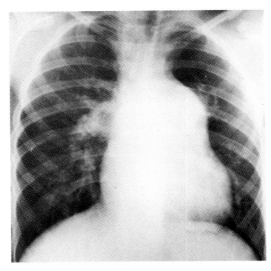

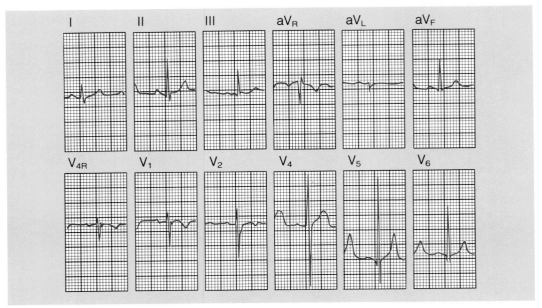

FIG. 3.7 *Posteroanterior chest film of a 12-year-old child reveals a large VSD and Eisenmenger's syndrome. The main and the central pulmonary arteries are markedly dilated, while the peripheral segmental branches appear attenuated. (Fig. 36-3, The Heart, 6th ed, p 593. Courtesy of the X-Ray Department, Henrietta Egleston Hospital for Children, Atlanta, Georgia)*

FIG. 3.8 *ECG of a seven-year-old child with a moderate-sized VSD shows large QRS complexes in leads V_4 and V_5. The mean QRS vector is to the left and posteriorly directed, suggesting left ventricular hypertrophy; the mean T vector is to the left and slightly posteriorly directed. (Redrawn; courtesy of the Electrocardiography Laboratory, Henrietta Egleston Hospital for Children, Atlanta, Georgia)*

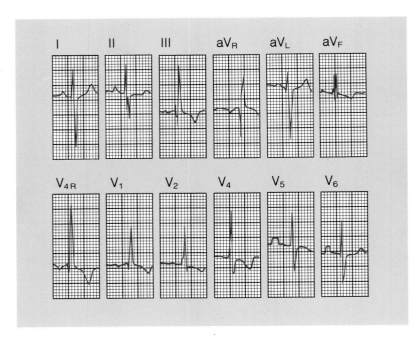

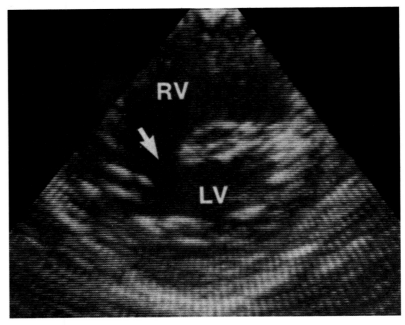

FIG. 3.9 *ECG of a seven-year-old child with an interventricular septal defect and Eisenmenger's syndrome shows evidence of right ventricular hypertrophy and prolonged QRS complexes. Standardization is normal in leads I, II, III, aV_R, aV_L, aV_F, and V_{4R} one half standardized in V_1, and one quarter standardized in leads V_2, V_4, V_5, and V_6. (Redrawn; courtesy of the Electrocardiography Laboratory, Henrietta Egleston Hospital for Children, Atlanta, Georgia)*

FIG. 3.10 *Cross-sectional echocardiography was performed in a patient with a large muscular VSD. The parasternal short-axis view through the left ventricle (LV) at the level of the papillary muscles shows that the defect (arrow) is located in the inferior portion of the septum near the cardiac apex (RV, right ventricle). (Reproduced with permission of the authors and publisher; see Figure Credits)*

CARDIAC CATHETERIZATION. The amount of left-to-right shunt may be identified by an increase in oxygen saturation in the right ventricle. When the defect is small, the right ventricular and the pulmonary arterial systolic pressures are normal. When the left-to-right shunt is large, the pulmonary arterial systolic pressure may approach systemic levels and the left atrial pressure may be elevated. When there is severe elevation of pulmonary arterial resistance, as in Eisenmenger's syndrome, the shunt becomes right-to-left or bidirectional.

Cardiac angiography and aortography are used to identify aortic regurgitation, patency of the arterial duct, location of the great arteries, and the number of defects (Fig. 3.12).

NATURAL HISTORY

About one-fourth of small interventricular defects close spontaneously within one and one-half years, one-half close in four years, and even more are closed at ten years (Alpert et al, 1979). With time some large defects become smaller, and a few may close.

Infants with large defects develop congestive heart failure. A small proportion develops subvalvar pulmonary stenosis, which produces a syndrome similar to tetralogy of Fallot.

Eisenmenger's syndrome is more likely to develop in patients beyond one year of age whose pulmonary systolic pressure is in excess of half of the systemic arterial pressure (Weidman et al, 1977).

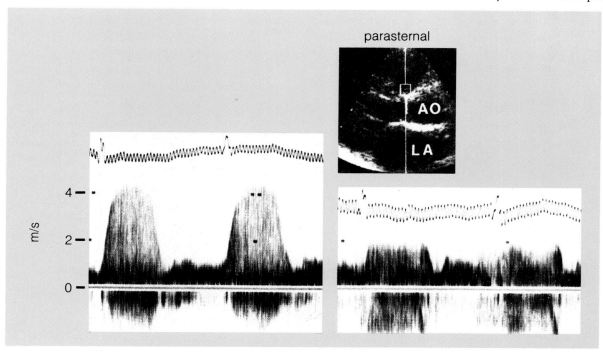

parasternal

FIG. 3.11 **Left,** *The high-velocity jet through a VSD toward the transducer is recorded with continuous-wave Doppler.* **Right,** *With pulsed Doppler the VSD can be localized. The maximal velocity gives a calculated pressure difference of 80 mmHg between the ventricles; the systolic blood pressure of 100 mmHg indicates a right ventricular systolic pressure of around 20 mmHG* (AO, *aorta;* LA, *left atrium*). *(Partially redrawn; reproduced with permission of the authors and publisher; see Figure Credits)*

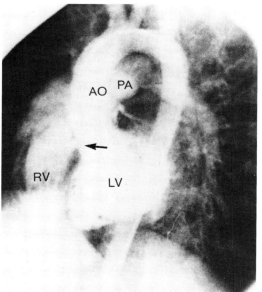

FIG. 3.12 *Left anterior oblique view of a left ventricular angiogram in a five-year-old child shows a small perimembranous VSD* (arrow). *(RV,* right ventricle; *LV,* left ventricle; *AO,* ascending aorta; *PA,* pulmonary artery). *(Fig. 36-4,* The Heart, *6th ed, p 594. Courtesy of the Cardiac Catheterization Laboratory, Henrietta Egleston Hospital for Children, Atlanta, Georgia)*

A small number of patients (less than 1%) develop aortic regurgitation, while about 10% develop endocarditis during the first 30 years of life (Weidman et al, 1977).

TREATMENT

An infant with VSD should be examined frequently in order to detect increasing cardiac volume overload. The ECG is used to identify those infants with elevation of the right ventricular systolic pressure.

Any patient exhibiting signs of heart failure should have catheterization and angiography; to plan treatment it is necessary to know the size of the shunt and the level of the systolic pulmonary arterial pressure. When heart failure is easy to manage, the infant may be treated medically with digoxin with hope that the defect will become smaller. When the pulmonary arterial systolic pressure is greater than half the systolic aortic pressure, the defect should be closed surgically.

Patients with small defects that persist into adulthood need no medical treatment except measures to prevent bacterial endocarditis. Currently there is no effective treatment for Eisenmenger's syndrome (Graham, 1979).

INDICATIONS FOR SURGERY

Surgery is indicated in infants with heart failure who do not respond satisfactorily to medical treatment and infants with pulmonary arterial systolic pressures that are more than half of the systolic aortic pressures. The child with a pulmonary-to-systemic blood flow ratio of greater than 1.8:1 should also have surgery. An enlarged heart or active symptomatology with a shunt of 1.4:1 in infants is an indication for surgery. The adult with a shunt of 1.4:1 should have surgical correction.

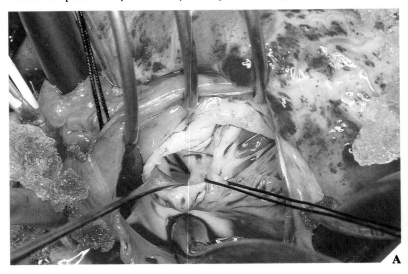
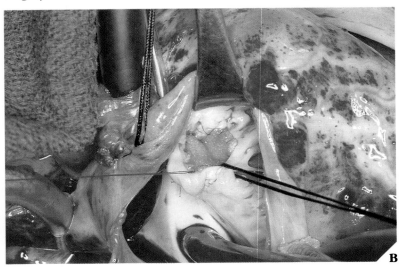

FIG. 3.13 (A) *Operative view of a perimembranous outlet VSD shows the characteristic location just beneath the commissure of the septal and the* anterior leaflets of the tricuspid valve. (B) *The Dacron patch has been sewn in with continuous and interrupted monofilament suture.*

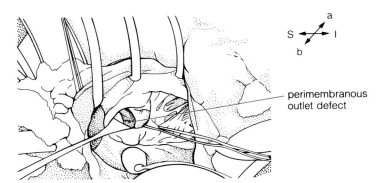
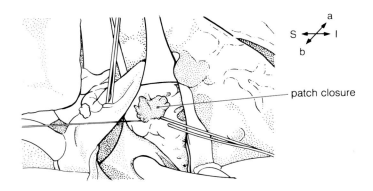

perimembranous outlet defect

patch closure

Unfortunately patients who develop Eisenmenger's syndrome are poor candidates for surgery. Surgery may be attempted in patients whose pulmonary vascular resistance is less than 11 units/m². (The reader is referred to Chapter 36, *The Heart,* 6th ed, pp 596–597, for further discussion of surgical management.)

SURGICAL PROCEDURE

The usual operative approach to a VSD is through a superoinferior incision in the right atrium. With gentle traction of the tricuspid valve most defects can be visualized well enough to effect the necessary repair. Repair of a typical perimembranous outlet defect located just under the junction of the septal and the anterior leaflets of the valve (Fig. 3.13) involves insertion of a low-porosity Dacron velour patch. Occasionally it is advantageous, or even necessary, to open the right

ventricle to obtain adequate exposure of the defect(s), especially with muscular defects in the outlet septum or doubly committed juxta-arterial defects (Fig. 3.14). Very rarely it is necessary to open the left ventricle; this approach has been recommended in cases of "Swiss-cheese" septum with multiple muscular defects in the trabecular portion of the septum.

Of vital importance to the surgeon is a clear understanding of the relationship of the borders of the defect(s) to the conduction tissues. The surgeon must accurately assess the anatomic type of VSD to locate quickly the conduction axis. In the case of a perimembranous inlet VSD the surgeon, having identified the anatomic type, knows that the penetrating bundle lies on his "right-hand" side; therefore the posteroinferior suture line is placed well away from the edge of the defect (Fig. 3.15). When a muscular inlet defect is involved, the conduction

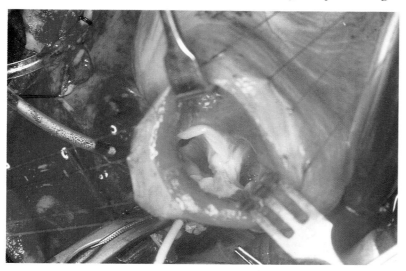

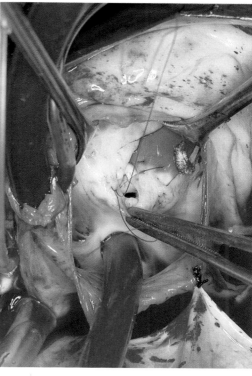

FIG. 3.15 *In this repair of a perimembranous inlet VSD the pledgeted suture is placed well away from the posteroinferior rim of the defect to avoid the conduction axis.*

FIG. 3.14 *Operative view of a doubly committed juxta-arterial VSD shows the muscular posteroinferior rim. (Reproduced with permission of the authors and publisher; see Figure Credits)*

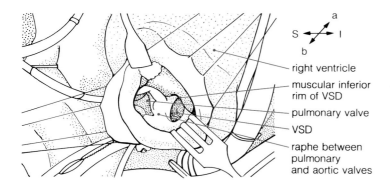

- right ventricle
- muscular inferior rim of VSD
- pulmonary valve
- VSD
- raphe between pulmonary and aortic valves

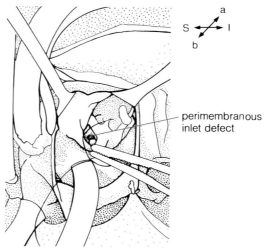

- perimembranous inlet defect

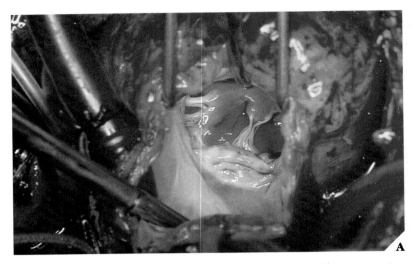 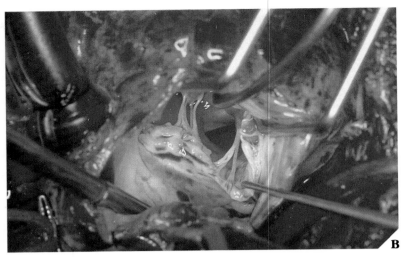

FIG. 3.16 (A) *In muscular inlet VSD a broad muscle bundle separates the defect from the membranous septum. The conduction tissue courses to the left of the defect as the surgeon views it through the tricuspid valve.* (B) *The muscular rim of the defect is located beneath the retracted septal leaflet of the tricuspid valve. (Reproduced with permission of the authors and publisher; see Figure Credits)*

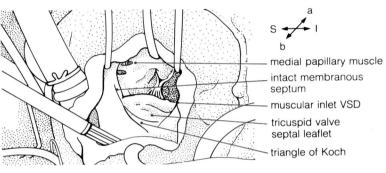 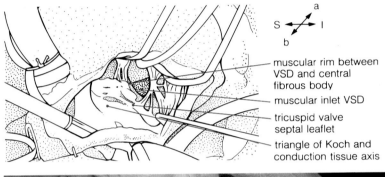

a
S ← → I
b

medial papillary muscle
intact membranous septum
muscular inlet VSD
tricuspid valve septal leaflet
triangle of Koch

a
S ← → I
b

muscular rim between VSD and central fibrous body
muscular inlet VSD
tricuspid valve septal leaflet
triangle of Koch and conduction tissue axis

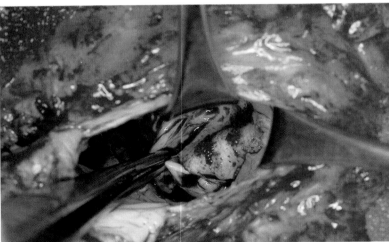 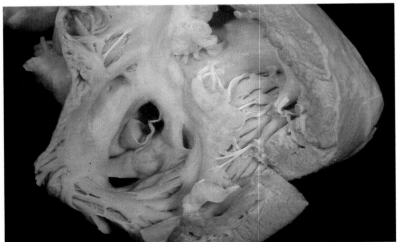

FIG. 3.17 *Operative view from the left ventricular aspect shows a Dacron patch placed three months earlier to close a VSD. The patch is almost completely incorporated into heart tissue.*

FIG. 3.18 *An interatrial communication within the oval fossa resulting from a deficiency of the floor of the fossa is a true septal defect. It is usually described as an ostium secundum defect, even though the floor of the fossa is made up of the primary atrial septum.*

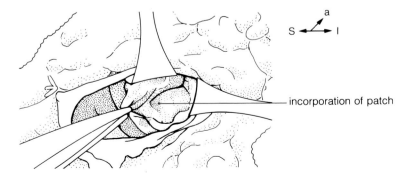 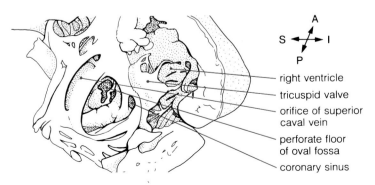

a
S ← → I

incorporation of patch

A
S ← → I
P

right ventricle
tricuspid valve
orifice of superior caval vein
perforate floor of oval fossa
coronary sinus

tissues are on the surgeon's "left-hand" side (Fig. 3.16).

In the majority of instances patch closure is necessary, although direct closure may occasionally be possible in smaller or narrower defects. Most surgeons prefer a low-porosity Dacron cloth, since it seals almost immediately while allowing for tissue growth. Within a few weeks it is incorporated into the heart tissue (Fig. 3.17). Providing there is no leakage along the edges of the patch, the patient has minimal risk of endocarditis.

ATRIAL SEPTAL DEFECT
DEFINITION AND PATHOLOGY

In each of the four types of interatrial communications there is a through-and-through opening between the left and the right atria (Edwards, 1966). Only those within the oval fossa, termed *ostium secundum* defects, are true septal defects (Fig. 3.18). Secundum defects range from patency of the oval foramen (Fig. 3.19A), through minimal to major deficiency of the floor of the fossa (Fig. 3.19B, C) to various

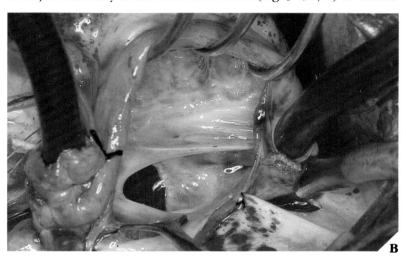

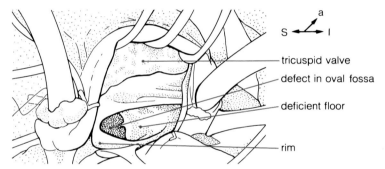

tricuspid valve
defect in oval fossa
deficient floor
rim

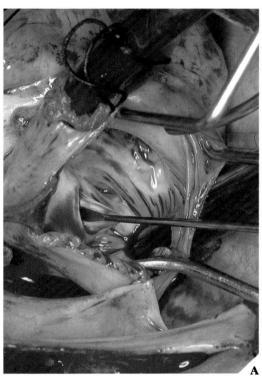

FIG. 3.19 *Operative views illustrate the morphologic variability of holes within the oval fossa.* (A) *Here probe patency of the fossa is demonstrated. When the probe is removed, the facility for shunting disappears.* (B) *In this view the floor of the fossa is insufficiently large to overlap the rim, resulting in a small defect.* (C) *When the entire floor of the fossa is deficient, a large hole is created.*

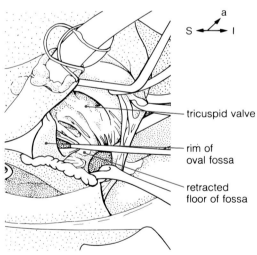

tricuspid valve
rim of oval fossa
retracted floor of fossa

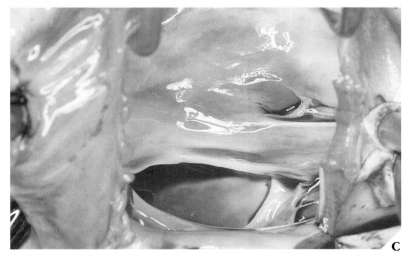

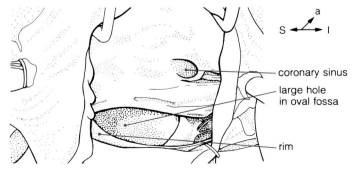

coronary sinus
large hole in oval fossa
rim

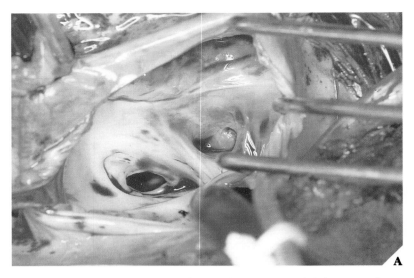

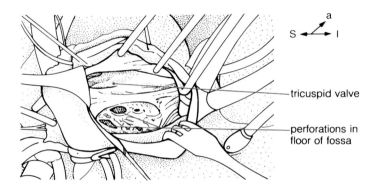

FIG. 3.20 *Holes in the fossa may be small (A) or large (B) because of perforations in the floor rather than deficiencies at its edge.*

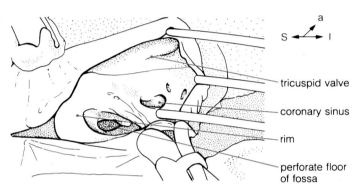

tricuspid valve

coronary sinus

rim

perforate floor of fossa

tricuspid valve

perforations in floor of fossa

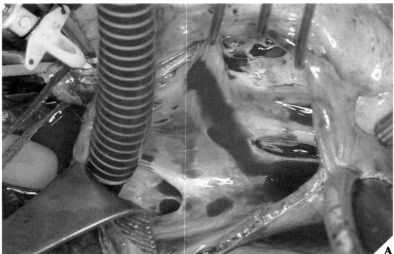

FIG. 3.21 *Operative views illustrate the anatomy of the sinus venosus defects in the mouth of the superior (A) and the inferior (B) caval veins. The*

oval fossa is intact in both hearts. Two pulmonary veins open into the right atrium in the superior defect.

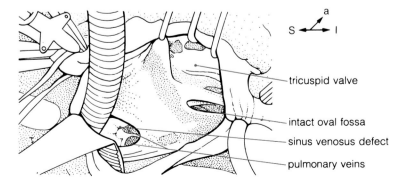

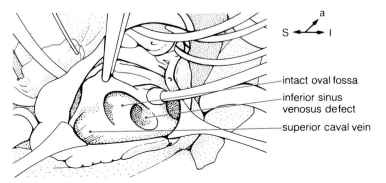

tricuspid valve

intact oval fossa

sinus venosus defect

pulmonary veins

intact oval fossa

inferior sinus venosus defect

superior caval vein

degrees of perforation of the floor (Fig. 3.20). The *sinus venosus* defect is an interatrial communication in the mouth of the superior (Fig. 3.21A) or inferior (Fig. 3.21B) caval veins, existing outside the environs of the oval fossa (Fig. 3.22). Anomalous entrance of one or more pulmonary veins into the right atrium occurs in most patients with this defect (see Fig. 3.21A). *Coronary sinus defects,* created at the mouth of the sinus because of unroofing of its atrial course, are very rarely found (Fig. 3.23). An atrial septal defect within the oval fossa

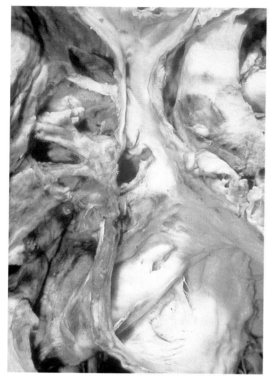

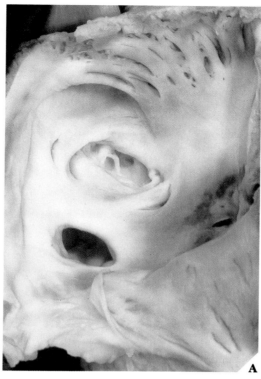

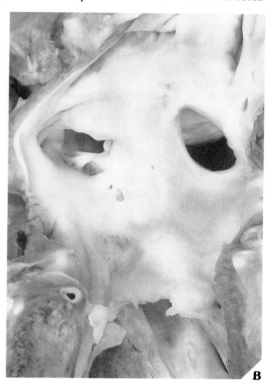

FIG. 3.22 *A sinus venosus defect is an interatrial communication in the mouth of the superior caval vein resulting from the biatrial connection of the superior caval and the right upper pulmonary veins. It is outside the confines of the true atrial septum (the environs of the oval fossa), although it unequivocally produces an interatrial defect. (Reproduced with permission of the authors and publisher; see Figure Credits)*

FIG. 3.23 *An interatrial communication through the mouth of the coronary sinus is viewed from the right (A) and the left (B) atrial aspects. The defect, which is outside the confines of the oval fossa, results from unroofing of the coronary sinus. There is a total lack of the party*

wall normally separating the coronary sinus from the left atrium (unroofed coronary sinus). Usually this lesion co-exists with a persistent left superior caval vein connected to the roof of the left atrium, but this anomalous venous connection is lacking in this particular heart.

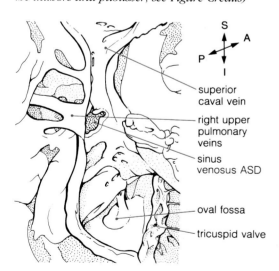

superior
caval vein

right upper
pulmonary
veins

sinus
venosus ASD

oval fossa

tricuspid valve

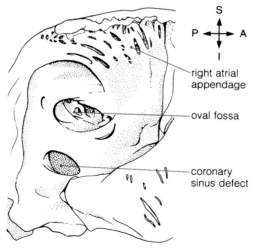

right atrial
appendage

oval fossa

coronary
sinus defect

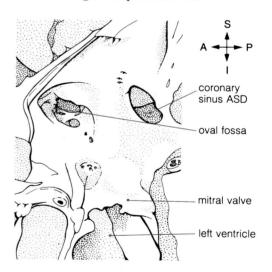

coronary
sinus ASD

oval fossa

mitral valve

left ventricle

associated with mitral stenosis is termed Lutembacher's syndrome. The ostium primum defect is an atrioventricular septal defect (see p. 3.18).

ABNORMAL PHYSIOLOGY

The ostium secundum type of septal defect produces a left-to-right shunt even though the left atrial pressure may be only a few millimeters of mercury higher than the pressure in the right atrium. This shunt may be large because the right atrium and the right ventricle offer little resistance to filling, and the tricuspid valve is large. Usually the pulmonary arterial system undergoes its normal change, tolerating a large increase in pulmonary blood flow with little rise in pulmonary arterial pressure. Some patients, however, develop pulmonary hypertension, reversal of the shunt, and arterial oxygen unsaturation; this state is termed Eisenmenger physiology. Mitral valve prolapse may occur.

The sinus venosus type of defect produces an abnormal physiologic state similar to that found with secundum-type defect. The abnormal physiology associated with Lutembacher's syndrome depends upon the severity of the mitral stenosis and the size of the atrial septal defect.

CLINICAL MANIFESTATIONS

Atrial septal defect is twice as common in females as males. It may be associated with Holt–Oram syndrome, Ellis–van Creveld syndrome, and thrombocytopenia–absent radius syndrome (Noonan, 1981).

SYMPTOMS

Most patients with secundum-type defects are asymptomatic until the fourth or fifth decade of life (Hamilton et al, 1979). Patients in the late teens and early 20s may experience fatigue and dyspnea. Atrial fibrillation, heart failure, and pulmonary hypertension may occur during or after the fourth decade of life. Endocarditis is rare.

The symptoms of patients with sinus venosus defects are similar to those of patients with ostium secundum defects.

PHYSICAL EXAMINATION

Patients with secundum defects may appear entirely normal, although some may have a slender build. An abnormal pulsation of the pulmonary trunk may be detected in the second intercostal space to the left of the sternum (the pulmonary artery area). A right ventricular lift of the left anterior precordium may be present. The second sound is

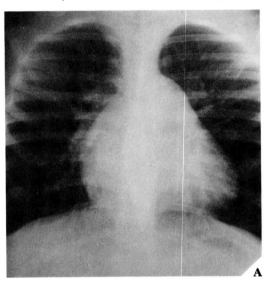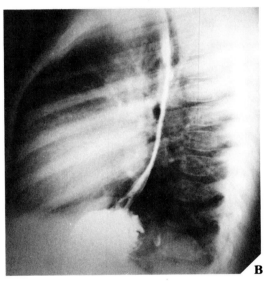

FIG. 3.24 **(A)** *Frontal chest radiograph of a four-year-old child with a secundum ASD, a large left-to-right shunt, and normal pulmonary arterial pressures shows that the aorta is small and the main pulmonary artery and its branches are large. The right ventricle appears to be large on the left lateral view* **(B)**. *(Fig. 36-9, The Heart, 6th ed, p 600. Courtesy of the X-Ray Department, Henrietta Egleston Hospital for Children, Atlanta, Georgia)*

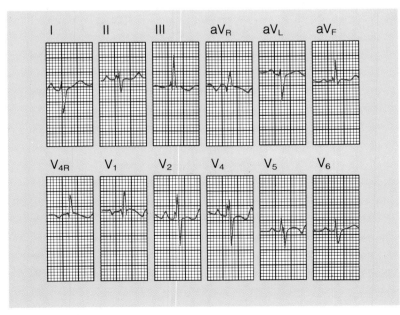

FIG. 3.25 *This ECG is from a five-year-old child with ostium secundum ASD. The mean QRS vector is directed to the right and anteriorly; the mean T vector is directed to the left and posteriorly. The configuration of the QRS complex in lead V_1 is rsR'. (Courtesy of the Electrocardiography Laboratory, Henrietta Egleston Hospital for Children, Atlanta, Georgia)*

almost always widely split; it remains so on inspiration and expiration. The pulmonary component of the second sound is usually normal or slightly increased in intensity. An opening snap of the tricuspid valve may be heard. There may be a diamond-shaped systolic murmur heard in the pulmonary area. A diastolic rumble due to increased blood flow through the tricuspid valve may be heard at the lower left sternal border. In adults this murmur may be mistaken for the murmur of mitral stenosis. The early systolic click and the late systolic murmur of mitral valve prolapse may be heard at the apex. Pulmonary valve regurgitation due to dilation of the pulmonary artery and pulmonary valve annulus may be detected in older patients even when the pulmonary arterial pressure is only slightly elevated.

The sinus venosus type of defect produces similar physical signs. When the pulmonary veins from the right upper lobe or middle lobe enter the superior caval vein and the atrial septal defect is small, the second heart sound may be abnormally split. However, the split may narrow on expiration and widen on inspiration.

LABORATORY STUDIES

CHEST RADIOGRAPHY. The chest film of a patient with an atrial septal defect shows a large pulmonary trunk, large pulmonary arterial branches, a small aorta, and right ventricular enlargement (Fig. 3.24).

ELECTROCARDIOGRAPHY. In the typical ECG of a secundum defect there is a right ventricular conduction delay with an rSr' or rSR configuration to the QRS complex in lead V_1 (Fig. 3.25). The PR interval may be long, and Wolff-Parkinson-White (WPW) configuration is occasionally seen.

ECHOCARDIOGRAPHY. The M-mode echocardiogram reveals evidence of volume overload of the right ventricle. The right atrium and the right ventricle are increased in size, and paradoxical motion of the ventricular septum is evident (Fig. 3.26).

The cross-sectional echocardiogram can identify a secundum-type defect with a sensitivity of approximately 90% (Fig. 3.27), while the

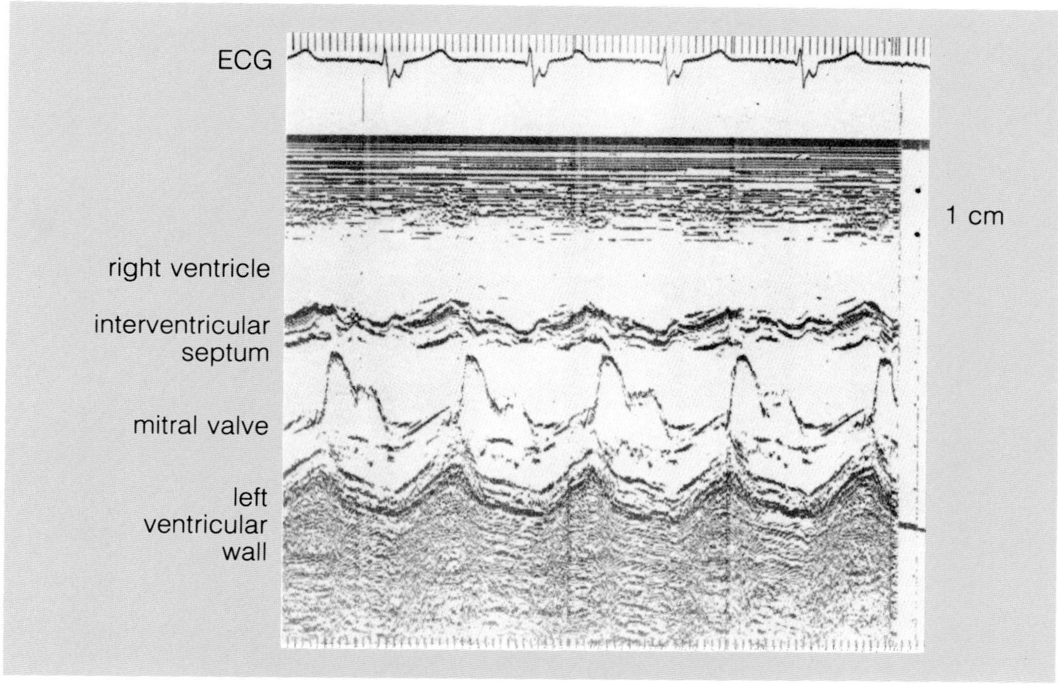

FIG. 3.26 *M-mode echocardiogram from a child with a secundum ASD demonstrates the increased right ventricular cavity dimension (2.4 cm end-diastolic diameter) and the anterior systolic motion of the interventricular septum characteristic of right ventricular diastolic overload.* (Fig. 36-10, The Heart, *6th ed, p 601*)

ECG

1 cm

right ventricle

interventricular septum

mitral valve

left ventricular wall

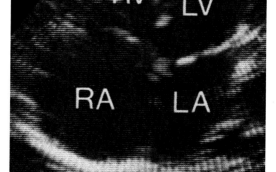

FIG. 3.27 *Cross-sectional echocardiography was performed in a patient with a large secundum ASD. The apical four-chamber view shows the enlarged right atrium (RA) and right ventricle (RV). The right ventricle forms the apex. An area of echocardiographic dropout is present in the midportion of the interatrial septum (LA, left atrium; LV, left ventricle). (Reproduced with permission of the authors and publisher; see Figure Credits)*

sinus venosus defect can be demonstrated in only 50% of patients (Shub et al, 1983).

CARDIAC CATHETERIZATION. Patients with secundum-type defects exhibit an increase in the oxygen saturation of the blood in the right atrium and the right ventricle; the pulmonary arterial systolic pressure is usually normal. Increase in pulmonary blood flow causes a small pressure gradient across the pulmonary valve. The level of pressure in the left and right atria is usually normal, with the left atrial pressure no more than 3 mmHg higher than the right atrial pressure.

The site of abnormal pulmonary venous connections may be identified by selective injection of contrast material. Aortography is used to identify a patent arterial duct, which may occur in some patients.

NATURAL HISTORY
Spontaneous closure of the secundum-type ASD is rare beyond infancy. A small percentage of these patients develop heart failure as infants, but almost all are asymptomatic and lead normal lives until adulthood.

Symptoms begin to appear in the 20s, and by age 40 most patients have dyspnea and fatigue (Hamilton et al, 1979). Severe pulmonary hypertension develops in a few patients in their 20s (Haworth, 1983). On rare occasions a patient may have a paradoxical embolus and brain abscess. Bacterial endocarditis is rare.

The natural history of a sinus venosus type of defect is similar to that of the secundum type.

TREATMENT
There is rarely a need for medical treatment in children and young adults with an ostium secundum or sinus venosus type ASD. Atrial fibrillation should be controlled with digitalis. Prophylaxis against infective endocarditis is usually not necessary in patients with isolated secundum defects.

INDICATIONS FOR SURGERY
Surgery is indicated in patients with an ostium secundum or sinus venosus defect when the shunt is 1.7–1 or greater. Surgical closure is

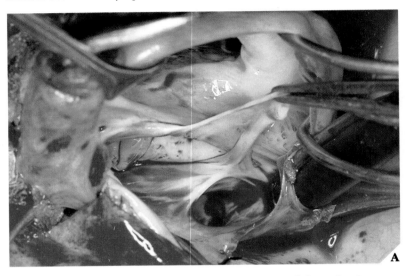

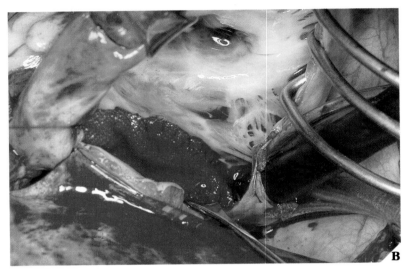

FIG. 3.28 **(A)** *An inferior sinus venosus ASD is exposed through a low lying posterior atrial incision that also exposes the venous drainage from the lower lobe of the right lung. The defect is opened into the oval fossa to allow broad communication with the left atrium.* **(B)** *A patch of low-poros-ity Dacron velour is inserted to direct the anomalous pulmonary venous return to the left atrium, leaving the inferior caval vein to drain into the right heart.*

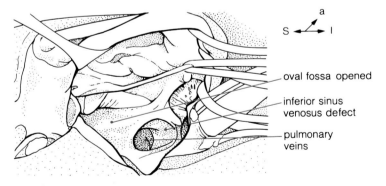

oval fossa opened

inferior sinus venosus defect

pulmonary veins

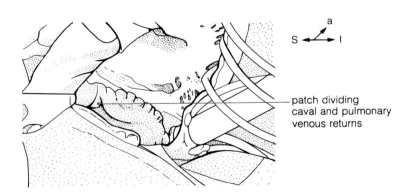

patch dividing caval and pulmonary venous returns

indicated if there is a shunt of 1.5–1 to 1.7–1, if right ventricular overload is recognized on physical examination, or if there is pulmonary hypertension. The defect should be closed prior to pregnancy. An adult with cardiac enlargement and a shunt of 2–1 with mild pulmonary hypertension should have surgery. (The reader is referred to Chapter 36, *The Heart,* 6th ed, pp 602–603, for further discussion of surgical management.)

SURGICAL PROCEDURE

In closure of atrial septal defects the incision in the atrial wall is tailored to accommodate the specific defect, particularly with the sinus venosus type. Either superior or inferior defects are likely to be associated with anomalous pulmonary venous connection, thereby requiring patch grafting to direct the anomalous venous return to the left atrium (Fig. 3.28). Because the anomalous pulmonary veins associated with a superior sinus venosus defect often involve the cavoatrial junction (Fig. 3.29A), it has been suggested that the atrial incision should be extended into the caval vein to facilitate repair. Because such an extension would greatly endanger the sinus node (Fig. 3.29B), it should be avoided if at all possible. Fortunately the majority of such defects can be corrected with an appropriately placed upper atrial incision (Fig. 3.29C).

Repair of secundum defects in the oval fossa depends on the ana-

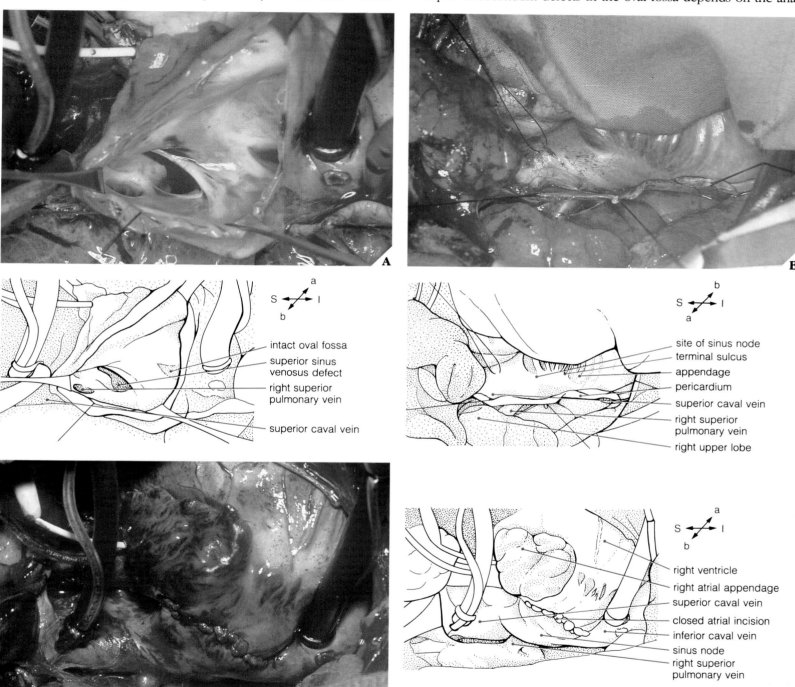

FIG. 3.29   (A) *In this operative view the superior aspect of the right atrium is opened to show a superior sinus venosus defect and anomalous veins draining into the cavoatrial junction.* (B) *The anomalous course of the right superior pulmonary vein and the site of the sinus node are clearly* visible. (C) *The incision used to gain access for repair of the sinus venosus defect is located well away from the site of the sinus node. (Reproduced with permission of the authors and publisher; see Figure Credits)*

tomic constraints. These defects may be closed by direct suture (Fig. 3.30), or with a large patch of Dacron (Fig. 3.31). It is important that the defect is closed without tension to avoid dehiscence as well as to minimize distortion of the sinus and atrioventricular nodes.

It should be kept in mind that oval fossa defects may accompany other intracardiac anomalies, such as atrioventricular septal defects (Fig. 3.32). The distinction between the defect in the atrial septum and the low-lying interatrial communication caused by deficiency of the atrioventricular septum is usually apparent.

ATRIOVENTRICULAR SEPTAL DEFECT
DEFINITION AND PATHOLOGY

A defect in the lower portion of the atrial septum and in the upper portion of the ventricular septum due to complete absence of the normal atrioventricular septal structures is termed an atrioventricular septal defect (AVSD), or sometimes endocardial cushion defect. The absence of atrioventricular septation results in a common atrioventricular junction guarded by a basically common valve. The left ventricular component of this valve is a three-leaflet structure; the so-

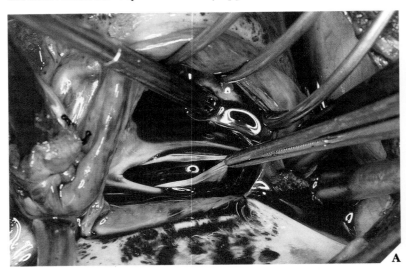
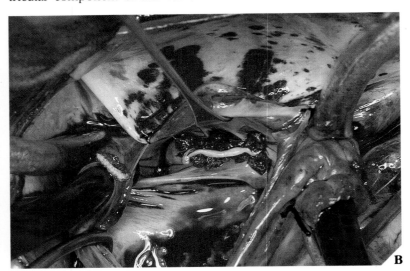

FIG. 3.30 *Closure of a narrow, relatively small secundum defect in the floor of the oval fossa* (**A**) *is accomplished with monofilament mattress sutures reinforced with Dacron pledgets* (**B**).

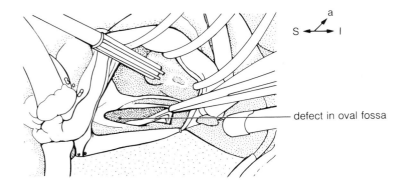
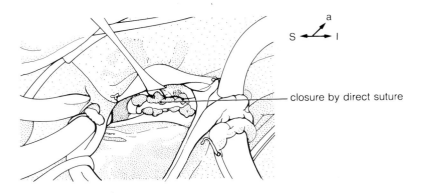

defect in oval fossa

closure by direct suture

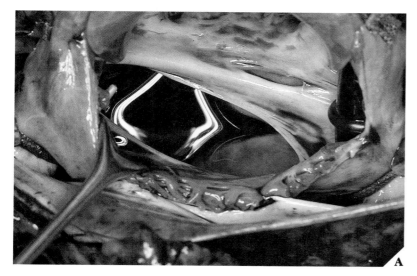
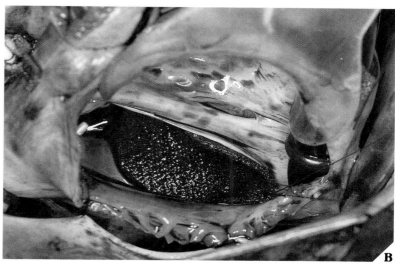

FIG. 3.31　(A) *The oval fossa is almost totally absent in this secundum defect. Direct closure would result in extreme tension on the suture line, inviting dehiscence and possible dysrhythmia secondary to distortion of the* conduction tissues. (B) *A large Dacron patch closes the defect without tension or distortion.*

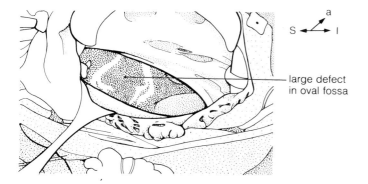

large defect
in oval fossa

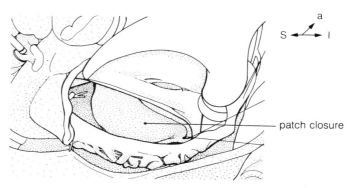

patch closure

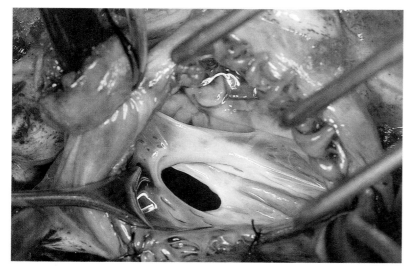

FIG. 3.32　*In this operative view an oval fossa atrial defect is seen in conjunction with an atrioventricular septal defect. The independent nature of these two lesions is clearly apparent.*

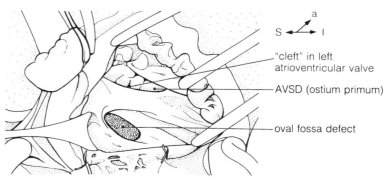

"cleft" in left
atrioventricular valve

AVSD (ostium primum)

oval fossa defect

called cleft (Fig. 3.33) represents the space between the two leaflets that are tethered in both ventricles, bridging the ventricular septum (Becker and Anderson, 1982).

There are several anatomic types of abnormalities. The *ostium primum* or *partial* type of defect (Fig. 3.34A) is characterized by a tongue of leaflet tissue that joins the facing surfaces of the bridging leaflets, dividing the basically common orifice into right and left components. The left valve then has a three-leaflet arrangement; the cleft is located between the left ventricular portions of the bridging leaflets. The leaflets themselves, together with the connecting tongue, are bound

to the septum as they bridge, so that shunting through the AVSD occurs exclusively at the atrial level.

The *complete* type (often termed common atrioventricular canal or common valve orifice) is characterized by a failure of the common junction to partition into separate atrioventricular orifices. The opening between the atria and the ventricles is thus protected by a common valve (Fig. 3.34B). The complete type is subdivided into three subgroups (Fig. 3.35). In *Type A* the superior bridging leaflet extends only marginally into the right ventricle; the commissure between the superior and the anterosuperior leaflets on the right ventricle is attached by

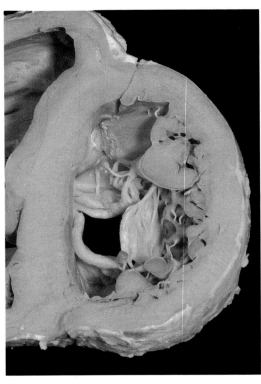

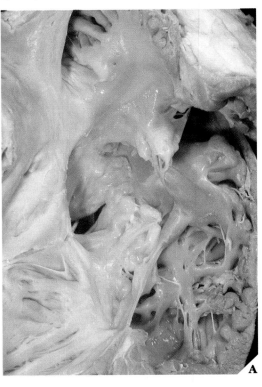

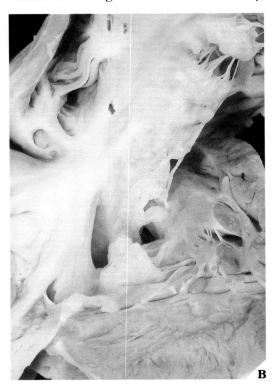

FIG. 3.33 *Short-axis section of an AVSD is viewed from beneath to show the trifoliate nature of the left atrioventricular valve. The abnormality in the mitral valve, frequently described as a cleft, is the space between the left ventricular components of the bridging leaflets. The left valve bears no resemblance to the mitral valve other than its residence within the left ventricle.*

FIG. 3.34 *The ostium primum (A) and the complete types of AVSD (B), which represent absence of the normal atrioventricular septal structures, have directly comparable morphology. The atrial septum is virtually intact in both hearts. In*

the primum defect the bridging leaflets guarding the common atrioventricular junction are joined by a connecting tongue, but they are separate structures in the heart with a common valve orifice.

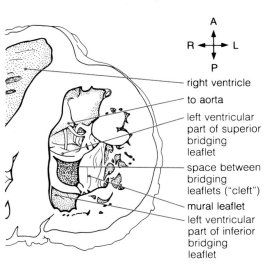

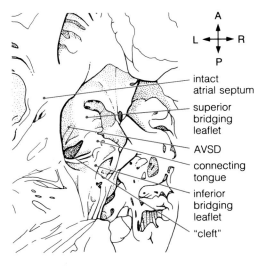

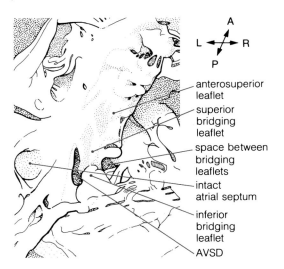

short cords to the ventricular septum. An interventricular connection is present between the bridging leaflets. In *Type B* the superior bridging leaflet extends further into the right ventricle. Cords from the leaflet are attached to an anomalous anterior papillary muscle in the right ventricle, but no cords attach to the ventricular septum. In *Type C* there is extensive bridging of the free-floating superior leaflet with diminution in size of the anterosuperior leaflet of the right ventricle. The commissure between the two is supported by the anterior papillary muscle of the right ventricle (Rastelli et al, 1968).

The AVSDs discussed above are the varieties most commonly seen in practice; however, there are many other defects that are associated with AVSDS. Often a narrowed left ventricular outflow tract with marked disproportion between the inlet and the outlet dimensions of the left ventricle is seen in conjunction with the three-leaflet arrangement of the left atrioventricular valve (Fig. 3.36).

ABNORMAL PHYSIOLOGY

The pulmonary arterial and the right ventricular pressures are normal or slightly elevated in patients with communication between the two atria but no shunt at the ventricular level; the pulmonary blood flow is also increased. These findings simulate those of a large ostium secundum ASD. In contrast the pulmonary arterial and the right ventricular pressures are usually elevated with a large VSD. The arrangement of the leaflets of the valves guarding the abnormal atrioventricular junction may cause severe regurgitation; blood may also be shunted from the left ventricle into the right atrium.

CLINICAL MANIFESTATIONS

About 3% of children with congenital heart disease have some type of AVSD; the female to male ratio is 1.3:1. About 50% or more of patients with the complete type have Down's syndrome (Fyler, 1980).

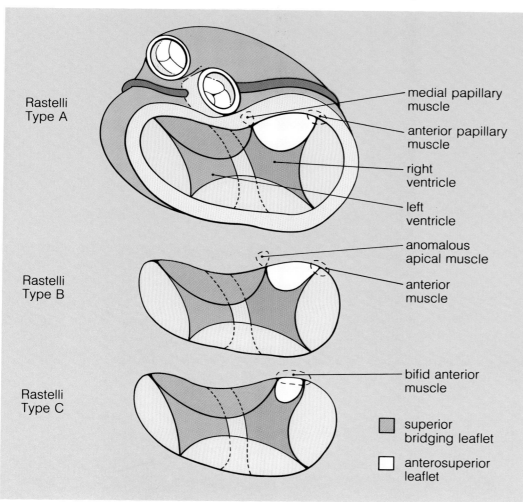

Rastelli
Type A

Rastelli
Type B

Rastelli
Type C

— medial papillary muscle

— anterior papillary muscle

— right ventricle

— left ventricle

— anomalous apical muscle

— anterior muscle

— bifid anterior muscle

▨ superior bridging leaflet

☐ anterosuperior leaflet

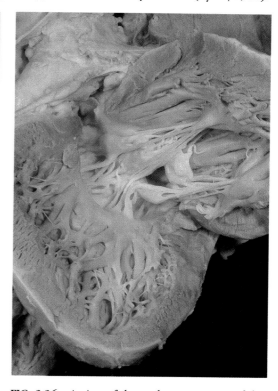

FIG. 3.36 *A view of the outlet component of the left ventricle in a heart with an AVSD shows the marked discrepancy between the inlet and the outlet dimensions along with the three-leaflet arrangement of the left atrioventricular valve.*

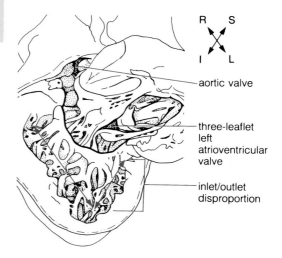

R S

I L

— aortic valve

— three-leaflet left atrioventricular valve

— inlet/outlet disproportion

FIG. 3.35 *This schematic drawing illustrates the variable extent of bridging of the superior leaflet in AVSD with common valve orifice. As the superior leaflet extends further into the right ventricle, the anterosuperior leaflet decreases in size. The* *commissure between the two is supported by a papillary muscle, which occupies a variable location within the right ventricle. (Redrawn; reproduced with permission of the authors and publisher; see Figure Credits)*

SYMPTOMS

Children with the partial type of AVSD are usually asymptomatic and simulate patients with secundum ASD, unless there is regurgitation through the left atrioventricular valve. Slight regurgitation may produce no symptoms, while severe regurgitation results in poor weight gain, fatigue, dyspnea, frequent upper respiratory infections, and heart failure.

Patients with the complete type of AVSD are often seriously ill and develop heart failure at an early age. If the defect is not treated surgically, death will occur in about half of patients during the first year of life.

PHYSICAL EXAMINATION

The abnormalities noted on physical examination of patients with partial defects are similar to patients with secundum ASDs, unless the arrangement of the left valve permits regurgitation. Accordingly when regurgitation is present, a systolic murmur is heard at the apex. When the regurgitation is severe, it also results in a diastolic rumble at the apex.

Patients with complete defects exhibit physical abnormalities similar to those found in patients with interventricular septal defects. There may be an anterior precordial lift and a large pulsation at the apex. A murmur of left or right valve regurgitation, which can be separated

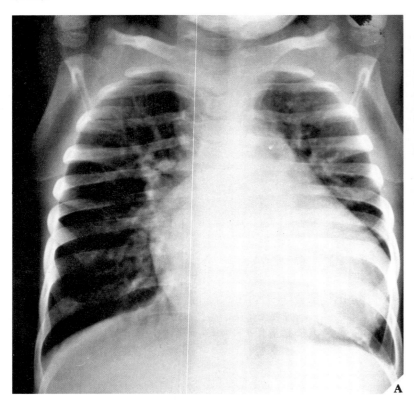 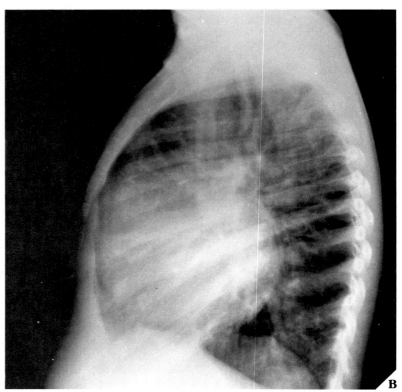

FIG. 3.37 (**A**) *Posteroanterior chest film of a 4-year-old child with a complete AVSD shows marked cardiac enlargement with increased pulmonary blood flow.* (**B**) *On the lateral view left atrial enlargement is evident.*

(Courtesy of the X-Ray Department, Henrietta Egleston Hospital for Children, Atlanta, Georgia)

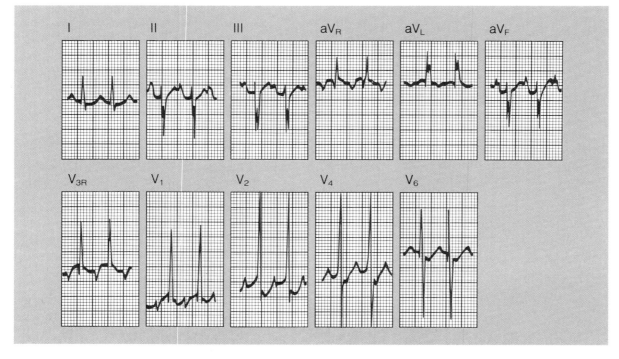

FIG. 3.38 *This ECG was obtained in an infant with a complete AVSD, a large left-to-right shunt, and severe pulmonary arterial hypertension. The superior mean QRS axis (−70°) is accompanied by first-degree heart block, biatrial abnormality, and biventricular hypertrophy. (Redrawn; Fig. 36-15, The Heart, 6th ed, p 607. Courtesy of the Electrocardiography Laboratory, Henrietta Egleston Hospital for Children, Atlanta, Georgia)*

from the murmur of VSD, may be detected. There is fixed splitting of the second sound. The pulmonary component of the second sound may be louder than normal, because pulmonary hypertension is commonly present.

CHEST RADIOGRAPHY. The partial lesion with regurgitation through the left atrioventricular valve is characterized by right and left ventricular hypertrophy, left atrial enlargement, and increased pulmonary blood flow (Fig. 3.37). The complete defect produces a very large heart with evidence of considerable increase in pulmonary blood flow.

ELECTROCARDIOGRAPHY. A partial defect without "mitral" regurgitation may be associated with right ventricular conduction delay, simulating the abnormality found with a secundum-type ASD. However, the mean QRS vector may be located to the left and superiorly.

Regurgitation through the left atrioventricular valve, when present, may produce left ventricular hypertrophy. First-degree heart block may be present.

A complete malformation may produce a long P-R interval, a wider-than-average QRS duration, biatrial abnormality, biventricular hypertrophy, and a mean QRS vector rotated to the left and anteriorly (Fig. 3.38).

ECHOCARDIOGRAPHY. A M-mode echocardiogram of a patient with a complete form of AVSD reveals an increase in right ventricular dimensions and anterior systolic movement of the ventricular septum, suggesting right ventricular diastolic overload of the right ventricle (Fig. 3.39).

A cross-sectional echocardiogram can detect an ASD and attachment of the bridging leaflets to the ventricular septum, thus demonstrating the AVSD (Fig. 3.40). In patients with the complete type of AVSD,

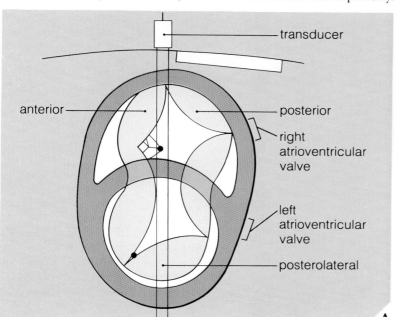

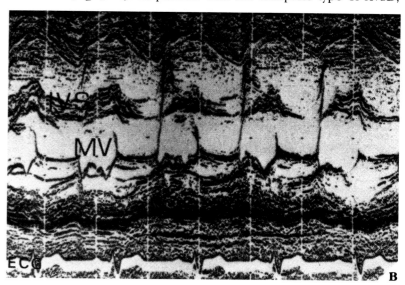

FIG. 3.39 (A) *This diagram represents a transverse cut of a heart with a complete form of AVSD. The orientation of the two bridging leaflets allows a diastolic movement at right angles to the interventricular septum, creating an echocardiographic hole between the anteroposterior leaflet of the right valve and the posterolateral cusp of the left valve.* (B) *In the M-mode echocardiogram an apparent common atrioventricular valve occupies the whole heart. The superimposition of the leaflet, together with the different degrees of atrioventricular valve septal overriding, may explain this picture. No echoes from the anteroseptal leaflet of the left valve are seen (MV, left atrioventricular valve; IVS, interventricular septum). (Partially redrawn; reproduced with permission of the authors and publisher; see Figure Credits)*

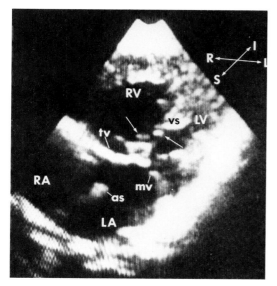

FIG. 3.40 *This cross-sectional echocardiogram in the apex view was obtained in a child with type A complete AVSD. The common anterior leaflet to the right (tv) and the left (mv) valves appears to be attached to the crest of the ventricular septum (vs) by multiple cords (arrows). The area of the ostium primum defect lies between the lowermost edge of the atrial septum (as) and the valve (RV, right ventricle; LV, left ventricle; RA, right atrium; LA, left atrium). (Reproduced with permission of the authors and publisher; see Figure Credits. Also, Fig. 36-17, The Heart, 6th ed, p 609)*

floating of the leaflets differentiates the atrial and the ventricular components of the lesion. Echoes taken in the short axis demonstrate the three-leaflet nature of the left valve, showing that the cleft is the space between the left ventricular components of the bridging leaflets. The extent of bridging of the superior leaflet into the right ventricle indicates the presence of subtypes A, B, and C as described by Rastelli and his colleagues (Rastelli et al, 1968) (see Fig. 3.35).

CARDIAC CATHETERIZATION.   There is an increase in oxygen saturation between the superior caval vein and the right atrium in patients with partial or complete types of AVSD. Whenever the right ventricular and the pulmonary systolic pressures exceed 60 mmHg in such patients, the possibility of a complete lesion must be considered. A complete defect produces nearly identical systolic pressures in the right ventricle, the pulmonary artery, and the systemic arterial system.

The left ventriculogram shows a characteristic gooseneck abnormality and shunting of blood from the left ventricle to the right ventricle (Fig. 3.41). Evidence of regurgitation through the left atrioventricular valve and shunting from the left ventricle to the right atrium may also be evaluated.

NATURAL HISTORY

A patient with an ASD located low in the atrial septum (ostium primum) with no regurgitation through the left atrioventricular valve has the same prognosis as the patient with a secundum defect. Such patients may have a trifoliate left valve that does not permit any regurgitation; they are then more susceptible to endocarditis than patients with secundum defects. When regurgitation is present, the prognosis is determined by its extent; heart failure may occur early in such patients. Infants with complete defects develop congestive heart failure and die unless surgical intervention is successful.

TREATMENT

Heart failure is managed with digitalis, diuretics, and drugs to decrease the afterload. Unfortunately medical management does not solve the problem of heart failure in such patients, and surgical treatment is usually required. Antibiotic prophylaxis against bacterial endocarditis is indicated for partial and complete defects.

Genetic counseling is indicated, because the risk of subsequent siblings having congenital heart disease is 2% (Nora and Nora, 1978).

INDICATIONS FOR SURGERY

The small infant with congestive heart failure and a large shunt at the ventricular level should undergo banding of the pulmonary trunk; excellent results have also been achieved using primary repair. The older infant with a complete defect who has heart failure and severe regurgitation through the left atrioventricular valve should have total correction.

SURGICAL PROCEDURE

To the cardiac surgeon operative repair of AVSDs is a challenging undertaking. Because the lesion lies literally at the center of the cardiac structure, the resultant defect(s) can have extremely complex consequences. To effect proper repair, the surgeon must understand that the atrioventricular valves in these cases are not simply deformed mitral and tricuspid valves to be corrected by sewing up the cleft. Instead they are unique structures conforming more or less to the underlying morphologic malformation; as such, they need to be repaired—or not repaired—accordingly.

Significant regurgitation from the left ventricle must be relieved (Fig. 3.42). The surgeon must always keep in mind that the cleft represents an integral part of the opening area of the valve; closing it improperly may create stenosis of the valve. In addition suturing the superior and the inferior bridging leaflets together may distort the closing mechanism, thereby creating regurgitation through the central portion of the orifice.

Another important point relates to the apical displacement of the atrioventricular valve mechanism. When it is necessary to incorporate the valves in the repair of the ventricular component of a complete AVSD, the unique positioning of the valves must be maintained. Attempting to reattach them at the anatomically correct position results in distortion and regurgitation.

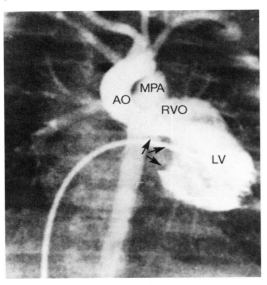

FIG. 3.41 *Posteroanterior view of the left ventricular angiogram from a child with complete AVSD demonstrates the characteristic gooseneck deformity* (arrows) *of the outflow tract of the left ventricle* (LV). *Opacification of the right ventricular outflow tract* (RVO) *and the pulmonary trunk* (MPA) *before, or in the absence of, atrial opacification reflects the presence of the interventricular communication* (AO, *aorta*). *(Fig. 36-20,* The Heart, *6th ed, p 610)*

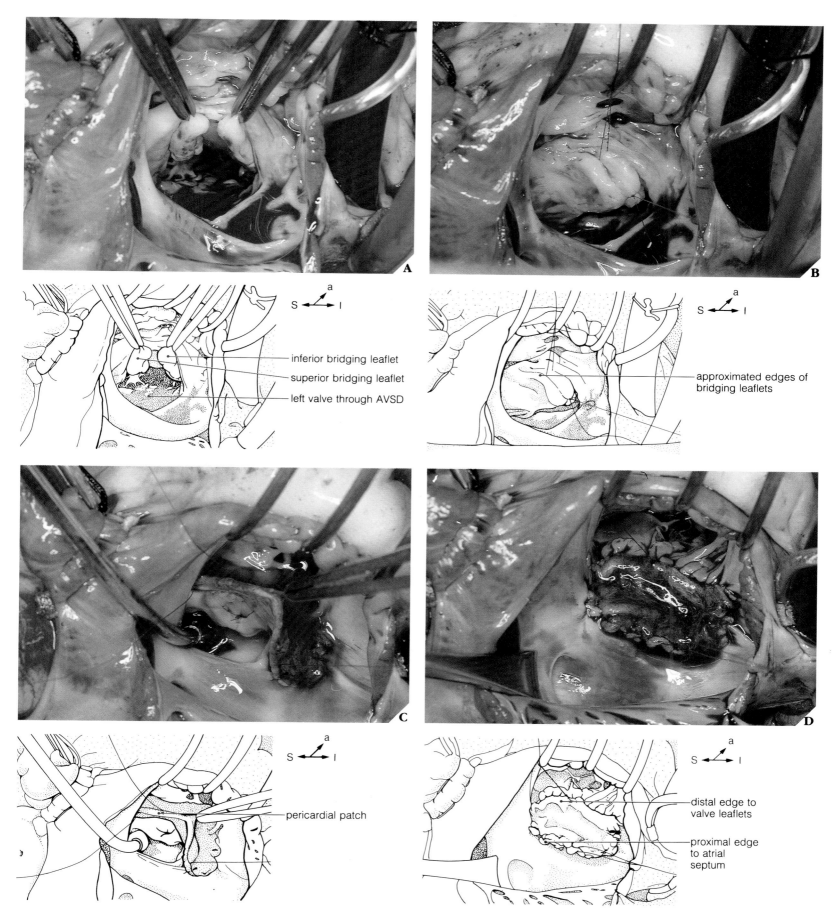

FIG. 3.42 *In surgical repair of an AVSD with left ventricular–right atrial shunting (A) the superior and inferior bridging leaflets are brought together to close the shunt (B). The edges of these leaflets are everted to avoid shortening. (C) The pericardial patch is sewn in place around the coronary sinus, diverting its orifice to the left side. (D) A section of pericardium is preferred in the event of continued valvar incompetence to minimize blood damage.*

The disposition of the conduction tissues is also crucial. Because the triangle of Koch is literally missing, the atrioventricular node is displaced posterolaterally nearer the orifice of the coronary sinus (Fig. 3.43). Therefore it is often judicious to extend the suture line so that the coronary sinus drains to the left side. Such a maneuver is not always required, but the surgeon should not hesitate to do this when necessary. The morphologic merit far outweighs the physiologic price paid by the patient.

When shunting through the septal defect is exclusively at the atrial level (partial or ostium primum defect), the surgeon, having repaired the left valve in appropriate fashion, simply closes the space between the lower edge of the atrial septum and the valve leaflets attached to the ventricular septum. Usually a pericardial patch is used. When there is a common orifice, as in the complete type of AVSD, there is almost always a ventricular component to the defect, which must also be closed. Debate continues as to whether this is best achieved using a single patch together with incision of the bridging leaflets or whether it is preferable to use separate atrial and ventricular patches. Currently mortality for repair of the partial defect is close to zero; for the common-orifice defect it is less than 10%. Problems still remain, however, with late development of regurgitation through the left atrioventricular valve. Improving knowledge of its anatomy suggests that this may be resolved in the near future.

TOTAL ANOMALOUS PULMONARY VENOUS CONNECTIONS
DEFINITION AND PATHOLOGY

Total anomalous pulmonary venous connection (TAPVC) is said to be present when all of the pulmonary veins enter the right atrium or a systemic vein rather than the left atrium. In this condition the pulmonary veins leave the lungs and join a common venous structure, which then terminates in a systemic venous location. Occasionally two or more veins terminate in the right atrium or a systemic vein. The sites of termination that are located above the diaphragm are the left innominate vein, the coronary sinus (Fig. 3.44), the right atrium, the superior caval vein (Fig. 3.45), and the azygos veins (Blake et al, 1965). The sites of termination that are located below the diaphragm are the portal vein, the venous duct, and the gastric vein (Fig. 3.46). The oval foramen is always present and patent.

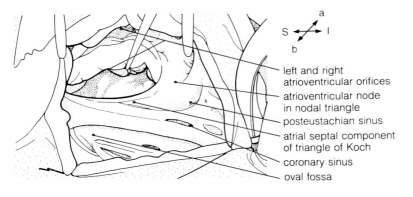

FIG. 3.43 *Because the triangle of Koch is missing in AVSD the conduction axis is displaced into the nodal triangle, as seen in this operative view. (Reproduced with permission of the authors and publisher; see Figure Credits)*

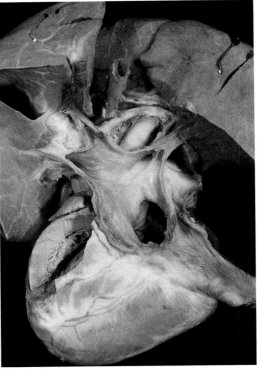

FIG. 3.44 *Total anomalous pulmonary venous connection to the coronary sinus can be seen in this heart dissected from behind.*

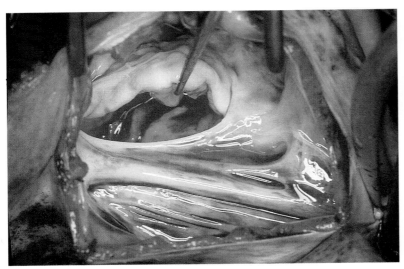

a

S ↔ I

b

left and right atrioventricular orifices
atrioventricular node in nodal triangle
posteustachian sinus
atrial septal component of triangle of Koch
coronary sinus
oval fossa

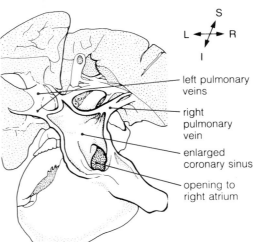

S

L ↔ R

I

left pulmonary veins

right pulmonary vein

enlarged coronary sinus

opening to right atrium

Rarely no major veins leave the common venous structure; in such cases small veins enter the esophageal wall. This condition is called atresia of the common pulmonary vein.

ABNORMAL PHYSIOLOGY

There must be a communication between the left and the right side of the heart in order for life to be sustained, since all of the blood from the pulmonary and the systemic circulations eventually returns to the right atrium. The systemic arterial oxygen saturation is low when there is an increase in pulmonary vascular resistance or when there is obstruction to the flow in the pulmonary veins (Gatham and Nadas, 1970).

CLINICAL MANIFESTATIONS
SYMPTOMS

Cyanosis in the infant is apparent. The symptoms of heart failure occur in the majority of patients by the age of three months. Most infants are thin and do not gain weight normally.

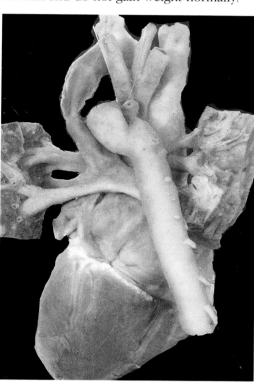

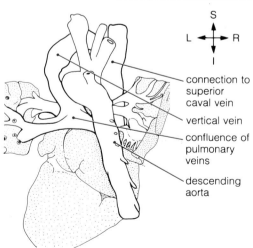

FIG. 3.45 *Total anomalous pulmonary venous connection to the superior caval vein can be seen in this heart viewed from behind. (Courtesy of Leon Gerlis, MD, Leeds, UK)*

connection to superior caval vein

vertical vein

confluence of pulmonary veins

descending aorta

PHYSICAL EXAMINATION

The infant is usually cyanotic and has an increased respiratory rate. The liver is large, and the jugular venous pulse is elevated. The right ventricular pulsation is hyperdynamic, and the second sound is abnormally split. The split remains during inspiration and expiration; the sound of pulmonary valve closure is usually abnormally loud. There may be a grade 2–3 systolic murmur heard at the left sternal border; a tricuspid diastolic rumble may be heard at the lower sternal border. A continuous murmur may be heard over the common venous structure. While the heart may not be large when the pulmonary veins are obstructed, pulmonary edema is present.

LABORATORY STUDIES

CHEST RADIOGRAPHY. The heart is usually enlarged with an increase in pulmonary blood flow; pulmonary edema may be present. When all of the venous blood enters the innominate vein, a characteristic radiographic contour is seen; it is usually described as the

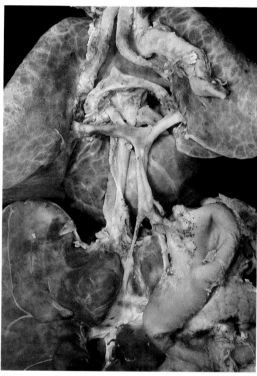

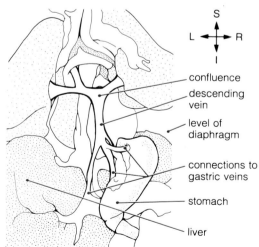

FIG. 3.46 *This heart dissected and viewed from behind shows totally anomalous infra-diaphragmatic pulmonary venous connection. The venous channel breaks up and terminates in the gastric veins.*

confluence

descending vein

level of diaphragm

connections to gastric veins

stomach

liver

"snowman" or "figure-of-eight" appearance (Fig. 3.47) (Keith et al, 1978).

ELECTROCARDIOGRAPHY. The ECG shows right atrial abnormality and right ventricular hypertrophy. There may be a qR pattern in the precordial leads.

ECHOCARDIOGRAPHY. The M-mode echocardiogram shows volume overload of the right ventricle when the pulmonary venous system is not obstructed. Signs of pulmonary hypertension may be present when the pulmonary veins are obstructed. The common venous structure may be seen behind the right atrium. Cross-sectional echocardiography may outline the site of drainage (Sahn et al, 1979).

CARDIAC CATHETERIZATION. The oxygen saturation is increased at the site of abnormal venous connection; similar saturations are found in all chambers of the heart. The right ventricular and the pulmonary arterial pressures are elevated. The pulmonary wedge pressure is elevated in patients who have obstruction of the pulmonary veins.

Pulmonary angiography usually reveals the abnormal venous connection. Contrast material may be injected into the common venous structure in order to identify the sites of termination and obstruction.

NATURAL HISTORY

Without treatment most patients with pulmonary hypertension and pulmonary venous obstruction die by the age of three months, while patients with pulmonary hypertension alone live longer. The usual clinical picture is heart failure and death within one year (Gatham and Nadas, 1970).

TREATMENT
Medical treatment is limited to the management of heart failure and respiratory infections.

INDICATIONS FOR SURGERY
Recent reports indicate that surgical mortality for repair of TAPVC has decreased, although it is still in the range of 11%–26% (Turley et al, 1980; Kirklin and Barratt–Boyes, 1986). Newborns or young infants with pulmonary edema or pulmonary venous obstruction should have surgery. Patients who fail to grow may require surgery, because they often have pulmonary hypertension.

SURGICAL PROCEDURE
Surgical correction of TAPVC usually entails the creation of a communication between the left atrium and the pulmonary venous system, the elimination of an abnormal venous connection to the systemic circulation, and closure of interatrial communication (Kirklin, 1973). The surgical anatomy and operative repair, as seen in a patient with supracardiac drainage into the innominate vein, are depicted in Figures 3.48 and 3.49. Long-term outlook is good for those who survive the surgical procedure.

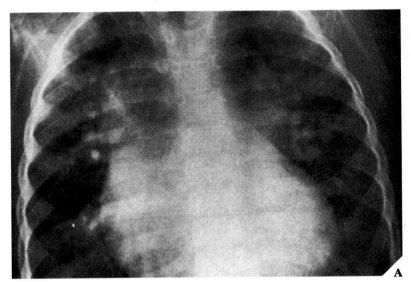

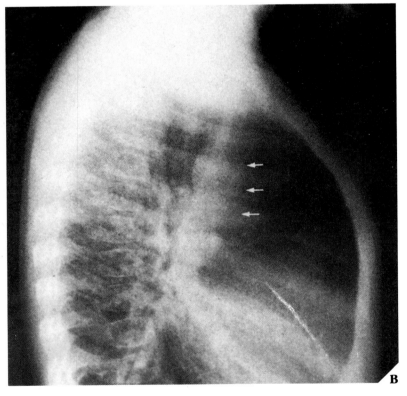

FIG. 3.47   (**A**) *Frontal chest film illustrates the typical "snowman" appearance of total anomalous pulmonary venous return to a left vertical vein. The pulmonary arterial vascularity is increased as the result of left-to-right shunting.* (**B**) *On the lateral view the density* (arrow) *anterior to the trachea represents the left vertical vein. No thymic tissue is present behind the sternum. (Reproduced with permission of the authors and publisher; see Figure Credits)*

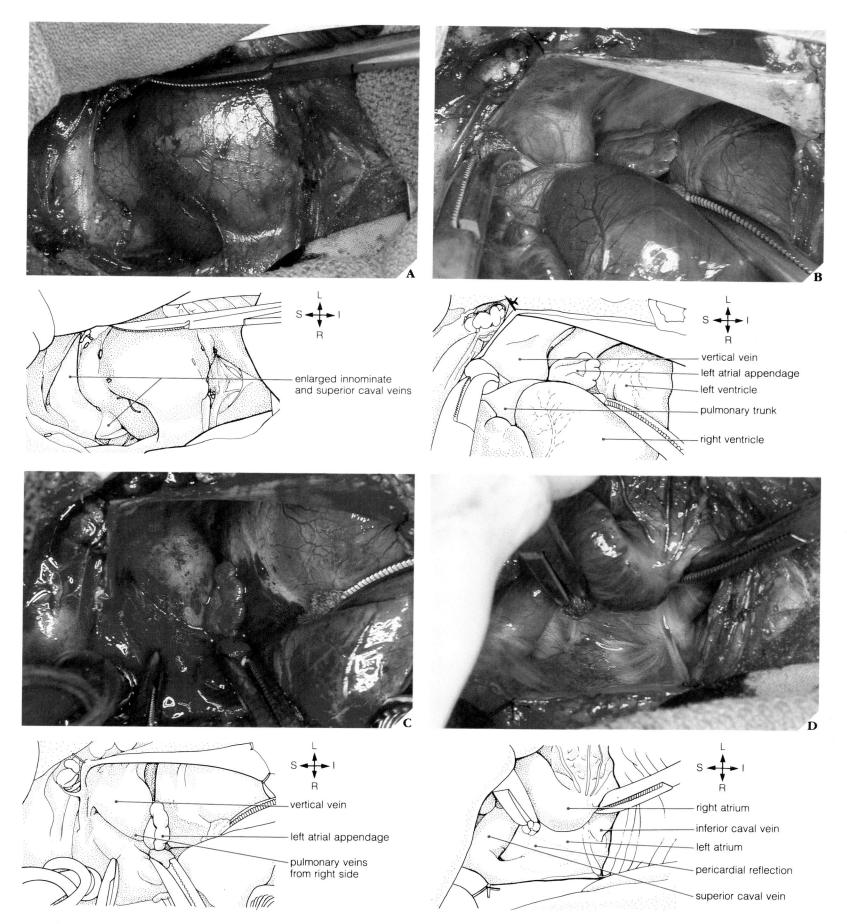

enlarged innominate
and superior caval veins

vertical vein
left atrial appendage
left ventricle
pulmonary trunk
right ventricle

vertical vein

left atrial appendage

pulmonary veins
from right side

right atrium

inferior caval vein

left atrium

pericardial reflection

superior caval vein

FIG. 3.48 (**A**) *In this operative view of a patient with total (bilateral and complete) anomalous pulmonary venous connection (TAPVC) draining into the innominate vein the extremely large innominate and superior caval veins are apparent.* (**B**) *On opening the pericardium and displacing the heart to the right, the confluence of the right and left veins is seen form-ing the vertical vein on the left.* (**C**) *Further dissection on cardiopulmonary bypass demonstrates the retropericardial course of the veins from the right side.* (**D**) *Retraction of the heart to the left demonstrates the lack of connection of the right-sided veins to the left atrium* (continued in Fig. 3.49, next page).

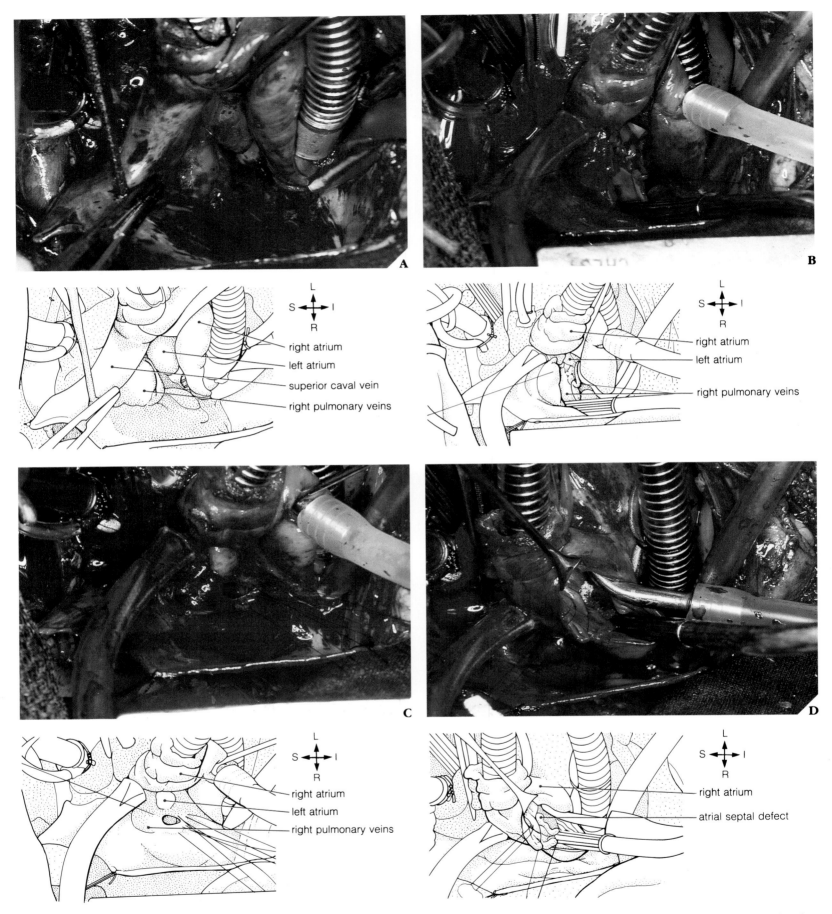

FIG. 3.49 *Repair of TAPVC* (continued). (**A**) *Retropericardial dissection demonstrates the right-sided veins in this area and their juxtaposition to the left atrial wall without attachment.* (**B**) *These two structures are joined us-* *ing fine monofilament sutures.* (**C**) *The final sutures are interrupted to facilitate growth of the anastomosis.* (**D**) *The atrial septal defect is closed through the right atrium.*

PATENT ARTERIAL DUCT
DEFINITION AND PATHOLOGY

In patent arterial duct (also termed patent ductus arteriosus) the arterial duct connects the pulmonary trunk and the aorta, running from the origin of the left pulmonary artery to the aorta just distal to the origin of the left subclavian artery (Fig. 3.50) (Edwards, 1979). The duct normally closes within three weeks of birth, becoming the arterial ligament (Fig. 3.51) (Wells, 1908).

A patent duct may be associated with coarctation of the aorta or ventricular septal defect. Patency of the duct may also be associated with conditions such as pulmonary atresia with intact ventricular septum. In such cases it is advantageous if the duct remains open; however, even when needed, it does tend to close.

ABNORMAL PHYSIOLOGY

The blood flows from the aorta through the duct to the pulmonary artery throughout the heart cycle, unless the pulmonary arterial vascular resistance is sufficiently elevated to alter this pattern. The left-to-right shunt may be small or large.

The blood flow through a high-resistance patent duct is small, causing little hemodynamic difficulty. The increased work of the left ventricle created by the increased volume is small; the pulmonary arteriolar resistance and the pulmonary arterial pressure are not elevated.

A large duct offers little resistance to blood flow; the pressure in the pulmonary artery is about the same as it is in the aorta. The volume load on the left ventricle is large, causing dilation and hypertrophy. Pulmonary congestion may develop, because the increased pressure in the left atrium and the pulmonary capillaries and the large pulmonary arterial blood flow develop at a time when the pulmonary arterioles are not fully capable of protecting the lungs. The patient with a moderate-sized or large duct may also have a right ventricle that becomes hypertrophic due to a pressure load created by pulmonary arteriolar vasoconstriction.

When the pulmonary vascular resistance equals or exceeds that of the systemic system, unsaturated blood is shunted from the pulmonary artery to the aorta. When this occurs, the feet may be more cyanosed as compared with the right hand.

CLINICAL MANIFESTATIONS

Patency of the arterial duct occurs more often in premature infants than in full-term babies, and more often in females than males. It is also common in infants whose mothers contracted rubella during the first trimester of pregnancy (Keith et al, 1978); males and females are equally affected in this case.

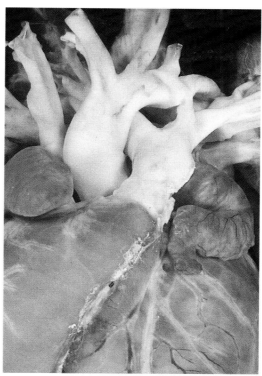

FIG. 3.51 *In this normal heart from a six-week-old infant the arterial duct constricts as it is transformed into the arterial ligament. The lumen is completely obliterated by this stage.*

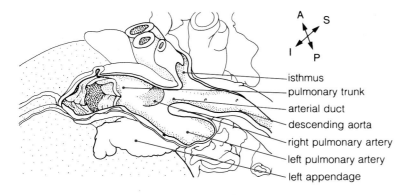

FIG. 3.50 *This heart with persistent patency of the arterial duct has been sectioned to replicate the view obtained by the echocardiographer from the suprasternal window. The duct is seen extending above the left pulmonary artery to the descending aorta.*

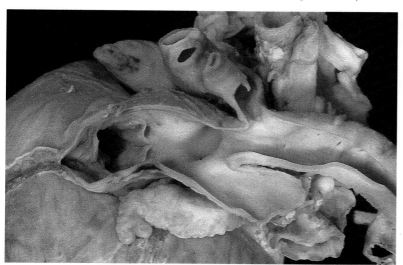

- isthmus
- pulmonary trunk
- arterial duct
- descending aorta
- right pulmonary artery
- left pulmonary artery
- left appendage

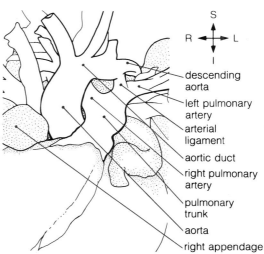

- descending aorta
- left pulmonary artery
- arterial ligament
- aortic duct
- right pulmonary artery
- pulmonary trunk
- aorta
- right appendage

SYMPTOMS

Patients with small left-to-right shunts through patent ducts have no symptoms, but they are subject to infective endarteritis. Patients with large left-to-right shunts may develop heart failure during the first few weeks of life. If heart failure does not develop at that age, it may not occur until after the third decade. Growth may be retarded. Premature infants may have the respiratory distress syndrome followed by heart failure.

PHYSICAL EXAMINATION

The peripheral arterial pulse may be brisk in full-term infants and children; the pulse pressure may be 45 mmHg or more. When the shunt is large, the apical impulse may be forceful and displaced to the left. A right ventricular lift may be prominent in infants with the respiratory distress syndrome and in children with pulmonary arterial hypertension.

The murmur varies with age, size of the shunt, and magnitude of the pulmonary arterial pressure and resistance. The typical murmur is heard in the second left intercostal space near the sternum and below the clavicle. The murmur is termed continuous, which implies that it builds up in systole, envelops the second sound, and trails off in diastole (Fig. 3.52). The second component of the second sound may be loud; however, the sound may also be masked by the peak intensity of the murmur. The diastolic component of the murmur may

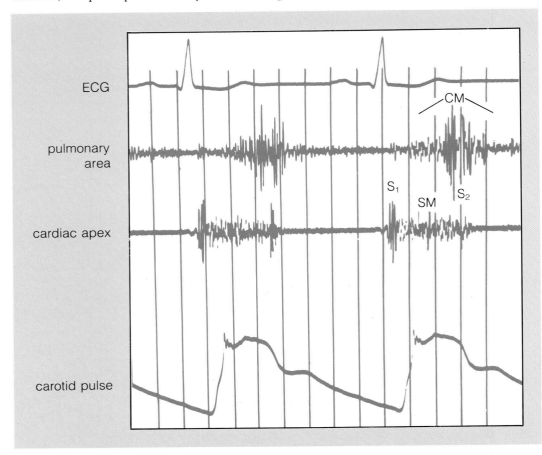

FIG. 3.52 *These phonocardiographic tracings were recorded in an 18-year-old female with a patent arterial duct. A continuous murmur (CM) present at the pulmonary area has its peak around the time of the second heart sound (S₂). A pansystolic murmur (SM) is also seen at the apex. It is due to mitral regurgitation associated with dilation of the left ventricle. (Redrawn; reproduced with permission of the authors and publisher; see Figure Credits)*

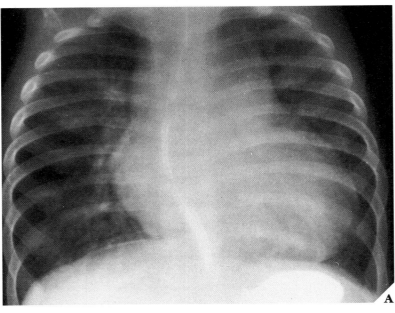

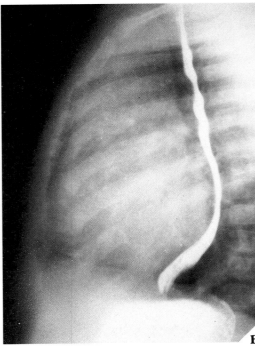

FIG. 3.53 *Chest radiographs of a one-month-old infant with a large patent arterial duct show on the posteroanterior view (A) moderate cardiac enlargement with increased pulmonary flow. (B) Lateral view shows right ventricular hypertrophy and marked left atrial enlargement. (Fig. 55-12, The Heart, 4th ed; see Figure Credits. Courtesy of the X-Ray Department, Henrietta Egleston Hospital for Children, Atlanta, Georgia)*

be faint or inaudible in newborns, in patients with pulmonary hypertension, and in patients with small shunts. Patients with moderate-sized left-to-right shunts may have a diastolic rumble at the apex. Patients with pulmonary hypertension may have a loud pulmonary valve closure sound followed by pulmonary valve regurgitation.

The continuous murmur of a patent arterial duct must be differentiated from the murmur of the normal venous hum and the murmurs associated with aortopulmonary septal defect, coronary arteriovenous fistula, or rupture of the sinus of Valsalva.

Cyanosis and clubbing of the toes and fingers of the left hand may be evident in patients in whom the shunt is reversed because of severe pulmonary hypertension.

LABORATORY STUDIES

CHEST RADIOGRAPHY. The chest film of a patient with a small patent arterial duct may be normal. When the duct permits a moderate-sized left-to-right shunt, slight cardiac enlargement, large pulmonary arteries, and a normal-sized aorta are evident (Fig. 3.53).

ELECTROCARDIOGRAPHY. The ECG of a patient with a small patent arterial duct may be normal. In contrast the patient with a moderate-sized left-to-right shunt may show an increase in QRS voltage, suggesting left ventricular enlargement (Fig. 3.54). The ECG in the presence of pulmonary hypertension often shows right ventricular hypertrophy.

ECHOCARDIOGRAPHY. M-mode echocardiography can be used to detect left atrial enlargement. The left ventricular dimension and the mean velocity of circumferential fiber shortening are increased.

Pulsed Doppler ultrasonography can be used to detect patent arterial duct, while continuous-wave Doppler can be used to measure the flow through it (Fig. 3.55) (Serwer et al, 1982).

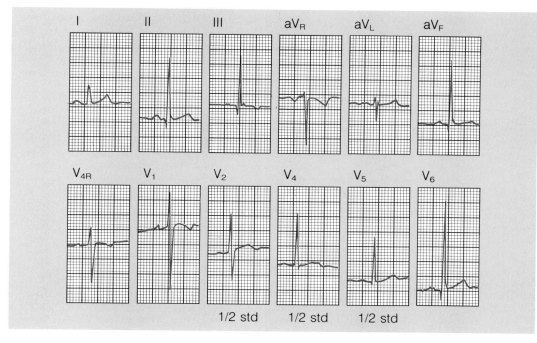

FIG. 3.54 *In this ECG of a 14-year-old child with a patent arterial duct the mean QRS vector is large. It is directed slightly posteriorly and slightly to the left, signifying left ventricular hypertrophy. The mean T vector is directed to the left and is flush with the frontal plane. Note that leads V$_2$, V$_4$, and V$_5$ are one half standardized. (Courtesy of the Electrocardiography Laboratory, Henrietta Egleston Hospital for Children, Atlanta, Georgia)*

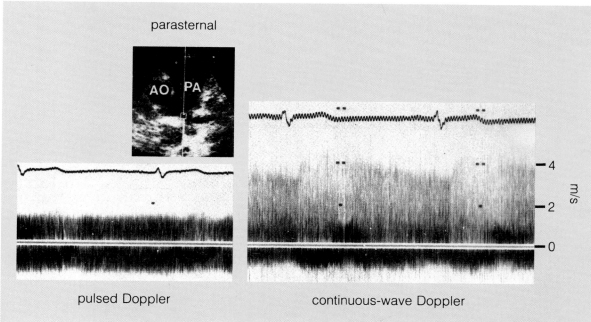

FIG. 3.55 *With a patent arterial duct and normal pulmonary arterial pressure continuous flow with high velocities into the pulmonary artery can be recorded. The velocity increases in systole and is highest at end-systole, when the pressure difference between the aorta (AO) and the pulmonary artery (PA) is greatest. With pulsed Doppler this flow is shown to originate at the bifurcation, but the recording in the direction of flow may no longer be clear because of aliasing. The flow velocity signal from the patent duct is less evident during systole, when flow into the pulmonary artery is seen as a darker band away from the transducer. (Partially redrawn; reproduced with permission of the authors and publisher; see Figure Credits)*

CARDIAC CATHETERIZATION. The arterial oxygen saturation is increased in the pulmonary artery, and the magnitude of the left-to-right shunt can be calculated. The pulmonary pressure is normal in patients with small or moderate-sized shunts, but it may be increased in patients with large shunts or pulmonary arteriolar disease. Aortography can be used to visualize the duct and the pulmonary arteries (Fig. 3.56).

NATURAL HISTORY

Patients may live a normal life span. The complications are infective endarteritis, heart failure, and the consequences of pulmonary hypertension. Bacterial endarteritis may occur regardless of the size of the duct. Heart failure related to ductal patency may cause death in premature or young infants. Pulmonary hypertension and reversal of shunt may lead to the complications of erythrocytosis, including cerebral thrombus.

TREATMENT

The incidence of patent arterial duct can be reduced by immunization against rubella and obstetrical measures to prevent prematurity.

Improvement of oxygenation and proper attention to fluid administration in the premature infant enhance the likelihood of closure. (Stevenson, 1977).The duct can be closed using inhibitors of prosta-

glandin synthesis, such as indomethacin and aspirin. This approach is used in newborn infants who weigh under 1750 g when other medical management is failing (Gersony et al, 1983). Transfemoral catheter closure of the duct with an Ivalon plug or a foam-covered hooked prosthesis has also been successful (Porstmann et al, 1971; Rashkind and Cuasco, 1979).

Heart failure is treated with digitalis and diuretics. Infective endarteritis may be prevented by the appropriate use of antibiotics.

INDICATIONS FOR SURGERY

The indications for surgery are uncontrollable heart failure in newborn or young infants, failure to grow adequately, and persistence of any size shunt after the first year of life (Gay et al, 1973). The presence of irreversible pulmonary vascular disease contraindicates surgery.

SURGICAL PROCEDURE

Operative interruption of the patent arterial duct remains as one of the most satisfying of all surgical undertakings. The important anatomic relationships are almost always predictable and the results are uniformly excellent. Various techniques have been successfully used to close arterial ducts. Traditionally longer, narrower ducts are closed by triple ligation (Fig. 3.57); short, broad ducts are closed by division

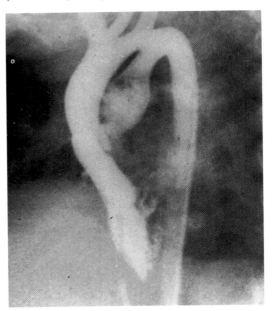
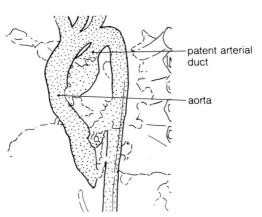

patent arterial duct

aorta

FIG. 3.56 *This left ventriculogram and aortogram was obtained in an 11-month-old child with mitral stenosis and a patent arterial duct. The left anterior oblique projection demonstrates the aorta and a large patent duct. Washout of contrast material within the duct results from right-to-left shunting. (Reproduced with permission of the authors and publisher; see Figure Credits. Courtesy of Robert M. Freedom, MD, Toronto, Ontario)*

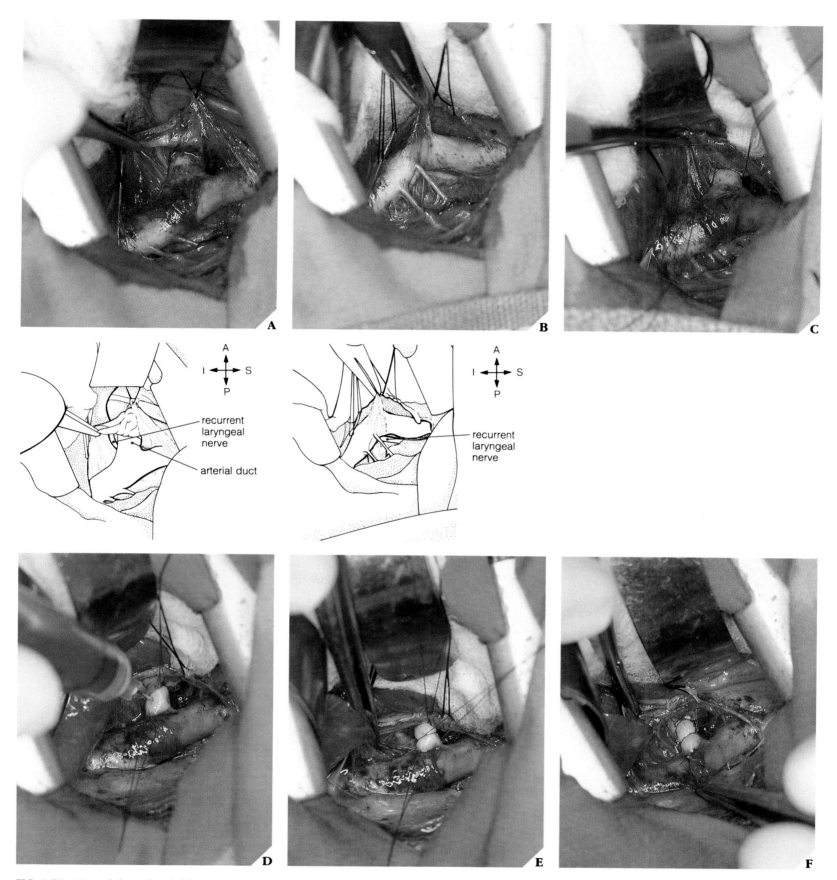

FIG. 3.57 *Viewed through a left lateral thoracotomy, the salient anatomic features of the arterial duct are apparent.* (**A**) *The recurrent laryngeal nerve is seen branching from the vagus nerve and curling beneath and around the arterial duct.* (**B**) *Displacement of the aorta shows the nerve in its course along the esophagus back into the cervical region.* (**C**) *Encircling sutures of monofilament material are placed on either end of the duct, taking small bites of the arterial wall to prevent central migration of these sutures.* (**D**) *After ligation the central portion is aspirated to ensure complete closure.* (**E,F**) *When this is accomplished, a third suture ligature is placed through the central portion of the cut.*

CONGENITAL HEART DISEASE

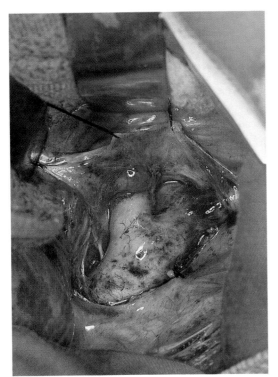

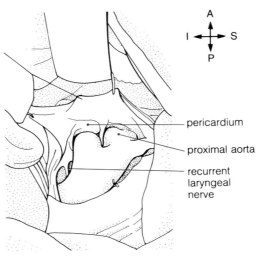

FIG. 3.58   A broad short patent arterial duct is seen through a left thoracotomy. The duct is approximately equal in size to the aortic arch and thus does not lend itself to simple ligation. The duct itself is differentiated from the arch by the lip of transparent pericardium extending over its anterior surface and by the recurrent laryngeal nerve coursing beneath it.

pericardium

proximal aorta

recurrent
laryngeal
nerve

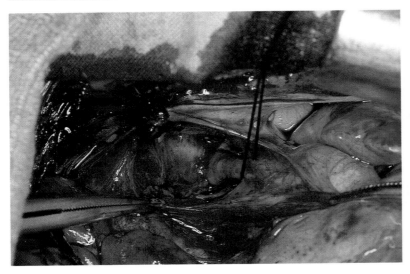

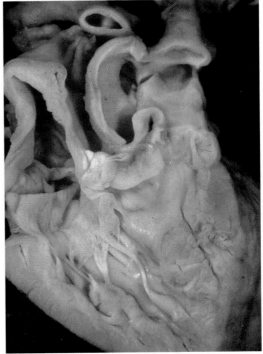

FIG. 3.60   This simulated paracoronal subcostal section of a heart shows an extensive communication between the ascending parts of the aorta and the pulmonary trunk; this lesion is usually termed an aortopulmonary window. The pulmonary and aortic valves are separate. (Reproduced with permission of the authors and publisher; see Figure Credits)

FIG. 3.59   A patent arterial duct is seen through a median sternotomy. The duct usually comes off the superior aspect of the pulmonary trunk, leading straight into the undersurface of the aorta. In this view the recurrent nerve is readily seen coursing beneath the duct and its aortic attachment. Simple ligation is usually all that is required under such circumstances.

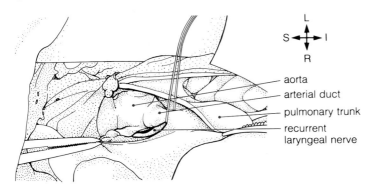

aorta

arterial duct

pulmonary trunk

recurrent
laryngeal nerve

aortopulmonary
window

pulmonary
trunk

aorta

pulmonary
valve

right ventricle

(Fig. 3.58). Either technique when properly applied is equally safe and effective.

With some regularity a patent arterial duct requires ligation in conjunction with other operative procedures. Usually the duct can be exposed quite well from a median sternotomy (Fig. 3.59).

AORTOPULMONARY SEPTAL DEFECT

In an aortopulmonary septal defect there is a communication between the aorta and pulmonary trunk just above the level of the arterial valves (Fig. 3.60). Most of the clinical features are similar to those described for patency of the arterial duct (see above). The murmur, however, is more often systolic than continuous, and it is usually located near the lower left sternal border rather than in the pulmonary area. The diagnosis is made by cardiac catheterization and angiography.

SINUS OF VALSALVA FISTULA

A posterior (noncoronary) sinus of Valsalva aneurysm may rupture into the right atrium, while a right coronary sinus of Valsalva aneurysm may rupture into the right ventricle (Sakakibara and Konno, 1962). Rupture may occur spontaneously or following trauma. Infective endocarditis may produce a fistula that causes a similar clinical picture

in addition to the characteristic signs of endocarditis.

The rupture may produce chest pain and pulmonary congestion. The murmur is continuous and is heard lower on the chest than is the murmur of a patent arterial duct. The murmur may be to-and-fro. The type of murmur is determined by the location of the fistula. Neck vein pulsation is abnormal when the sinus ruptures into the right atrium. Aneurysm of the right sinus is commonly associated with a ventricular septal defect. The exact diagnosis is usually confirmed by cardiac catheterization and angiography, although the clinical features are virtually diagnostic (Meyer et al, 1975).

CORONARY ARTERIOVENOUS FISTULA

The reader is referred to the discussion (below) under "Anomalies of the Coronary Arteries."

COARCTATION OF THE AORTA
DEFINITION AND PATHOLOGY

Coarctation of the aorta is a term applied to the narrowing of the aorta almost always localized in the region of the arterial duct (Clagett et al, 1954). The lesion may be an isolated shelf (Fig. 3.61), a waist lesion (Fig. 3.62), or a more elongated tubular narrowing of a segment of

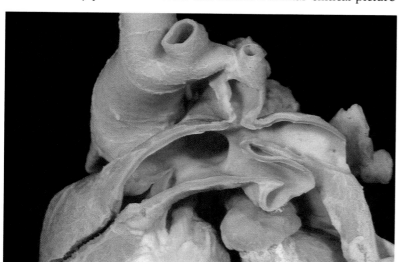

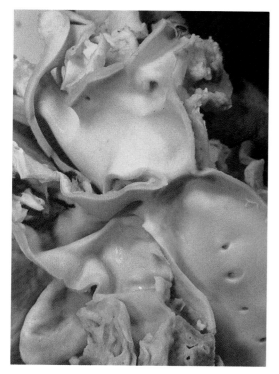

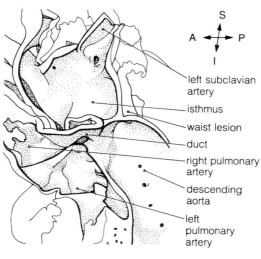

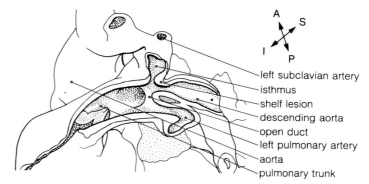

FIG. 3.61   *This heart specimen with preductal coarctation has been sectioned to replicate the view obtained by the echocardiographer from the suprasternal window. The coarctation shelf is continuous with the wall of the arterial duct, and it is composed of ductal tissue.*

left subclavian artery
isthmus
shelf lesion
descending aorta
open duct
left pulmonary artery
aorta
pulmonary trunk

FIG. 3.62   *In this specimen coarctation with an open arterial duct is due to a waist lesion in the immediate preductal position. The narrowing is an infolding of the aortic wall rather than a discrete intraluminal shelf (see Fig. 3.61).*

left subclavian artery
isthmus
waist lesion
duct
right pulmonary artery
descending aorta
left pulmonary artery

the aortic arch (Fig. 3.63). Collateral circulation in coarctation usually occurs when the arterial duct is closed.

Coarctation may be associated with left ventricular endocardial fibroelastosis, subendocardial fibrosis (Fig. 3.64), patent arterial duct, ventricular septal defect (VSD) (Fig. 3.65), bicuspid valve (in almost half of cases) (Fig. 3.66), subaortic obstruction, complete transposition, double-outlet right ventricle with subpulmonary VSD (the Taussig–Bing anomaly) (Fig. 3.67), aberrant right subclavian artery, or anomalies of the mitral valve, particularly the parachute deformity. Coarctation also accompanies those lesions with univentricular atrioventricular connection to the left ventricle, such as double-inlet or tricuspid atresia, in which there is a discordant ventriculoarterial connection and a restrictive VSD.

ABNORMAL PHYSIOLOGY

The systolic and the diastolic blood pressures are elevated above normal levels in the arms. The systolic blood pressure is less in the legs than it is in the arms, while the diastolic pressure is near or slightly lower than normal. In some cases the blood pressure is normal in the upper extremities and decreased in the lower extremities. The elevated pressure is due to a combination of mechanical obstruction and humoral factors (Parker et al, 1982).

CLINICAL MANIFESTATIONS

Almost half of patients with Turner's syndrome have coarctation of the aorta. Approximately half of infants with coarctation experience heart failure during the first few months of life. About 20% of patients with severe heart failure and coarctation have isolated coarctation, about 20% have a patent arterial duct, and about one half have a VSD (Fyler, 1980). The male to female ratio is 3:1 in patients with isolated coarctation and 1:1 when other lesions are present.

SYMPTOMS

The symptomatic infant may have heart failure with dyspnea, difficulty in feeding, and poor weight gain. Older patients are usually asymptomatic, although a child may complain of intermittent claudication of the legs. The symptoms of heart failure may occur after age 40. Endarteritis or endocarditis may occur at any age.

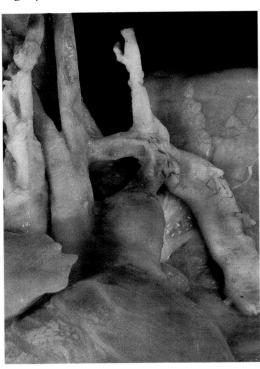

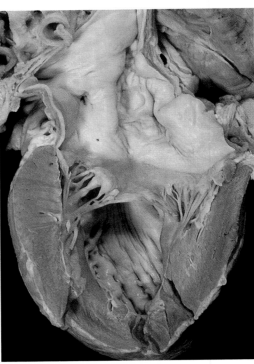

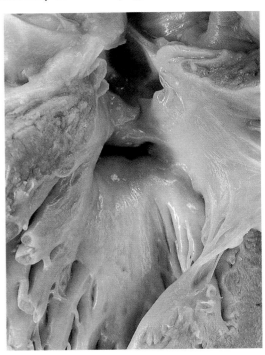

FIG. 3.63   *This heart with discrete coarctation in preductal location (not shown) also has severe tubular hypoplasia of the segment of aortic arch between the left common carotid and the left subclavian arteries.*

FIG. 3.64   *This heart from a five-year-old child who died with severe, unoperated aortic coarctation with a closed arterial duct is dissected to show the left atrium and ventricle. There is extensive hypertrophy of the left ventricle with marked subendocardial fibrosis.*

FIG. 3.65   *This heart is sectioned to show the left ventricular aspect of a malalignment VSD. The outlet septum is deviated into the left ventricle, thus producing subaortic obstruction. Severe preductal coarctation is also exhibited.*

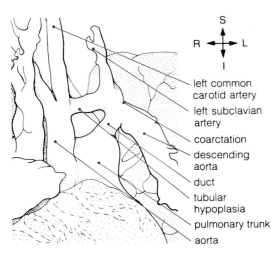

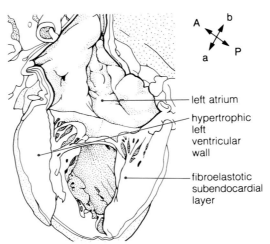

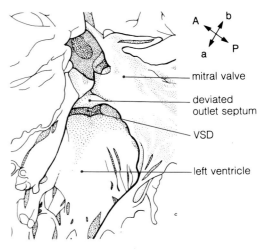

PART II: DISEASES OF THE HEART

PHYSICAL EXAMINATION

The infant may exhibit signs of heart failure. The murmur of coarctation (see below) may not be audible until heart failure is improved. There may be murmurs related to associated defects.

Older children and adults may exhibit more characteristic signs of coarctation of the aorta. The trunk may reveal more muscular development than the lower extremities. There may be signs of Turner's syndrome (ovarian agenesis) in female patients. The blood pressure may be normal or only slightly elevated in the arms. A lower pressure in one arm compared with the other suggests that the corresponding subclavian artery arises below the coarctation. The blood pressure is less in the legs than it is in the arms in patients with coarctation, whereas normally it is higher in the legs than in the arms; the latter is true because the size of the muscles in the legs of the normal person produces a cushion around the arteries. One third of patients have no hypertension, and two thirds have slight-to-moderate elevation of blood pressure. It is important to record the blood pressure in the arms after exercise because this may produce an abnormal elevation of pressure when compared with normal patients.

There is a prominent arterial pulsation noted in the neck. Palpation of the apex impulse of the left ventricle may suggest left ventricular hypertrophy. The femoral arterial pulsations may be diminished or absent, and collateral arterial vessels may be seen and palpated in the intercostal spaces in the back.

The aortic component of the second sound may be increased in intensity; an early systolic click at the apex suggests the presence of a bicuspid aortic valve.

The systolic murmur of coarctation is best heard in the interscapular region; it may be faint or inaudible anteriorly. Continuous murmurs are usually heard over the collateral vessels on the back in older children and adults. A bicuspid aortic valve may cause a systolic murmur and the murmur of aortic regurgitation. The murmurs due to associated conditions, such as VSD or a patent arterial duct, may also be heard.

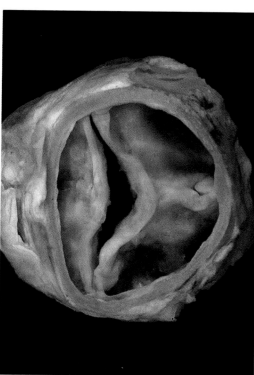

FIG. 3.66 *A bifoliate (bicuspid) aortic valve viewed from above clearly shows the raphe suggesting fusion of the right and left coronary leaflets. The valve is also thickened and stenotic.*

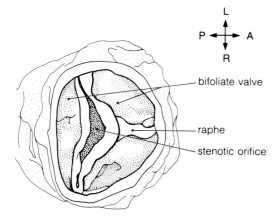

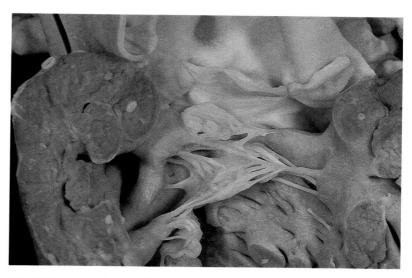

FIG. 3.67 *An overview of the right ventricle and great arteries in this heart reveals a double-outlet right ventricle with subpulmonary VSD (the Taussig–Bing malformation). This anomaly is seen in association with restrictive subaortic infundibulum.*

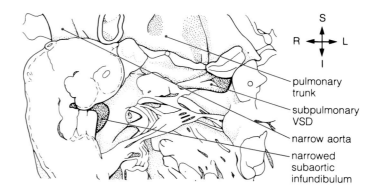

LABORATORY STUDIES

CHEST RADIOGRAPHY. The chest film of the infant with heart failure shows cardiac enlargement and, when there is an associated duct or VSD, an increase in pulmonary blood flow. The aortic arch gives the appearance of the figure *3* and the barium-filled esophagus resembles the letter *E*. Rib notching is seen after the age of eight years (Fig. 3.68). The proximal portion of the aorta is enlarged, especially when there is aortic stenosis due to a bicuspid aortic valve.

ELECTROCARDIOGRAPHY. The ECG in an infant with heart failure may show a right atrial abnormality, right ventricular hypertrophy, or biventricular hypertrophy; the T waves may be inverted in the left precordial leads. The ECGs of older children and adults may be normal (Fig. 3.69) or they may show left atrial abnormality, left ventricular hypertrophy, and left anterior hemiblock.

ECHOCARDIOGRAPHY. Left ventricular function can be assessed

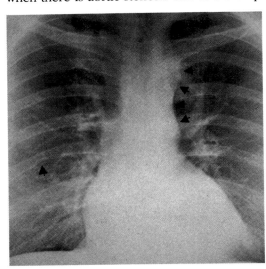

FIG. 3.68 *Note the large notch in the seventh posterior rib* (right arrow) *in the chest film of this adult with coarctation of the aorta. The vascularity is normal with a normal-sized left ventricular contour* (right middle arrows). *The transverse aortic arch and the upper descending thoracic aorta are distorted. The findings regarding the thoracic aorta in this case cannot be differentiated from those of an aortic dissection. The notched rib is the premier radiographic finding in the differential. Note what is probably the precoarctation aortic dilation* (right upper arrow), *as well as what is probably a postcoarctation dilation of the aorta* (right lower arrow). *(Reproduced with permission of the authors and publisher; see Figure Credits)*

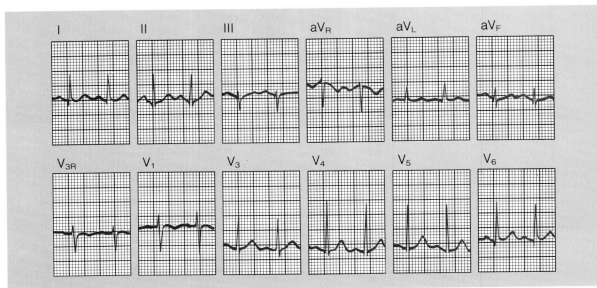

FIG. 3.69 *This ECG of an eight-year-old girl with coarctation of the aorta is normal, as is often the case with this anomaly. Blood pressure in the arms was 170/110 mmHg. Early in life the ECG may show right ventricular hypertrophy; later in life, with sufficient hypertension and aortic valve stenosis, the ECG may show left ventricular hypertrophy. (Redrawn; reproduced with permission of the authors and publisher; see Figure Credits)*

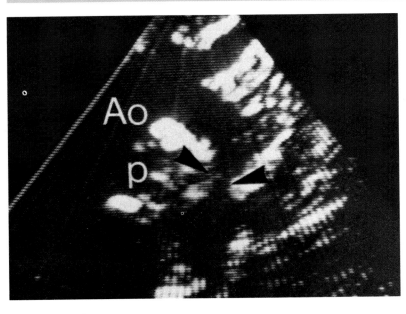

FIG. 3.70 *Cross-sectional echocardiography was performed on a patient with coarctation of the aorta. On the suprasternal notch long-axis view an area of narrowing is seen just beyond the origin of the left subclavian artery* (arrows). *Post-stenotic dilation of the descending aorta is apparent* (Ao, *aorta*; p, *right pulmonary artery*). *(Reproduced with permission of the authors and publisher; see Figure Credits)*

using M-mode echocardiography. The coarctation itself can be viewed with cross-sectional echocardiography; associated defects may also be visualized (Fig. 3.70)

CARDIAC CATHETERIZATION.
A systolic pressure difference may be detected between the left ventricle and the femoral artery, although this difference may not be present when there is a large VSD or arterial duct. Other defects, such as aortic valve stenosis or regurgitation, VSD, or arterial duct, may be detected. Aortography reveals the exact site and length of the coarctation (Fig. 3.71).

NATURAL HISTORY
About 20% of infants with heart failure have coarctation of the aorta. Most of these babies respond to medical treatment, including digitalis; as collateral circulation develops, the signs of heart failure gradually decrease. Some patients, particularly those with associated defects, require surgery in infancy. Re-stenosis occurs in some patients operated on at this age irrespective of the type of surgery employed.

Older patients with hypertension may have rupture of the aorta, rupture of a berry aneurysm in the brain, endocarditis, or heart failure. Because of this, surgery is indicated early during childhood. The blood pressure returns to normal in most patients following surgery, but it may remain elevated without renal disease or re-stenosis of the coarc-

tation site. This postoperative hypertension seems to occur less frequently in patients who are operated on early in childhood (Maron, 1979).

TREATMENT
Medical therapy includes advice regarding the prevention of infective endocarditis and the treatment of heart failure. The medical management of hypertension may be needed. Balloon dilation angioplasty of the coarcted segment has been used for both native coarctation and re-stenosis. Since the technique works by rupturing the aortic media and in some cases aneurysms develop, it seems wiser to reserve balloon dilation for cases of re-stenosis (Lock et al, 1983).

INDICATIONS FOR SURGERY
The infant with heart failure may need surgical correction of the aorta if the response to medical measures is unsatisfactory. Asymptomatic children with coarctation should be operated on before the age of six years (Sehested, 1978).

SURGICAL PROCEDURE
The operative approach to coarctation is through a left thoracotomy. Even on the chest wall one may encounter large collateral vessels that require individual ligation (Fig. 3.72). Within the chest other collaterals

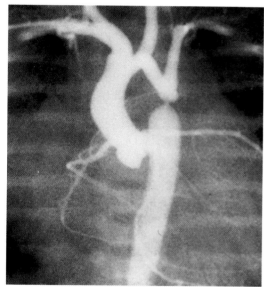

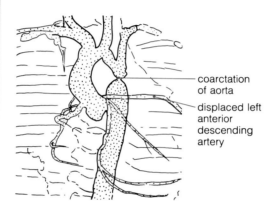

coarctation of aorta

displaced left anterior descending artery

FIG. 3.71 *In this patient contrast material was injected through a catheter inserted from the right subclavian artery. On the frontal view tight coarctation of the aorta is present distal to the left subclavian artery. The segment of the arch as far proximally as the innominate artery is mildly hypoplastic. Mild post-stenotic dilation is present beyond the coarctation. The left anterior descending coronary artery branch is displaced by an enlarged left ventricle. (Reproduced with permission of the authors and publisher; see Figure Credits. Courtesy of Robert M. Freedom, MD, Toronto, Ontario)*

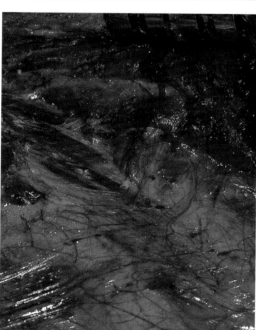

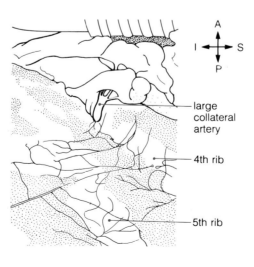

A

I ◄►S

P

large collateral artery

4th rib

5th rib

FIG. 3.72 *In this surgical repair of coarctation of the aorta in an 18-year-old patient the large collateral arteries are seen coursing beneath the ribs and communicating with the intercostal muscle.*

are apparent including the internal thoracic artery (IMA) (Fig. 3.73), the intercostal arteries (Fig. 3.74), and enlarged bronchial arteries. Abbott's artery (Hamilton and Abbott, 1928) is occasionally encountered proximal to the coarctation (Fig. 3.75); it may cause troublesome bleeding. The arterial duct or ligament is most commonly found in close proximity to the coarctation, and it usually requires division when the coarctation is resected (Fig. 3.76). Care must also be exercised to avoid damage to the vagus and the recurrent laryngeal nerves.

An end-to-end anastomosis is usually used to repair the aorta. It is best to resect as little aorta as possible (Fig. 3.77), although it may be neces-

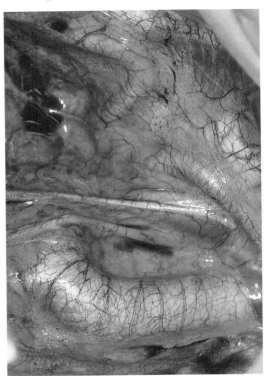

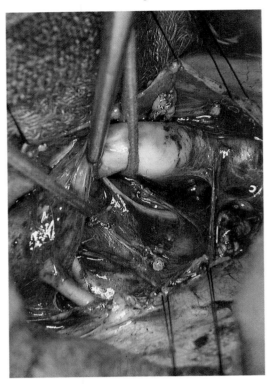

FIG. 3.73 *Operative view through a left thoracotomy for repair of coarctation of the aorta shows an extremely enlarged left subclavian artery giving rise to a dilated and tortuous internal thoracic artery (IMA).*

FIG. 3.74 *Large intercostal arteries are seen in close proximity to the area of coarctation in this operative view. The recurrent laryngeal nerve passes just behind the proximal aorta.*

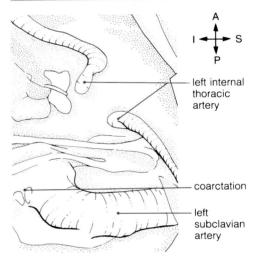

left internal thoracic artery

coarctation

left subclavian artery

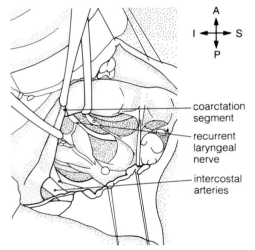

coarctation segment

recurrent laryngeal nerve

intercostal arteries

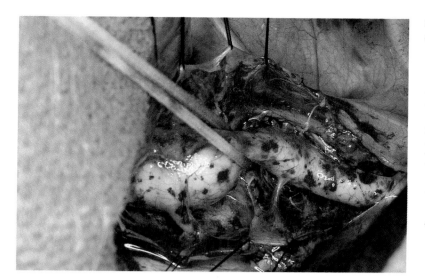

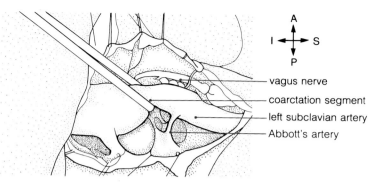

FIG. 3.75 *Abbott's artery arises proximal to the area of coarctation on this operative view.*

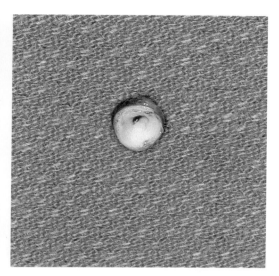

vagus nerve
coarctation segment
left subclavian artery
Abbott's artery

A
I — S
P

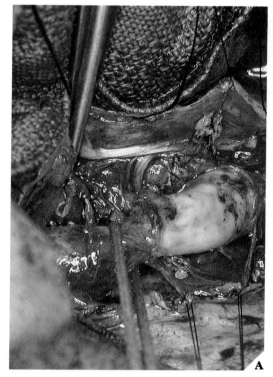

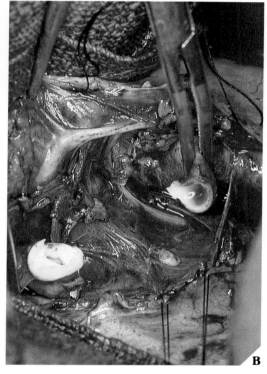

A

B

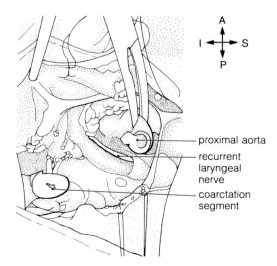

FIG. 3.77 *This short coarcted segment was removed from the patient depicted in Figure 3.76. The extreme narrowness of the lumen is caused by the shelflike projection of the coarctation tissue.*

FIG. 3.76 (**A**) *In this operative view a coarctation is seen in close proximity to the arterial ligament. The recurrent laryngeal nerve here courses around the ligament.* (**B**) *The aorta is transected* *and the ligament is divided, while the narrow segment of coarctation is still in place. The course of the recurrent laryngeal nerve can now be easily identified.*

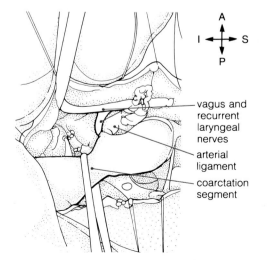

A
I — S
P

vagus and recurrent laryngeal nerves
arterial ligament
coarctation segment

A
I — S
P

proximal aorta
recurrent laryngeal nerve
coarctation segment

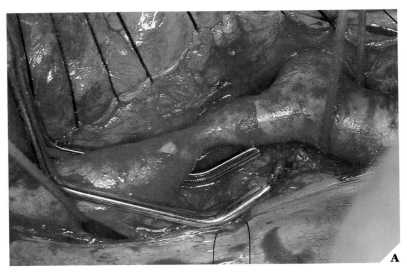

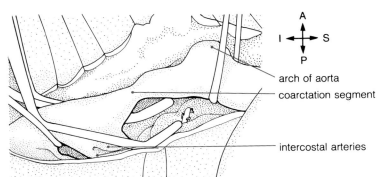

arch of aorta

coarctation segment

intercostal arteries

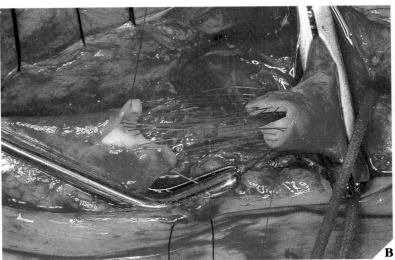

A

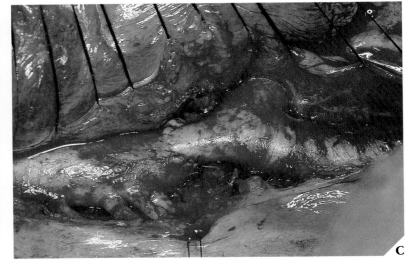

B

C

FIG. 3.78 (A) *In this surgical repair of coarctation of the aorta a vascular clamp is applied to avoid occluding important collateral vessels.* (B) *The anterior and posterior interior wall of the inferior segment and the posterior wall of the superior segment of aorta are incised to enlarge the* anastomosis. *Continuous monofilament suture is used to close the posterior row.* (C) *The anterior aspect of the anastomosis is completed with interrupted sutures.*

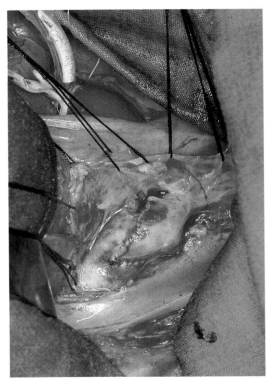

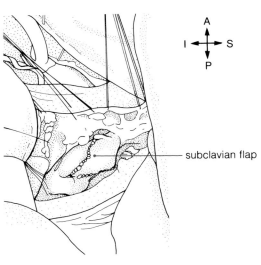

subclavian flap

FIG. 3.79 *Coarctation repair in a newborn is accomplished using the subclavian flap technique. The pulmonary artery was temporarily banded during the procedure because of the presence of a concomitant ventricular septal defect.*

sary to tailor the anastomosis to achieve the widest possible opening (Fig. 3.78). In children under one year of age the subclavian artery may be used as an inlay flap to enlarge the aorta (Fig. 3.79). This is particularly useful in the unusual situation in which the narrow segment lies between the subclavian and left carotid arteries (Fig. 3.80).

AORTIC STENOSIS IN THE YOUNG

Congenital heart disease is the usual cause of aortic valve stenosis in infants and children and it may be the cause in adults. Certain features of this condition in children justify a separate discussion on the subject. (See Chapter 4 for a discussion of aortic valve stenosis in adults.)

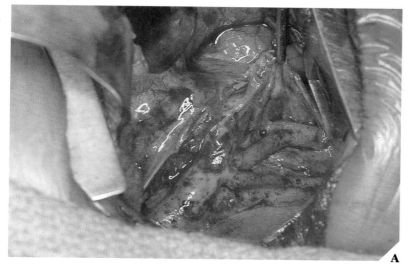

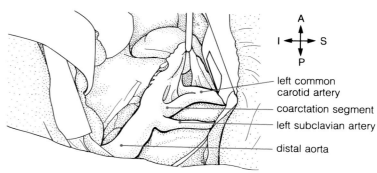

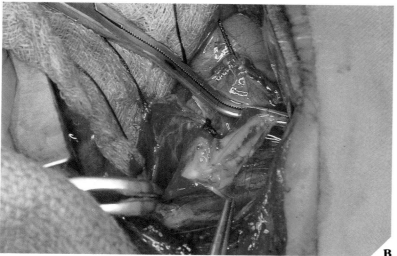

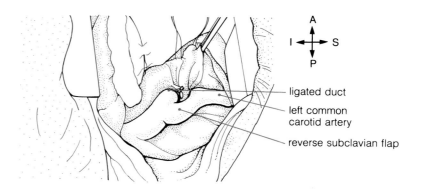

FIG. 3.80 *In the surgical repair of a coarctation occurring between the left subclavian and the left common carotid arteries (A) the subclavian artery is divided and the coarcted segment of the aorta is opened (B). The* *subclavian vessel is used as a flap graft to enlarge the narrowed segment. (C) The completed repair shows the subclavian flap in place.*

DEFINITION AND PATHOLOGY

Aortic stenosis, or left ventricular outflow tract obstruction, can be divided into three types: valvar, including bicuspid (see Fig. 3.66) and unicuspid (Fig. 3.81) variants; subvalvar, including shelf-like (Fig. 3.82) or muscular (Fig. 3.83) variants; or supravalvar, including hourglass (Fig. 3.84), hypoplastic, and membranous variants. Valvar congenital stenosis is common, whereas the other types of obstruction are rare. Left ventricular hypertrophy and endocardial fibroelastosis may be present, and a bicuspid aortic valve is common. Coarctation of the aorta is the most commonly associated defect.

ABNORMAL PHYSIOLOGY

The reader is referred to the discussion of abnormal physiology of aortic valve stenosis in adults in Chapter 4.

CLINICAL MANIFESTATIONS
SYMPTOMS

The majority of children are asymptomatic even when the stenosis is severe, but dyspnea, fatigue, syncope, angina, and sudden death may occur.

Infants with severe stenosis develop heart failure within the first few weeks of life; this is considered a medical emergency. Those with less severe stenosis may develop heart failure during the first six months of life.

Children with subvalvar stenosis are usually asymptomatic. The syndrome is recognized because of a systolic murmur, often thought to be due to a ventricular septal defect. Although subvalvar stenosis may be due to development of a fibrous shelf, obstruction may also be caused by muscular hypertrophy. This condition is known as asymmetric septal hypertrophy, or when more extensive, as idiopathic hypertrophic subaortic stenosis. This condition is usually part of the hypertrophic cardiomyopathy. This occurs more commonly in males; older children and adults with this condition have syncope, angina, and heart failure.

Patients with supravalvar aortic stenosis have symptoms that are similar to those with valvar or subvalvar aortic stenosis except that heart failure in the newborn is rare.

PHYSICAL EXAMINATION

Peripheral arterial pulses may be diminished in infants with severe aortic valve stenosis. When severe heart failure is present, a murmur may not be detected. Older children and adults may have a systolic thrill in the aortic area, a sustained apex impulse during systole, an aortic ejection click at the apex, an atrial gallop, a diminished aortic

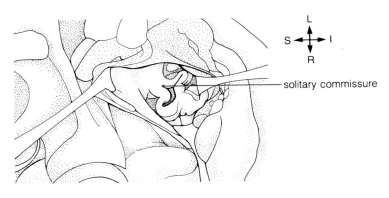

FIG. 3.81 *Operative view shows a unicuspid, unicommissural, and stenotic aortic valve.*

solitary commissure

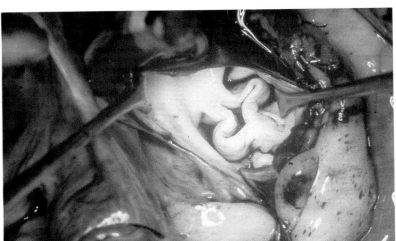

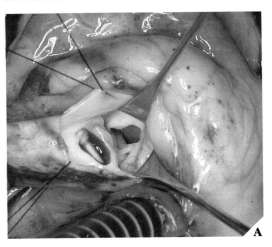

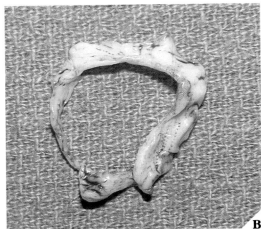

A   B

FIG. 3.82 **(A)** *Operative view through the aortic valve shows subvalvar aortic stenosis produced by a fibrous shelf.* **(B)** *The resected shelf encircled the outflow tract.*

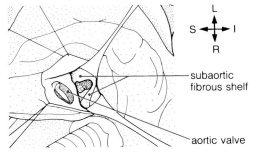

subaortic fibrous shelf

aortic valve

valve closure sound, paradoxical splitting of the second sound, and a diamond-shaped, systolic murmur in the aortic area. A murmur of aortic regurgitation may be detected.

The systolic murmur of subvalvar aortic stenosis is often mistaken for that of a ventricular septal defect. The discrete, shelf-like type of subvalvar obstruction causes aortic regurgitation in one half of cases. An aortic ejection click is not heard, and when aortic regurgitation is present, a two-peaked pulse is palpated in the carotid artery. (The muscular type of subvalvar stenosis—hypertrophic cardiomyopathy—is discussed in Chapter 6.)

One type of supravalvar aortic stenosis may be familial, transmitted as an autosomal-dominant trait. Another type, usually called Williams syndrome, occurs sporadically; it is characterized by supravalvar aortic stenosis, characteristic facies (high forehead, epicanthic folds, and underdeveloped bridge of the nose and mandible), hypercalcemia, and mental retardation. Peripheral pulmonary artery stenoses may be found in both types of supravalvar aortic stenosis.

LABORATORY STUDIES

CHEST RADIOGRAPHY. The heart of a patient with valvar aortic stenosis is usually of normal size, although there may be post-stenotic dilation of the aorta.

The chest film of a patient with subvalvar aortic stenosis is usually normal. The left ventricle may become prominent, but post-stenotic dilation of the aorta does not occur.

The chest x-ray film of a patient with supravalvar aortic stenosis is usually normal, and post-stenotic dilation of the aorta does not occur.

ELECTROCARDIOGRAPHY. Symptomatic infants with valvar aortic stenosis may show biventricular hypertrophy. The ECG may be normal in older children and adults with mild stenosis, but it usually shows various stages of left ventricular hypertrophy when the stenosis is severe.

The ECG of a patient with the shelf-like type of subvalvar aortic stenosis may be similar to the ECG seen in patients with valvar stenosis.

The ECG of the muscular variety of aortic stenosis associated with idiopathic cardiac hypertrophy usually reveals left ventricular hypertrophy; the ST-T waves may be bizarre. The QRS complex may be typical of the WPW phenomenon (see Chapter 6).

The ECG of supravalvar aortic stenosis may reveal left ventricular hypertrophy. Right ventricular hypertrophy may also be present in patients with peripheral stenoses of the pulmonary arteries.

ECHOCARDIOGRAPHY. M-mode and cross-sectional echocardio-

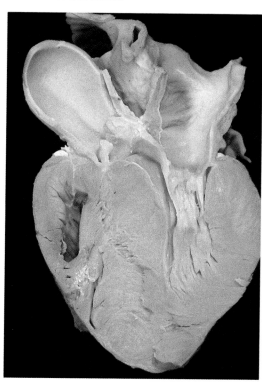

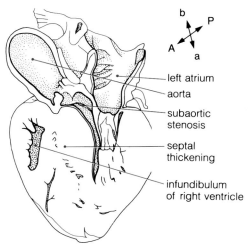

FIG. 3.83 *This simulated parasternal long-axis section shows how hypertrophic cardiomyopathy produces severe asymmetric thickening of the ventricular septum, which results in subaortic obstruction.*

left atrium
aorta
subaortic stenosis
septal thickening
infundibulum of right ventricle

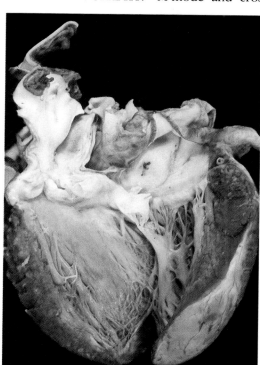

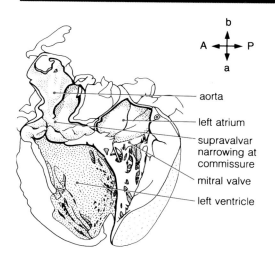

FIG. 3.84 *This heart photographed from the left ventricular aspect shows severe narrowing of the aortic outflow at the level of the commissural ridge, an example of the hourglass variant of supravalvar aortic stenosis.*

aorta
left atrium
supravalvar narrowing at commissure
mitral valve
left ventricle

graphic studies reveal the obstructive lesions in patients with valvar, subvalvar, and supravalvar aortic stenosis (Fig. 3.85).

Doppler studies permit an assessment of the systolic pressure gradient across discrete forms of left ventricular outflow tract obstruction.

CARDIAC CATHETERIZATION. Complete right and left heart catheterization should be performed on symptomatic infants with left ventricular outflow tract obstruction in order to determine the cardiac output and to identify the systolic pressure gradient across the obstruction. Associated lesions may also be discovered at cardiac catheterization. Older children and adults who exhibit only a murmur and have no symptoms may be studied initially with noninvasive means. The visualization of the left ventricular anatomy by left ventriculography and aortography may be useful and coronary arteriography is essential in adult patients to identify the presence or absence of coronary disease.

NATURAL HISTORY

Most infants with severe valvar aortic stenosis develop heart failure within the first year of life (Moss et al, 1977). One third of patients with less severe stenosis gradually develop a greater left ventricular–aortic pressure gradient; the ECG may reveal more left ventricular hypertrophy, and heart failure may develop. Syncope or sudden death may occur as complications of valvar aortic stenosis. Infective endocarditis is always a threat even with slight valve stenosis.

The infant with subvalvar aortic stenosis rarely develops heart failure (Wright et al, 1983); older children and adults may have syncope, arrhythmias, and sudden death. Endocarditis occurs rarely.

The complications of supravalvar aortic stenosis are similar to those of valvar aortic stenosis.

TREATMENT

Patients with heart failure should be treated with digitalis and diuretics, and prophylaxis against bacterial endocarditis is always necessary. Asymptomatic patients with little clinical evidence of difficulty must be followed carefully; Doppler studies have become important in this regard.

Balloon dilation of valvar aortic stenosis has been accomplished, but this procedure is still experimental and should only be done within strict research protocol (Lababidi et al, 1984).

INDICATIONS FOR SURGERY

Infants with heart failure must be treated surgically. Young patients with valvar aortic stenosis may have a valvotomy (Ellis and Kirklin, 1962). Patients who have had lifesaving valvotomies may need valve replacement when they are older. Older patients with symptoms of heart failure, syncope, a ventricular–aortic peak systolic pressure gradient of 75 mmHG, or a valve area of 0.5 cm²/m² should have valve replacement.

Patients who are symptomatic due to fixed, shelf-like subvalvar stenosis should have surgery. Surgery is also indicated in patients whose systolic pressure gradient across the membrane is 30 mmHg or greater. Patients with the muscular type of subvalvar stenosis may need myectomies if medical management is not successful in relieving angina or syncope.

The indications for surgery for supravalvar stenosis are the same as for valvar aortic stenosis. Coronary ostial involvement may require special attention at the time of surgery.

SURGICAL PROCEDURE

In congenital valvar stenosis in infants the valve can often be opened at one or more of the fused commissures (Fig. 3.86). Because the orifice is so small, even an opening of a few millimeters can be lifesaving. It is important not to create aortic regurgitation; this complication may occur if one attempts to open a rudimentary commissure, or if the incision in a true commissure is carried further than 1–1.5 mm of the aortic attachment.

A subaortic ring can often be removed intact (see Fig. 3.82B), ensuring complete relief of the outflow obstruction. This procedure is performed through the aortic root while the valve cusps are retracted (Fig. 3.87). Blunt dissection allows one to peel the ring off its attachments with minimal risk of detaching the mitral valve apparatus or damaging the conduction tissues.

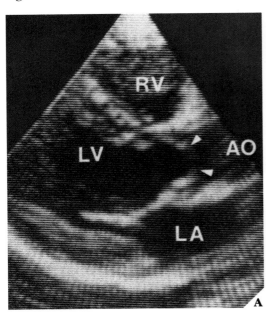

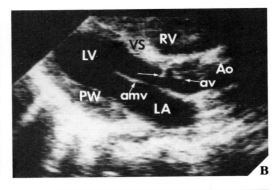

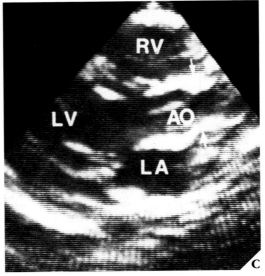

FIG. 3.85 *Cross-sectional echocardiograms in the parasternal long-axis view in three patients with aortic stenosis.* (**A**) *In aortic valve stenosis the aortic valve cusps* (arrows) *are thickened and domed with diminished cusp separation* (AO, *aorta;* LA, *left atrium;* LV, *left ventricle;* RV, *right ventricle*). (**B**) *In discrete, fibrous subvalvar aortic stenosis a thin, discrete shelf* (unlabeled arrow) *is seen attached to the interventricular septum* (VS) *in the left ventricular* (LV) *outflow tract immediately below the aortic valve* (av) (PW, *posterior left ventricular wall;* amv, *anterior leaflet of the mitral valve*). (**C**) *In supravalvar aortic stenosis an hourglass-type constriction is seen on the external aspects of the aorta* (arrows) *with a corresponding narrowing of the aortic lumen.* (**A,C:** *Reproduced with permission of the authors and publisher; see Figure Credits.* **B:** *Fig. 36-37,* The Heart, *6th ed, p 640)*

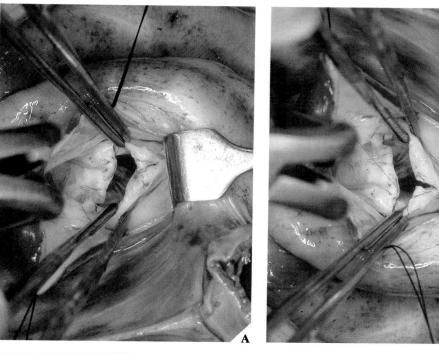

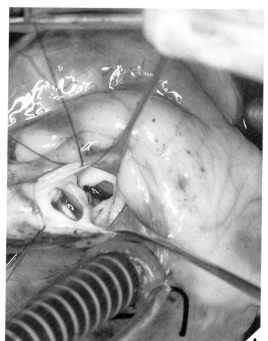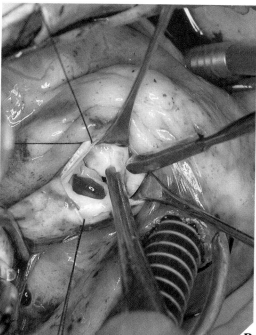

FIG. 3.86 (A) Operative view shows congenital bicuspid aortic valvar stenosis in an infant. (B) The fused commissure has been divided to within 1.5 mm of the aortic wall.

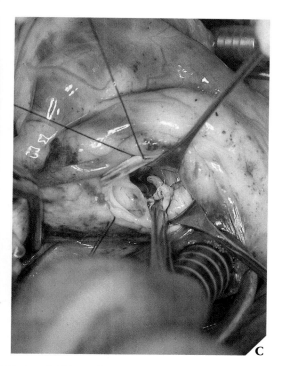

FIG. 3.87 (A) In surgical repair of a congenital subvalvar aortic stenosis the subvalvar shelf is seen through the retracted aortic valve. (B) The thickened fibromuscular shelf is grasped with forceps and teased away from the ventricular septal wall. (C) Careful blunt dissection avoids inadvertent detachment of the area of aortic–mitral continuity, minimizing danger to the conduction tissues.

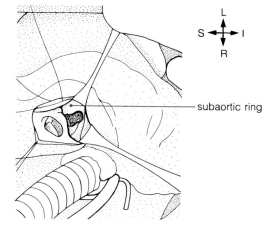

subaortic ring

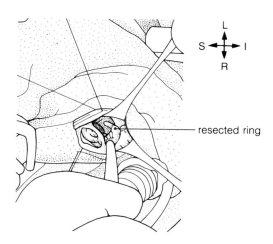

resected ring

Supravalvar aortic stenosis, whether localized or diffuse, requires enlargement of the ascending aorta proximal and distal to the constriction; a pericardial patch is the most useful material for this purpose (Fig. 3.88). There is no evidence that the double- or triple-flanged patch is superior in relieving the obstruction of the supravalvar type of aortic obstruction.

AORTIC ATRESIA

Aortic atresia exists when the aortic valve is not patent; the atretic part of the aorta is proximal to the origin of the coronary arteries. The ascending aorta is hypoplastic and usually tapers as it nears the heart, although it is often bulbous at the origin of the coronary arteries. The left ventricular cavity is almost always small, and the mitral valve is

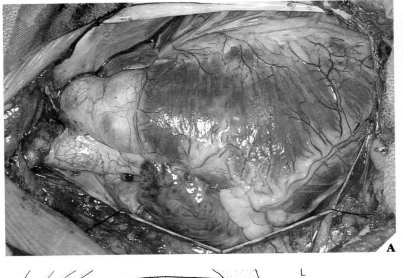

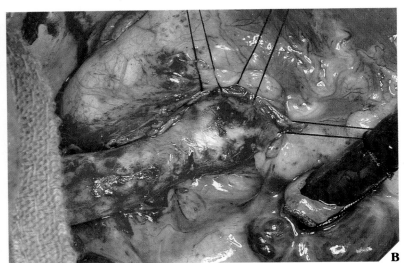

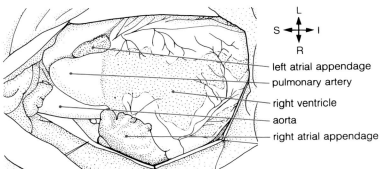

left atrial appendage
pulmonary artery
right ventricle
aorta
right atrial appendage

pulmonary artery
right carotid artery
aorta

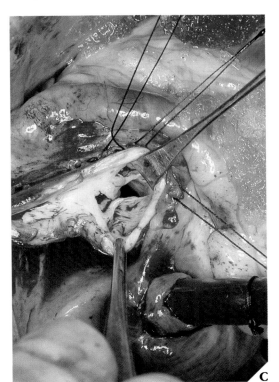

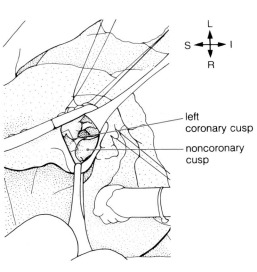

left coronary cusp
noncoronary cusp

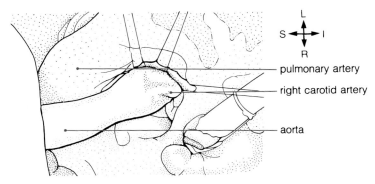

FIG. 3.88 (A) Operative view of the heart in repair of supravalvar aortic stenosis shows the small aortic root in comparison with the normal-sized pulmonary artery. (B) The supravalvar constriction is more apparent with further dissection. (C) A vertical incision extended well down into the noncoronary sinus shows the markedly constricted ring with the particularly narrow left coronary sinus (continued).

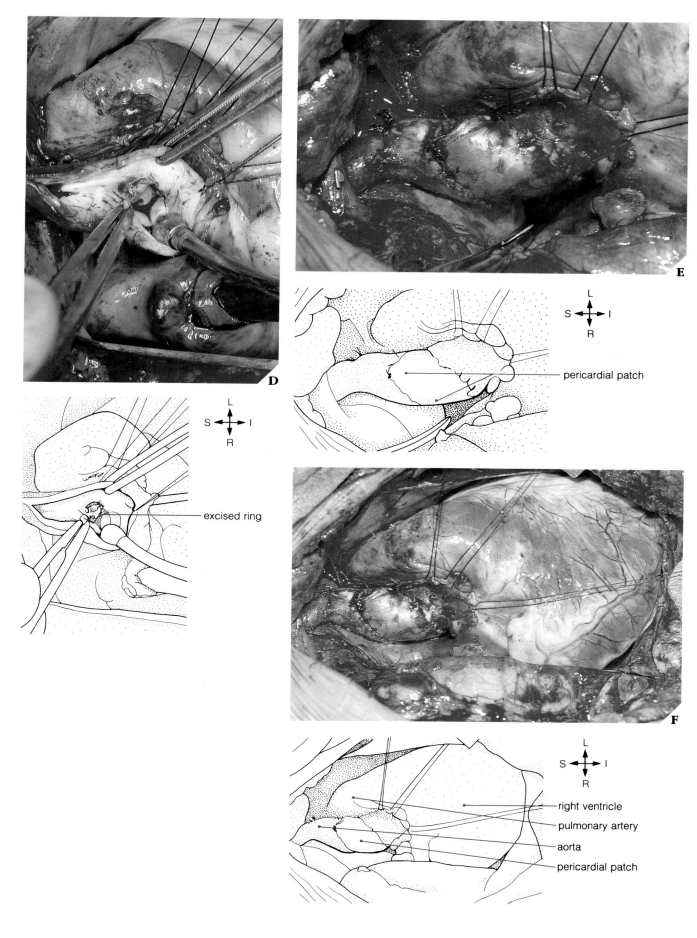

FIG. 3.88 (continued)
(D) *This bar of
tissue, resembling an
exaggeration of the
aortic bar, is excised
from within the
aorta, freeing up the
attachments of the
left coronary cusp to
allow full excursion.
(E) Resection of the
bar, together with in-
sertion of a helical
pericardial patch, en-
larges the aorta. (F)
The aorta is now ap-
proximately the same
size as the pulmo-
nary artery (compare
with parts A and B).*

D

E

peridardial patch

excised ring

F

right ventricle

pulmonary artery

aorta

pericardial patch

CONGENITAL HEART DISEASE

hypoplastic or atretic (Fig. 3.89). The right ventricular cavity is large with a thickened wall. Patency of the oval foramen may permit a left-to-right shunt that is usually restrictive. Occasionally there is a connection between a pulmonary vein and a systemic vein. The arterial duct is usually patent. Very rarely aortic atresia may be found with a ventricular septal defect, a large left ventricle, and a normal-sized mitral valve (Fig. 3.90).

This condition is the major cause of cardiac death during the first two weeks of life. The infant, more often male than female, may become suddenly cyanotic, and may exhibit severe respiratory distress.

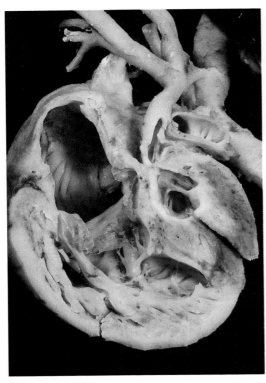
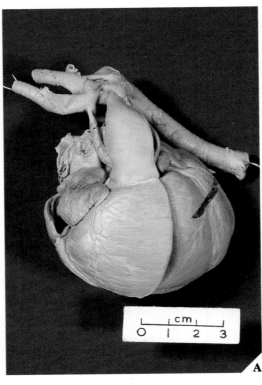
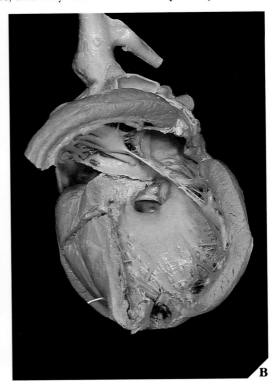

FIG. 3.89 *This simulated four-chamber long-axis section shows the typical findings of aortic atresia with an intact ventricular septum, a hypoplastic left ventricle with fibroelastic wall, and mitral stenosis—the so-called hypoplastic left heart syndrome.*

FIG. 3.90 *This heart shows a rare form of aortic atresia (A) characterized by a good-sized left ventricle due to the coexisting ventricular septal defect (B).*

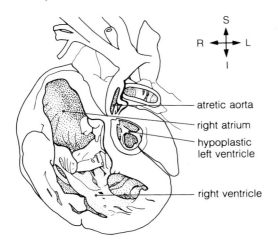

atretic aorta
right atrium
hypoplastic left ventricle
right ventricle

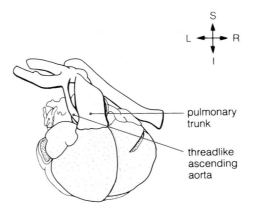

pulmonary trunk
threadlike ascending aorta

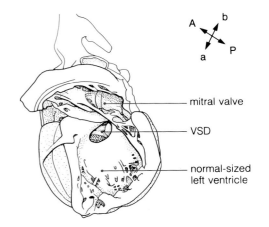

mitral valve
VSD
normal-sized left ventricle

Signs of heart failure may be present; the peripheral pulse is weak, while the apex impulse is strong. Heart failure may be detected on the chest film, while the ECG usually shows right ventricular hypertrophy (Fig. 3.91). The echocardiogram is diagnostic because the aortic root is small or absent (Fig. 3.92). Data collected by cardiac catheterization and angiography are confirmatory.

This condition is almost always fatal. Prostaglandin-E helps maintain patency of the duct. While surgical palliation is quite difficult, staged procedures have been successfully performed. The surgeon creates complex shunts in an effort to increase blood flow into the aorta.

CONGENITAL AORTIC REGURGITATION

Isolated aortic regurgitation may be associated with bicuspid aortic valve or abnormal aortic valve leaflets, which may be rudimentary, dysplastic, or tethered (Fig. 3.93). It may also accompany cystic medial necrosis of the aorta, as in Marfan's syndrome (Roberts et al, 1981; Hashimoto et al, 1984). These conditions should be considered whenever the murmur of isolated aortic regurgitation is heard in a young child. The exact etiology is determined by cardiac catheterization and angiography. Surgery is indicated for patients with symptoms of heart failure or evidence of left ventricular dysfunction.

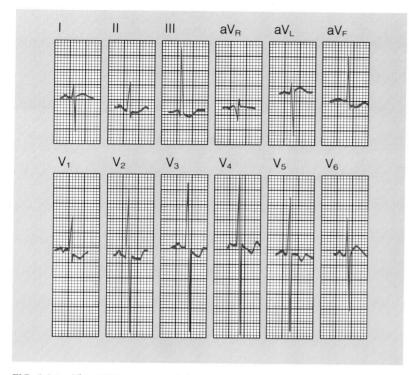

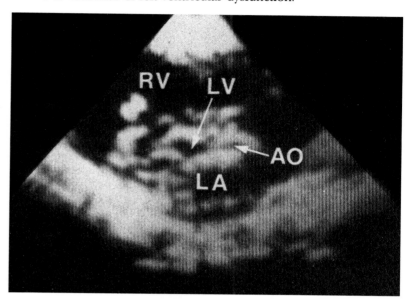

FIG. 3.92 *Cross-sectional echocardiogram in the parasternal long-axis view is from a newborn with aortic and mitral atresia. The ascending aorta (AO) is diminutive; the left ventricle (LV) has a slitlike cavity and is extremely hypertrophic. The right ventricle (RV) is enlarged (LA, left atrium). (Reproduced with permission of the authors and publisher; see Figure Credits)*

FIG. 3.91 *This ECG was recorded in a male infant who survived for four weeks with aortic atresia and endocardial fibroelastosis. The P waves in leads I and II are slightly bifid despite the presence of a small left atrium. The QRS electrical axis points downward and to the right. Right ventricular hypertrophy is manifested by the tall R wave in lead V$_1$ and the deep wave in V$_6$. The large RS complexes in central precordial leads suggest biventricular hypertrophy; at postmortem the left ventricle had a thick wall but a very small cavity with marked endocardial fibroelastosis. (Redrawn; reproduced with permission of the authors and publisher; see Figure Credits)*

FIG. 3.93 *This aortic valve is regurgitant because of the tethering of one of its leaflets.*

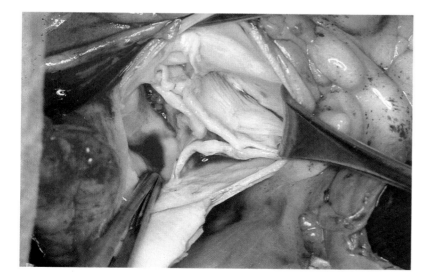

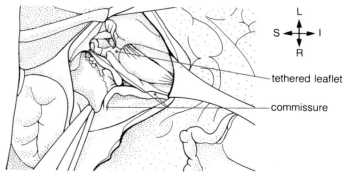

PULMONARY STENOSIS WITH INTACT VENTRICULAR SEPTUM
DEFINITION AND PATHOLOGY

Isolated congenital *pulmonary valve stenosis,* when seen in infancy, is usually due to a small opening at the top of a dome-shaped structure (Fig. 3.94) (White et al, 1950), and less often is due to valvar dysplasia (Fig. 3.95) (Edwards, 1979). *Supravalvar stenosis* may also occur; it may be localized, segmental, diffuse, or due to multiple peripheral pulmonary artery stenoses. *Subvalvar stenosis* commonly occurs at the infundibular level of the right ventricle, but it may also occur in hypertrophic cardiomyopathy. (The reader is referred to Chapters 4 and 6 for further discussion.)

ABNORMAL PHYSIOLOGY

While the area of the normal pulmonary orifice at birth is about 0.5 cm^2, it increases with age until it reaches about 2 cm^2/m^2. The valve orifice area must be decreased 60% to produce a significant obstruction in blood flow.

With pulmonary stenoses the right ventricular systolic pressure is usually greater than the pulmonary arterial systolic pressure. The pressure in the right ventricle may be 240 mmHg or higher.

The significance of a right ventricle–pulmonary artery gradient must always be assessed in the light of the pulmonary blood flow. When the pulmonary arterial blood flow is normal, a right ventricle–pulmonary artery gradient of less than 50 mmHg is considered to rep-

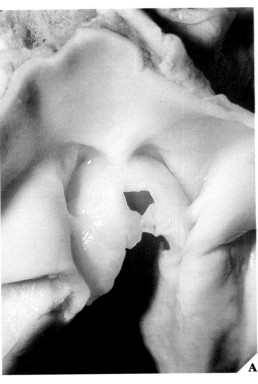
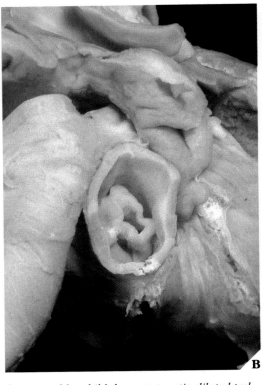
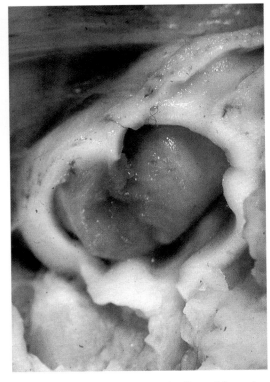

FIG. 3.94 (A) *This heart specimen shows a dome-shaped stenosis of an initially three-leaflet pulmonary valve from a neonate. (B) In this example of domed stenosis of the pulmonary valve*

from an older child the post-stenotic dilated pulmonary trunk is cut away to show the rubbery valve leaflets.

FIG. 3.95 *Severely dysplastic leaflets of the pulmonary valve, as seen in this specimen, produce stenosis as a consequence of their sheer bulk.*

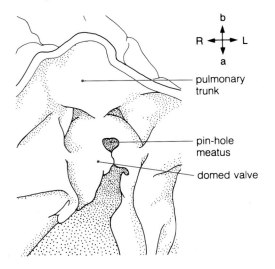
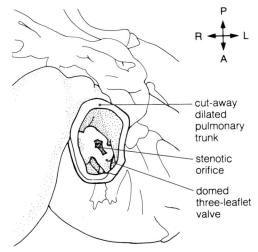
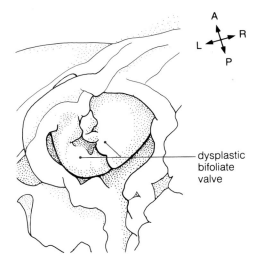

resent mild stenosis. A gradient greater than 100 mmHg indicates severe stenosis.

When the right ventricle fails, right ventricular end-diastolic and right atrial mean pressures are increased. The oval foramen may open, and a right-to-left shunt may develop, producing arterial oxygen unsaturation and cynosis. Stagnant cyanosis may occur in patients with poor cardiac output without right-to-left shunts because of the increased extraction of oxygen from the blood in the capillaries of the skin.

CLINICAL MANIFESTATIONS
SYMPTOMS
Many patients with right ventricular outflow tract obstruction may be asymptomatic, but some have dyspnea and fatigue. Young infants may have symptoms of heart failure (Freed et al, 1973).

PHYSICAL EXAMINATION
Patients with dysplastic pulmonary valves may be short with low-set ears and mental retardation; this is termed Noonan syndrome (Noonan, 1968). Cyanosis is uncommon except in patients with an interatrial communication and severe pulmonary valve obstruction (Lucas et al, 1962).

An a wave may be seen in the deep jugular venous pulse of patients with pulmonary valve stenosis. Right ventricular hypertrophy may be detected as an anterior lift located to the left of the midsternal area; a systolic thrill may be felt in the pulmonary area. An early systolic click may be heard in patients with dome-shaped valves, but it may not be heard with severe stenosis or dysplastic valves. An atrial gallop may be present. The pulmonary closure sound is delayed; it may be inaudible when there is severe stenosis. A loud diamond-shaped, sys-

tolic murmur is heard in the pulmonary area. The more severe the stenosis, the later the murmur peaks in systole. With severe stenosis the murmur may mask aortic valve closure.

Subvalvar stenosis may occur as a part of idiopathic cardiac hypertrophy. The systolic murmur may be heard in such patients, but an ejection click is not audible. An atrial gallop may be heard.

Supravalvar pulmonary stenosis may be found in patients with Noonan's syndrome, the congenital rubella syndrome, and Williams' syndrome (hypercalcemia, typical facies, mental retardation, and dental abnormalities). The symptoms and the physical findings are similar to those of valvar stenosis, except there is no ejection click and the second sound may be normal. Systolic murmurs may be heard on the back when there are peripheral pulmonary arterial stenoses. A continuous murmur may be heard over the back when a diastolic gradient accompanies the pulmonary branch stenosis.

LABORATORY STUDIES
CHEST RADIOGRAPHY   Since the heart size is usually normal, a huge heart indicates a critical state. The right ventricle may appear large in the left lateral view. Usually the pulmonary trunk and its left branch are dilated, and the right pulmonary artery is normal-sized (Fig. 3.96). Pulmonary blood flow may be decreased when there is a right-to-left shunt at the atrial level. The pulmonary trunk is not dilated in patients with subvalvar or supravalvar stenosis.

ELECTROCARDIOGRAPHY.   Right ventricular hypertrophy and a right atrial abnormality are seen in the ECG of a patient with pulmonary valve stenosis (Fig. 3.97). Patients with dysplasia of the pulmonary valve may have a superiorly located mean QRS vector (Koretzky et al, 1969).

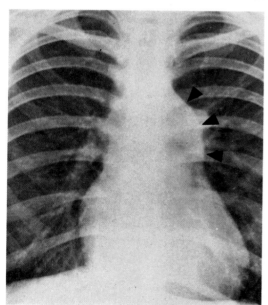

FIG. 3.96 *In this chest radiograph of a patient with pulmonary valve stenosis, the pulmonary trunk is enlarged* (arrows) *with normal pulmonary vascularity. (Reproduced with permission of the authors and publisher; see Figure Credits)*

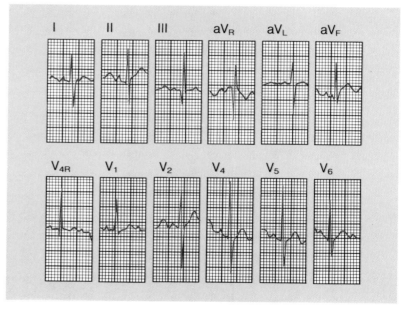

FIG. 3.97 *In this ECG of a seven-month-old infant with pulmonary valve stenosis the P waves are pointed, and the mean QRS vector is directed slightly to the right and anteriorly. The mean T vector is directed to the left and slightly anteriorly. These abnormalities signify right ventricular hypertrophy. (Courtesy of the Electrocardiography Laboratory, Henrietta Egleston Hospital for Children, Atlanta, Georgia)*

ECHOCARDIOGRAPHY. There is an exaggeration of the maximal a wave depth of the pulmonary valve recorded with inspiration in patients with moderate-to-severe pulmonary valve stenosis. Presystolic opening of the valve may occur (Weyman et al, 1975).

Abnormalities associated with valvar (Fig. 3.98), and infundibular (Fig. 3.99) pulmonary stenoses can be differentiated with cross-sectional echocardiography.

CARDIAC CATHETERIZATION. In patients with valvar stenosis the right ventricular systolic pressure is elevated, and there is a pressure gradient across the pulmonary valve. When the stenosis is severe, it may be unwise to pass the cardiac catheter into the pulmonary trunk. The arterial oxygen saturation is normal, unless there is a right-to-left shunt at the atrial level.

Subpulmonary stenosis may be detected by analyzing the right ventricular pressure curves in pull-back pressure tracings, since the gradient occurs within the right ventricle. It is important to exclude associated congenital heart defects.

Suprapulmonary stenoses produce systolic pressure differences across obstructions throughout the pulmonary arteries. The pulse pressure may be wide in the pulmonary trunk, and the right ventricular systolic pressure is elevated.

Valvar, subvalvar, and supravalvar pulmonary stenoses, including stenosis of branches of the pulmonary artery, produce characteristic abnormalities that can be identified by right ventricular and pulmonary arterial angiography (Fig. 3.100). Doming of the pulmonary valve is not seen in patients with dysplasia of the valve.

NATURAL HISTORY

Patients with mild-to-moderate pulmonary valve stenosis have good prognoses; only a few progress to severe obstruction (Nadas, 1977), which may produce heart failure and early death in young infants and adults (Mody, 1975); patients are subject to infective endocarditis. Paradoxical emboli may occur through a patent oval foramen, and brain abscess is possible.

Patients with subvalvar pulmonary stenosis have good survival curves.

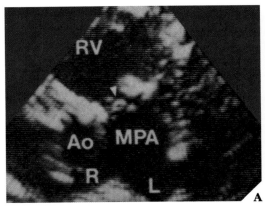

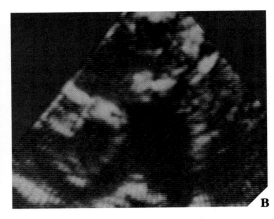

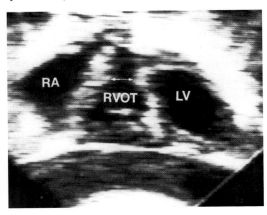

FIG. 3.98   *Cross-sectional echocardiograms in the parasternal short-axis view were obtained through the base of the heart in diastole (A) and systole (B) from a patient with severe pulmonary valve stenosis. The pulmonary valve (arrow) is thickened, and the annulus is severely narrowed.*

There is post-stenotic dilation of the pulmonary trunk (MPA) (Ao, aorta; L, left pulmonary artery; R, right pulmonary artery; RV, right ventricle). (Reproduced with permission of the authors and publisher; see Figure Credits)

FIG. 3.99   *Cross-sectional echocardiogram in the subxiphoid coronal view (L-4) of the right ventricular outflow tract (RVOT) shows a narrowed infundibular area (arrows) associated with pulmonary stenosis. The right ventricular outflow tract is small compared with the left ventricle (LV), only a portion of which is seen from this view (RA, right atrium). (Reproduced with permission of the authors and publisher; see Figure Credits)*

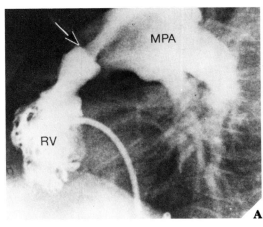

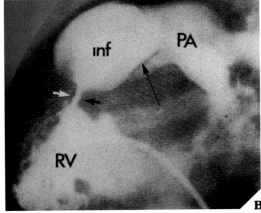

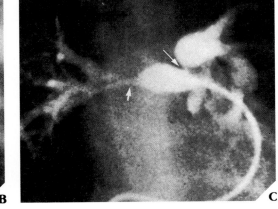

FIG. 3.100   **(A)** *Lateral view of a right ventricular (RV) angiogram demonstrates the typical features of valvar pulmonary stenosis. The pulmonary valve (arrow) is domed, and a narrow jet of contrast enters the dilated pulmonary trunk (MPA).* **(B)** *This lateral right ventriculogram demonstrates very severe stenosis (white and black arrows) at the level of the ostium of the infundibulum (inf) in this patient with congenital isolated infundibular pulmonary stenosis. The subarterial infundibular chamber and the pulmonary trunk (PA) are dilated. The pulmonary valve (long black* arrow) *is slightly thickened.* **(C)** *Injection of contrast medium into a pulmonary artery shows a focal stenosis at the origin of the left pulmonary artery (long arrow) and a more diffuse stenosis of the right pulmonary artery (short arrow). (A: Fig. 36-44, The Heart, 6th ed, p 656; courtesy of the Cardiac Catheterization Laboratory, Henrietta Egleston Hospital for Children, Atlanta, Georgia. B,C: Reproduced with permission of the authors and publishers; see Figure Credits)*

Patients with supravalvar stenosis usually have a stable course; however, the artery distal to the obstruction may rupture or thrombose, and infective arteritis is possible.

TREATMENT

Heart failure should be treated with digitalis and diuretics; infective endocarditis should be prevented.

INDICATIONS FOR SURGERY

Heart failure in an infant with pulmonary valve stenosis should prompt early surgical intervention or balloon dilation. Cyanosis or a right ventricular systolic pressure above systemic levels are indications for immediate pulmonary valvotomy. Asymptomatic infants and children with a right ventricular systolic pressure of 70 mmHg or a right ventricle–pulmonary artery gradient of 50 mmHg or more should have elective surgery or catheter dilation during childhood (Nadas, 1977).

The indications for surgical intervention in patients with subvalvar stenosis are similar to those listed for valvar stenosis, except when the condition is part of hypertrophic cardiomyopathy, which complicates the problem considerably (see Chapter 6).

The indications for surgical correction of supravalvar stenosis are similar to those for valve stenosis. However, the surgery itself may not be possible, since distal pulmonary stenosis is not readily assessable.

SURGICAL PROCEDURE

Although there have been successful attempts at balloon angioplasty of congenitally stenotic pulmonary valves, surgical intervention remains the most effective means of correcting this problem. In the operative repair of valvar pulmonary stenosis the tethered commissures are dissected from the wall of the artery and then opened (Fig. 3.101). This produces a widely patent orifice with minimal regurgitation. The supravalvar region may also be stenotic, particularly with a dysplastic valve (Fig.

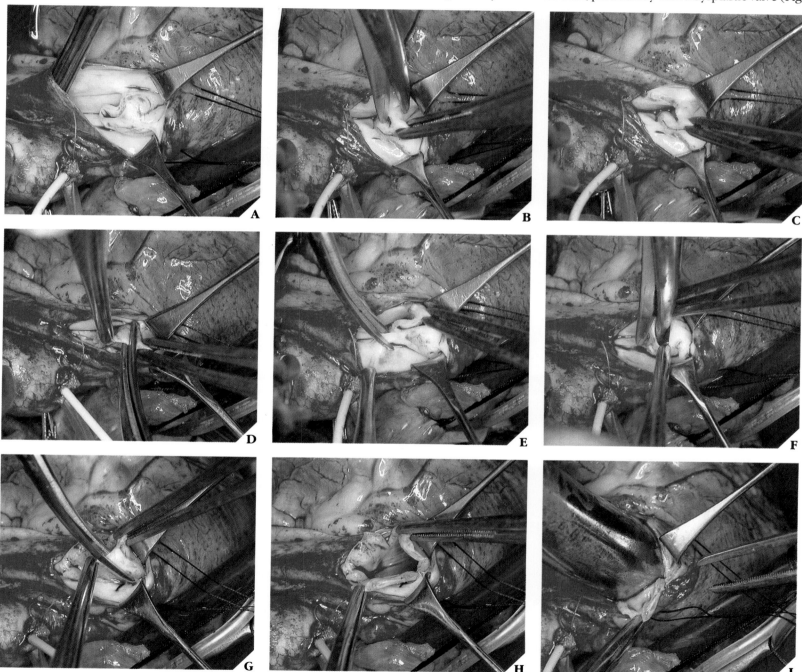

FIG. 3.101   (A–I) *Operative views show a step-by-step correction of congenital valvar pulmonary stenosis. Tethering at each commissure results in a narrow orifice that is displaced distally in the pulmonary trunk. Each of* these commissures can be dissected from the wall of the artery and then divided. This opens the valve orifice quite adequately, producing minimal pulmonary regurgitation.

3.102). Pulmonary arterial stenosis may be repaired with a pericardial patch if the stenosis is proximal to the hilum of the lung. The surgical treatment of subvalvar pulmonary stenosis entails the surgical removal of the obstructing subvalvar muscle.

CONGENITAL PULMONARY VALVE REGURGITATION

Congenital pulmonary valve regurgitation may be associated with pulmonary valve stenosis, pulmonary hypertension, anomalies of the pulmonary valve, or absence of the leaflets of the pulmonary valve. The latter may be present in patients with tetralogy of Fallot or VSD (Fig. 3.103).

When the pulmonary arterial pressure is elevated, the murmur of pulmonary valve regurgitation immediately follows the second sound; it is high-pitched and decrescendo. When there is normal or low pulmonary arterial pressure, the murmur of pulmonary regurgitation does not begin immediately after the second sound, and it is lower-pitched than expected for pulmonary regurgitation due to pulmonary hypertension.

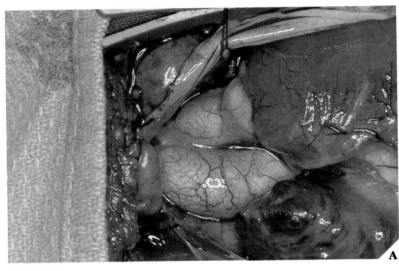

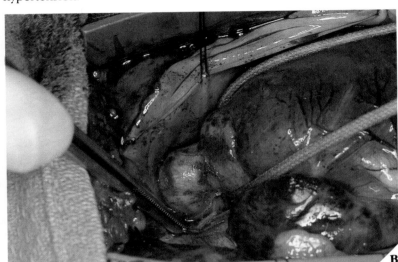

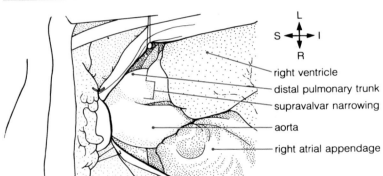

- right ventricle
- distal pulmonary trunk
- supravalvar narrowing
- aorta
- right atrial appendage

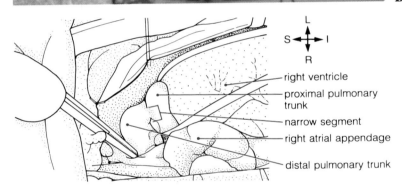

- right ventricle
- proximal pulmonary trunk
- narrow segment
- right atrial appendage
- distal pulmonary trunk

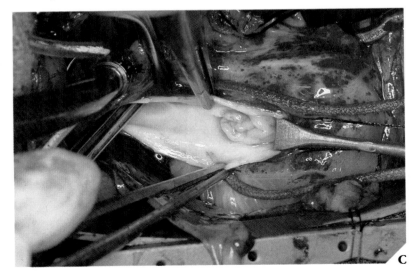

FIG. 3.102 (A) *In this initial operative view supravalvar pulmonary stenosis is evident.* (B) *A section of the pulmonary trunk is exposed to demonstrate its waisting.* (C) *The opened pulmonary trunk shows a very dysplastic pulmonary valve; its distal attachments correspond to the area of pulmonary truncal narrowing.*

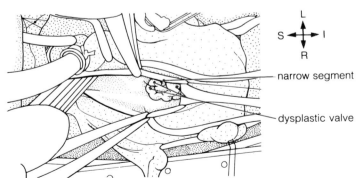

- narrow segment
- dysplastic valve

The diagnosis can be determined by the Doppler technique; other anomalies may be identified by cardiac catheterization.

The absence of the pulmonary valve leaflets produces heart failure, and surgical treatment is frequently indicated for this condition.

See above for discussion of treatment of pulmonary valve stenosis and the multiple causes of pulmonary hypertension.

CONGENITAL MITRAL STENOSIS
DEFINITION AND PATHOLOGY

The obstructing lesion of congenital mitral stenosis may be located within the left atrium; this is termed the supravalvar ring (Fig. 3.104). Two major types of stenotic lesions are located at or below the mitral valve: a dysplastic mitral valve (Fig. 3.105) and the so-called parachute

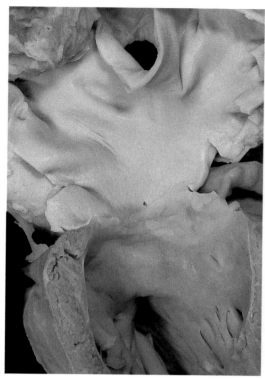

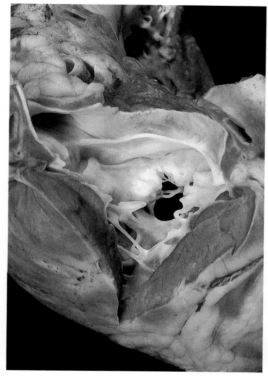

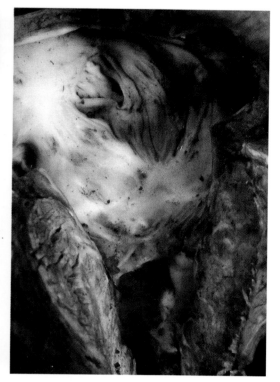

FIG. 3.103   *In so-called absence of the leaflets of the pulmonary valve, the leaflets are represented by rudimentary fragments at the ventricular arterial junction, shown here in a patient with VSD. Note the dilation of the pulmonary arteries.*

FIG. 3.104   *A supravalvar mitral ring is seen in the left atrium of a heart with double-inlet left ventricle.*

FIG. 3.105   *A dysplastic, stenotic, and miniaturized mitral valve is seen in this heart with aortic atresia and intact ventricular septum.*

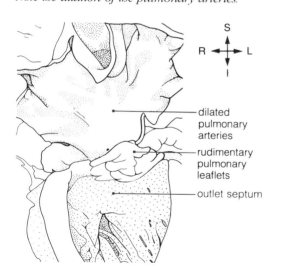

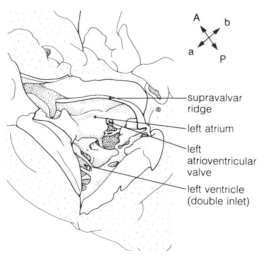

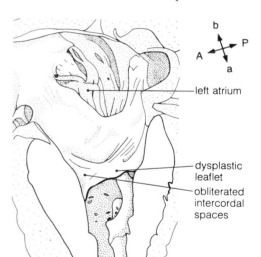

deformity (Fig. 3.106) (Collins–Nakai et al, 1977). The Shone syndrome is significant in this setting; it consists of a stenosing ring of the left atrium, parachute mitral valve, subaortic stenosis, and the coarctation of the aorta (Shone et al, 1963).

ABNORMAL PHYSIOLOGY

The obstructing lesions produce left atrial and pulmonary venous hypertension when there is a diastolic pressure gradient between the left atrium and the left ventricle. The significance of a small gradient may not be appreciated when pulmonary blood flow is decreased or when there is a large atrial septal defect. The pulmonary arterial pressure and the pulmonary arteriolar resistance become elevated.

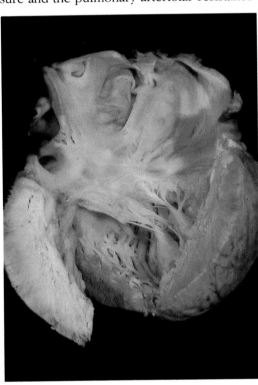

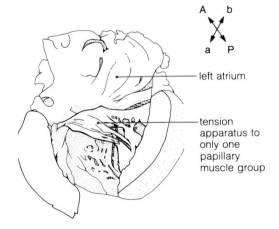

left atrium

tension apparatus to only one papillary muscle group

FIG. 3.106 *A mitral valve with absence of the anterolateral papillary muscle is seen in the setting of classic tricuspid atresia. All of the tension apparatus inserts into the remaining posteromedial muscle. This arrangement is one form of the so-called parachute deformity, although some use this term to describe hearts in which there is fusion of the left ventricular papillary muscles.*

CLINICAL MANIFESTATIONS

This rare condition is usually associated with other defects and is often recognized only at cardiac catheterization. It occurs more often in males.

SYMPTOMS

During the second year of life the patient may have dyspnea on effort, fatigue, and episodes suggesting acute pulmonary edema. Repeated respiratory tract infections are common.

The first heart sound may be louder than normal at the apex, and an opening snap may be heard. A low-pitched, diastolic rumble may be heard at the apex, and the murmurs of other defects may be

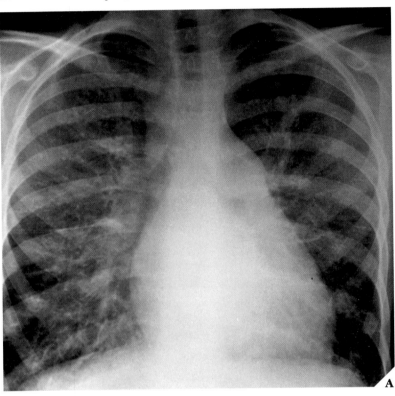

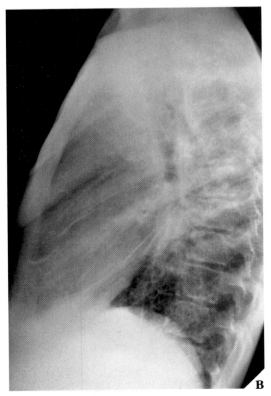

FIG. 3.107 *Chest radiographs were obtained in a seven-year-old male with congenital mitral stenosis. (A) Posteroanterior film shows a large pulmonary trunk, but the enlarged left atrium is barely seen. (B) On the lateral view right ventricular hypertrophy is evident. (Courtesy of the X-Ray Department, Henrietta Egleston Hospital for Children, Atlanta, Georgia)*

detected. When there is decreased pulmonary blood flow, the rumble of mitral stenosis may not be heard.

LABORATORY STUDIES

CHEST RADIOGRAPHY. The chest film may show Kerley B lines, left atrial enlargement, and right ventricular hypertrophy (Fig. 3.107).

ELECTROCARDIOGRAPHY. The ECG shows a left atrial abnormality and right ventricular hypertrophy (Fig. 3.108).

ECHOCARDIOGRAPHY. The M-mode echocardiogram can be used to detect left ventricular inflow obstruction. Cross-sectional echocardiography can be used to identify the abnormality of the mitral valve and left atrium. A supravalvar mitral ring (Fig. 3.109A), congenital mitral valve stenosis (Fig. 3.109B), and a parachute mitral valve (Fig. 3.109C) can all be differentiated by echocardiography.

CARDIAC CATHETERIZATION. A diastolic pressure gradient across the mitral valve is diagnostic, but it may not be appreciated when the

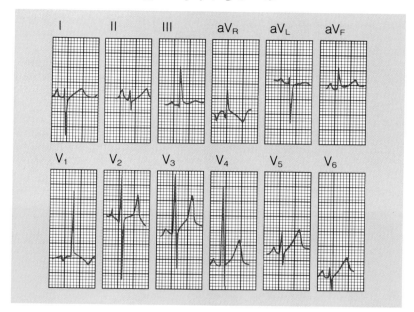

FIG. 3.108 *This ECG was obtained from a two-year-old girl with congenital mitral stenosis. Tall, peaked P waves of right atrial abnormality are present in leads I, II, and V₂. The QRS electrical axis is directed markedly to the right. The tall, monophasic R wave in lead V₁ and the deep S wave in V₆ reflect right ventricular hypertrophy. The large RS complexes in V₂ and V₃ suggest biventricular hypertrophy, possibly caused by coexisting coarctation of the aorta. (Redrawn; reproduced with permission of the authors and publisher; see Figure Credits. Courtesy of James J. Acker, MD, Knoxville, Tennessee)*

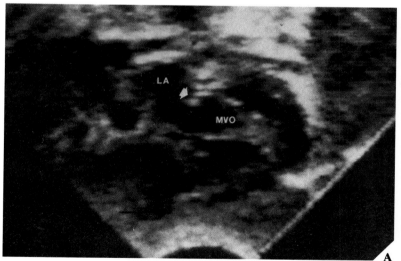

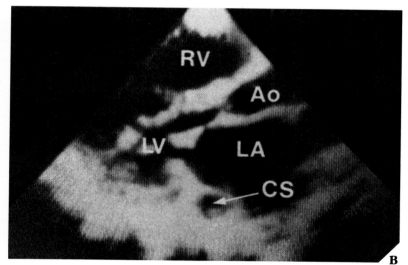

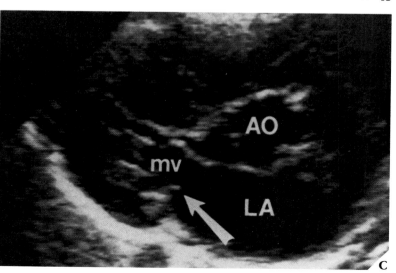

FIG. 3.109 *Cross-sectional echocardiographic differentiation of congenital mitral stenosis. (A) A subxiphoid long-axis view in a patient with supravalvar mitral ring shows the membrane extending as a shelf from the mitral annulus (arrow) (LA, left atrium; MVO, mitral valve). (B) Parasternal long-axis view from a 13-year-old female with congenital mitral valve stenosis shows thickened mitral valve leaflets and the enlarged left atrium (LA). The right ventricle (RV) is enlarged because of long-standing pulmonary hypertension. The coronary sinus (CS) is enlarged because of a persistent left superior caval vein draining into the coronary sinus (Ao, aorta; LV, left ventricle). (C) Parasternal long-axis view from a patient with supravalvar mitral ring shows the membrane (arrow) extending as a shelf from the mitral annulus. This finding is associated with parachute mitral valve (mv). (Reproduced with permission of the authors and publisher; see Figure Credits)*

pulmonary blood flow is diminished or when there is an atrial septal defect. The pulmonary arterial pressure is elevated, and other congenital defects may be identified. Left atrial and left ventricular angiography may reveal the abnormalities.

NATURAL HISTORY

The clinical course is one of deterioration as a result of progressive stenosis and increasing pulmonary congestion.

TREATMENT

Medical treatment consists of the use of digitalis and diuretics, restriction of activity, and the treatment of respiratory tract infections.

INDICATIONS FOR SURGERY

Surgery is necessary in these patients, although the surgical risk is high. Operative intervention ranges from mitral valve replacement, often two or more times as the child grows older, to valvoplasty, which is difficult to perform.

MITRAL ATRESIA

Mitral atresia may be due to an imperforate valve (Fig. 3.110), but more often it is due to the absence of the left atrioventricular con-

nection (Fig. 3.111) (Gittenberger–de Groot et al, 1984). The arterial trunks are normally positioned in half the cases. Mitral atresia is commonly associated with aortic atresia; pulmonary stenosis or atresia may also occur. The blood usually exits the left atrium through the oval foramen or through a vein that connects to a systemic vein.

Infants with no pulmonary stenosis or a small oval foramen experience heart failure. The right ventricle is hyperdynamic, and a continuous murmur may be produced as blood rushes through the restrictive oval foramen. A diastolic flow rumble is heard at the end of the sternum. When pulmonary stenosis is present, the symptoms and signs are similar to those occurring with tetralogy of Fallot. Cyanosis is usually slight; it may be intense when there is pulmonary atresia, although this is a rare combination.

The chest film shows pulmonary congestion when pulmonary stenosis is absent or the oval foramen is small (Fig. 3.112). The left atrium may not be enlarged.

The ECG shows right atrial abnormality and right ventricular hypertrophy. Echocardiography is very useful in identifying the absence of the mitral valve (Rigby et al, 1982).

Cardiac catheterization and angiography reveal a communication between the left and right atria, left atrial hypertension, and evidence of associated defects.

Medical treatment is not adequate, and surgical techniques are only

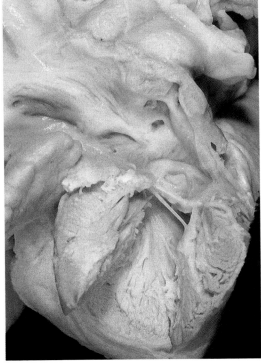

FIG. 3.110 *An imperforate mitral valve may produce mitral atresia in the setting of a concordant atrioventricular connection.*

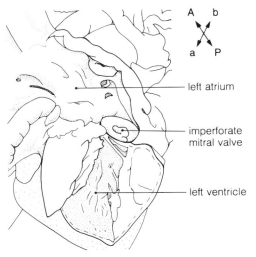

A b
a P

left atrium

imperforate mitral valve

left ventricle

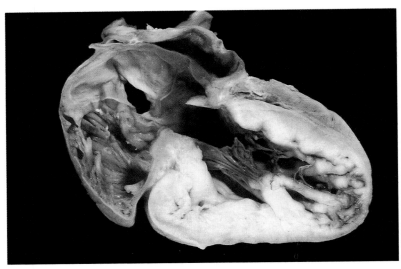

FIG. 3.111 *Absence of the left atrioventricular connection is associated with the connection of the right atrium to a dominant right ventricle in the presence of a rudimentary and grossly hypoplastic left ventricle. The muscular floor of the left atrium is blind-ending, hence producing an alternative pattern of mitral atresia (see Fig. 3.110).*

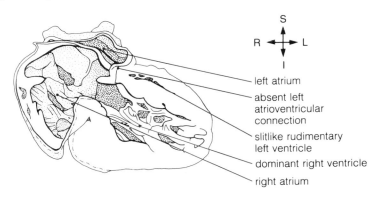

S
R ← → L
I

left atrium

absent left atrioventricular connection

slitlike rudimentary left ventricle

dominant right ventricle

right atrium

palliative. The atrial septal communication can be enlarged, and the pulmonary blood flow may be adjusted by pulmonary arterial banding or the production of systemic-to-pulmonary shunts as needed (Mickell et al, 1980).

CONGENITAL MITRAL REGURGITATION

Congenital mitral regurgitation may be part of, or secondary to, some other congenital heart defects, or it may be due to a primary mitral valve abnormality. Regurgitation through a left-sided atrioventricular valve may be part of an atrioventricular septal defect (atrioventricular canal malformation) or congenitally corrected transposition; however, the left valve is not then of mitral morphology. True mitral regurgitation may be associated with fibroelastosis, aortic stenosis, coarctation of the aorta, anomalous origin of the left coronary artery from the pulmonary artery, Marfan's syndrome, and mucopolysaccharidosis (Krovetz et al, 1965). Primary causes include isolated clefts of the valve leaflets (Fig. 3.113), myxomatous degeneration of the valve, absence

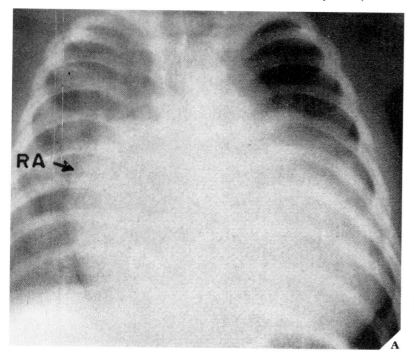

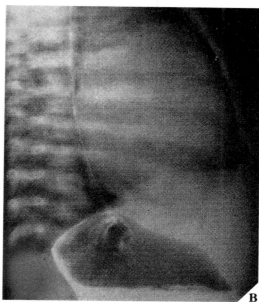

FIG. 3.112 (A) *On the frontal film of a patient with coexistent aortic and mitral valve atresia, there is marked cardiac enlargement, including right atrial (RA) and right ventricular enlargement. (B) Right lateral view confirms the considerable cardiac enlargement. (Reproduced with permission of the authors and publisher; see Figure Credits)*

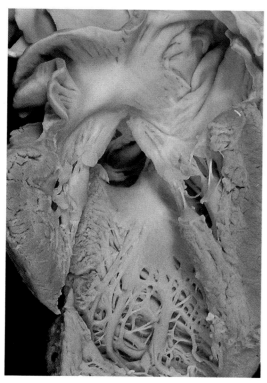

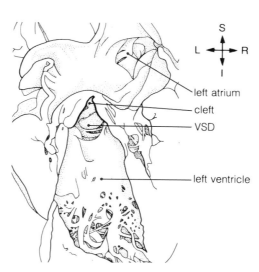

left atrium
cleft
VSD

left ventricle

FIG. 3.113 *A cleft in the anterior (aortic) leaflet of the mitral valve points toward the outflow tract of the left ventricle. In this example the cleft points toward a ventricular septal defect in the setting of double-outlet right ventricle with subpulmonary defect (the Taussig–Bing malformation). This isolated cleft of the mitral valve bears no resemblance to the so-called cleft found in the setting of the trifoliate left valve of an atrioventricular septal defect (see Figs. 3.33, 3.36).*

of leaflets, valve holes, duplication of the valve orifice (Fig. 3.114), and abnormal attachments of the papillary muscle and tendinous cords. Rheumatic fever may cause mitral regurgitation. Rheumatic fever occurs rarely in the United States and almost never under the age of five years. The patient may complain of symptoms of heart failure.

A systolic murmur can be heard at the apex and when the regurgitation is great, a diastolic rumble may be heard at the apex. The second sound is widely split, but it narrows with expiration. The closure sound of the pulmonary valve is loud when pulmonary hypertension is present.

The chest film reveals enlargement of the left ventricle and the left atrium. The ECG shows left ventricular hypertrophy and a left atrial abnormality. The echocardiogram may reveal many of the abnormalities associated with this condition as well as primary mitral valve lesions (Fig. 3.115).

Cardiac catheterization and angiography reveal the various conditions that may cause mitral regurgitation. These techniques may also be used to identify the size of the left atrium and the left ventricle and the regurgitant volume.

Patients may tolerate this condition for many years; severe mitral regurgitation, however, produces heart failure and arrhythmias. Therapy for heart failure may be useful, but some patients require mitral valvoplasty and annuloplasty. When this is not possible, valve replacement may be necessary.

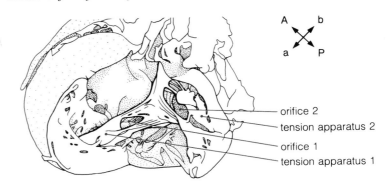

FIG. 3.114 *In this heart, photographed from the left ventricular aspect, duplication of the tension apparatus of the mitral valve appears along with double orifice of the leaflets.*

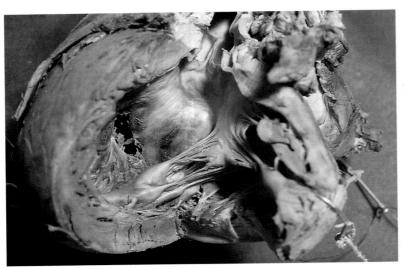

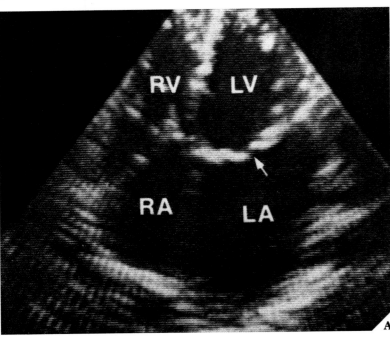

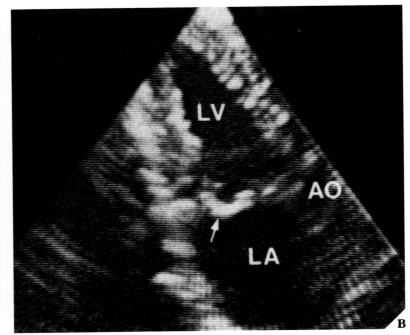

FIG. 3.115 *These cross-sectional echocardiograms were obtained from a patient with significant mitral valve prolapse and mitral regurgitation. (A) In the apical four-chamber view a slight posterior displacement (arrow) of the mitral leaflets into the left atrium (LA) is seen. The left atrium and the left ventricle (LV) are dilated (RA, right atrium; RV, right ventricle). (B) On the apical long-axis view the mitral valve prolapse, which occurs in a predominantly superior direction (arrow), is more obvious. The mitral valve is thickened, and the left atrium and left ventricle are dilated (AO, aorta). (Reproduced with permission of the authors and publisher; see Figure Credits)*

COR TRIATRIATUM
(DIVISION OF AN ATRIAL CHAMBER)
DEFINITION AND PATHOLOGY

The most common type of divided atrium exists when a muscular structure separates the left atrium into two chambers, upper and lower. Obviously a hole must be present in the abnormal septum, but it may be of pinhole dimensions (Fig. 3.116). The size of the hole determines the degree of pulmonary venous obstruction.

There may be a defect in the atrial septum that communicates between the upper compartment of the left and the right atria. Additional associated conditions include connection of the pulmonary vein to a systemic vein, tetralogy of Fallot, and pulmonary stenosis. The right atrium may also be divided by persistence of the valves of the embryonic venous sinus (eustachian and thebesian valves).

CLINICAL MANIFESTATIONS

In this rare defect patients are usually considered to be normal at birth. Later there may be evidence of pulmonary venous congestion, such as dyspnea, orthopnea, or weight gain.

A prominent right ventricular lift may be detected, and the pulmonary component of the second sound may be increased in intensity. While diagnostic murmurs may not be present, the murmur of pulmonary regurgitation may be heard. Rarely a continuous murmur may be heard across the obstructed septum located in the left atrium.

There may be slight cardiac enlargement, the pulmonary trunk may be prominent, and there may be evidence of pulmonary congestion and pulmonary edema.

The ECG shows the mean QRS vector rotated to the right and anteriorly, signifying right ventricular hypertrophy. Right atrial abnormality may be noted in the P waves. The abnormal atrial septum may be identified by cross-sectional echocardiography (Fig. 3.117A), and high-velocity flow may be demonstrated by the Doppler technique (Fig. 3.117B).

Cardiac catheterization reveals elevation of pulmonary arterial wedge pressure and pulmonary arterial hypertension. The lower chamber of the left atrium may be entered through an oval foramen; the pressure recorded there is low. The abnormal septum within the left atrium may be visualized by angiography.

FIG. 3.116 *In this heart a fibromuscular partition divides the left atrium; the communication between the atrial compartments is of pinhole dimensions.*

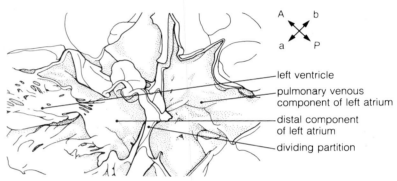

left ventricle

pulmonary venous component of left atrium

distal component of left atrium

dividing partition

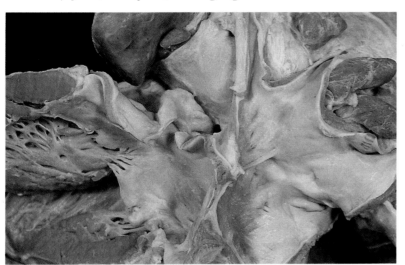

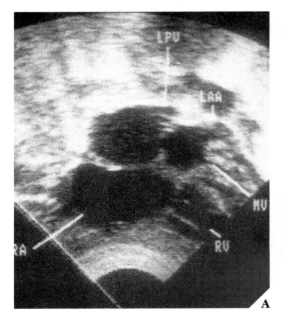

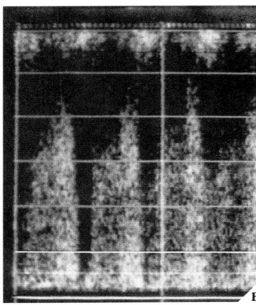

FIG. 3.117 **(A)** *Apical four-chamber view of a cross-sectional echocardiogram from a patient with cor triatriatum shows the membrane lying across the left atrium (LAA) between the mitral annulus and the lower left pulmonary vein (LPV).* **(B)** *High-velocity flow distal to this membrane is demonstrated by the Doppler technique (RV, right ventricle; RA, right atrium; MV, mitral valve). (Reproduced with permission of the authors and publisher; see Figure Credits)*

NATURAL HISTORY

There is progressive pulmonary venous hypertension, severe pulmonary congestion, and right-sided heart failure.

TREATMENT

Whereas digitalis and diuretics may be useful, they do not solve the problem of cor triatriatum. Surgical removal of the abnormal septum located within the left atrium should be carried out without delay.

DEFINITION AND PATHOLOGY

The right atrioventricular connection is completely absent in most patients with tricuspid atresia (Fig. 3.118). A few patients have imperforate valves, usually in the setting of Ebstein's malformation (Fig. 3.119). A right-to-left shunt must be present for the patient to survive. An atrial septal defect or a patent oval foramen is present, and a ventricular septal defect (VSD) (Fig. 3.120) usually permits blood to

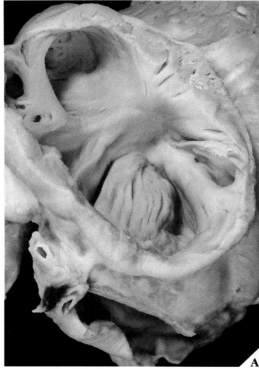
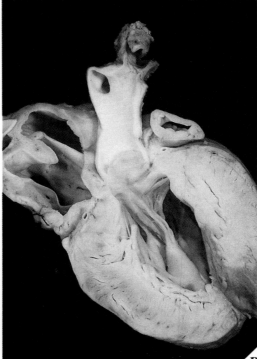
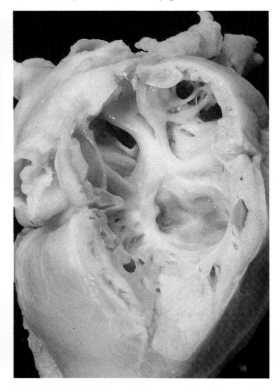

FIG. 3.118 *Classic tricuspid atresia is almost always due to complete absence of the right atrioventricular connection. As viewed from the right atrium (A), the atrial chamber is blind-ending with a muscular floor. The so-called dimple points to the left ventricular outflow tract, as shown in the simulated four-chamber section*

(B). *This view also shows the atrioventricular groove tissue interposing between the atrial floor and the ventricular mass. The rudimentary right ventricle is anterosuperiorly located and is not seen in this section. (B: Reproduced with permission of the authors and publisher; see Figure Credits)*

FIG. 3.119 *This view of the posterior aspect of the right atrioventricular junction shows the much rarer variant of tricuspid atresia produced by an imperforate tricuspid valve in the setting of Ebstein's malformation. (Reproduced with permission of the authors and publisher; see Figure Credits)*

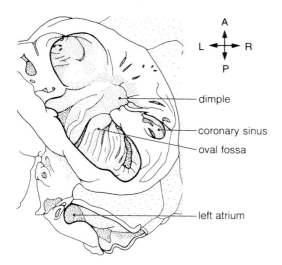
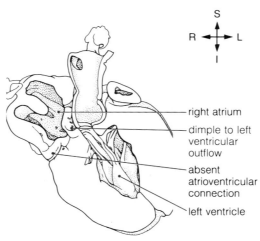
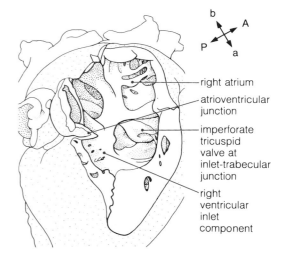

enter a rudimentary right ventricle. The blood flow from the ventricular mass is then determined by its ventriculoarterial connection, which is usually concordant. When the ventriculoarterial connection is discordant, as in transposition, coarctation is usually present and a restrictive VSD produces subaortic obstruction (Tandon et al, 1974; Rao, 1980).

ABNORMAL PHYSIOLOGY

The right atrial pressure is higher than the left atrial pressure, producing a prominent a wave in the right atrium. Blood in the left ventricle is always desaturated. With concordant ventriculoarterial connections pulmonary blood flow is decreased, because the right ventricle, the pulmonary artery, or the VSD is small. In such cases an arterial duct may be present to deliver desaturated blood to the lungs. When the great arteries are discordantly connected (transposed), blood flow to the lungs may be increased.

CLINICAL MANIFESTATIONS
SYMPTOMS

Two different clinical pictures may occur. When the great arteries are concordantly connected, cyanosis is present from birth. Paroxysmal hypoxic spells may occur; squatting is evident at a later age. When the VSD is large and the right ventricle and the pulmonary trunk are also large, pulmonary blood flow is increased. An increase in pulmonary

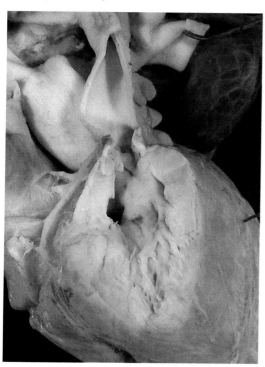

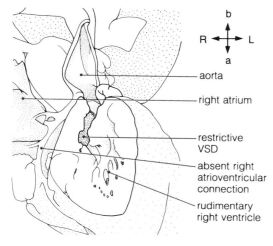

- aorta
- right atrium
- restrictive VSD
- absent right atrioventricular connection
- rudimentary right ventricle

FIG. 3.120 *Discordant ventriculoarterial connection (transposition) and a restrictive VSD are seen in the rudimentary right ventricle from a case of tricuspid atresia. The heart also exhibits severe isthmic hypoplasia and coarctation.*

blood flow also occurs when the great arteries are discordantly connected. This leads to symptoms of heart failure with slight cyanosis.

PHYSICAL EXAMINATION

Severe or slight cyanosis may be present; clubbing of the fingers appears later in the first year of life. A prominent a wave is seen in the internal jugular veins, and the liver may be enlarged. When there is a VSD and decreased pulmonary blood flow, the second sound is single. A systolic murmur may be heard to the left of the midsternal region, or there may be no murmur. When there is an increase in pulmonary blood flow, the apex impulse is forceful and the second sound is split. A loud systolic murmur and a thrill may be best heard in the left midsternal area; a diastolic rumble may be heard at the apex. Signs of heart failure may be present.

LABORATORY STUDIES

CHEST RADIOGRAPHY. The heart is usually normal in size; however, it may be enlarged in patients with an increase in pulmonary arterial blood flow. The right heart border is straight because of the small right ventricle. The blood flow to the lungs is usually diminished. However, when the VSD and the right ventricle are large or when the great arteries are transposed, the blood flow to the lungs is increased (Fig. 3.121).

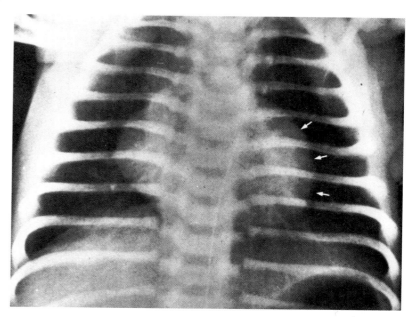

FIG. 3.121 *Chest radiograph of an infant with tricuspid atresia shows decreased pulmonary arterial vascularity and cardiomegaly. The prominent right lower cardiac border results from the enlarged right atrium. The very round prominent left cardiac border results from enlargement of left ventricle (arrows). When the ventricular septal defect is large or there is associated discordant ventriculoarterial connection, blood flow to the lungs is increased. However, the pulmonary blood flow is diminished in most patients with tricuspid atresia. (Reproduced with permission of the authors and publisher; see Figure Credits)*

ELECTROCARDIOGRAPHY. The ECG usually shows left ventricular hypertrophy (mean QRS vector located between 0° and −90°) and right atrial abnormality (Fig. 3.122). When the great arteries are transposed, the mean QRS axis is located between 0° and +90° (Dick et al, 1975).

ECHOCARDIOGRAPHY. M-mode echocardiography usually reveals a rudimentary right ventricle; the tricuspid valve is not seen (Solinger et al, 1976). Cross-sectional echocardiography reveals absence of the right atrioventricular connection and many of the associated defects (Fig. 3.123) (Houston et al, 1977).

CARDIAC CATHETERIZATION. The right atrial pressure is abnormally elevated, and it is higher than the left atrial pressure. The catheter passes from the right atrium into the left atrium; the right ventricle cannot be entered through the tricuspid valve. With normally related great arteries the pulmonary pressure and flow depend on the size of the VSD, the right ventricle, the pulmonary artery, and the pulmonary valve. Accordingly the pulmonary blood flow may be diminished or increased. When there is no VSD, pulmonary blood flows via an arterial duct or, rarely, aortopulmonary collateral arteries. When the great arteries are transposed, the catheter may enter the pulmonary trunk from the left ventricle. Angiocardiography usually reveals the entire anatomy (Fig. 3.124).

NATURAL HISTORY

Cyanosis is evident in most of the infants at birth. It usually progresses with closure of the arterial duct or as the VSD becomes smaller (Rao, 1977). About one half of patients die by six months of age, about two thirds die by one year of age, and 90% die by ten years of age. Life

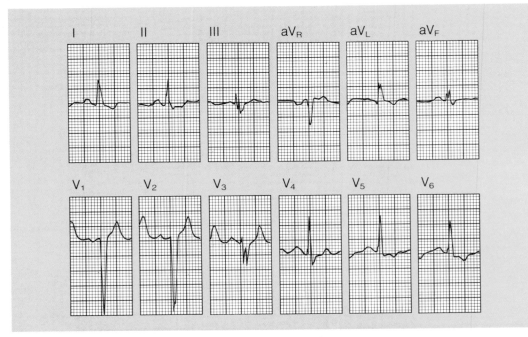

FIG. 3.122 *Left ventricular hypertrophy is evident in this ECG from a 31-year-old woman with congenital tricuspid atresia, who survived because of atrial and ventricular septal defects. The P waves are large; the mean QRS vector is directed to the left and posteriorly because the right ventricle is small and the left ventricle is large. The mean T vector is located to the right and anteriorly. (Redrawn; courtesy of the Electrocardiography Laboratory, Emory Hospital and Emory Clinic, Atlanta, Georgia)*

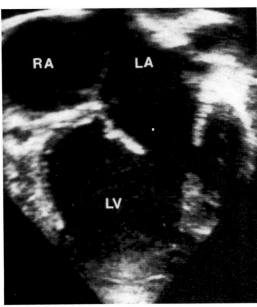

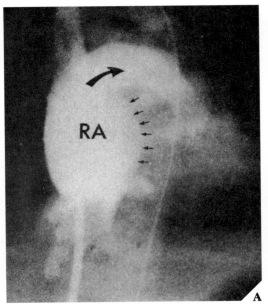

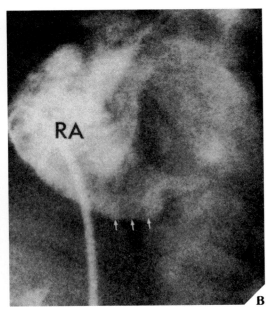

FIG. 3.123 *Cross-sectional echocardiogram in the apical four-chamber view of a patient with tricuspid atresia shows that a single atrioventricular valve—the mitral valve—is present (LA, left atrium; LV, left ventricle; RA, right atrium). (Reproduced with permission of the authors and publisher; see Figure Credits)*

FIG. 3.124 *(A) This selective right atriogram in the frontal projection is from a patient with tricuspid atresia and right-to-left atrial shunting through a sinus venosus–type atrial septal defect (curvilinear arrow). The remainder of the atrial septum is intact (small black arrows). (B) In the hepatoclavicular projection the right atriogram demonstrates the smooth floor of the right atrium (RA, white arrows). (Reproduced with permission of the authors and publisher; see Figure Credits)*

expectancy is longer when there is moderate blood flow to the lungs. Hypoxia and its complications are the most common cause of death, but heart failure may occur. When pulmonary atresia is present, the life expectancy is three months.

TREATMENT

Hypoxia and cyanosis of the newborn may be treated with prostaglandin E_1 to maintain a patent arterial duct, but relief is temporary. Hypoxic episodes may be treated as described for tetralogy of Fallot (see p. 3.74). Patients with heart failure may be treated with digitalis and diuretics. Balloon atrial septostomy may help.

INDICATIONS FOR SURGERY

Severe hypoxia in an infant with tricuspid atresia requires prompt surgical treatment to produce a systemic-to-pulmonary arterial shunt.

Patients with transposed great arteries and heart failure should have banding of the pulmonary trunk.

SURGICAL PROCEDURE

There are four procedures used for palliation (Weinberg, 1980; Trusler et al, 1978): the Blalock–Taussig or a similar shunt; the Glenn procedure, in which the superior caval vein and the right pulmonary artery are anastomosed; banding of the pulmonary trunk; and balloon atrial septostomy or surgical atrioseptectomy.

The more definitive operation, which is performed later in life, is a modified Fontan procedure that directs blood from the right atrium through an anastomosis either into the pulmonary arteries or the rudimentary right ventricle (Fig. 3.125) (Fontan and Baudet, 1971). The reported operative mortality is about 4%.

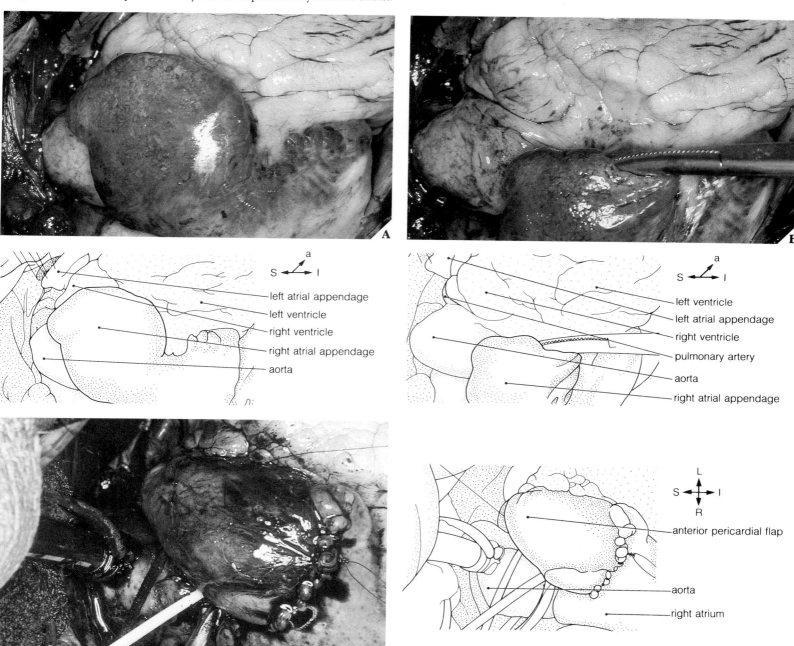

FIG. 3.125 (A) Operative view shows the markedly dilated right atrial appendage in a five-year-old child with classic tricuspid atresia. (B) Retraction of the atrial appendage uncovers the rudimentary right ventricle leading to a normal-sized pulmonary artery. (C) The appendage is opened to provide a posterior flap connecting the right atrium to the pulmonary artery distal to the competent pulmonary valve. The anterior wall of this tunnel is made up of a free pericardial graft.

TRICUSPID REGURGITATION

Isolated disease of the tricuspid valve producing regurgitation is rare. Tricuspid regurgitation may be observed in patients with Ebstein's disease, complete atrioventricular septal defect, or dysplasia of several valves (Bharati and Lev, 1973). Dysplasia of only the tricuspid valve may occur; in this condition there is poor development of the valve and its tendinous cords (Becker et al, 1971).

Infants with isolated tricuspid regurgitation may experience heart failure. An abnormal parasternal lift and a loud systolic murmur are detected in the same location. A diastolic rumble may be heard at the lower left sternal border, and the murmur of an arterial duct may be heard.

The chest film shows a large heart with decreased pulmonary blood flow. The ECG shows large P waves, right ventricular hypertrophy, or right bundle branch block. The echocardiogram reveals right ventricular dilation.

Cardiac catheterization discloses a right-to-left shunt at the atrial level and right ventricular pressures that are normal or moderately

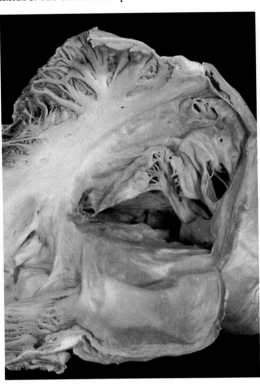

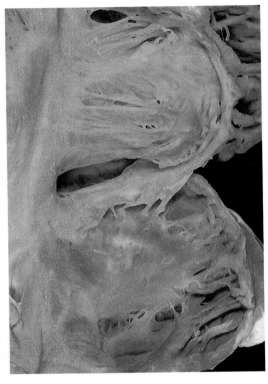

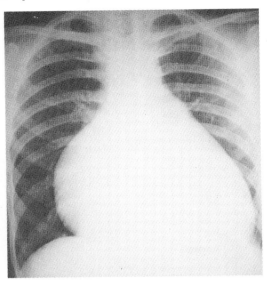

FIG. 3.128 *This chest radiograph of a 12-year-old boy with Ebstein's malformation shows marked cardiomegaly and diminished pulmonary flow. (Fig. 36-67, The Heart, 6th ed, p 679. Courtesy of the X-Ray Department, Henrietta Egleston Hospital for Children, Atlanta, Georgia)*

FIG. 3.126 *The right atrial aspect of the right atrioventricular junction in this example of Ebstein's malformation shows a normal focal attachment of the anterosuperior leaflet of the tricuspid valve with marked downward displacement of the septal and the mural leaflets.*

FIG. 3.127 *The atrial aspect of the abnormal right atrioventricular junction in this example of Ebstein's malformation shows linear attachment of the grossly abnormal anterosuperior leaflet of the tricuspid valve. The valve is consequently much more deformed than that shown in Figure 3.126.*

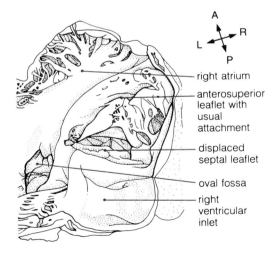

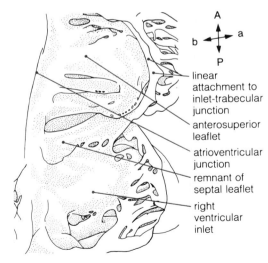

elevated. The right atrial pressure curve shows a large V wave of tricuspid regurgitation. Right ventricular angiography shows a large right ventricle and right atrium. When the pulmonary artery cannot be entered, it is not possible to determine if it is because the valve does not open or pulmonary atresia is present. Angiographic techniques have been developed to separate these two conditions (Freedom et al, 1978).

Patients with isolated tricuspid valve regurgitation often die soon after birth (Barr et al, 1974). If they survive this early period, their condition usually improves.

Medical management consists of treatment of heart failure and hypoxia.

The surgical treatment of isolated tricuspid regurgitation is not possible early after birth. If the child recovers to some degree, it may be possible to perform annuloplasty, commissural plication, or tricuspid valve replacement at an older age. (See the previous discussion of the surgical correction of tricuspid regurgitation associated with other anomalies.)

EBSTEIN'S MALFORMATION
DEFINITION AND PATHOLOGY

The basic pathologic defect in Ebstein's malformation is downward displacement of the dysplastic tricuspid valve leaflets into the right ventricle. The right atrium is large, and the functional component of the right ventricle is smaller than normal (Lev et al, 1970). The annular attachment of the anterosuperior leaflet of the valve is normally positioned, while the mural (inferior) and septal leaflets are attached to the right ventricle below the atrioventricular junction. The papillary muscle and cords are abnormally formed, but the major variant in morphology depends on whether the diseased edges of the leaflets are attached in focal (Fig. 3.126) or linear (Fig. 3.127) fashion. Linear attachment produces much more severe anatomic derangement. There is almost always an additional atrial septal defect.

ABNORMAL PHYSIOLOGY

The compliance of the right ventricle is decreased, and tricuspid regurgitation is usually present. These abnormalities may lead to a right-to-left shunt at the atrial level (Kumar et al, 1971).

CLINICAL MANIFESTATIONS
SYMPTOMS

Infants develop symptoms of heart failure and cyanosis, while older children and adults may be asymptomatic or may have dyspnea on effort (Watson, 1974). Patients with Ebstein's malformation have palpitation due to supraventricular tachycardia; syncope and sudden death may occur.

PHYSICAL EXAMINATION

Infants are usually cyanotic; older children and adults may exhibit clubbing of the fingers and toes. A small percentage of patients have no right-to-left shunt, and therefore have no cyanosis.

Palpation of the precordium may not reveal abnormal pulsations, but the liver may be enlarged. The jugular venous pulse reflects the presence of tricuspid regurgitation. The first sound is loud and abnormally split. The second sound is also abnormally split. Atrial and ventricular gallop sounds are heard. Murmurs of tricuspid regurgitation or stenosis may be detected.

LABORATORY STUDIES

CHEST RADIOGRAPHY. The chest film may be normal in mild cases, but it usually shows a large heart. The right atrium is large, and pulmonary blood flow is diminished. The radiograph often resembles that of pericardial effusion (Fig. 3.128).

ELECTROCARDIOGRAPHY. Large P waves are commonly present. The P-R interval may be long, and right bundle branch block is common (Fig. 3.129). The Wolff-Parkinson-White syndrome is present in 10% of patients (Watson, 1974).

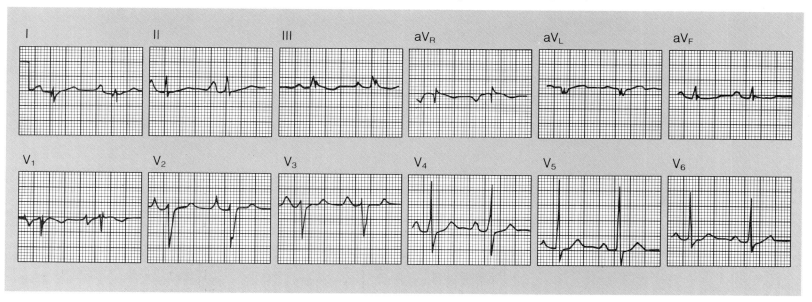

FIG. 3.129 *In this ECG of a 20-year-old male with Ebstein's malformation extremely large P waves and intraventricular conduction delay are evident. The P-R interval is 0.20 second. The P waves suggest right atrial abnormality. (Redrawn; reproduced with permission of the authors and publisher; see Figure Credits)*

ECHOCARDIOGRAPHY. The echocardiographic abnormalities are specific for Ebstein's malformation (Fig. 3.130). The tricuspid valve is large, and its closure is delayed when compared to mitral valve closure (Giuliani et al, 1979).

CARDIAC CATHETERIZATION. Because patients with Ebstein's malformation are prone to arrhythmias, they are at greater risk of having an arrhythmia during cardiac catheterization. Death can occur during cardiac catheterization. Tricuspid regurgitation and right-to-left shunts may be recognized. A right ventricular pressure curve is not recorded at the usual location but at the apex and right ventricular outflow tract.

An angiogram of the right ventricle shows abnormal valve morphology and tricuspid regurgitation (Fig. 3.131).

NATURAL HISTORY

Ebstein's malformation is a serious abnormality; half of patients who are recognized as having the disease die early in infancy (Giuliani et al, 1979). Those who survive and are identified later in life often die in early adult life. Mild cases probably go unrecognized.

TREATMENT

Heart failure and cardiac arrhythmias are treated with appropriate drugs with variable success.

INDICATIONS FOR SURGERY

Surgical treatment has improved remarkably in recent years. Patients with uncontrollable heart failure, paradoxical emboli, or severe cyanosis are candidates for surgery. Arrhythmias may continue after the abnormal hemodynamics are corrected. Troublesome arrhythmias are not an indication for surgery, except when other surgical procedures for the interruption of accessory conduction pathways are required.

SURGICAL PROCEDURE

The procedures include plication of the atrialized portion of the right ventricle, tricuspid valvoplasty or replacement, and the Fontan pro-

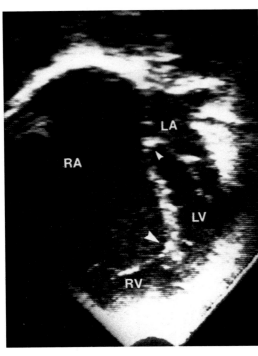

FIG. 3.130   *Cross-sectional echocardiogram in the apical four-chamber view of Ebstein's malformation shows marked displacement of septal tricuspid attachment to the interventricular septum (large arrow) relative to the attachment of the mitral leaflet (small arrow). The right atrium (RA) is very large and includes the atrialized portion of the right ventricle (RV) (LA, left atrium; LV, left ventricle). (Reproduced with permission of the authors and publisher; see Figure Credits)*

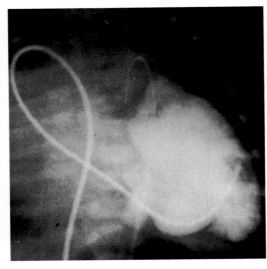

FIG. 3.131   *Frontal projection of a right ventriculogram, obtained by injecting contrast material into the functional right ventricle, shows the position of the tricuspid valve annulus overlying the left spinal margin. The notch formed by the displaced anterior tricuspid valve leaflet is demonstrated. Note the dilated and smooth-walled atrialized portion of the right ventricle. (Reproduced with permission of the authors and publisher; see Figure Credits. Courtesy of Robert M. Freedom, MD, Toronto, Ontario)*

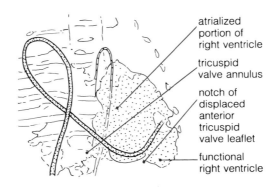

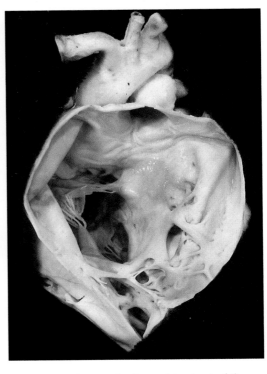

FIG. 3.132   *As seen in the outlet aspect of the right ventricle in a heart exhibiting Uhl's anomaly, the wall of the right ventricle is composed only of the apposed epicardial and endocardial layers because of complete absence of the myocardial layer. However, the trabeculations on the septal surface of the ventricle are normally formed.*

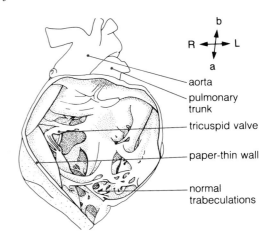

cedure (see Fig. 3.125). Surgical treatment for arrhythmias can be achieved at the same operation for correction of the valve lesion.

UHL'S MALFORMATION

Uhl's malformation is a condition characterized by an atrophic and fibrotic right ventricle with normal tricuspid and pulmonary valves (Fig. 3.132) (Gasul et al, 1960).

Chest pain and syncope related to exertion are common. There is a prominent a wave in the neck veins, a quiet precordium, a widely split second sound, and a systolic murmur heard over the precordium. The heart is large when viewed on the chest radiograph. The P waves are large in the ECG with diminished right ventricular QRS forces. A Qr configuration of the QRS is often seen in the midprecordial leads. The echocardiogram shows dilation of the right ventricle, delayed closure of the tricuspid valve, and diastolic opening of the pulmonary valve. Cardiac catheterization reveals a large a wave and a right-to-left shunt at the atrial level. An echocardiogram or angiogram that shows a large right ventricle excludes Ebstein's malformation.

Most patients die of heart failure or arrhythmia. Right ventricular thrombi have been seen at autopsy.

Treatment consists of managing the heart failure, arrhythmias, and hypoxia. Most surgical procedures have failed although Fontan's operation (see Fig. 3.125) may possibly be helpful.

TETRALOGY OF FALLOT
DEFINITION AND PATHOLOGY

The four abnormalities that comprise the tetralogy of Fallot (Fig. 3.133) are a large ventricular septal defect (VSD), origination of the aorta from both ventricles above the septal deficiency, infundibular right ventricular outflow tract obstruction, and right ventricular hypertrophy (Edwards, 1979).

ABNORMAL PHYSIOLOGY

The VSD is usually about the size of the aortic valve, and both are larger than the right ventricular outflow tract. Accordingly the systolic pressure is the same in the right and the left ventricles and the aorta, but it is lower than normal in the pulmonary trunk. When the resistance to pulmonary blood flow is great, there is a right-to-left shunt and cyanosis. When the resistance to pulmonary blood flow is not high, the pulmonary blood flow may be normal or increased, and the arterial oxygen saturation may be normal; this clinical picture is termed the acyanotic tetralogy of Fallot. When the right ventricular outflow tract obstruction is very severe, pulmonary blood flow may also occur through collateral arteries or a patent arterial duct, which may close, producing a further reduction of the pulmonary blood flow. The right ventricular infundibular stenosis may gradually increase; it also transiently increases with physical maneuvers or with drugs that increase contractility.

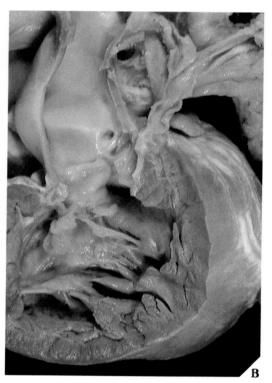

FIG. 3.133 (A) A simulated paracoronal subcostal section of a heart with tetralogy of Fallot shows a perimembranous VSD, muscular subpulmonary obstruction as a consequence of anterocephalad deviation of the outlet septum, overriding of the aortic valve, and marked right ventricular hypertrophy. (B) The right ventricular aspect of this heart shows muscular pulmonary atresia in the setting of tetralogy of Fallot. There is a perimembranous VSD, and the confluent pulmonary arteries are fed through an arterial duct.

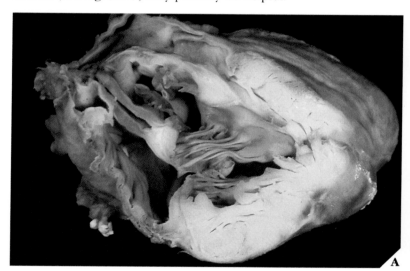

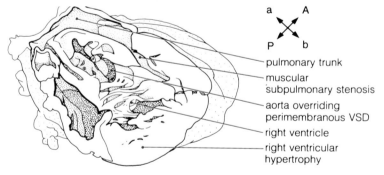

a A
P b

- pulmonary trunk
- muscular subpulmonary stenosis
- aorta overriding perimembranous VSD
- right ventricle
- right ventricular hypertrophy

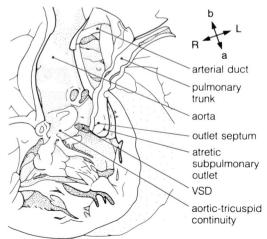

b L
R a

- arterial duct
- pulmonary trunk
- aorta
- outlet septum
- atretic subpulmonary outlet
- VSD
- aortic-tricuspid continuity

Children with tetralogy of Fallot may develop dyspnea and faintness after exercise. These symptoms are relieved by assuming the squatting position, which increases peripheral arterial resistance, decreases the right-to-left shunt, and increases pulmonary blood flow.

Hypoxic episodes may be caused by a decrease in peripheral arterial resistance, which decreases pulmonary blood flow. These spells may also be due to any stimulus causing a dynamic increase in the infundibular muscular obstruction.

CLINICAL MANIFESTATIONS
SYMPTOMS

Infants with tetralogy of Fallot are usually discovered because of cyanosis, although all patients with the condition are not cyanotic. Patients may become more cyanotic as the arterial duct closes and as they grow older. A few patients have a left-to-right shunt at birth, but with increasing infundibular stenosis they develop a right-to-left shunt. Tetralogy of Fallot is the cause of cyanosis in 75% of children who are older than two years (Keith et al, 1978).

Infants have hypoxic spells that can result in syncope and death (Morgan et al, 1965). Children have dyspnea on effort, which is relieved by squatting.

PHYSICAL EXAMINATION

Cyanosis is usually present except in patients with acyanotic tetralogy of Fallot (see above). Clubbing occurs after three or four months of age, but heart failure rarely occurs.

There is an anterior lift of the precordium, suggesting right ventricular hypertrophy. A systolic murmur is usually heard to the left of the midsternal area. The murmur ends before the second sound, which is usually single because the pulmonary closure sound is not heard. The murmur of an arterial duct may be heard until the duct closes.

LABORATORY STUDIES

CHEST RADIOGRAPHY. The heart size is not increased, but the configuration is abnormal because of the small pulmonary trunk. The right ventricle appears large on the lateral radiograph. The aortic arch is on the right side in one quarter of patients. Blood flow to the lungs is diminished (Fig. 3.134).

ELECTROCARDIOGRAPHY. The ECG shows right ventricular hypertrophy and a right atrial abnormality (Fig. 3.135). When the mean QRS vector is directed far to the right or superiorly, it is likely that an additional defect is present.

ECHOCARDIOGRAPHY. The M-mode echocardiogram shows abrupt ending of the septum below the overriding aorta. Right ventricular hypertrophy, a narrow outflow tract, and a dilated aorta are evident (Fig. 3.136). Cross-sectional echocardiography is even more useful. These techniques are also effective in excluding other conditions.

CARDIAC CATHETERIZATION. The right and the left ventricular pressures are equal, and the right atrial pressure is normal. The pulmonary arterial pressure is usually low, but it may be normal. A hypoxic spell may be precipitated when the cardiac catheter occludes a small right ventricular outflow tract. Pull-back pressure recordings identify the level of right ventricular outflow tract obstructions. There is a right-to-left shunt at the ventricular level, and the peripheral arterial blood oxygen saturation is diminished.

Right and left ventriculography and coronary arteriography are valuable tools used to identify anomalies of the coronary arteries (Fig. 3.137).

NATURAL HISTORY

Severe cyanosis and hypoxic spells indicate a poor prognosis (Bonchek et al, 1973). Patients develop polycythemia and cerebral thromboses; thrombi in the pulmonary arteries, brain abscess, and infective endocarditis may also occur (Ferencz, 1960). Without surgical treatment about 25% of infants die during the first year, 50% die by the age of three years, and 75% die by the age of ten years. Only a small percentage live beyond age 30; a few case reports describe patients beyond this age (Bertranaou et al, 1978). The natural history and deaths at an early age are profoundly influenced by surgical intervention (see below).

TREATMENT

Hypoxic spells are treated by placing the infant in the knee–chest position and administering oxygen, morphine, sodium bicarbonate,

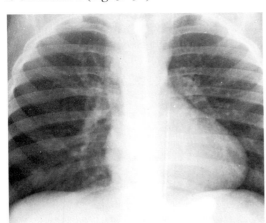

FIG. 3.134 *Chest film of a three-year-old boy with tetralogy of Fallot demonstrates a boot-shaped heart with a right aortic arch and mildly diminished pulmonary flow. (Fig. 36-51, The Heart, 6th ed, p 664. Courtesy of the X-Ray Department, Henrietta Egleston Hospital for Children, Atlanta, Georgia)*

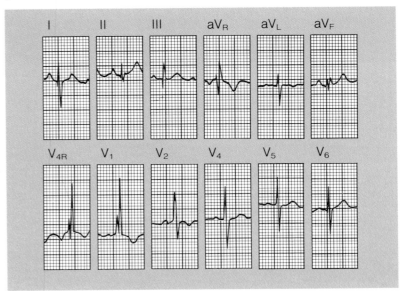

FIG. 3.135 *In this ECG from a three-year-old boy with tetralogy of Fallot the P waves are prominent, and right ventricular hypertrophy is apparent. (Courtesy of the Electrocardiography Laboratory, Henrietta Egleston Hospital for Children, Atlanta, Georgia)*

and propranolol. Viscosity can be diminished by withdrawing blood and transfusing fresh plasma. Dehydration should be avoided; iron deficiency must be treated with iron supplements. Any infection must be treated promptly, and prophylactic antibiotics should be used in an attempt to prevent endocarditis. In the newborn infant the administration of prostaglandin E_1 may help keep the arterial duct open until surgery can be performed (Heymann and Rudolph, 1977).

INDICATIONS FOR SURGERY

Prompt surgical intervention is indicated for the severely cyanotic infant. Surgical treatment is indicated for children who have increasing symptoms with hematocrits approaching 65%. Elective surgery may be performed in early childhood.

There are several approaches to the surgical treatment of this condition; the choice depends on the size of the child, the precise nature

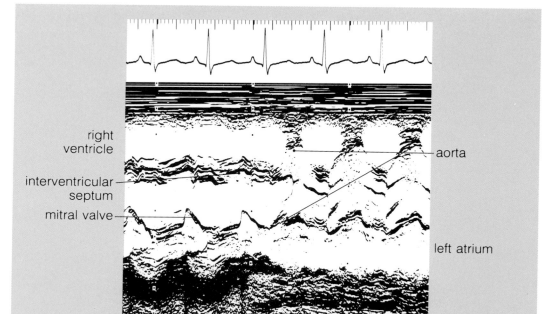

FIG. 3.136 *M-mode echocardiogram in a child with tetralogy of Fallot demonstrates aortic override of the interventricular septum and aortic–mitral valve continuity. (Fig. 36-52, The Heart, 6th ed, p 664. Courtesy of the Electrocardiography Laboratory, Henrietta Egleston Hospital for Children, Atlanta, Georgia)*

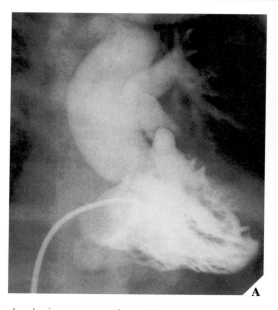
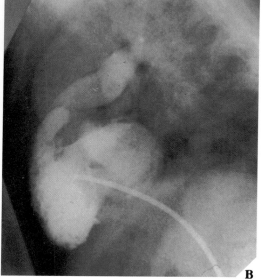

FIG. 3.137 **(A)** *In a patient with tetralogy of Fallot the cranially tilted frontal projection of a right ventriculogram shows hypertrophy of this chamber. There is opacification of both the aorta and the pulmonary trunk; the left pulmonary artery is better visualized. The pulmonary valve is obviously stenotic, and it is higher than the aortic valve.* **(B)** *Left long-axial oblique projection demonstrates the anterosuperiorly deviated outlet septum with the small pulmonary trunk supported above the right ventricular infundibulum. The stenotic pulmonary valve can be seen. Right-to-left shunting is evident through the ventricular septal defect, which is located inferior to the malaligned outlet septum. (Reproduced with permission of the authors and publisher; see Figure Credits. Courtesy of Robert M. Freedom, MD, Toronto, Ontario)*

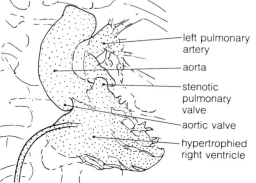
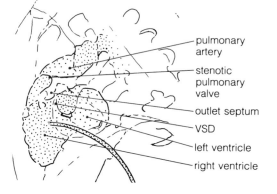

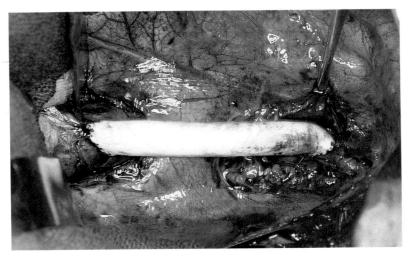

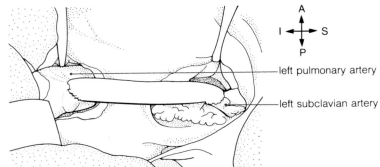

FIG. 3.138 *This operative view through a left lateral thoracotomy shows a modified Blalock–Taussig shunt performed in a patient with tetralogy of Fallot. The 6-mm diameter Gortex graft joins the uninterrupted left subclavian artery to the left pulmonary artery.*

left pulmonary artery

left subclavian artery

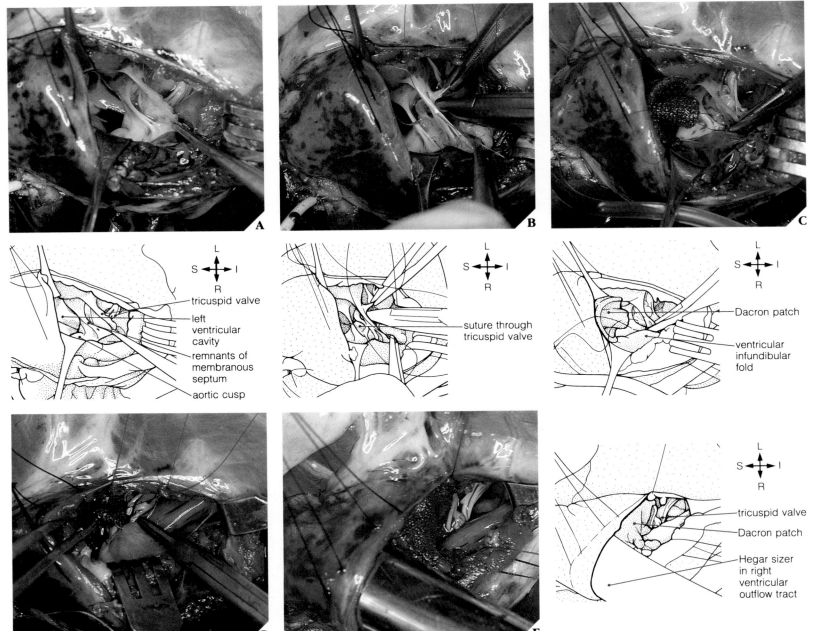

tricuspid valve

left ventricular cavity

remnants of membranous septum

aortic cusp

suture through tricuspid valve

Dacron patch

ventricular infundibular fold

tricuspid valve

Dacron patch

Hegar sizer in right ventricular outflow tract

FIG. 3.139 (**A**) *Repair of a tetralogy of Fallot is viewed through the opened right ventricular outflow tract. The very large perimembranous outlet VSD can be seen just beneath the junction of the anterior and the septal leaflets of the tricuspid valve.* (**B**) *These leaflets are used to anchor the patch in the area where the conduction tissue is most vulnerable.* (**C**) *Pledgeted sutures are placed from the right atrial aspect of the valve tissue through the valve into the Dacron patch material.* (**D**) *The suture line is then brought up along the ventricular infundibular fold across to the anteriorly displaced outlet septum.* (**E**) *The pulmonary valve orifice is entirely adequate as sized by a Hegar dilator.*

PART II: DISEASES OF THE HEART

of the anomalies and capabilities of the medical center. The modified Blalock–Taussig shunt is an anastomosis between the subclavian and the pulmonary arteries using a Gortex graft (Fig. 3.138). This increases the amount of unsaturated blood that goes to the lung (Guyton et al, 1983; Kirklin et al, 1977). Total correction is desirable, either at the first operation or later after a palliative procedure has been performed. The operative risk of total correction is less than 10%, and the long-term results are excellent.

SURGICAL PROCEDURE

The complete correction of tetralogy of Fallot (Fig. 3.139) is a complex undertaking, but one that has met with considerable success in properly selected patients. It is almost always necessary to patch the characteristically large VSD, being appropriately cautious in the area of the conduction tissues. Division and resection of the large muscle bundles in the right ventricular outflow tract may be all that is required to relieve the right ventricular outflow obstruction. Regularly, how-

ever, a patch is necessary (Fig. 3.140) to avoid unacceptably high right ventricular pressures. Generally it is believed that the right ventricle tolerates a volume load better than excessive pressures, so that the lack of pulmonary stenosis has been purchased with resultant pulmonary regurgitation. Clearly one must try to minimize both the volume and pressure load, when possible.

PULMONARY ATRESIA WITH VENTRICULAR SEPTAL DEFECT

Atresia of the pulmonary trunk may occur with an intact ventricular septum or in the presence of a VSD. The latter lesion may be found with various ventriculoarterial connections, such as complete transposition or double-outlet right ventricle, but most frequently it is seen in the setting of the tetralogy of Fallot (Fig. 3.141). The small cordlike remnant of the pulmonary trunk arises from the right ventricle. The atresia may involve the subpulmonary infundibulum and a short por-

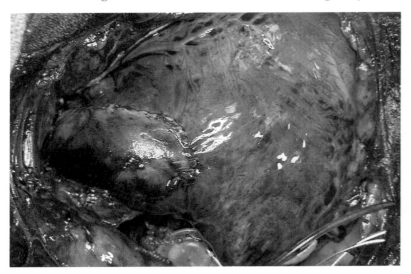

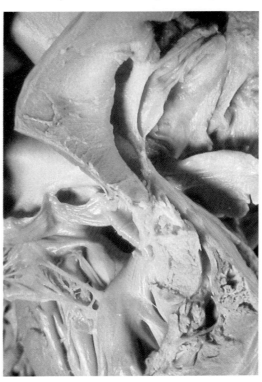

FIG. 3.141   *Dissection of the right ventricle in this case of pulmonary atresia with VSD shows the morphology of a severe case of tetralogy of Fallot.*

FIG. 3.140   *As seen in this operative view, a patient with tetralogy of Fallot requires outflow tract patching. Pericardium is entirely satisfactory patch material, having superior handling and hemostatic properties.*

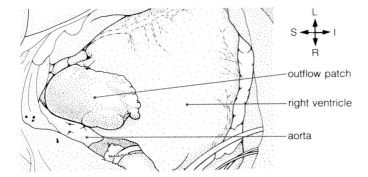

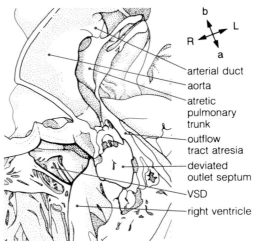

tion of the pulmonary trunk; rarely it may be due to an imperforate valve membrane. The pulmonary trunk distal to the atretic area may be patent, or the pulmonary arteries may be discontinuous or even absent. Pulmonary blood supply may flow through an arterial duct, but more usually it is supplied by multiple systemic–pulmonary collateral arteries (Fig. 3.142).

The clinical picture is that of severe tetralogy of Fallot (see p. 3.73). The condition is often erroneously called pseudotruncus arteriosus; it is more accurate to consider the usual anomaly as a variant of tetralogy of Fallot.

The clinical manifestations, including the finding in the chest film and ECG, are similar to those produced by severe tetralogy of Fallot. The pulmonary trunk cannot be entered at cardiac catheterization, and contrast material does not directly enter the pulmonary arteries when the right ventricle is injected. The VSD can be identified.

When the distal pulmonary arteries can be visualized by injecting the contrast material into the aorta or collateral vessels, it is possible to place a Blalock–Taussig shunt between the systemic arterial system and the pulmonary arteries. It is important surgically to identify the connections of all the bronchopulmonary segments, since these may be supplied from different sources.

COMPLETE TRANSPOSITION OF THE GREAT ARTERIES
DEFINITION AND PATHOLOGY

The pulmonary trunk arises from the left ventricle and the aorta arises from the right ventricle in the setting of a concordant atrioventricular connection (Figs. 3.143, 3.144). Other abnormalities must be present for the patient to survive, including VSD (Fig. 3.145), found in one

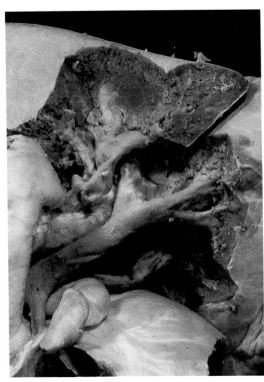

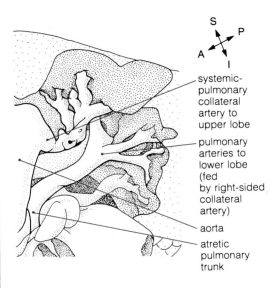

S
P
A
I

systemic-
pulmonary
collateral
artery to
upper lobe

pulmonary
arteries to
lower lobe
(fed
by right-sided
collateral
artery)

aorta

atretic
pulmonary
trunk

FIG. 3.142 *This dissection shows the origins of pulmonary arterial supply to the left lung in a patient with pulmonary atresia and VSD. The upper lobe is supplied by one systemic–pulmonary collateral artery, while another systemic–pulmonary collateral on the right side anastomoses with confluent intrapericardial pulmonary arteries supplying the lower part of the left lung.*

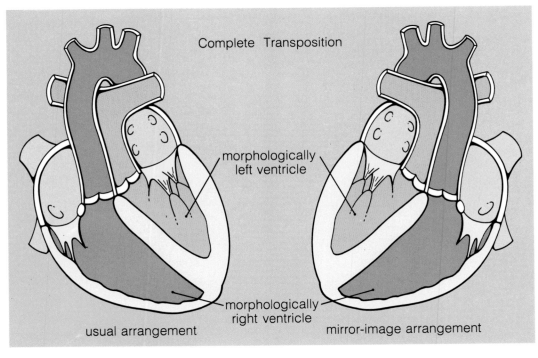

Complete Transposition

morphologically
left ventricle

morphologically
right ventricle

usual arrangement

mirror-image arrangement

FIG. 3.143 *This diagram shows the chamber connections that create the combination best described as complete transposition. This condition may be found with usually arranged (solitus) and mirror-image (inversus) atrial chambers, but not with atrial isomerism.*

third of patients, an atrial septal defect, or patency of the arterial duct (Paul, 1983). Other associated abnormalities include pulmonary valve stenosis, subpulmonary stenosis (Fig. 3.146), aneurysm of the ventricular septum, and adherence of the anterior (pulmonary) leaflet of the mitral valve to the ventricular septum.

ABNORMAL PHYSIOLOGY

Patients with complete transposition are able to survive because of the patent oval foramen, VSD, or patent arterial duct. The physiologic derangement depends on the type and severity of these associated defects.

CLINICAL MANIFESTATIONS

The condition is two to three times more common in males than in females. Complete transposition occurs in slightly less than 10% of children who are recognized as having congenital heart disease; about one third of the untreated patients die within the first week of life (Paul, 1983).

SYMPTOMS

The physician and parents note the infant's discomfort due to hypoxia and heart failure.

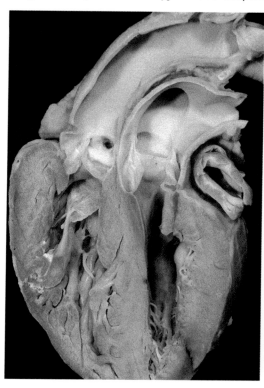

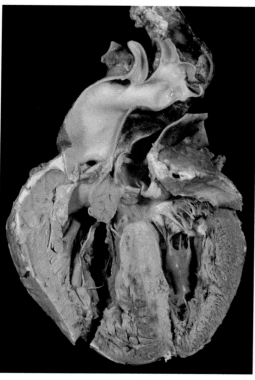

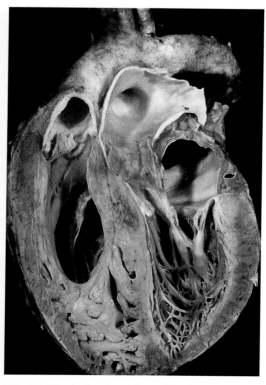

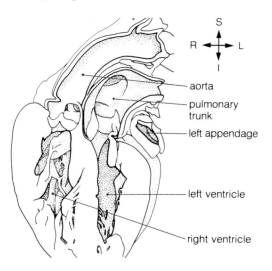

FIG. 3.144 *A simulated four-chamber long-axis section through the ventricular outlets shows the discordant ventriculoarterial connection that, combined with a concordant atrioventricular connection, is the hallmark of complete transposition of the great arteries.*

aorta
pulmonary trunk
left appendage
left ventricle
right ventricle

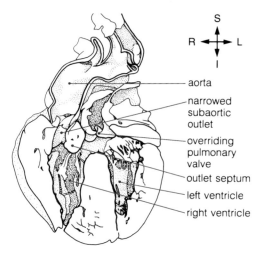

FIG. 3.145 *A subpulmonary VSD in the setting of complete transposition has a completely muscular right ventricular margin. The overriding pulmonary valve and the narrowed subaortic outflow tract arise as the consequence of malalignment of the outlet septum. This lesion can be considered as one variant of the Taussig–Bing malformation (see Figs. 3.113, 3.167).*

aorta
narrowed subaortic outlet
overriding pulmonary valve
outlet septum
left ventricle
right ventricle

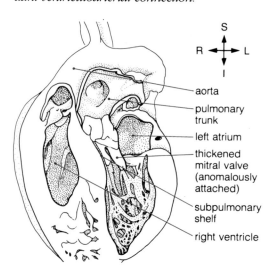

FIG. 3.146 *A simulated four-chamber section through the ventricular outlets shows severe subpulmonary obstruction in the setting of complete transposition of the great arteries. A discrete subpulmonary fibrous shelf that coexists with an anomalous attachment of the anterolateral papillary muscle of the mitral valve is the cause of the obstruction. A similar shelf produces subaortic obstruction if found in the setting of concordant ventriculoarterial connection.*

aorta
pulmonary trunk
left atrium
thickened mitral valve (anomalously attached)
subpulmonary shelf
right ventricle

PHYSICAL EXAMINATION

The infant with an intact ventricular septum or a small VSD has intense cyanosis; breathing difficulty is apparent. An anterior precordial lift may be present. The first sound is loud and the second sound is split, signifying the presence of aortic and pulmonary valves. Murmurs may not be heard.

Cyanosis may be slight when a large VSD is present; these patients may have signs of heart failure and difficulty in breathing. The right and the left ventricular pulsations are prominent. The sound of closure of the pulmonary valve is audible. A systolic murmur is usually present to the left at the lower end of the sternum; a diastolic rumble may be heard at the apex.

LABORATORY STUDIES

CHEST RADIOGRAPHY. The chest film of a patient with complete transposition and an intact ventricular septum is shown in Fig. 3.147. The pulmonary flow may appear normal, but it is usually increased. The shadow of the great arteries may appear narrow due to the displaced pulmonary trunk. The heart is large, giving an egg-on-side appearance. On the chest film of a patient with a large interventricular septal defect the pulmonary blood flow is increased, the shadow of the great arteries is narrow, and the heart is large (egg-on-side appearance) (Fig. 3.148).

ELECTROCARDIOGRAPHY. The abnormalities in the ECG vary with the age of the patient and the existence of interventricular septal defect. When the infant with transposed great arteries has an intact ventricular septum, the P waves may be tall. Abnormal right ventricular forces develop toward the end of the first week of life. Upright T waves in leads V_1 and V_{3R} signify that right ventricular hypertension is present. Older infants have right ventricular hypertrophy (Fig. 3.149). When the patient has a large VSD, ECG shows biatrial abnormalities and biventricular hypertrophy.

ECHOCARDIOGRAPHY. Cross-sectional echocardiography reveals the origination of pulmonary trunk from the left ventricle and the aorta from the right ventricle (Fig. 3.150). Associated lesions can also be identified.

FIG. 3.147 *On this chest film of a three-week-old infant with complete transposition a VSD is probably absent or very small, and the main pulmonary artery segment is not seen. There is slight cardiac enlargement with a narrow mediastinum. (Reproduced with permission of the authors and publisher; see Figure Credits)*

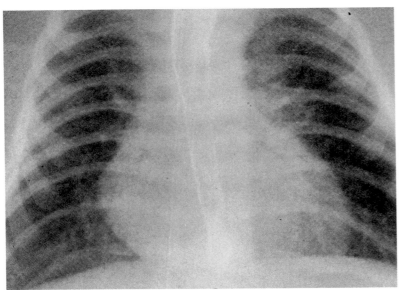

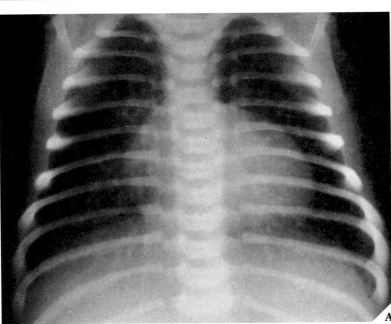

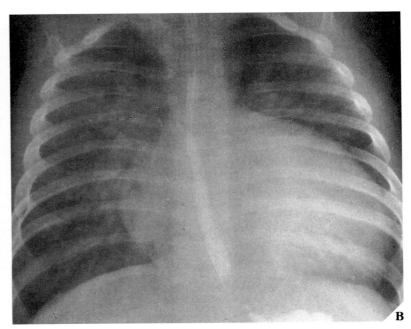

FIG. 3.148 *Chest radiographs of an infant with complete transposition and a large VSD were obtained at age one month (A) and at age five months (B). Marked cardiac enlargement and pulmonary plethora developed during the four-month interval, as pulmonary vascular resistance decreased and pulmonary arterial blood flow increased. The egg-on-side con-tour of the heart and the narrow cardiac base characteristic of complete transposition are evident in both films. (Fig. 55-2, The Heart, 4th ed; see Figure Credits. Courtesy of the X-Ray Department, Henrietta Egleston Hospital for Children, Atlanta, Georgia)*

CARDIAC CATHETERIZATION. Systemic arterial oxygen saturation may be extremely low in patients without a VSD, but only slightly low in patients with a large VSD. The oxygen saturation in the pulmonary artery is always higher than in a systemic artery. The right ventricular systolic pressure is at systemic levels, as is the left ventricular pressure if a large VSD, patent arterial duct, or pulmonary valve stenosis is present. Angiography outlines the associated abnormalities (Fig. 3.151).

Cardiac catheterization should be performed on a patient suspected of having complete transposition. Atrial septostomy should be performed if the atrial septum is intact.

NATURAL HISTORY

Without treatment 50% of patients with complete transposition die during the first month of life, and 90% die within the first year. Patients with intact ventricular septum die of hypoxia and its complications; patients with a large VSD die of heart failure and pulmonary vascular disease (Gutgesell et al, 1979; Newfeld et al, 1979). Patients with a VSD and pulmonary valve stenosis have the best prognosis.

Corrective procedures have improved the survival of many patients with complete transposition, but results are far from satisfactory. Several new problems seem to follow surgical treatment (see below).

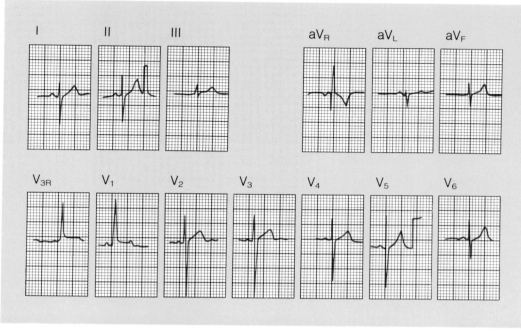

FIG. 3.149 *The salient features of the ECG from an infant with complete transposition are the dominant S_1 and R/S_{aV_F}-right axis deviation. There is also a dominant R wave in V_1 and an S wave in V_5 and V_6; this is interpretable as right ventricular hypertrophy. The T wave in V_1 is also upright. (Redrawn; reproduced with permission of the author and publisher; see Figure Credits)*

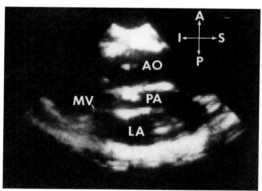

FIG. 3.150 *Both great arteries are visualized in the cross-sectional echocardiogram in the parasternal long-axis view from a patient with complete transposition and intact ventricular septum. The pulmonary trunk (PA) is identified posterior to the aorta (AO) by its sharp posterior angulation around the superior aspect of the left atrium (LA) (MV, mitral valve). (Reproduced with permission of the authors and publisher; see Figure Credits; also, Fig. 36-73, The Heart, 6th ed, p 693)*

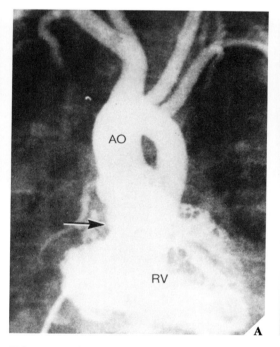

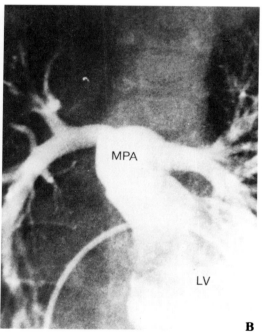

FIG. 3.151 *(A) Posteroanterior view of the right ventricular angiogram from a patient with complete transposition and intact ventricular septum demonstrates that the aorta (AO) arises from the heavily trabeculated right ventricle (RV) above a subaortic infundibulum (arrow). (B) On the left ventricular angiogram the pulmonary trunk (MPA) can be seen arising from the smooth-walled left ventricle (LV). (Fig. 36-74, The Heart, 6th ed, p 693. Courtesy of the Cardiac Catheterization Laboratory, Henrietta Egleston Hospital for Children, Atlanta Georgia)*

TREATMENT

Heart failure may be treated with digitalis, and hypoxia is managed with balloon atrial septostomy; however, medical treatment is only transiently satisfactory.

INDICATIONS FOR SURGERY

If balloon atrial septostomy is not adequate as determined by cross-sectional echocardiography, and the systemic arterial P_{O_2} does not rise to above 30 mmHg, it may be necessary to surgically create a larger interatrial opening in patients without a VSD. There is an in-creasing trend to refer such patients for immediate corrective surgery. Prostaglandin E_1 is also recommended to maintain a patent arterial duct (Paul, 1983). If these treatments fail, a systemic-to-pulmonary arterial shunt or total correction (Mustard or Senning procedure, or arterial switch operation) may be necessary.

Patients with a large VSD and pulmonary hypertension may require banding of the pulmonary trunk, with the recognition that a more definitive procedure will be necessary later. Many physicians believe it is wise to use palliative procedures early and more corrective procedures later in the first year of life.

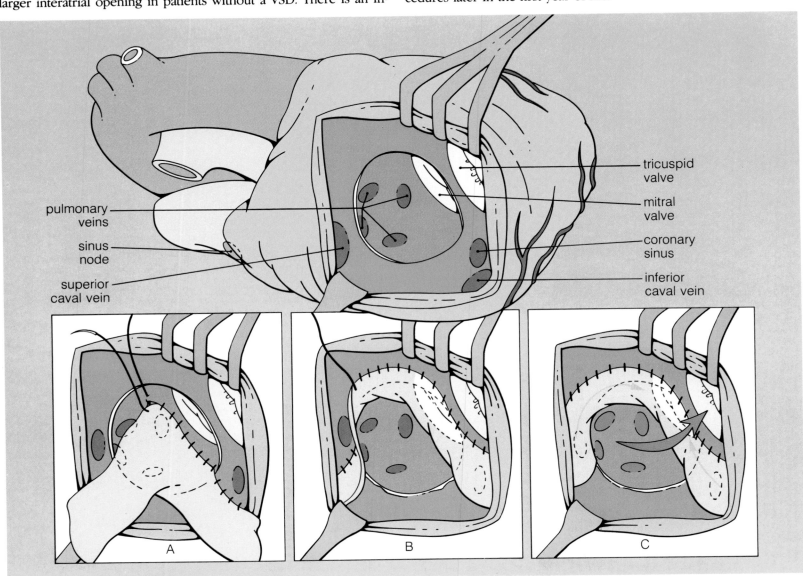

FIG. 3.152 *This schematic representation shows the crucial stages in the Mustard procedure for repair of complete transposition.* (**A**) *After the atrial septum is resected, a baffle, usually made of pericardium and shaped in a trouser pattern, is sewn to direct the systemic veins to the mitral valve and the pulmonary veins to the tricuspid valve. This is accomplished by sewing the waist of the trousers to the distal remnant of the atrial septum; the left leg is taken around the orifice of the inferior caval vein.* (**B**) *The suture line takes the right leg around the orifice of the superior caval vein.* (**C**) *The completed baffle has the crotch of the trousers sewn to the left margin of the left atrium beneath the orifices of the pulmonary veins. Systemic venous blood now runs through the legs of the trousers to the left ventricle, and pulmonary venous blood runs across the crotch of the legs to the right ventricle, thus correcting the discordant ventriculoarterial connection.*

SURGICAL PROCEDURE

Surgical correction of complete transposition is an evolving story. For some years the best hope for long-term survival of patients with transposition has been the successful execution of a venous switch operation. Such an operation is usually performed at three to six months of age in the patient who has previously undergone a palliative atrial septostomy. Earlier operation is possible but not advantageous, unless inadequate palliation is achieved in the newborn period. Hospital survival and long-term benefit are essentially the same regardless of the particular technique used to effect the venous rerouting, so the decision to use either the Mustard (Fig. 3.152) or the Senning (Fig. 3.153) technique depends on the personal preference of the surgeon.

Another important chapter in the treatment of complete transpo-

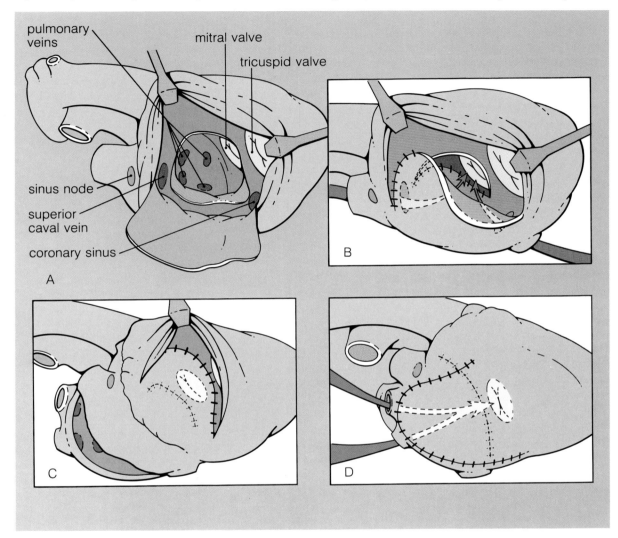

FIG. 3.153 *This schematic diagram depicts the steps in the Senning procedure for redirection of blood at the atrial level to correct the circulation of complete transposition. (A) The initial right atrial incision is made with care to avoid the sinus node and its blood supply; another incision liberates the atrial septum from its distal insertion at the atrioventricular junction. Should the septum itself be deficient because of prior balloon septostomy, it is reconstituted with a prosthetic patch. (B) The proximal edge of the right atrial incision is sewn down to the distal margin of the cut made to liberate the atrial septum. (C) Dissection of Waterston's groove then permits an incision to be made into the left atrium; the distal margin of the atrial septum is sewn to the left margin of the mitral valve beneath the orifices of the pulmonary veins. These procedures create the pathways to carry the systemic venous return (except from the coronary sinus) into the left ventricle. (D) The pathway to carry pulmonary venous return into the tricuspid valve is then completed by sewing the distal edge of the right atrial incision to the margin of the left atrial incision. Unlike the Mustard procedure, the Senning operation uses the patient's own tissues in the repair (apart from the patch that reconstitutes the atrial septum).*

sition began with the first successful application of an arterial-switch technique (Fig. 3.154) by Jatene and his colleagues (Jatene et al, 1976). Several groups have reported successful application of this technique with various modifications in newborn children. In spite of the apparent advantages it is not yet certain that this technique will enjoy the widespread applicability and long-term success achieved with the venous-switch operation (Quaegebeur et al, 1986).

Considering the severe anatomic and physiologic derangement affecting these patients, corrective surgery has been remarkably successful. Nevertheless it must be recognized that certain problems may continue and new ones may develop after operation. Venous obstruction, pulmonary and/or systemic, and conduction disturbances are the principal problems following venous-switch surgery. Of course the major objection to these operations remains the questionable fate of a right ventricle subjected to a systemic workload over many years. A major advantage of the arterial-switch technique is that it obviates this problem. Only the passage of time will reveal the extent of this problem and whether the arterial-switch operation is the answer to it.

CONGENITALLY CORRECTED TRANSPOSITION

The great arteries are transposed in the setting of a discordant atrioventricular connection. The pulmonary trunk arises from the morphologically left ventricle, which in turn is connected to the right atrium. The aorta arises from the morphologically right ventricle, which is connected to the left atrium (Fig. 3.155). The mitral valve is usually located on the right side along with the left ventricle (Fig. 3.156A), and the tricuspid valve is located on the left side with the right ventricle (Fig. 3.156B). The course of the coronary arteries is arranged in mirror-image fashion.

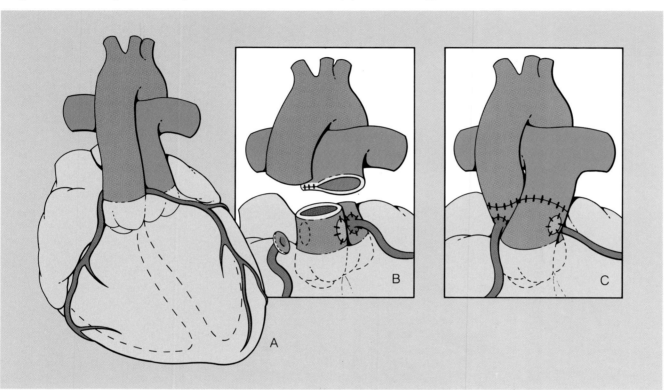

FIG. 3.154 *This schematic diagram depicts the procedures involved in the correction of complete transposition at the arterial level, the so-called arterial-switch procedure. (A) In the original arrangement the aorta, connected to the right ventricle and supporting the coronary arteries, is anterior and to the right of the pulmonary trunk, which emerges from the left ventricle. (B) In the initial steps of the operative procedure the arterial trunks are transected. The extensive pulmonary segment is plicated to match its size to that of the aortic root; it thus becomes the pulmonary outflow from the right ventricle. The coronary arteries, together with a button of arterial wall, are removed from this root, and the openings are closed with prosthetic material. The left coronary artery is reattached to the original root of the pulmonary trunk, soon to become the aortic outlet from the left ventricle. (C) In the completed procedure the right coronary artery has also been reattached to the old pulmonary root, which, with its reconnection to the aorta, is now the aortic root complete with coronary arteries. The old aortic outlet from the right ventricle now supplies the pulmonary trunk and is devoid of coronary arteries. The advantage of this procedure is that the ventricles now drive their appropriate circulation, since the discordant ventriculoarterial connection has been corrected at the arterial level.*

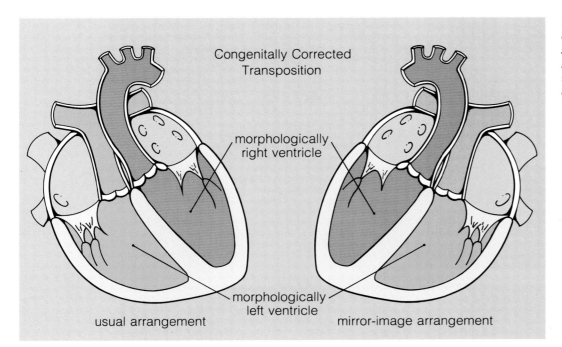

Congenitally Corrected
Transposition

morphologically
right ventricle

morphologically
left ventricle

usual arrangement

mirror-image arrangement

FIG. 3.155 *This diagram shows the chamber connections producing the combination best described as congenitally corrected transposition. Like complete transposition, this lesion may exist with usually arranged or mirror-image atrial chambers, but not with atrial isomerism.*

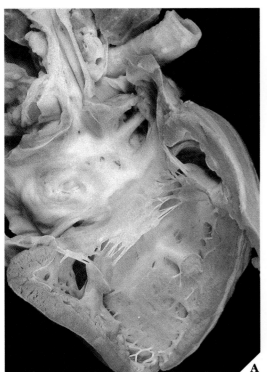

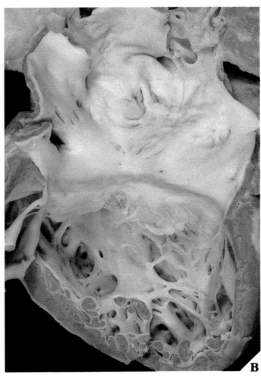

A

B

FIG. 3.156 *The discordant atrioventricular connection that is the hallmark of congenitally corrected transposition is shown here in the setting of a heart with the usual atrial arrangement. (A) The right atrium is connected to the right-sided, morphologically left ventricle, while the left atrium is connected to the left-sided, morphologically right ventricle (B).*

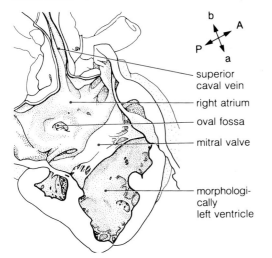

b

A

P

a

superior
caval vein

right atrium

oval fossa

mitral valve

morphologically
left ventricle

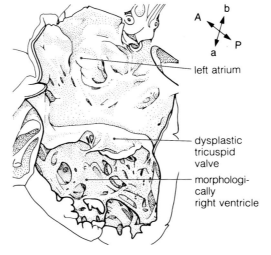

b

A

P

a

left atrium

dysplastic
tricuspid
valve

morphologically
right ventricle

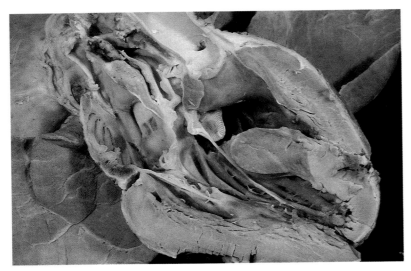

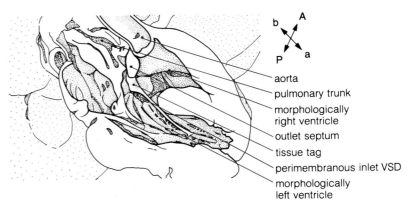

FIG. 3.157 A simulated paracoronal subcostal section of a heart shows a perimembranous inlet VSD along with subpulmonary obstruction due to fibrous tissue tags in a heart with congenitally corrected transposition.

aorta
pulmonary trunk
morphologically right ventricle
outlet septum
tissue tag
perimembranous inlet VSD
morphologically left ventricle

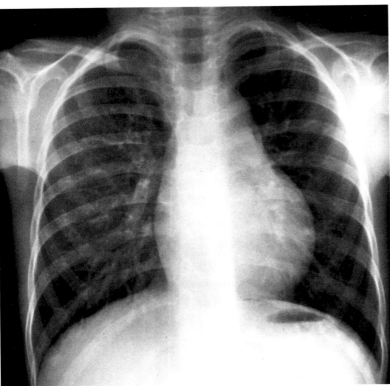

FIG. 3.158 On the posteroanterior chest radiograph of a patient with congenitally corrected transposition of the great vessels note the straight upperleft heart border. This is produced by the aorta originating from the systemic ventricle, which, in corrected transposition, is the anatomic right ventricle. (Courtesy of the X-Ray Department, Henrietta Egleston Hospital for Children, Atlanta, Georgia)

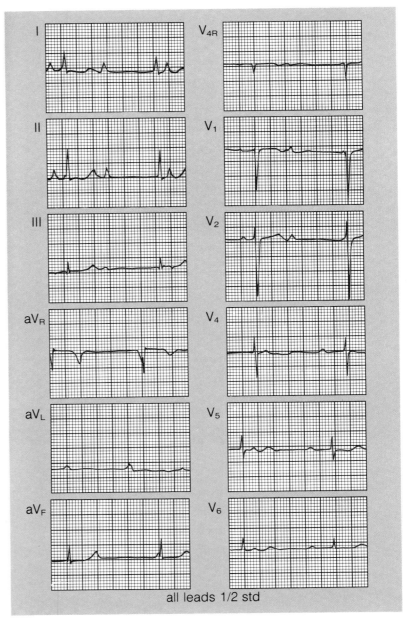

all leads 1/2 std

FIG. 3.159 On the ECG of a six-year-old patient with congenitally corrected transposition of the great arteries Q waves are evident at V_{4R}, and the R waves are small at V_1. Complete atrioventricular block is present; the ventricular rate is about 50 per minute, and the atrial rate is 85 per minute. (Courtesy of the Electrocardiography Laboratory, Henrietta Egleston Hospital for Children, Atlanta, Georgia)

PART II: DISEASES OF THE HEART

A VSD is usually present (Fig. 3.157). An Ebstein-like malformation may be seen in the left-sided, morphologically right ventricle where the tricuspid valve is located. Pulmonary stenosis or atresia is also commonly present (see Fig. 3.157) (Ruttenberg, 1983). When pulmonary stenosis and an interventricular septal defect are present, the condition hemodynamically resembles tetralogy of Fallot. Other serious anomalies are common. Atrioventricular conduction abnormalities may be present, and evidence of the existence of the condition may be detected before delivery.

The second sound may be louder than usual, because the aortic valve is located nearer the chest wall than it is normally. Murmurs depend on the associated defects that are present. Therefore when a patient appears to have tetralogy of Fallot but the second component of the second sound is loud, congenitally corrected transposition should be considered.

A straight upper-left heart border representing the contour of the transposed aorta is a characteristic finding on the chest film (Fig.

3.158). The ECG often shows atrioventricular block including complete heart block, with Q waves in the right precordial leads (Fig. 3.159). Cross-sectional echocardiography enables identification of the morphology of the abnormally connected right and left ventricles, the pulmonary trunk and the aorta, and the nature and number of associated defects (Fig. 3.160).

Cardiac catheterization may also identify many of the associated abnormalities, and ventricular angiograms are characteristic (Fig. 3.161).

The natural history depends on the associated defects. Many of the defects can be corrected by surgery, but there is a question as to the capability of the morphologically right ventricle to maintain a normal cardiac output throughout a complete and normal lifespan.

Correctable defects should be treated when the indications for surgical intervention arise. A permanent cardiac pacemaker is occasionally needed, even though intracardiac electrical mapping decreases the occurrence of surgical damage to the conduction system.

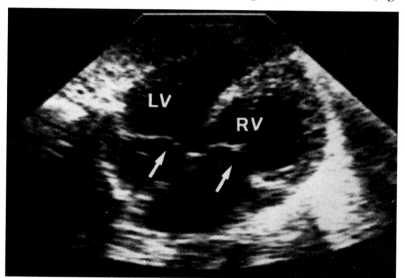

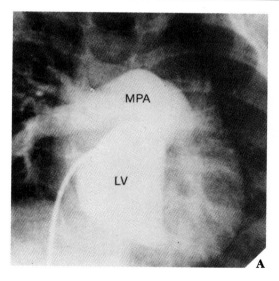 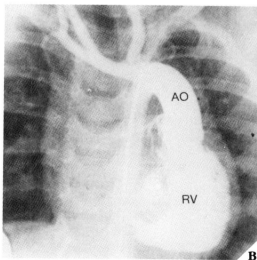

FIG. 3.160 *This cross-sectional echocardiogram in the apical four-chamber view from an infant shows congenitally corrected transposition (ventricular inversion with L-transposition of the great arteries). In a normal heart the right-sided atrioventricular valve is closer to the apex than the left-sided atrioventricular valve, but in ventricular inversion the opposite is true (arrows) (LV, morphologically left ventricle; RV, morphologically right ventricle). (Reproduced with permission of the authors and publisher; see Figure Credits)*

FIG. 3.161 *(A) As seen on the posteroanterior view of the left ventricular (LV) angiogram in a child with corrected transposition of the great arteries, the pulmonary trunk (MPA) arises from the smooth-walled left ventricle, which receives the systemic venous blood. (B) On the posteroanterior view of the right ventricular (RV) angiogram the ascending aorta (AO) arises to the left of the pulmonary trunk from the more heavily trabeculated right ventricle, which receives the pulmonary venous blood. The ventricular septum, seen here perpendicular to the frontal plane, is intact. (Fig. 36-81, The Heart, 6th ed, p 702. Courtesy of the Cardiac Catheterization Laboratory, Henrietta Egleston Hospital for Children, Atlanta, Georgia)*

DOUBLE-INLET VENTRICLE
DEFINITION AND PATHOLOGY

Double-inlet ventricle exists when both atrial chambers are connected to the same ventricle, either through two separate valves or a common atrioventricular valve. This condition is commonly referred to as single ventricle, an erroneous term for the lesion since in most examples two ventricles are arranged in dominant and rudimentary fashion. Thus the most common example is double-inlet left ventricle in the presence of a rudimentary right ventricle, usually with a discordant ventriculoarterial connection (Fig. 3.162), but sometimes with a concordant ventriculoarterial connection, the so-called Holmes heart (Fig. 3.163). Less frequently there is a double-inlet right ventricle with a rudimentary left ventricle; this variant is usually found with a double outlet from the dominant right ventricle (Fig. 3.164). Least common is a double inlet to a solitary ventricle of indeterminate morphology. Of necessity this last variant is found with either a double or a single

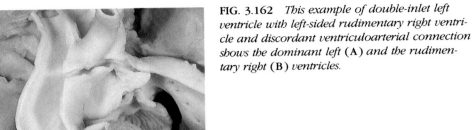

FIG. 3.162 *This example of double-inlet left ventricle with left-sided rudimentary right ventricle and discordant ventriculoarterial connection shows the dominant left (A) and the rudimentary right (B) ventricles.*

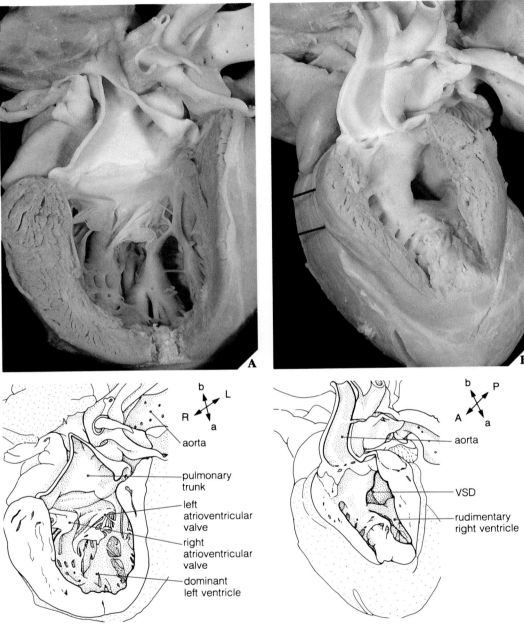

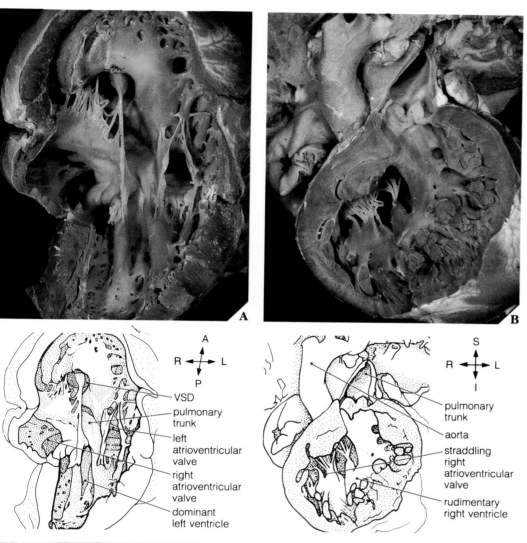

FIG. 3.163 *The dominant left (A) and the rudimentary right (B) ventricles are exposed in this example of double-inlet left ventricle with right-sided rudimentary right ventricle and concordant ventriculoarterial connections (the so-called Holmes heart). There is minimal straddling of the right atrioventricular valve.*

VSD
pulmonary trunk
left atrioventricular valve
right atrioventricular valve
dominant left ventricle

A
R ← → L
P

pulmonary trunk
aorta
straddling right atrioventricular valve
rudimentary right ventricle

S
R ← → L
I

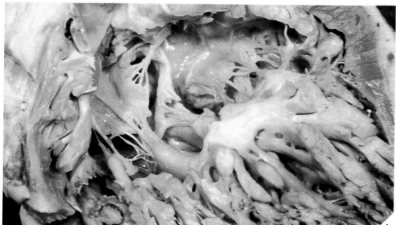
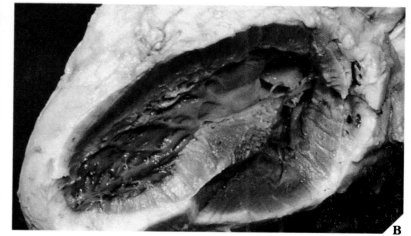

FIG. 3.164 *A double inlet and a double outlet from a dominant right ventricle (A) are seen in the presence of a rudimentary left ventricle found in left-sided and posteroinferior position (B). There is straddling and overriding of the mitral valve.*

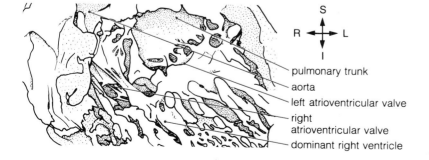
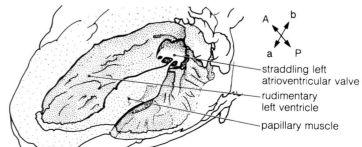

pulmonary trunk
aorta
left atrioventricular valve
right atrioventricular valve
dominant right ventricle

S
R ← → L
I

straddling left atrioventricular valve
rudimentary left ventricle
papillary muscle

A b
a P

outlet from the solitary ventricle (Fig. 3.165). Associated malformations are frequent; and they include a VSD in those patients with two ventricles, subatrial outflow tract obstruction, and malformation of the atrioventricular valves.

ABNORMAL PHYSIOLOGY

Because of the double inlet there is obligatory mixing of blood within the dominant or solitary ventricle, and hence some degree of cyanosis. This can be mitigated to some degree by preferential streaming through the heart, which is determined by the ventricular morphology, the relationship of the VSD (if present) to the atrioventricular valves, and the ventriculoarterial connection. Pulmonary stenosis, if present, protects the pulmonary circulation. If the pulmonary outflow is unobstructed, there is increased pulmonary flow. Often the aortic flow is reduced in the most common variant of double-inlet left ventricle, because there is a discordant ventriculoarterial connection and a restrictive VSD (see Fig. 3.162).

CLINICAL MANIFESTATIONS

The condition is uncommon, occurring in less than 1% of patients with congenital heart disease. It is now recognized with increasing frequency, however, due to better identification by cross-sectional echocardiography, and the figure indicating the frequency of recognition may need to be revised upwards in future years. It occurs equally in males and females, and it is frequent in patients with visceral heterotaxy (isomerism).

SYMPTOMS

The symptoms depend on the associated lesions. Patients with right atrial isomerism (asplenia) are dominated by the associated pulmonary atresia and total anomalous pulmonary venous connection; they present early with intense cyanosis. Others with severe subaortic stenosis present in neonatal life with shock. Patients with balanced pulmonary flow may not have symptoms immediately at birth, but most present within the first year of life with a murmur or failure to thrive.

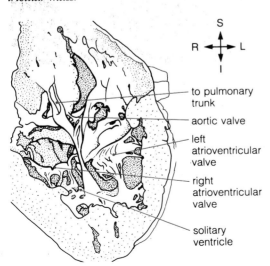

FIG. 3.165 *A double inlet and a double outlet are found in a solitary and indeterminate ventricle. It was not possible to find any evidence of a second rudimentary ventricle within the ventricular mass.*

to pulmonary trunk
aortic valve
left atrioventricular valve
right atrioventricular valve
solitary ventricle

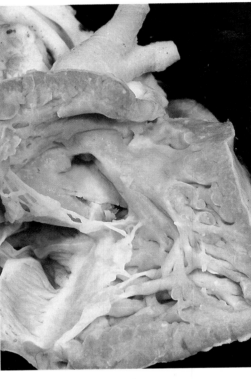
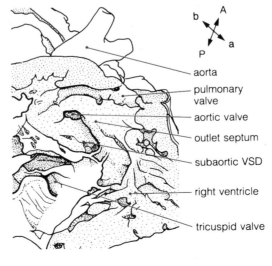

FIG. 3.166 *The right ventricular aspect of double-outlet right ventricle shows a subaortic VSD, normally related great arteries, and bilaterally complete infundibular structures.*

aorta
pulmonary valve
aortic valve
outlet septum
subaortic VSD
right ventricle
tricuspid valve

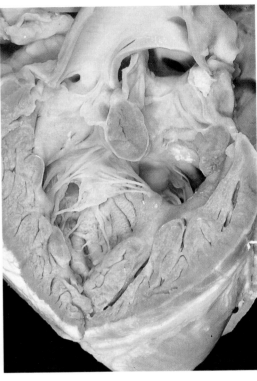
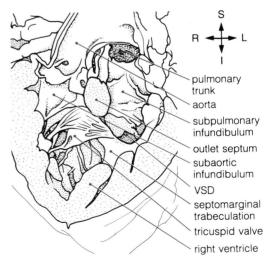

FIG. 3.167 *The right ventricular aspect of this heart shows a double-outlet right ventricle with subpulmonary VSD, the aorta anterior and to the right, and bilaterally complete infundibular structures. This combination is known as the Taussig–Bing anomaly (see Figs. 3.113, 3.145).*

pulmonary trunk
aorta
subpulmonary infundibulum
outlet septum
subaortic infundibulum
VSD
septomarginal trabeculation
tricuspid valve
right ventricle

PHYSICAL EXAMINATION

The presence of cyanosis depends on the associated lesions. Most patients have murmurs that are related to the precise morphology present.

LABORATORY STUDIES

CHEST RADIOGRAPHY. Findings on chest films depend on the associated lesions. Patients with atrial isomerism have the characteristic bronchial arrangement of this condition; patients with right isomerism are likely to have radiographic signs of total anomalous pulmonary venous connection. Some, but not all, patients have enlarged hearts, while the state of pulmonary blood flow is related to the presence or absence of pulmonary obstruction. There are no specific radiographic features for double-inlet ventricle.

ELECTROCARDIOGRAPHY. The ECG shows no specific features for double-inlet ventricle, although if the patient is known to have this condition, the tracing may give strong clues as to the nature of the dominant ventricle. Thus patients with double-inlet left ventricle have dominant left ventricular forces, while those with double-inlet right ventricle have ECG tracings showing evidence of right ventricular hypertrophy. Patients with atrial isomerism may show abnormal P waves, particularly an abnormal axis in left isomerism or evidence of dual sinus nodes in right isomerism.

ECHOCARDIOGRAPHY. Echocardiography is diagnostic for double-inlet ventricle. M-mode tracings showing two valves without any intervening septal structure are highly suggestive, although large VSDs may produce similar features. Cross-sectional techniques are more reliable. The key to diagnosis is the demonstration that a ventricular septum is present but does not separate the atrioventricular junctions. Therefore finding the septum anterior to both valves is diagnostic of double-inlet left ventricle, while discovery of the septum posterior to the valves indicates double-inlet right ventricle. Failure to find any septum suggests double-inlet to a solitary and indeterminate ventricle. Cross-sectional echocardiography should also permit diagnosis of the associated lesions.

CARDIAC CATHETERIZATION. Unless there is marked streaming, the oxygen saturation is the same in both great arteries. Ventricular pressures may be equal between dominant and rudimentary ventricles, but usually the VSD is restrictive. Gradients may also be demonstrated across abnormal atrioventricular or arterial valves. Angiography, particularly angled views, demonstrates well the ventricular morphology, the degree of ventricular dominance, the ventriculoarterial connections, and the associated lesions.

NATURAL HISTORY

It is difficult to be precise about natural history, because until recently most patients were not identified until they had survived the first year of life. Now that the diagnosis is often made at birth, it is known that patients with these lesions have a poor prognosis, particularly when it is found in the setting of right atrial isomerism. These patients do poorly irrespective of surgical treatment. The majority of those without isomerism need surgery in the first year of life to ensure survival. If left untreated surgically, only a very few patients reach adult life. Surgical treatment therefore is recommended even if results are less than perfect.

TREATMENT

Medical therapy is instituted where necessary to control heart failure or to correct acidosis, but successful treatment in the majority of cases is surgical.

INDICATIONS FOR SURGERY

Because the prognosis is poor (see above), surgical treatment should be implemented.

SURGICAL PROCEDURE

Initial treatment is palliative: banding to control excessive blood flow, shunting to augment diminished pulmonary flow, and reconstructive procedures on the aortic arch to offset the existence of coarctation and related lesions. It may also be necessary as a palliative measure to enlarge a restrictive VSD that impedes adequate aortic flow. This procedure, however, carries a very high risk; it may be preferable in these circumstances to create an aortopulmonary septal defect. If the patient survives such palliative procedures, which currently occurs in the majority of cases, the options for further corrective surgery are septation of the dominant or the solitary ventricle, or construction of a conduit in a modified Fontan procedure. Very few cases are suitable for the septation procedure, whereas the majority are candidates for the modified Fontan operation. It necessitates closure of the right atrioventricular valve (or the right component of a common valve) and construction of a conduit or anastomosis between the isolated right atrium and the pulmonary arteries. In well selected patients the overall mortality for this procedure is now less than 10% with good short- and intermediate-term follow-up.

DOUBLE-OUTLET RIGHT VENTRICLE
DEFINITION AND PATHOLOGY

This abnormality is said to be present when more than 50% of both great arteries arise from the morphologically right ventricle. There is usually a VSD, which is subaortic in two thirds of the patients (Fig. 3.166) and subpulmonary (the Taussig–Bing malformation) (Fig. 3.167) in 20% of patients. The VSD is related to both great arteries (doubly committed) in 3%, while it is unrelated to either great artery in the remainder (Hagler et al, 1983). Pulmonary valve stenosis occurs in over 50% of patients. Atrial septal defect, subaortic stenosis, and coarctation of the aorta are also common, while mitral valve obstruction may occur (Hagler et al, 1983; Zamora et al, 1975).

ABNORMAL PHYSIOLOGY

There is a right-to-left shunt from the right ventricle to the aorta and a left-to-right shunt through the VSD. When pulmonary stenosis is present, there is preferential flow out through the aorta. Arterial oxygen desaturation varies from slight to severe depending on the associated abnormalities.

CLINICAL MANIFESTATIONS

This condition is uncommon, occurring in 0.5% of patients with congenital heart disease. It occurs equally in males and females, and it is sometimes associated with the trisomy-18 syndrome.

SYMPTOMS

The symptoms of patients with subaortic VSDs are similar to the symptoms of patients with large VSDs. Congestive heart failure occurs early, but cyanosis may not be evident. Patients with subaortic ventricular defects in addition to pulmonary valve stenosis have natural histories similar to those with tetralogy of Fallot. Patients with subpulmonary VSDs without pulmonary valve stenosis have natural histories similar to patients with complete transposition with large VSDs without pulmonary valve stenosis.

PHYSICAL EXAMINATION

Cyanosis depends on the presence of other anomalies. A loud systolic murmur due to the VSD is heard in the midsternal area.

LABORATORY STUDIES

CHEST RADIOGRAPHY. The heart is enlarged, and pulmonary blood flow is increased in those patients without pulmonary valve stenosis. The abnormalities on chest film of a patient with double-outlet right ventricle associated with pulmonary stenosis and subaortic VSD may stimulate those of tetralogy of Fallot. Although the heart is usually larger in the former, the aortic arch may be located on the right, as it often is in patients with tetralogy of Fallot.

In patients with subpulmonary septal defects without pulmonary stenosis the pulmonary trunk is large, lying next to the aorta rather than behind it. This separates the condition from complete transposition, which it may otherwise simulate.

ELECTROCARDIOGRAPHY. The ECG shows right ventricular hypertrophy and right atrial abnormality. The mean QRS vector may be located superiorly in patients with subaortic septal defects who have no pulmonary stenosis.

ECHOCARDIOGRAPHY. The diagnosis of double-outlet right ventricle is determined by cross-sectional echocardiography when 50% of both arteries arise from the morphologically right ventricle and, in all cases, when there is mitral–semilunar valve discontinuity (Fig. 3.168) (Hagler et al, 1981).

CARDIAC CATHETERIZATION. The oxygen saturation is increased in the right ventricle, and it is lower in the pulmonary arteries than it is in the aorta in patients with subaortic septal defects. It is lower in the aorta than it is in the pulmonary arteries in patients with subpulmonary septal defects. The pressures in the right ventricle, the aorta, and the left ventricle are usually equal. The pressure in the left ventricle may be higher than the pressure in the right ventricle when the VSD is small and restrictive. Anomalies of the mitral, the aortic, and the pulmonary valves may be identified.

Angiography of the right and the left ventricles shows the VSD and the origin of the great arteries (Fig. 3.169). An aortogram is necessary

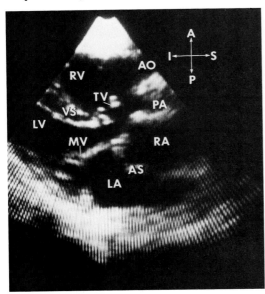
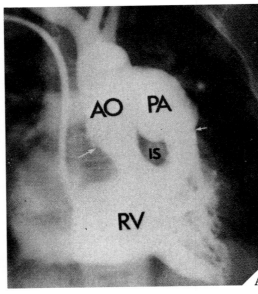
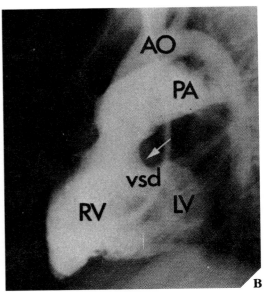

FIG. 3.168 *Cross-sectional echocardiogram in the parasternal long-axis view from a patient with double-outlet right ventricle and VSD shows that the aorta* (AO) *and the pulmonary trunk* (PA) *both arise from the right ventricle* (RV) *in a parallel orientation anterior to the ventricular septum* (VS). *There is no continuity between the posterior aortic wall and the mitral valve* (MV) (TV, *tricuspid valve;* LV, *left ventricle;* RA, *right atrium;* LA, *left atrium;* AS, *atrial septum*). *(Reproduced with permission of the authors and publisher; see Figure Credits. Also, Fig. 36-78,* The Heart, *6th ed, p 698)*

FIG. 3.169 *Right ventriculograms* (RV) *in a patient with double-outlet right ventricle, side-by-side great arteries, and subaortic VSD show on the frontal view* (**A**) *that the aorta* (AO) *lies to the right of the pulmonary trunk* (PA) *and that bilateral muscular infundibulums, with the outlet septum* (is), *separate the two semilunar outflow tracts. The semilunar valves* (arrows) *are at the same level.* (**B**) *The lateral right ventriculogram*

shows both great arteries originating from the morphologically right ventricle; the posterior morphologically left ventricle fills via the subaortic VSD (vsd). *The anterior walls of the aorta and the pulmonary trunk are in about the same plane. The VSD lies below a muscular bar* (arrow) *that prevents mitral–semilunar valve fibrous continuity. (Reproduced with permission of the authors and publisher; see Figure Credits)*

PART II: DISEASES OF THE HEART

to rule out an arterial duct, and a coronary arteriogram is needed to rule out coronary anomalies.

NATURAL HISTORY

Patients with double-outlet right ventricle without pulmonary stenosis develop severe heart failure or pulmonary arteriolar vascular disease, and usually die during the first year of life. When pulmonary stenosis is present, patients may die of increasing hypoxia. If the VSD gradually decreases in size, the patient may die.

TREATMENT

Heart failure may be treated with drugs, and hypoxia may be improved with oxygen; however, medical treatment is unsatisfactory.

INDICATIONS FOR SURGERY

Most patients with double-outlet right ventricle should have surgical correction. Infants without pulmonary stenosis should have banding of the pulmonary trunk. There is a trend now with improved surgery to correct the hearts of such infants between the ages of three and twelve months. The Taussig–Bing malformation is managed at a young age by banding and the creation of an atrial septal defect with total correction later in life. Systemic-to-pulmonary shunts are used in patients with decreased pulmonary blood flow with total correction later in life.

SURGICAL PROCEDURE

Operative options may be quite limited in this complex malformation. In a retrospective analysis of 63 hearts with double-outlet right ventricles and concordant atrioventricular connections, it was determined that more than one third did not lend themselves to corrective surgery of any type (Wilcox et al, 1981). Twenty-five cases (40%) appeared to be amenable to correction using an intracardiac baffle to channel left ventricular flow to the aorta. The remaining 15 hearts were thought to need more complex procedures, such as a venous or an arterial switch (see Figs. 3.152, 3.154) or modifications of these procedures. If one considers these 63 hearts to be fairly representative of the spectrum of malformations falling under the diagnosis of double-outlet right ventricle, it is not surprising that the operative mortality in a large series of such patients may be as high as 25%–35%. Two variables are of critical importance to operative success: the relationship of the VSD to the aorta, and the presence of associated cardiac anomalies. Thus when one is dealing with patients with subaortic septal defects and no other anomalies, it is reasonable to expect survival figures to approach those of isolated ventricular defect. However, when septal defect and the aorta are remote from each other or when subaortic or subpulmonary stenosis or an associated atrioventricular defect is also present, then the results are correspondingly less satisfactory.

DOUBLE-OUTLET LEFT VENTRICLE
DEFINITION AND PATHOLOGY

In this rarely encountered condition the aorta and the pulmonary trunk arise entirely or predominately from the left ventricle (Fig. 3.170). VSD, pulmonary stenosis, and tricuspid valve abnormalities may also be present (Van Praagh et al, 1983).

CLINICAL MANIFESTATIONS

The clinical manifestations vary according to the associated lesions. Angiography is necessary to separate this malformation from clinically similar conditions, such as tetralogy of Fallot, tricuspid atresia, or complete transposition.

TREATMENT

Surgical experience is limited because the condition is so rare (Villani et al, 1979). A systemic-to-pulmonary arterial shunt can be created when there is pulmonary stenosis. In other cases the VSD and the subpulmonary outlet may be closed, and a right ventricle–pulmonary artery conduit with a valve may be created. If right ventricular hypoplasia or tricuspid valve disease is present, a right atrium–pulmonary artery conduit may be used (Fontan-type procedure). With this procedure it may be necessary to close the tricuspid valve orifice and an atrial septal defect if present.

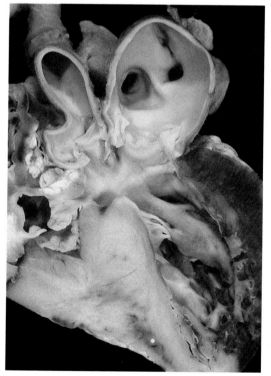

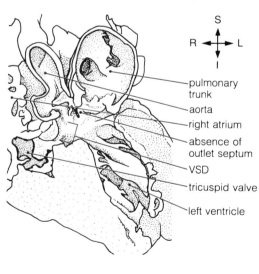

FIG. 3.170 *A simulated four-chamber long-axis section through the ventricular outlets of this heart shows a double outlet from the left ventricle.*

S
R ← → L
I

- pulmonary trunk
- aorta
- right atrium
- absence of outlet septum
- VSD
- tricuspid valve
- left ventricle

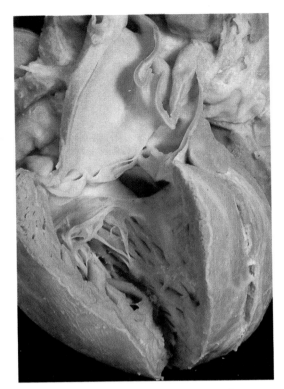

FIG. 3.171 *The right ventricular aspect of this heart exposes a common arterial trunk. The common truncal valve overrides a subarterial VSD with a muscular posterointerior rim. The pulmonary arteries arise from a short confluent channel that originates from the common trunk (type 1).*

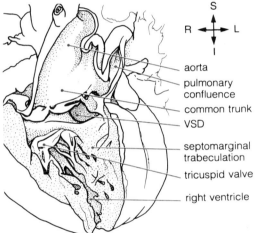

S
R — L
I

aorta
pulmonary confluence
common trunk
VSD
septomarginal trabeculation
tricuspid valve
right ventricle

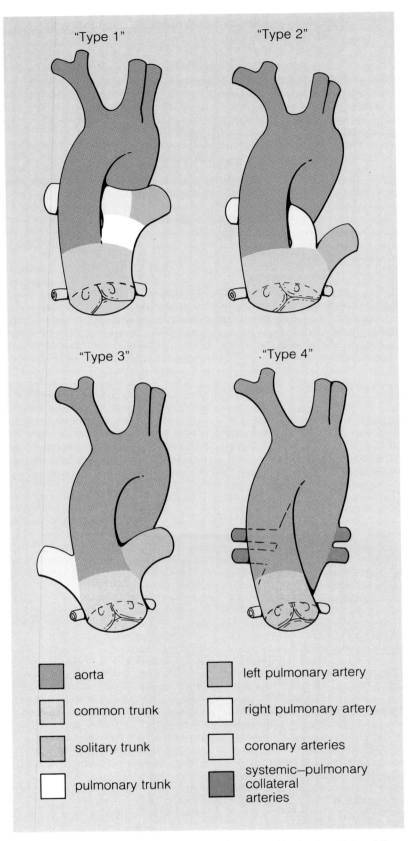

"Type 1"   "Type 2"

"Type 3"   ."Type 4"

aorta   left pulmonary artery

common trunk   right pulmonary artery

solitary trunk   coronary arteries

pulmonary trunk   systemic–pulmonary collateral arteries

FIG. 3.172 *This diagram demonstrates the variability in the origin of the pulmonary arteries from a common arterial trunk; four types are conventionally described. The so-called type 4 is not strictly a common trunk, since the intrapericardial pulmonary arteries are completely absent, and blood supply to the lungs is derived from systemic–pulmonary collateral arteries and supplied directly to intraparenchymal branches. While it can be argued embryologically that the trunk in this circumstance is common, it could also be an aorta. It is preferable to describe it simply and accurately as a solitary arterial trunk.*

COMMON ARTERIAL TRUNK
DEFINITION AND PATHOLOGY

When a single artery leaves the heart through a common valve above a VSD to supply the systemic, pulmonary, and coronary arteries, it is labeled a common arterial trunk or truncus arteriosus (Fig. 3.171). There are four types of common arterial trunks (Fig. 3.172). The first type (see Fig. 3.171) is characterized by partial separation of the common trunk, so that a vestige of the pulmonary trunk is present; the pulmonary arteries pass to the lungs from this vestige. In the second variant the right and the left pulmonary arteries arise separately from the posterior portion of the common trunk. The third type is rare; characteristically the right and the left pulmonary arteries arise from the lateral aspects of the common trunk (Collett and Edwards, 1949). The fourth type, also the most controversial, is characterized by a solitary trunk with total absence of the intrapericardial pulmonary arteries. The argument centers on whether the solitary trunk in this setting is an aorta or a common trunk. It is probably best described simply as a solitary arterial trunk; clinically it is considered an example of pulmonary atresia with VSD (see above).

A common trunk can be identified when it can be shown that the coronary arteries, the aorta, and the pulmonary arteries arise directly from it. Other abnormalities are associated with this defect. Obstructive lesions, in particular interruption of the arch (Fig. 3.173), may occur in the aortic pathway from the trunk. The descending aorta is then supplied through the arterial duct. A right aortic arch occurs in about 20% of patients, and a single coronary artery occurs in 5%. Branches of the right coronary artery may traverse the anterior wall of the right ventricle (Anderson et al, 1978). One of the pulmonary arteries may be absent. The truncal valve may be abnormal with two to five leaflets (Gelband et al, 1972).

ABNORMAL PHYSIOLOGY

Patients with common arterial trunks (types 1, 2, 3) have an increase in pulmonary blood flow, because the contents of the right and the left ventricles are expelled into the common conduit from which the pulmonary arteries arise. There is a slight decrease in P_{O_2}.

Type 4 presents more usually as pulmonary atresia with a VSD. The condition of patients with duct-dependent blood supply is more precarious than that of patients in whom the blood supply is through the bronchial arteries. The collateral arteries give surprisingly good blood supply during the neonatal period. Fortunately this congenital anomaly is rare.

CLINICAL MANIFESTATIONS
SYMPTOMS

The symptoms and the signs of a common arterial trunk depend on the amount of pulmonary blood flow. Most patients have an increase in pulmonary blood flow. Heart failure may be severe, and poor growth is evident during the first few weeks of life. Patients with solitary trunks are severely hypoxic and die early in life.

PHYSICAL EXAMINATION

Cyanosis may be noted in patients with type 1, 2, or 3 common arterial trunk; it is more severe when the pulmonary arteries are small. The systemic arterial pulsation may be prominent. An abnormal parasternal lift may be noted, and the apex impulse may be large. The second heart sound is single, and a systolic click may be detected. A systolic murmur may be heard in the third and the fourth intercostal spaces near the left sternal border. Truncal regurgitation is commonly heard. A continuous murmur may be heard over the lung fields due to the torrential increase in pulmonary arterial blood flow.

FIG. 3.173 *In this heart with a common arterial trunk the descending aorta is supplied from the common trunk via an arterial duct. The interruption of the aortic arch is between the left common carotid and the left subclavian arteries.*

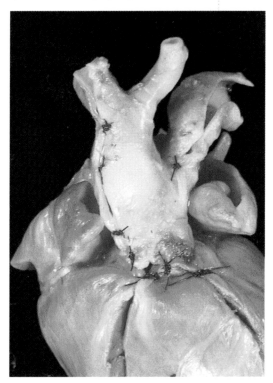

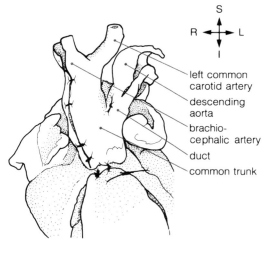

left common carotid artery

descending aorta

brachio-cephalic artery

duct

common trunk

LABORATORY STUDIES

CHEST RADIOGRAPHY. The chest film reveals a large heart, a large arterial trunk, and increased pulmonary blood flow. A right aortic arch is common (Fig. 3.174). In rare cases the pulmonary arteries are small, the heart may be only slightly enlarged, and the pulmonary blood flow may be normal or decreased.

ELECTROCARDIOGRAPHY. The ECG shows increased QRS voltage and biventricular hypertrophy (Fig. 3.175).

ECHOCARDIOGRAPHY. Two separate arterial valves cannot be recorded, and the left atrium may be enlarged. Otherwise the M-mode echocardiogram is similar to that of tetralogy of Fallot. Cross-sectional echocardiography can distinguish between these diagnoses when the pulmonary arterial origin is visualized (Fig. 3.176).

CARDIAC CATHETERIZATION. Bidirectional shunting and systemic arterial oxygen desaturation are observed. When the pulmonary arteries are small, the oxygen desaturation may be severe. An effort must be made to advance the catheter into both pulmonary arteries. Pulmonary hypertension is usually present, and the pulmonary vascular resistance must be determined.

Right ventricular angiography is used to identify the VSD and to visualize the arterial trunk and the pulmonary arteries. Angiographic study of a solitary arterial trunk reveals no central pulmonary arteries; the lungs are supplied through large systemic-to-pulmonary collateral arteries.

NATURAL HISTORY
The majority of children with common arterial trunk, if untreated surgically, die before the age of one year of heart failure and severe pulmonary vascular disease. A few have complications of erythrocytosis and endocarditis. Patients with small pulmonary arteries live longer.

TREATMENT
Medical treatment is limited to drug therapy for heart failure and hypoxia.

INDICATIONS FOR SURGERY
Infants with heart failure should have corrective surgery during the first few months of life. Banding of the pulmonary arteries is used by some surgeons, followed sometime later with more definitive surgery. Other surgeons prefer to correct the anomalies to the greatest extent possible at the first operation.

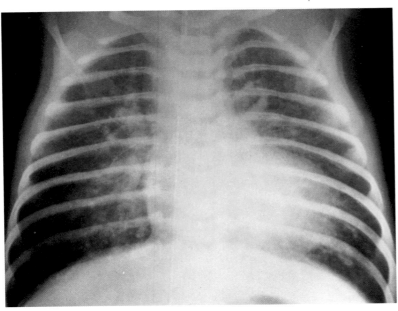

FIG. 3.174 *Posteroanterior chest radiograph of an infant with common arterial trunk shows mild cardiomegaly, increased pulmonary vascular markings, and a right aortic arch. (Fig. 36-113, The Heart, 5th ed; see Figure Credits. Courtesy of the X-Ray Department, Henrietta Egleston Hospital for Children, Atlanta, Georgia)*

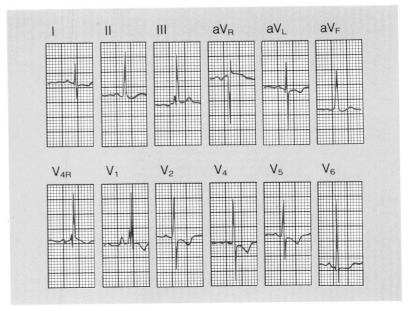

FIG. 3.175 *In this ECG of a three-year-old child with common arterial trunk the P waves are prominent and peaked in lead V_1, suggesting right atrial abnormality. The mean QRS vector is vertical and anteriorly directed. The QRS complex is large. The mean T vector is directed inferiorly and posteriorly. (Courtesy of the Electrocardiography Laboratory, Henrietta Egleston Hospital for Children, Atlanta, Georgia)*

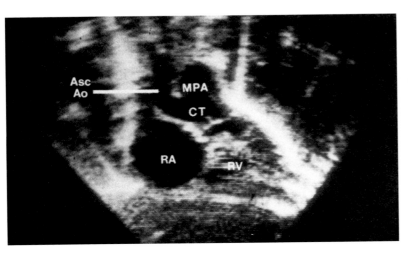

FIG. 3.176 *Cross-sectional echocardiogram in the subxiphoid long-axis view (L-3) from a patient with common arterial trunk and an interrupted aortic arch shows that the pulmonary artery segment is large and the ascending aorta (Asc Ao) is small. No transverse aortic arch can be seen from any view, since the ascending aorta ends at the left carotid branch (CT, common trunk; MPA, pulmonary trunk; RA, right atrium; RV, right ventricle). (Reproduced with permission of the authors and publisher; see Figure Credits)*

The type of surgery performed depends on the anatomy of the pulmonary arteries, the pulmonary arterial pressure and the degree of pulmonary vascular disease. Accordingly the surgeon has three options: pulmonary artery banding; removal of the pulmonary arteries from the trunk with anastomosis to a valve-containing conduit that is anastomosed to the right ventricle, closure of the VSD, and correction of the truncal regurgitation with a valve; or a systemic-to-pulmonary shunt when the pulmonary arteries are small and restrictive.

SURGICAL PROCEDURE

The technical aspects of operating on patients with common arterial trunk have been greatly facilitated by the use of improved conduits. The ease of insertion and the lack of postoperative bleeding recommend the use of fresh-frozen allografts when available; Figure 3.177 illustrates the anatomic abnormalities associated with a common arterial trunk. The condition was corrected by using a conduit such as described above.

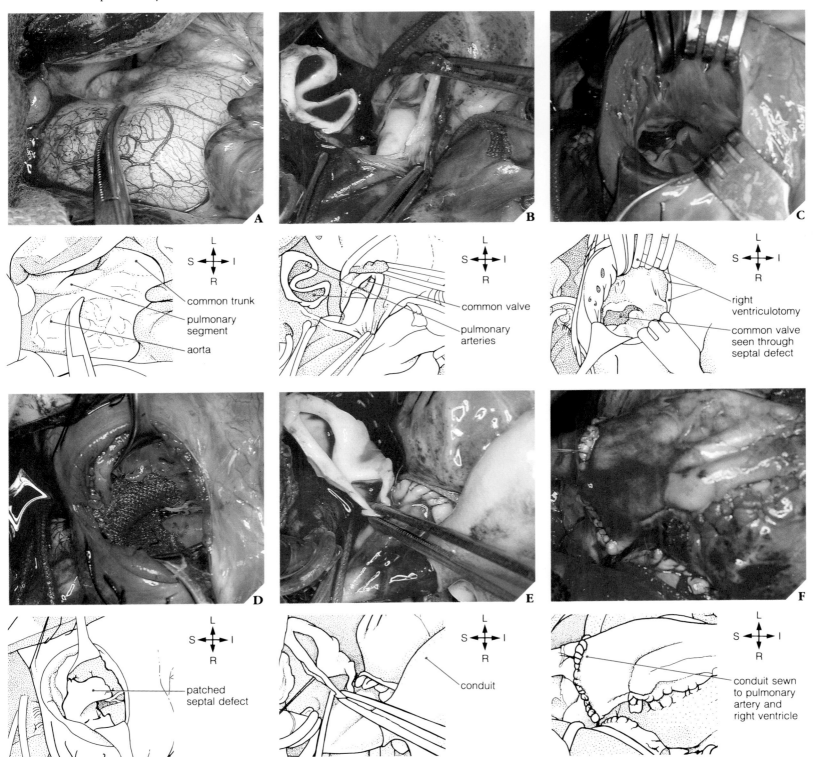

FIG. 3.177   (A) *In repair of a common arterial trunk, as seen through a median sternotomy, the common trunk arises from the base of the heart. The short segment of pulmonary trunk is behind and to the left of the aorta.* (B) *When this is divided, the two pulmonary arterial branches are readily seen.* (C) *Incision into the right ventricular wall allows visualiza-* *tion of the common valve through the VSD.* (D) *The septal defect is patched, isolating the right ventricular chamber.* (E) *Careful measurement of the conduit is necessary to avoid kinking.* (F) *Distal and proximal anastomoses are then effected using continuous monofilament sutures.*

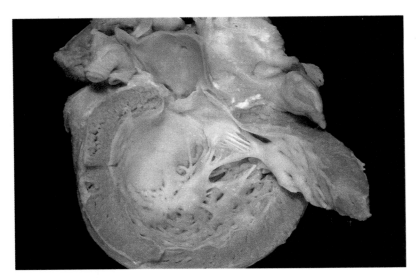

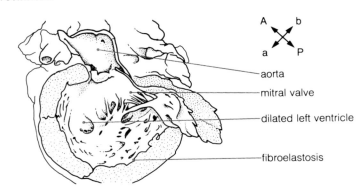

FIG. 3.178 *The left ventricle is large in the dilated form of endocardial fibroelastosis.*

aorta

mitral valve

dilated left ventricle

fibroelastosis

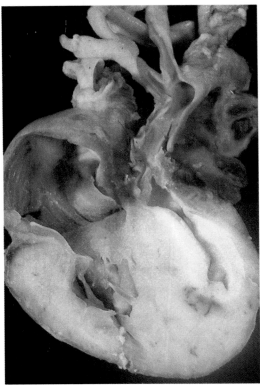

FIG. 3.179 *The much rarer variant of primary constricted endocardial fibroelastosis of the left ventricle is shown in this simulated four-chamber long-axis section. The subaortic outflow tract is patent. This type of constricted fibroelastosis is more usually found in the setting of aortic atresia and intact ventricular septum.*

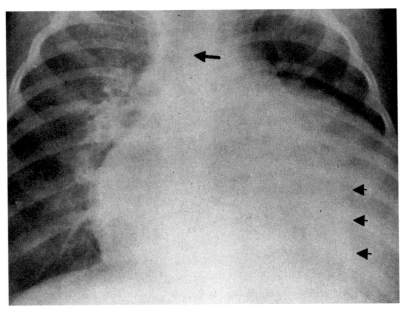

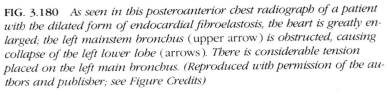

FIG. 3.180 *As seen in this posteroanterior chest radiograph of a patient with the dilated form of endocardial fibroelastosis, the heart is greatly enlarged; the left mainstem bronchus (upper arrow) is obstructed, causing collapse of the left lower lobe (arrows). There is considerable tension placed on the left main bronchus. (Reproduced with permission of the authors and publisher; see Figure Credits)*

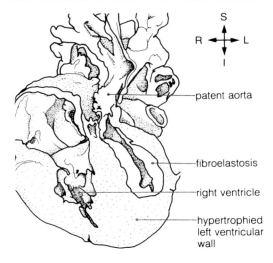

patent aorta

fibroelastosis

right ventricle

hypertrophied left ventricular wall

PART II: DISEASES OF THE HEART

ENDOCARDIAL FIBROELASTOSIS
DEFINITION AND PATHOLOGY

Fibroelastosis is the proliferation of elastic and collagenous fibers in the endocardial region of the heart. Predominately the left ventricle tends to be involved and may be *dilated* or *contracted.*

The left ventricular cavity may be large, and the myocardial wall may be thick. This *dilated type* of endocardial fibroelastosis (Fig. 3.178) may be primary or secondary. Conditions associated with the secondary variety are aortic valve stenosis, coarctation of the aorta, anomalous origin of the coronary arteries from the pulmonary trunk, and left-to-right shunts. In the *contracted type* the left ventricle cavity may be smaller than normal (Fig. 3.179). This condition may occasionally be associated with aortic atresia.

ABNORMAL PHYSIOLOGY

The abnormal physiology is determined by the associated lesions. When no other lesions are present, the heart may be large in the dilated variety; heart failure may be present, and there is a decrease in left ventricular compliance.

CLINICAL MANIFESTATIONS

Fibroelastosis that is unassociated with other congenital lesions (primary fibroelastosis) occurs in infancy. The incidence is about 1% in the population of patients with congenital heart disease. It occurs more often in males than females with a ratio of about 1.5:1. When heart failure seems out of proportion to the severity of coarctation of the aorta or aortic stenosis, fibroelastosis may be a factor.

SYMPTOMS

Patients have symptoms of heart failure, including grunting respirations, cough, and weakness. A respiratory infection may precipitate heart failure.

PHYSICAL EXAMINATION

The abnormalities found on physical examination depend on the associated lesions (secondary fibroelastosis). The patient, however, has signs of heart failure whether the condition is primary or secondary. Rales may be heard in the lungs, and the liver may be large. The heart is large in the dilated type, and gallop rhythm is present.

LABORATORY STUDIES

CHEST RADIOGRAPHY.   The heart is greatly enlarged in the dilated variant of the disease (Fig. 3.180).

ELECTROCARDIOGRAPHY.   The ECG shows left ventricular hypertrophy (Fig. 3.181); left atrial or biatrial abnormalities may also be seen. Tall T waves in the midprecordial leads should suggest carnitine deficiency, which may result in fibroelastosis (Tripp et al, 1981). Low voltage may be present on rare occasion.

ECHOCARDIOGRAPHY.   Cross-sectional echocardiography (Fig. 3.182) may show a dilated left ventricle that contracts poorly in the primary dilated type of fibroelastosis, or a small left ventricular cavity in the contracted type.

CARDIAC CATHETERIZATION.   Cardiac catheterization reveals an elevated left ventricular diastolic pressure and elevated left atrial and pulmonary wedge pressures. Left ventriculography shows a dilated left ventricle with poor contractility in the dilated type of fibroelastosis. The left ventricular cavity is small in the contracted type.

NATURAL HISTORY

This disease is serious. Many patients die early in life, the majority during the first year. Decongestive measures may help increase survival. Patients who survive until the age of five have a chance of long-

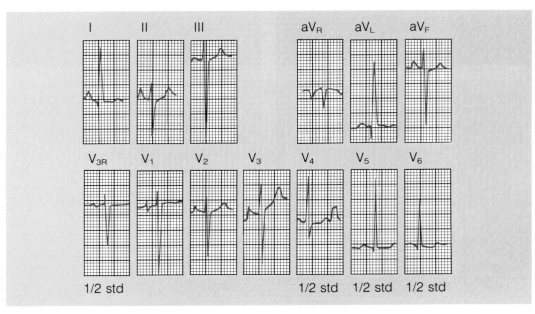

FIG. 3.181   *The salient feature of this ECG from an infant with endocardial fibroelastosis is leftward deviation of the mean QRS vector. There is also a deep S wave in lead V₁ and a very tall R wave in leads V₅ and V₆, which is interpretable as left ventricular hypertrophy. (Redrawn; reproduced with permission of the authors and publisher; see Figure Credits)*

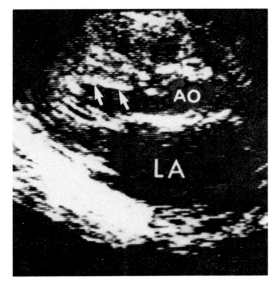

FIG. 3.182   *Parasternal long-axis cross-sectional echocardiogram from a patient with subendocardial fibroelastosis shows that the ventricular cavity is small, and a dense rim of echo-producing material surrounds the endocardial surface of the ventricle* (arrows) (AO, *aorta;* LA, *left atrium*). *(Reproduced with permission of the authors and publisher; see Figure Credits)*

term survival; however, it is not definite whether these patients have fibroelastosis or myocarditis, since the diagnosis is only confirmed at autopsy. This condition may be complicated by the occurrence of systemic emboli.

TREATMENT

Patients with heart failure should be treated with digitalis and diuretics; respiratory infections should be promptly treated. The careful management of these patients leads to an improved survival. There is no surgical treatment except cardiac transplantation in selected patients.

AORTIC ARCH ANOMALIES

There are many anomalies of the aortic arch; important examples are a double arch (Fig. 3.183) and retroesophageal origin of one subclavian artery (Fig. 3.184). The latter anomaly may coexist with interruption of a segment of the arch (Fig. 3.185); the descending aorta is then supplied by an arterial duct. The symptoms and the signs of aortic arch abnormalities are determined by the impingement upon adjacent structures, particularly the trachea and the esophagus. If symptoms are present, it is necessary to divide surgically a segment of the encircling arteries (Figs. 3.186, 3.187).

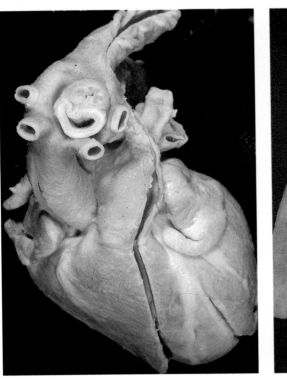

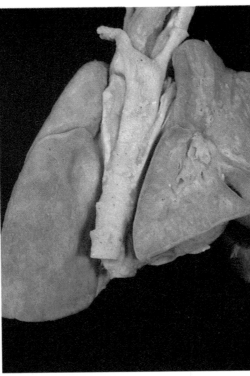

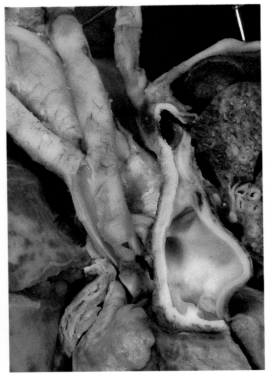

FIG. 3.183 *A complete double aortic arch encircles the tracheoesophageal pedicle. Each arch gives rise to a subclavian and a carotid artery; there is a central descending aorta.*

FIG. 3.184 *Retroesophageal origin of the right subclavian artery is seen in the setting of a left-sided aortic arch and a right-sided descending aorta in this specimen, photographed from behind.*

FIG. 3.185 *Interruption of the aortic arch between the left common carotid and the left subclavian arteries is seen in association with retroesophageal origin of the right subclavian artery from the descending aorta, which is fed through an arterial duct from the pulmonary trunk.*

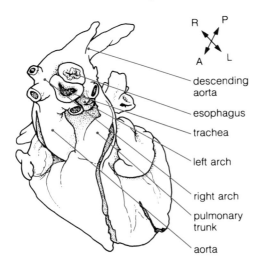

descending aorta

esophagus

trachea

left arch

right arch

pulmonary trunk

aorta

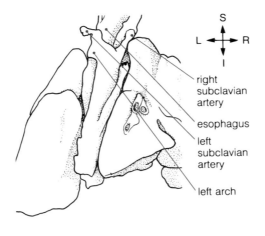

right subclavian artery

esophagus

left subclavian artery

left arch

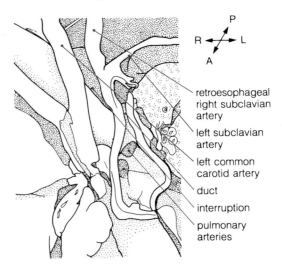

retroesophageal right subclavian artery

left subclavian artery

left common carotid artery

duct

interruption

pulmonary arteries

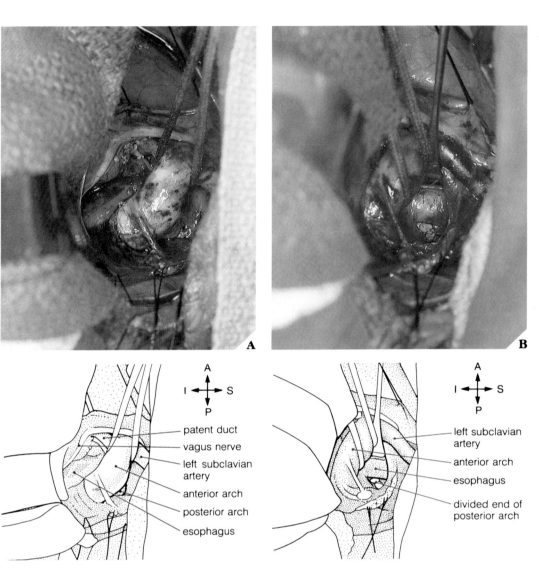

patent duct
vagus nerve
left subclavian artery
anterior arch
posterior arch
esophagus

left subclavian artery
anterior arch
esophagus
divided end of posterior arch

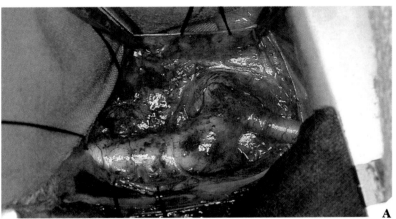

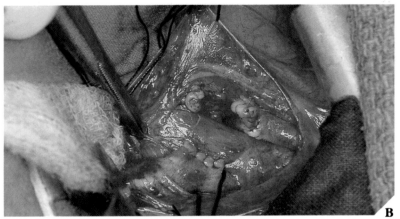

FIG. 3.187 *In another example of a double aortic arch encircling the esophagus* (A) *the anterior segment is divided to relieve the obstruction* (B).

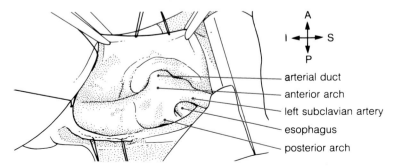

arterial duct
anterior arch
left subclavian artery
esophagus
posterior arch

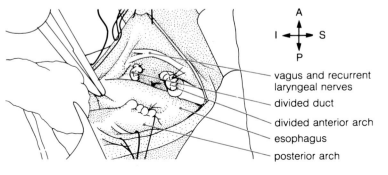

vagus and recurrent laryngeal nerves
divided duct
divided anterior arch
esophagus
posterior arch

CONGENITAL HEART DISEASE

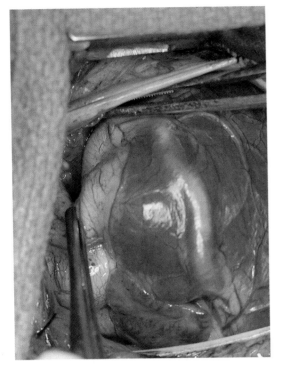

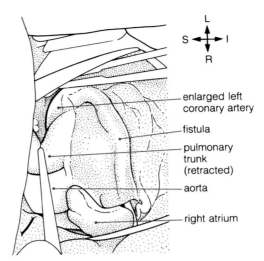

FIG. 3.188 *Operative view shows a large fistula extending between the enlarged left coronary artery and the cavity of the right ventricle.*

enlarged left coronary artery

fistula

pulmonary trunk (retracted)

aorta

right atrium

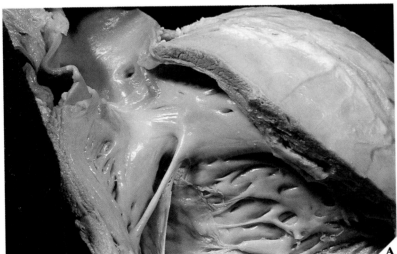

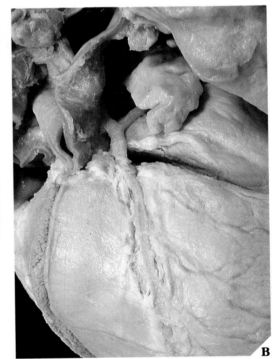

FIG. 3.189 *In this example of anomalous origin of the left coronary artery from the pulmonary trunk the opened pulmonary trunk (A) reveals the coronary orifice, and the course of the artery can be seen (B). (Courtesy of A. Smith, MD, Liverpool, UK)*

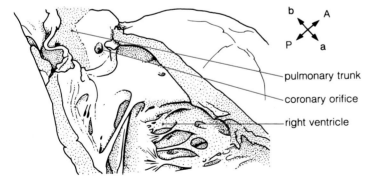

pulmonary trunk

coronary orifice

right ventricle

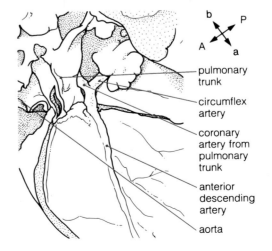

pulmonary trunk

circumflex artery

coronary artery from pulmonary trunk

anterior descending artery

aorta

PART II: DISEASES OF THE HEART

ANOMALIES OF THE CORONARY ARTERIES

Many anomalies of the coronary arteries have been identified since the advent of coronary arteriography. Only two anomalies are discussed here: coronary arteriovenous fistula (Fig. 3.188) and origin of the left coronary artery from the pulmonary trunk (Figs. 3.189, 3.190).

A coronary arteriovenous fistula is usually recognized by the presence of a continuous murmur over the precordium below the area where the murmur of a patent arterial duct is usually heard. Left ventriculography and coronary arteriography confirm the diagnosis (Fig. 3.191).

When the left coronary artery arises from the pulmonary trunk (see Fig. 3.189), the patent may develop myocardial damage (see Fig. 3.190). The ECG may show myocardial infarction (Fig. 3.192). An infant may appear to be in pain from the effort of sucking a bottle. The ECG may

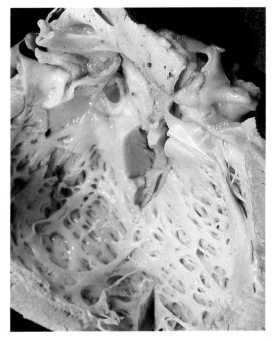

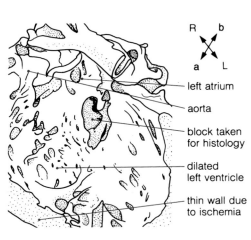

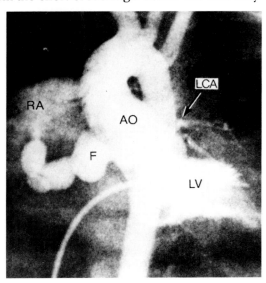

FIG. 3.191 *Posteroanterior view of a left ventricular* (LV) *angiogram in a child shows a coronary arteriovenous fistula* (F) *from the left coronary artery* (LCA) *to the right atrium* (RA) (AO, *aorta*). (*Fig. 36-149,* The Heart, *5th ed; see Figure Credits*)

FIG. 3.190 *This dilated and ischemic left ventricle is found in the setting of anomalous origin of the left coronary artery from the pulmonary trunk. (Courtesy of A. Smith, MD, Liverpool, UK)*

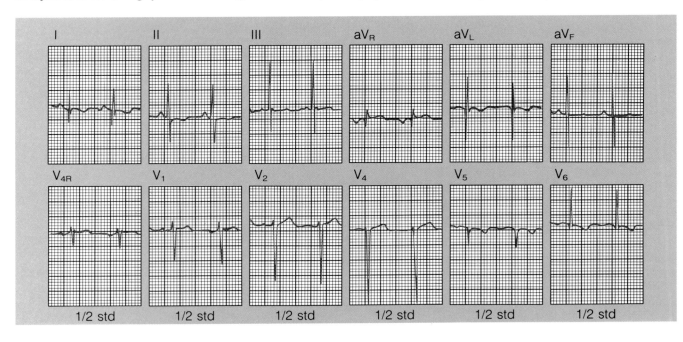

FIG. 3.192 *Twelve-lead ECG in an infant whose left coronary artery originates from the pulmonary trunk demonstrates the pattern of anterolateral infarction (chest leads recorded at one half standard voltage). (Redrawn; Fig. 36-86,* The Heart, *6th ed, p 709)*

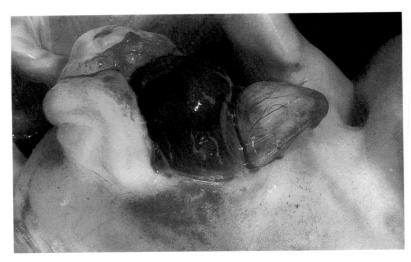

FIG. 3.193 *An extrathoracic heart (ectopia cordis) was found along with exomphalos in a fetus; the heart also exhibits tricuspid atresia.*

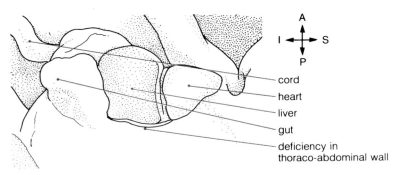

cord
heart
liver
gut
deficiency in
thoraco-abdominal wall

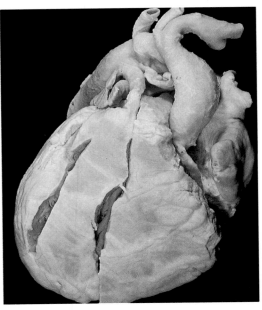

FIG. 3.194 *This anatomically normal heart was dissected from an individual with mirror-image arrangement of all the organs but with no cardiac abnormalities. The heart was positioned within the right chest, its apex pointing to the right. There is mirror-image atrial arrangement, and the pulmonary trunk is anterior and to the right of the aorta.*

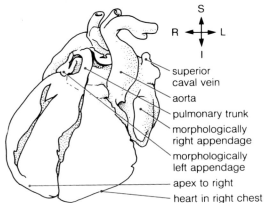

superior
caval vein
aorta
pulmonary trunk
morphologically
right appendage
morphologically
left appendage
apex to right
heart in right chest

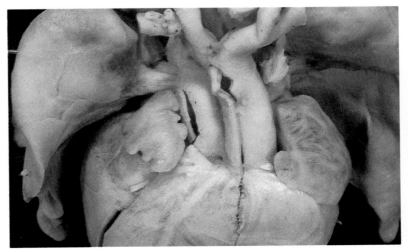

FIG. 3.195 *This specimen, viewed from the anterior aspect of the base of the heart, was obtained from an individual with mirror-image atrial arrangement and complete transposition. The heart was located in the right chest with its apex pointing to the right; the aorta is anterior and to the left of the pulmonary trunk.*

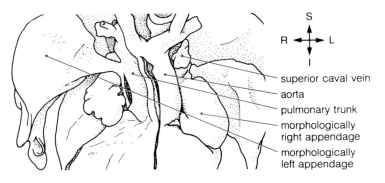

superior caval vein
aorta
pulmonary trunk
morphologically
right appendage
morphologically
left appendage

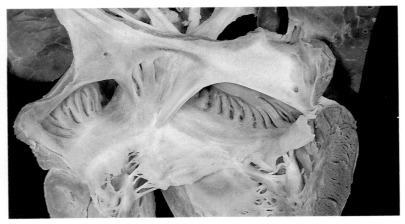

FIG. 3.196 *The internal aspect of the common atrial chamber of an individual with right atrial isomerism and congenital asplenia shows the bilateral terminal crests, each giving rise to obvious pectinate muscles. There is a double inlet to a dominant left ventricle through a common atrioventricular valve.*

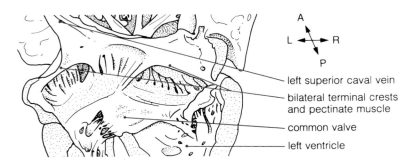

left superior caval vein
bilateral terminal crests
and pectinate muscle
common valve
left ventricle

show ST-segment displacement during the episode (see Fig. 3.192). Endocardial fibroelastosis may also be present in such patients. Both these types of coronary anomalies may be corrected by surgery.

MALPOSITION OF THE HEART

The normally positioned heart lies in the left chest with its apex pointing to the left. Malposition exists whenever the heart is located elsewhere or its apex points other than to the left. The extreme malposition is an extrathoracic heart, or ectopia cordis (Fig. 3.193). Other malpositions occur either with abnormal arrangements of the entire body organs, abnormal connections of the cardiac segments, or an extracardiac deformity that shifts the heart within the chest. The best known abnormal organ arrangement is mirror-image arrangement, or situs inversus. It is exceedingly rare to find this condition with a completely normal heart (Fig. 3.194). More usually there is either

complete (Fig. 3.195) or corrected transposition. Much more common than mirror-image arrangement are the two abnormal arrangements associated with the splenic disorders, asplenia and polysplenia. These syndromes of visceral heterotaxy are best analyzed in terms of right (Fig. 3.196) or left (Fig. 3.197) atrial isomerism. The thoracic organs (lungs and bronchi) also show evidence of right or left isomerism (Fig. 3.198). The abnormal chamber connection most usually associated with abnormal cardiac position is congenitally corrected transposition, but double-inlet ventricle is also associated with an abnormal location of the heart. Pulmonary problems, such as pneumothorax, may distort the position of the heart. Hypoplasia of one lung characteristically is associated with a right-sided heart in the scimitar syndrome. Cardiac malposition is not a diagnosis in its own right, but it indicates the likelihood of intracardiac lesions. Each case must be assessed on its own merits.

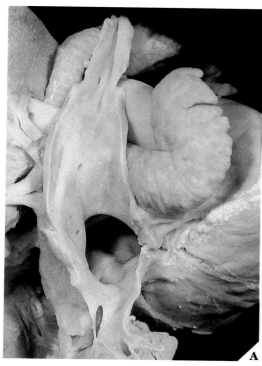
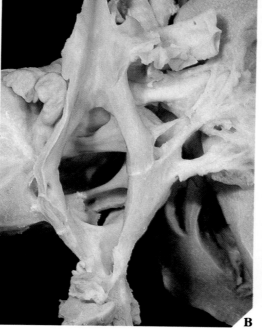
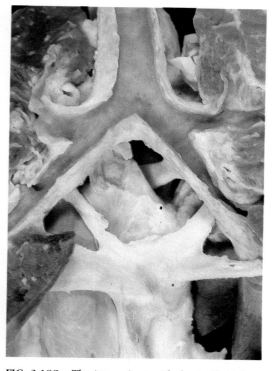

FIG. 3.197 *The right (A) and left (B) aspects of the atrial chambers of bilaterally left morphology from an individual with left atrial isomerism*

show the bilateral superior caval veins, each connecting to their respective atria in the fashion of a persistent left superior caval vein.

FIG. 3.198 *The isomeric morphologically right bronchi, seen here from the posterior aspect, were found in an individual with right atrial isomerism and congenital asplenia. The pulmonary veins have an anomalous connection to the midline aspect of the common atrial chamber, which anteriorly had two appendages of right morphology.*

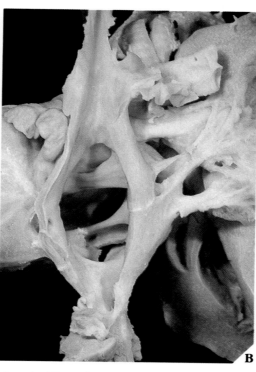

S
P ← → A
I

right-sided superior caval vein

right-sided morphologically left appendage

right pulmonary veins

coronary sinus

hepatic vein

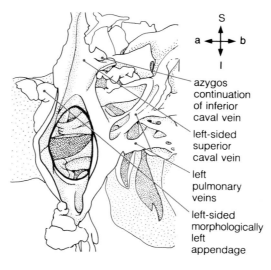

S
a ← → b
I

azygos continuation of inferior caval vein

left-sided superior caval vein

left pulmonary veins

left-sided morphologically left appendage

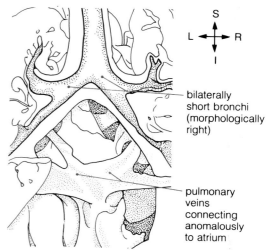

S
L ← → R
I

bilaterally short bronchi (morphologically right)

pulmonary veins connecting anomalously to atrium

REFERENCES

Alpert BS, Cook DH, Varghese PJ, Rowe RD (1979) Spontaneous closure of small ventricular septal defects: 10-year follow-up. *Pediatrics* 63:204.

Anderson KR, McGoon DC, Lie JT (1978) Surgical significance of the coronary arterial anatomy in truncus arteriosus communis. *Am J Cardiol* 41:76.

Barr PA, Celermajer JM, Bowdler JD, Cartmill TB (1974) Severe congenital tricuspid incompetence in the neonate. *Circulation* 49:962.

Becker AE, Anderson RH (1982) Atrioventricular septal defects: What's in a name? *J Thorac Cardiovasc Surg* 83:461.

Becker AE, Becker MJ, Edwards JE (1971) Pathologic spectrum of dysplasia of the tricuspid valve. Features in common with Ebstein's malformations. *Arch Pathol* 91:167.

Bertranaou EG, Blackstone EH, Hazelrig JB, Turner ME Jr, Kirklin JW (1978) Life expectancy without surgery in tetralogy of Fallot. *Am J Cardiol* 42:458.

Bharati S, Lev M (1973) Congenital poly-valvular disease. *Circulation* 47:575.

Blake HAR, Hall J, Manion WC (1965) Anomalous pulmonary venous return. *Circulation* 32:406.

Bonchek LI, Starr A, Sunderland CO, Menashe VD (1973) Natural history of tetralogy of Fallot in infancy: Clinical classification and therapeutic implications. *Circulation* 48:386.

Capelli H, Andrade JL, Somerville J (1983) Classification of the site of ventricular septal defect by 2-dimensional echocardiography. *Am J Cardiol* 51:1474.

Clagett OT, Kirklin JW, Edwards JE (1954) Anatomic variations and pathologic changes in 124 cases of coarctation of the aorta. *Surg Gynecol Obstet* 98:103.

Collett RW, Edwards JE (1949) Persistent truncus arteriosus: A classification according to anatomic types. *Surg Clin North Am* 29:1245.

Collins–Nakai RL, Rosenthal A, Castaneda AR, Bernhard WF, Nadas AS (1977) Congenital mitral stenosis: A review of 20 years' experience. *Circulation* 56:1039.

Dick M, Fyler DC, Nadas AS (1975) Tricuspid atresia: Clinical course in 101 patients. *Am J Cardiol* 36:327.

Edwards JE (1979) Classification of congenital heart disease in the adult, in Roberts WC (ed): *Congenital Heart Disease in Adults, Cardiovasc Clin* series 10/1. Philadelphia, FA Davis Company, p 1.

Edwards JE (1966) The pathology of atrial septal defect. *Semin Roentgenol* 1:24.

Ellis FH Jr, Kirklin JW (1962) Congenital valvular aortic stenosis: Anatomic findings and surgical technique. *J Thorac Surg* 43:199.

Ferencz C (1960) The pulmonary vascular bed in tetralogy of Fallot: I. Changes associated with pulmonary stenosis. *Bull Johns Hopkins Hosp* 106:81.

Fontan F, Baudet E (1971) Surgical repair of tricuspid atresia. *Thorax* 26:240.

Freed MD, Rosenthal A, Bernhard WF, Litwin SB, Nadas AS (1973) Critical pulmonary stenosis with diminutive right ventricle in neonates. *Circulation* 48:875.

Freedom RM, Culham G, Moes F, Olley PM, Rowe RD (1978) Differentiation of functional and structural pulmonary atresia: Role of angiography. *Am J Cardiol* 41:914.

Fyler DC (1980) Report of the New England regional infant cardiac program. *Pediatrics* 65(suppl 2):375.

Gasul BM, Lendrum BL, Arcilla RA (1960) Congenital aplasia or marked hypoplasia of the myocardium of the right ventricle (Uhl's anomaly). *Circulation* 22:752.

Gatham GE, Nadas AS (1970) Total anomalous pulmonary venous connection. Clinical and physiologic observations of 75 pediatric patients. *Circulation* 42:143.

Gay JH, Daily WJR, Meyer BHP, Trump DS, Cloud DT, Moltham ME (1973) Litigation of the patent ductus arteriosus in premature infants: Report of 45 cases. *J Pediatr Surg* 8:677.

Gelband H, Van Meter S, Gersony WM (1972) Truncal valve abnormalities in infants with persistent truncus arteriosus. A clinicopathologic study. *Circulation* 45:397.

Gersony WM, Peckman GJ, Ellison RC, Miettinen OS, Nadas AS (1983) Effects of indomethacin in premature infants with patent ductus arteriosus: Results of a national collaborative study. *J Pediatr* 102:895.

Gittenberger–de Groot AC, Wenink ACG (1984) Mitral artresia. Morphological details. *Br Heart J* 51:252.

Giuliani ER, Fuster V, Brandenburg RO, Mair DD (1979) Ebstein's anomaly: The clinical features and natural history of Ebstein's anomaly of the tricuspid valve. *Mayo Clin Proc* 54:163.

Graham TP Jr (1979) The Eisenmenger reaction and its management, in Roberts WC (ed): *Congenital Heart Disease in Adults*. Philadelphia, FA Davis Company, p 531.

Gutgesell HP, Garson A, McNamara DG (1979) Prognosis for the newborn with transportation of the great arteries. *Am J Cardiol* 44:96.

Guyton RA, Owens JE, Waumett JD, Dooley KJ, Hatcher CR Jr, Williams WH (1983) The Blalock-Taussig shunt: Low risk, effective palliation, and pulmonary artery growth. *J Thorac Cardiovasc Surg* 85:917.

Hagler DJ, Ritter DG, Puga FJ (1983) Doublet-outlet right ventricle, in Adams FH, Emmanouilides GC (eds): *Moss' Heart Disease in Infants, Children, and Adolescents*. Baltimore, Williams & Wilkins, p 351.

Hagler DJ, Tajik AJ, Seward JB, Mair DD, Ritter DG (1981) Double-outlet right ventricle, wide-angle two-dimensional echocardiographic observations. *Circulation* 63:419.

Hamilton WT, Haffajee CE, Dalen JE, Dexter L, Nadas AS (1979) Atrial septal defect sedundum: Clinical profile with physiologic correlates in children and adults, in Roberts WC (ed): *Congenital Heart Disease in Adults*. Philadelphia, FA Davis Company, p 267.

Hamilton WF, Abbott ME (1928) Coarctation of aorta of adult type; complete obliteration of descending arch at insertion of ductus in boy of 14; bicuspid aortic valve; impending rupture of the aorta; cerebral death; statistical study and historical retrospect of 200 recorded cases, with autopsy, of stenosis or obliteration of descending arch in subjects above age of 2 years. *Am Heart J* 3:381.

Hashimoto R, Miyamura H, Eguchi S (1984) Congenital aortic regurgitation in a child with a tricuspid non-stenotic aortic valve. *Br Heart J* 51:358.

Haworth SG (1983) Pulmonary vascular disease in secundum atrial septal defect in childhood. *Am J Cardiol* 51:265.

Heymann MA, Rudolph AM (1977) Ductus arteriosus dilatation by prostaglandin E_1 in infants with pulmonary atresia. *Pediatrics* 59:325.

Hoffman JIE, Christianson R (1978) Congenital heart disease in a cohort of 19,502 births with long-term follow up. *Am J Cardiol* 42:641.

Houston AB, Gregory NL, Coleman EN (1977) Two-dimensional sector scanner echocardiography in cyanotic congenital heart disease. *Br Heart J* 39:1076.

Jatene AD, Fontes VF, Paulista TP, et al (1976) Anatomic correction of transposition of the great vessels. *J Thorac Cardiovasc Surg* 72:364.

Keith JD, Rowe RD, Vlad P (1978) *Heart Disease in Infancy and Childhood*, 3rd ed. New York, Macmillan.

Kirklin JW (1973) Surgical treatment for total anomalous pulmonary venous connection in infancy, In Barratt–Boyes BG (ed), *Heart Disease in Infancy: Diagnosis and Surgical Treatment*. Edinburgh, Churchill Livingstone, p 89.

Kirklin JW, Bargeron LM Jr, Pacifico AD (1977) The enlargement of small pulmonary arteries by preliminary palliative operations. *Circulation* 56:612.

Kirklin JW, Barratt–Boyes DG (1986) *Cardiac Surgery*. New York, John Wiley and Sons, p 513.

Koretzky ED, Moller JH, Korns ME, Schwartz CJ, Edwards JE (1969) Congenital pulmonary stenosis resulting from dysplasia of valve. *Circulation* 40:43.

Krovetz LJ, Lorincz AE, Schiebler GL (1965) Cardiovascular manifestations of the Hurler syndrome. Hemodynamic and angiocardiographic observations in 15 patients. *Circulation* 31:132.

Kumar AE, Fyler DC, Miettinen OS, Nadas AS (1971) Ebstein's anomaly. Clinical profile and natural history. *Am J Cardiol* 28:84.

Lababidi Z, Wu J, Walls JT (1984) Percutaneous balloon aortic valvuloplasty: Results in 23 patients. *Am J Cardiol* 53:194.

Lev M, Liberthson RR, Joseph RH, et al (1970) The pathologic anatomy of Ebstein's disease. *Arch Pathol* 90:334.

Lock JE, Bass JL, Amplatz K, Fuhrman BP, Castaneda–Zuniga W (1983) Balloon dilation angioplasty of aortic coarctations in infants and children. *Circulation* 68:109.

Lucas RV Jr, Varco RL, Lillehei CW, Adams P Jr, Anderson RC, Edwards JE (1962) Anomalous muscle bundle of the right ventricle. Hemodynamic consequences and surgical considerations. *Circulation* 25:443.

Maron BJ (1979) Coarctation of the aorta in the adult, in Roberts WC (ed): *Congenital Heart Disease in Adults*. Philadelphia, FA Davis, p 311.

Meyer J, Wukasch DC, Hallman GL, Cooley DA (1975) Aneurysm and fistula of the sinus of Valsalva: Clinical considerations and surgical treatment in 45 patients. *Ann Thorac Surg* 19:170.

Mickell JJ, Mathews RA, Park SC, Lenox CC, Fricker FJ (1980) Left atrioventricular valve atresia: Clinical management. *Circulation* 61:123.

Mitchell SC, Korones SB, Berendes HW (1971) Congenital heart disease in 56,109 births: Incidence and natural history. *Circulation* 43:323.

Mody MR (1975) The natural history of uncomplicated valvular pulmonic stenosis. *Am Heart J* 90:317.

Morgan BC, Guntheroth WG, Bloom RS, Fyler DC (1965) A clinical profile of paroxysmal hyperpnea in cyanotic congenital heart disease. *Circulation* 31:66.

Moss AJ, Adams FH, Emmanouilides GC (1977) *Heart Disease in Infants, Children, and Adolescents*, 2nd ed. Baltimore, Williams & Wilkins.

Nadas AS (ed) (1977) Pulmonary stenosis, aortic stenosis, ventricular septal defect: Clinical course and indirect assessment (Report from the Joint Study on the Natural History of Congenital Heart Defects). *Circulation* 56(Suppl 1):1.

Nadas AS, Fyler DC (1972) *Pediatric Cardiology,* 3rd ed. Philadelphia, WB Saunders.

Newfeld EA, Paul MH, Muster AJ, Idriss FS (1979) Pulmonary vascular disease in transposition of the great vessels and intact ventricular septum. *Circulation* 59:525.

Noonan JA (1981) Syndromes associated with cardiac defects, in Engle MA, Brest AN (eds): *Pediatric Cardiovascular Disease.* Philadelphia, FA Davis Company, p 97.

Noonan JA (1968) Hypertelorism with Turner phenotype: A new syndrome with associated congenital heart disease. *Am J Dis Child* 116:373.

Nora JJ, Nora AH (1978) *Genetics and Counseling in Cardiovascular Diseases.* Springfield, IL, Charles C. Thomas.

Ostman–Smith I, Silverman NH, Oldershaw P, Lincoln C, Shinebourne EA (1984) Cor triatriatum sinistrum. Diagnostic features on cross-sectional echocardiography. *Br Heart J* 51:211.

Parker FB Jr, Streeten DHP, Farrell B, Blackman MS, Sondheimer HM, Anderson GH Jr (1982) Preoperative and postoperative renin levels in coarctation of the aorta. *Circulation* 66:513.

Paul MH (1983) Transposition of the great arteries, in Adams FH and Emmanouilides GC (eds): *Moss' Heart Disease in Infants, Children, and Adolescents.* Baltimore, Williams & Wilkins, p 296.

Porstmann W, Wierny L, Warnke H, Gerstberger G, Romaniuk PA (1971) Catheter closure of patent ductus arteriosus: 62 cases treated without thoracotomy. *Radiol Clin North Am* 9:203.

Quaegebeur JM, Rohmer J, Ottenkamp J, et al (1986) The arterial switch operation: An eight-year experience. *J Thorac Cardiovasc Surg* 92:361.

Rao PS (1980) A unified classification for tricuspid atresia. *Am Heart J* 99:799.

Rao PS (1977) Natural history of the ventricular septal defect in tricuspid atresia and its surgical implications. *Br Heart J* 39:276.

Rashkind WJ, Cuasco CC (1979) Transcatheter closure of patent ductus arteriosus: Successful use in a 3.5 kilogram infant. *Pediatr Cardiol* 1:3.

Rastelli GC, Kirklin JW, Titus JL (1968) Anatomic observations on complete form of persistent common atrioventricular canal with septal reference to atrioventricular valves. *Mayo Clin Proc* 41:296.

Rigby ML, Gibson DG, Joseph MC, et al (1982) Recognition of imperforate atrioventricular valves by two-dimensional echocardiography. *Br Heart J* 47:329.

Roberts WC, Morrow AG, McIntosh CL, Jones M, Epstein SE (1981) Congenitally bicuspid aortic valve causing severe, pure aortic regurgitation without superimposed infective endocarditis. *Am J Cardiol* 47:206.

Ruttenberg HD (1983) Corrected transposition (L-transposition) of the great arteries and splenic syndromes, in Adams FH, Emmanouilides GC (eds): *Moss' Heart Disease in Infants, Children, and Adolescents.* Baltimore, Williams & Wilkins, p 333.

Sahn DJ, Allen HD, Lange LW, Goldberg SJ (1979) Cross-sectional echocardiographic diagnosis of the sites of total anomalous pulmonary venous drainage. *Circulation* 60:1317.

Sakakibara S, Konno S (1962) Congenital aneurysm of the sinus of Valsalva. Anatomy and classification. *Am Heart J* 63:405.

Sehested J (1978) Evaluation of optimum time for surgical repair of coarctation of the aorta. *Surg Gynecol Obstet* 146:593.

Serwer GA, Armstrong BE, Anderson PAW (1982) Continuous wave Doppler ultrasonographic quantitation of patent ductus arteriosus flow. *J Pediatr* 100:297.

Shone JD, Sellers RD, Anderson RC, Adams P Jr, Lillehei CW, Edwards JE (1963) The developmental complex of "parachute mitral valve," supravalvular ring of left atrium, subaortic stenosis, and coarctation of the aorta. *Am J Cardiol* 11:714.

Shub C, Dimopoulos IN, Seward JB, et al (1983) Sensitivity of two-dimensional echocardiography in the direct visualization of atrial septal defect utilizing the subcostal approach: Experience with 154 patients. *J Am Coll Cardiol* 3:127.

Solinger R, Elbl F, Minhas K (1976) Echocardiography: Its role in the severely ill infant. *Pediatrics* 57:543.

Stevenson JG (1977) Fluid administration in the association of patent ductus arteriosus complicating respiratory distress syndrome. *J Pediatr* 90:257.

Tandon R, Edwards JE (1974) Tricuspid atresia. A reevaluation and classification. *J Thorac Cardiovasc Surg* 67:530.

Tripp ME, Katcher ML, Peters HA, et al (1981) Systemic carnitine deficiency presenting as familial endocardial fibroelastosis. A treatable cardiomyopathy. *N Engl J Med* 305:385.

Trusler GA, Williams WG (1978) Long-term results of shunt procedures of tricuspid atresia. *Ann Thorac Surg* 25:312.

Turley K, Tucker WY, Ullyot DJ, Ebert PA (1980) Total anomalous pulmonary venous connection in infancy: Influence of age and type of lesion. *Am J Cardiol* 45:921.

Van Praagh R, Weinberg PM (1983) Double-outlet left ventricle, in Adams FH, Emmanouilides GC (eds): *Moss' Heart Disease in Infants, Children, and Adolescents.* Baltimore, Williams & Wilkins, p 370.

Villani M, Lipscombe S, Ross DN (1979) Double-outlet left ventricle: How should we repair it? *J Cardiovasc Surg* 20:413.

Watson H (1974) Natural history of Ebstein's anomaly of the tricuspid valve in childhood and adolescence: An international coopertive study of 505 cases. *Br Heart J* 36:417.

Weidman WH, Blount SG Jr, Dushane JW, Gersony WM, Hayes CJ, Nadas AS (1977) Clinical course in ventricular septal defect. *Circulation* 56(suppl 1):56.

Weinberg PM (1980) Anatomy of tricuspid atresia and its relevance to current forms of surgical therapy. *Am Thorac Surg* 29:306.

Wells HG (1908) Persistent patency of the ductus arteriosus. *Am J Med Sci* 136:381.

Weyman AE, Dillon JC, Fiegenbaum H, Change S (1975) Echocardiographic differentiation of infundibular from valvar pulmonary stenosis. *Am J Cardiol* 36:21.

White PD, Hurst JW, Fennell RH (1950) Survival to the age of 75 years with congenital pulmonary stenosis and patent foramen ovale. *Circulation* 2(4):558.

Wilcox BR, Ho SY, Macartney FJ, Becker AE, Gerlis LM, Anderson RH (1981) The surgical anatomy of double-outlet right ventricle with situs solitus and atrial ventricular concordance. *J Thorac Cardiovasc Surg* 82:405.

Wright GB, Keane JF, Nadas AS, Bernard WF, Castaneda AR (1983) Fixed subaortic stenosis in the young: Medical and surgical course in 83 patients. *Am J Cardiol* 52:830.

Zamora R, Moller JH, Edwards JE (1975) Double-outlet right ventricle. Anatomic types and associated anomalies. *Chest* 68:672.

FIGURE CREDITS

FIG. 3.10 From Silverman NH, Snider AR: *Two-Dimensional Echocardiography in Congenital Heart Disease.* Norwalk, CT, Appleton-Century-Crofts, 1982, p 78.

FIG. 3.11 (A,B) From Hatle L, Angelsen B: *Doppler Ultrasound in Cardiology.* Philadelphia, Lea & Febiger, 1985, p. 237.

FIG. 3.14 From Wilcox BR, Anderson RH: *Surgical Anatomy of the Heart.* New York, Raven Press, 1985, p 6.9.

FIG. 3.16 (A,B) From Wilcox BR, Anderson RH: *Surgical Anatomy of the Heart.* New York, Raven Press, 1985, p 6.8.

FIG. 3.22 From Becker AE, Anderson RH: *Cardiac Pathology.* New York, Raven Press, 1983, p 10.14.

FIG. 3.27 From Silverman NH, Snider AR: *Two-Dimensional Echocardiography in Congenital Heart Disease.* Norwalk, CT, Appleton-Century-Crofts, 1982, p 68.

FIG. 3.29 (A–C) From Wilcox BR, Anderson RH: *Surgical Anatomy of the Heart.* New York, Raven Press, 1985, p 6.3.

FIG. 3.35 From Wilcox BR, Anderson RH: *Surgical Anatomy of the Heart.* New York, Raven Press, 1985, p. 6.13.

FIG. 3.39 Partially redrawn from Lundstrom N-R: *Pediatric Echocardiography— Cross Sectional, M-Mode and Doppler.* Amsterdam, Elsevier/North-Holland Biomedical Press, 1980, p 193.

FIG. 3.40 From Hagler DJ, Tajik AJ, Seward JB, Mair DD, Ritter DG: Real-time wide-angle sector echocardiography: Atrioventricular canal defects. *Circulation* 59:140, 1979; with permission of the American Heart Association, Inc.

FIG. 3.43 From Wilcox BR, Anderson RH: *Surgical Anatomy of the Heart.* New York, Raven Press, 1985, p 6.11.

FIG. 3.47 (A,B) From Freedom RM, Culham JAG, Moes CAF: *Heart Disease.* New York, Macmillan, 1984, p 272.

FIG. 3.52 Redrawn from Tavel ME: *Clinical Phonocardiography and External Pulse Recording.* Chicago, Year Book Medical Publishers, 1972, p 143.

FIG. 3.53 (A,B) From Brinsfield DE, Plauth WH Jr: Clinical recognition and medical management of congenital heart disease, in Hurst JW (ed): *The Heart,* 4th ed. New York, McGraw-Hill, 1978, p 848.

FIG. 3.55 Partially redrawn from Hatle L, Angelsen B: *Doppler Ultrasound in Cardiology.* Philadelphia, Lea & Febiger, 1985, p 222.

FIG. 3.56 From Freedom RM, Culham JAG, Moes CAF: *Heart Disease.* New York, Macmillan 1984, p 458.

FIG. 3.60 From Becker AE, Anderson RH: *Cardiac Pathology.* New York, Raven Press, 1983, p 15.2.

FIG. 3.68 From Elliott LP, Schiebler GL: *The X-Ray Diagnosis of Congenital Heart Disease in Infants, Children, and Adults.* Springfield, IL, Charles C Thomas, 1979, p 231.

FIG. 3.69 Redrawn from Gooch AS, Maranhao V, Goldberg H: *Congenital Heart Disease.* Philadelphia, FA Davis, 1969, Fig. 13.

FIG. 3.70 From Silverman NH, Snider AR: *Two-Dimensional Echocardiography in Congenital Heart Disease.* Norwalk, CT, Appleton-Century-Crofts, 1982, p 110.

FIG. 3.71 From Freedom RM, Culham JAG, Moes CAF: *Heart Disease*. New York, Macmillan, 1984, p 466.

FIG. 3.85 (A,C) From Silverman NH, Snider AR: *Two-Dimensional Echocardiography in Congenital Heart Disease*. Norwalk, CT, Appleton-Century-Crofts, 1982, p 100, 108.

FIG. 3.91 Redrawn from Perloff JK: *The Clinical Recognition of Congenital Heart Disease*. Philadelphia, WB Saunders, 1978, p 748.

FIG. 3.92 From Silverman NH, Snider AR: *Two-Dimensional Echocardiography in Congenital Heart Disease*. Norwalk, CT, Appleton-Century-Crofts, 1982, p 190.

FIG. 3.96. From Elliott LP, Schiebler GL: *The X-ray Diagnosis of Congenital Heart Disease in Infants, Children and Adults*. Springfield, IL, Charles C Thomas, 1979, p 248.

FIG. 3.98 (A,B) From Silverman NH, Snider AR: *Two-Dimensional Echocardiography in Congenital Heart Disease*. Norwalk, CT, Appleton-Century-Crofts, 1982, p 113.

FIG. 3.99 From Williams RG, Bierman FZ, Sanders SP: *Echocardiographic Diagnosis of Cardiac Malformations*. Boston, Little, Brown, 1986, p 104.

FIG. 3.100 (B,C) From Freedom RM, Culham JAG, Moes CAF: *Heart Disease*. New York, Macmillan, 1984, p 255.

FIG. 3.108 Redrawn from Perloff JK: *The Clinical Recognition of Congenital Heart Disease*. Philadelphia, WB Saunders, 1978, p 161.

FIG. 3.109 (A,C) From Williams RG, Bierman FZ, Sanders SP: *Echocardiographic Diagnosis of Cardiac Malformations*. Boston, Little, Brown, 1986, p 114.

FIG. 3.109 (B) From Silverman NH, Snider AR: *Two-Dimensional Echocardiography in Congenital Heart Disease*. Norwalk, CT, Appleton-Century-Crofts, 1982, p 120.

FIG. 3.112 (A,B) From Eliot RS, Shone JD, Kanjuh VI, Ruttenberg HD, Carey LS, Edwards JE: Mitral atresia. A study of 32 cases. *Am Heart J* 70:16, 1965.

FIG. 3.115 (A,B) From Silverman NH, Snider AR: *Two-Dimensional Echocardiography in Congenital Heart Disease*. Norwalk, CT, Appleton-Century-Crofts, 1982, p 128.

FIG. 3.117 (A,B) From Williams RG, Bierman FZ, Sanders SP: *Echocardiographic Diagnosis of Cardiac Malformations*. Boston, Little, Brown, 1986, p 119.

FIG. 3.118 (B) From Becker AE, Anderson RH: *Cardiac Pathology*. New York, Raven Press, 1983, p 11.19.

FIG. 3.119 From Becker AE, Anderson RH: *Cardiac Pathology*. New York, Raven Press, 1983, p 11.19.

FIG. 3.121 From Gedgaudas E, Moller JH, Castaneda-Zuniga WR, Amplatz K: *Cardiovascular Radiology*. Philadelphia, WB Saunders, 1985, p 161.

FIG. 3.123 From Williams RG, Bierman FZ, Sanders SP: *Echocardiographic Diagnosis of Cardiac Malformations*. Boston, Little, Brown, 1986, p 100.

FIG. 3.124 (A,B) From Freedom RM, Culham JAG, Moes CAF: *Heart Disease*. New York, Macmillan, 1984, p 86.

FIG. 3.129 Redrawn from Goldfarb MS, Lutz JF, Hurst JW: Patient No. 4, in Hurst JW (ed): *Clinical Essays on the Heart*, vol 4. New York, McGraw-Hill, 1984, p 26.

FIG. 3.130 From Williams RG, Bierman FZ, Sanders SP: *Echocardiographic Diagnosis of Cardiac Malformations*. Boston, Little, Brown, 1986, p 95.

FIG. 3.131 From Freedom RM, Culham JAG, Moes CAF: *Heart Disease*. New York, Macmillan, 1984, p 114.

FIG. 3.137 (A,B) From Freedom RM, Culham JAG, Moes CAF: *Heart Disease*. New York, Macmillan, 1984, p 179.

FIG. 3.147 From Elliott LP, Schiebler GL: *The X-Ray Diagnosis of Congenital Heart Disease in Infants, Children, and Adults*. Springfield, IL, Charles C Thomas, 1979, p 332.

FIG. 3.148 (A,B) From Brinsfield DE, Plauth WH Jr: Clinical recognition and medical management of congenital heart disease, in Hurst JW (ed): *The Heart*, 4th ed. New York, McGraw-Hill, p 835.

FIG. 3.149 Redrawn from Fink BW: *Congenital Heart Disease: A Deductive Approach to Its Diagnosis*. Chicago, Year Book Medical Publishers, 1985, p 115.

FIG. 3.150 From Hagler DJ, Tajik AJ, Seward JB, Mair DD, Ritter DG: Wide-angle two-dimensional echocardiographic profiles of conotruncal abnormalities. *Mayo Clin Proc* 55:73, 1980.

FIG. 3.160 From Lintermans JP: *Two-Dimensional Echocardiography in Infants and Children*. Dordrecht, Martinus Nijhoff, 1986, p 129.

FIG. 3.168 From Hagler DJ, Tajik AJ, Seward JB, Mair DD, Ritter DG: Double-outlet right ventricle, wide-angle, two-dimensional echocardiographic observations. *Circulation* 63:419, 1981; with permission of the American Heart Association, Inc.

FIG. 3.169 (A,B) From Freedom RM, Culham JAG, Moes CAF: *Heart Disease*. New York, Macmillan, 1984, p 558.

FIG. 3.174 From Plauth WH Jr, Nugent EW, Schlant RC, Edwards JE, Williams WH, Kirklin JW: The pathology, abnormal physiology, clinical recognition, and medical and surgical treatment of congenital heart disease, in Hurst JW (ed): *The Heart*, 5th ed. New York, McGraw-Hill, 1982, p 774.

FIG. 3.176 From Williams RG, Bierman FZ, Sanders SP: *Echocardiographic Diagnosis of Cardiac Malformations*. Boston, Little, Brown, 1986, p 186.

FIG. 3.180 From Elliott LP, Schiebler GL: *The X-Ray Diagnosis of Congenital Heart Disease in Infants, Children, and Adults*. Springfield, IL, Charles C Thomas, 1979, p 215.

FIG. 3.181 Redrawn from Fink BW: *Congenital Heart Disease: A Deductive Approach to Its Diagnosis*. Chicago, Year Book Medical Publishers, 1985, p 183.

FIG. 3.182 From Weyman AE: *Cross-Sectional Echocardiography*. Philadelphia, Lea & Febiger, 1982, p 328.

FIG. 3.191 From Plauth WH Jr, Nugent EW, Schlant RC, Edwards JE, Williams WH, Kirklin JW: The pathology, abnormal physiology, clinical recognition, and medical and surgical treatment of congenital heart disease, in Hurst JW (ed): *The Heart*, 5th ed. New York, McGraw-Hill, 1982, p 822.

4
VALVAR HEART DISEASE

J. Willis Hurst, MD
Charles E. Rackley, MD
Anton E. Becker, MD
Benson R. Wilcox, MD
SELECTION OF
CLINICAL ILLUSTRATIONS ASSISTED BY
Scott J. Pollack, MD

AORTIC VALVE STENOSIS*
ETIOLOGY AND PATHOLOGY

Aortic valve stenosis may result from a variety of conditions. Congenital abnormalities, such as bicuspid aortic valve with a small annulus and unicuspid aortic valve, usually produce symptoms early in life (see Chapter 3). Occasionally such malformations may become manifest in adulthood (Fig. 4.1). In older patients rheumatic heart disease (Fig. 4.2) and isolated calcific disease of the elderly (Fig. 4.3) are the most common pathologic conditions. In the latter situation approximately half of patients have an underlying congenitally bicuspid aortic valve without hypoplasia (Fig. 4.4), while the remainder have a trifoliate aortic valve (Fig. 4.5). Calcification of the valve eventually occurs in all types of stenosis, including the congenital forms that first become symptomatic in adulthood (Pomerance, 1972; Edwards, 1979).

ABNORMAL PHYSIOLOGY

The size of the aortic orifice is normally 2–3 cm². Stenosis of the aortic valve creates resistance to ejection, and a pressure gradient develops during systole between the left ventricle and the aorta. The elevated left ventricular pressure produces a pressure overload on the left ventricle, which remodels itself by increasing the thickness of the left ventricular wall—a process known as concentric hypertrophy (Kennedy et al, 1968). Dilation of the left ventricular cavity does not occur until myocardial contractility is depressed (Rackley and Hood, 1976).

The left ventricular end-diastolic pressure becomes elevated in patients with aortic stenosis. Atrial contraction then contributes to the left ventricular diastolic volume of blood that is subsequently ejected during left ventricular systole (Stott et al, 1970). Left ventricular compliance decreases, thus contributing to elevated left ventricular end-diastolic pressure. This eventually leads to left atrial enlargement.

Eventually the sustained left ventricular pressure load leads to dilation of the left ventricle and decreased contractility of the myocar-

*Abstracted with permission of the authors and publisher from Rackley CE, Edwards JE, Wallace RB, Katz NM: Aortic valve disease, Chapter 37, pp 729–754, in Hurst JW (ed): *The Heart,* 6th ed. New York, McGraw-Hill, 1986. Figures reproduced in this section from the above chapter, other chapters in *The Heart,* or other sources are also reprinted with permission of the authors and publishers. For the full bibliographic citations of the sources of figures and tables other than the above chapter, see Figure Credits at the end of this chapter.

dium (Dodge and Baxley, 1969). Myocardial ischemia may occur due to restricted coronary blood flow to the hypertrophied myocardium.

CLINICAL MANIFESTATIONS

Aortic stenosis is more common in males than females. A congenital origin should be considered in young patients with isolated aortic stenosis. Middle-aged patients who have aortic stenosis in association with mitral valve disease usually have a rheumatic etiology, regardless of a history of rheumatic fever. Middle-aged patients with isolated aortic stenosis may have congenital biscuspid aortic valve disease. Elderly patients may have nonrheumatic, noncongenital, calcific aortic stenosis.

SYMPTOMS

Patients experience symptoms late in the course of the disease, including angina pectoris, dyspnea due to heart failure, syncope, and sudden death.

ANGINA PECTORIS. Angina pectoris is the most common symptom of aortic stenosis (Rotman et al, 1971). Life expectancy is about five years after the development of myocardial ischemia. Coronary atherosclerosis is often present in adult patients with aortic stenosis even when no symptoms are present. Myocardial ischemia occurs due to restriction of myocardial blood flow by the stenosis and left ventricular oxygen consumption is greater than normal due to the increase in left ventricular muscle mass. Oxygen availability is also decreased at the left ventricular subendocardial level as a result of an increase in systolic wall stress in that region (Hood et al, 1969).

DYSPNEA. The survival period is about two years for adults with aortic stenosis who have dyspnea due to heart failure (Baker and Sommerville, 1959).

SYNCOPE. Syncope is a common symptom in patients with aortic stenosis. It may be the first symptom noted by the patient, often occurring after exertion (Flamm et al, 1967). Survival is about three to four years in patients with syncope.

SUDDEN DEATH. Sudden death is the feared event in patients with severe aortic stenosis; it occurs in about 3%–5% of asymptomatic patients. The mechanisms responsible for syncope are undoubtedly

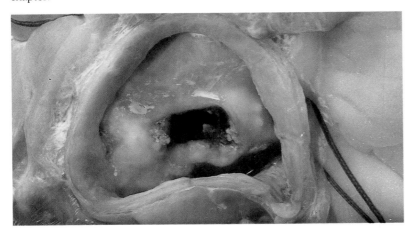

FIG. 4.1 *This example of aortic valve stenosis in an adult is due to a congenitally malformed valve, most likely unicuspid in nature.*

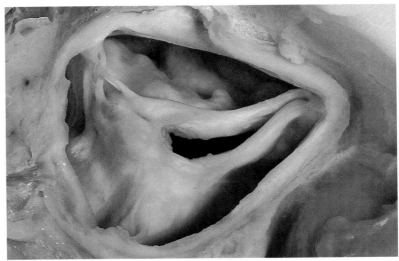

FIG. 4.2 *An example of rheumatic aortic valve stenosis shows marked commissural fusion and fibrotic leaflets with calcifications. In such instances pathologic studies almost always reveal an affected mitral valve, which is not necessarily clinically manifest.*

responsible for sudden death; however, the final pathophysiologic pathway is usually a cardiac arrhythmia.

PHYSICAL EXAMINATION

In severe aortic stenosis the pulse pressure becomes narrowed and the upstroke of the arterial pulse is slow. This diminished amplitude with delayed pulse peak has been described as pulsus parvus et tardus.

While the apex impulse may not be displaced laterally, the duration of the impulse may be prolonged. The left atrial contribution to left ventricular filling may be detected, and a systolic thrill may be felt in the second intercostal space near the sternum and in the neck.

The auscultatory findings in valvar aortic stenosis include a diamond-shaped systolic murmur, a decrease in intensity of aortic valve closure (A_2), faint aortic regurgitation, and paradoxical splitting of the second sound. In young patients a systolic ejection sound may be heard best at the apex (Hancock, 1966). The systolic murmur may be higher pitched at the apex in older patients; it usually radiates into the neck or, rarely, laterally to the apical area. Accordingly it may be difficult

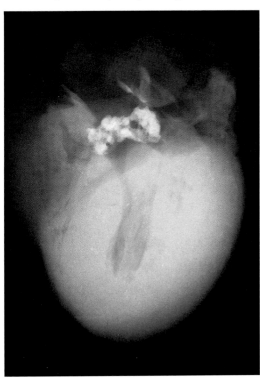

FIG. 4.3 *Postmortem x-ray film of a heart demonstrates isolated calcific aortic stenosis.*

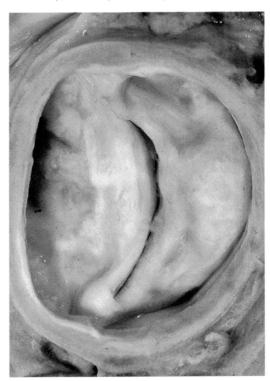

FIG. 4.4 *Isolated calcific stenosis is seen in association with a congenitally bicuspid aortic valve. (Reproduced with permission of the authors and publisher; see Figure Credits)*

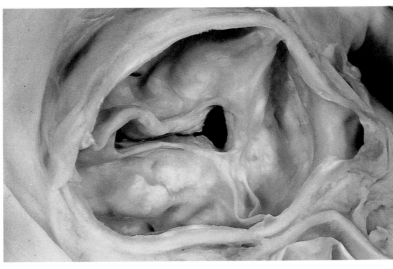

FIG. 4.5 *This example of isolated aortic valve stenosis is caused by a trileaflet aortic valve.*

to separate the murmur of aortic stenosis from carotid artery bruits, which occur commonly in the elderly (Crawley et al, 1978). The murmur may not be heard or it may be misjudged as unimportant in patients with severe pulmonary emphysema, severely diminished cardiac output, or mitral stenosis.

LABORATORY STUDIES

CHEST RADIOGRAPHY.   Early in the course of the disease the chest film may show a normal-sized heart (Klatte et al, 1962), although later the heart may become enlarged. Post-stenotic dilation of the aorta, calcification of the aortic valve (best seen on the lateral view), and a slightly enlarged left atrium may be seen on the radiograph (Fig. 4.6).

ELECTROCARDIOGRAPHY.   The electrocardiogram (ECG) shows evidence of left ventricular hypertrophy. The QRS voltage is often increased, and the mean T vector eventually comes to lie 180° away from the mean QRS vector. There may be a left atrial abnormality (Fig. 4.7).

ECHOCARDIOGRAPHY.   Aortic valve stenosis may be differentiated by echocardiography from nonvalvar types of left ventricular outflow

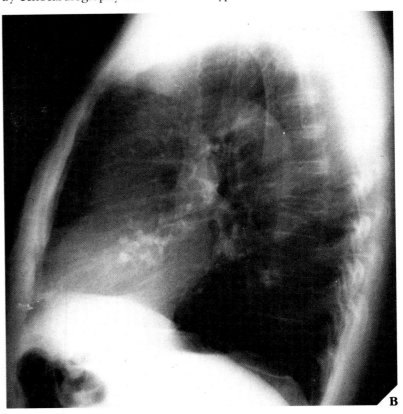

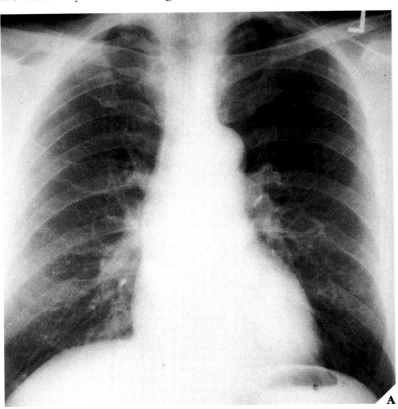

FIG. 4.6   **(A)** *Posteroanterior view of the chest in a 62-year-old male with calcific aortic stenosis shows a normal-sized heart with a slightly enlarged ascending aorta.* **(B)** *Lateral view reveals considerable calcification of the* aortic valve. (Courtesy of Robert G. Sybers, MD, and Wade H. Shuford, MD, Atlanta, Georgia)

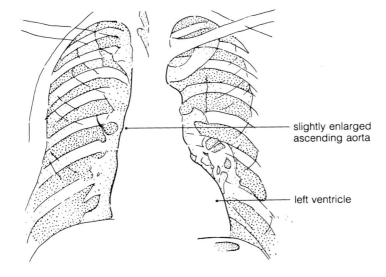

slightly enlarged
ascending aorta

left ventricle

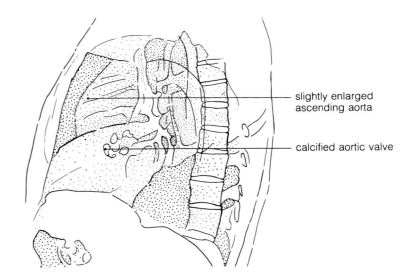

slightly enlarged
ascending aorta

calcified aortic valve

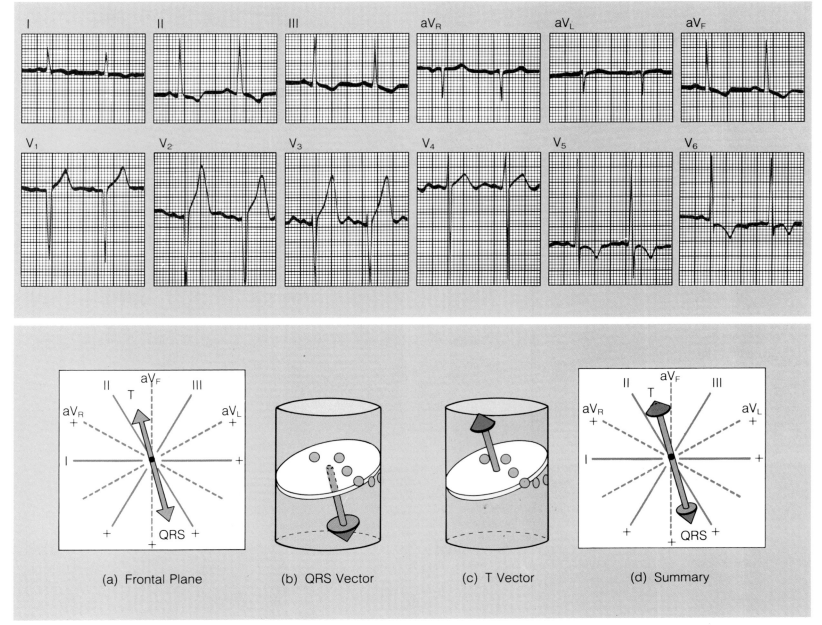

| I | II | III | aV$_R$ | aV$_L$ | aV$_F$ |

| V$_1$ | V$_2$ | V$_3$ | V$_4$ | V$_5$ | V$_6$ |

(a) Frontal Plane   (b) QRS Vector   (c) T Vector   (d) Summary

FIG. 4.7 *ECG obtained in a 32-year-old patient with calcific aortic stenosis illustrates left ventricular hypertrophy.* (**a**) *The QRS complex is largest in lead II, slightly positive in lead I, and negative in lead aV$_L$. QRS complexes of this nature can be represented by a mean vector directed to the right of the positive limb of lead II. The T wave is slightly negative in lead I, large and negative in leads II, III, and aV$_F$, and positive in lead aV$_L$. Accordingly the mean T vector is directed to the right of the negative limb of lead aV$_F$ but to the left of a perpendicular to lead aV$_L$. (**b,c**) Shown here is the spatial orientation of the mean QRS and T vectors. The mean QRS is rotated 50° posteriorly, because the transitional pathway passes between the* V$_4$ *and* V$_5$ *positions. The mean T vector is tilted 50° anteriorly, because the transitional pathway passes between the* V$_4$ *and* V$_5$ *positions. Note the increased magnitude of the QRS complexes. (**d**) Final summary figure shows the spatial arrangement of the vectors. The mean QRS vector is directed downward and posteriorly, and the mean T vector is directed to the right and anteriorly; the spatial QRS–T angle is 180°. These findings are characteristic of left ventricular hypertrophy associated with an abnormally wide QRS–T angle. The mean QRS vector is vertically directed and may be related to the thin, long-chested build of the patient. (Redrawn; reproduced with permission of the authors and publisher; see Figure Credits)*

tract obstruction, such as idiopathic hypertrophic subaortic stenosis (Reigenbaum, 1976). Thickening, calcification, decreased mobility of the aortic valve leaflets, and the degree of left ventricular hypertrophy can all be detected on the echocardiogram (Fig. 4.8). Left ventricular function can be estimated from chamber dimensions, estimates of end-diastolic and end-systolic volumes, and the ejection fraction. A bicuspid aortic valve can also be identified (Radford et al, 1976). A systolic separation of the aortic leaflets of less than 8 mm detected by

cross-sectional echocardiography in long-axis sections is predictive of severe aortic stenosis.

The systolic pressure gradient across the aortic valve can be determined using the Doppler technique (Fig. 4.9). This appears to be an acceptable method of following the pressure gradient across the aortic valve, although the results may not be as accurate as determining the gradient by cardiac catheterization. The Doppler technique is more accurate, when compared with the gradient determined by cardiac

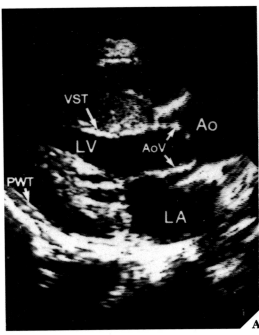 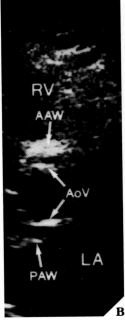 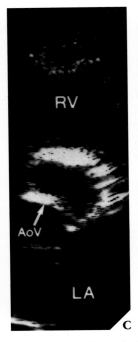 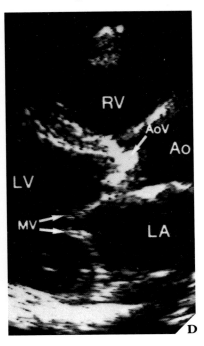

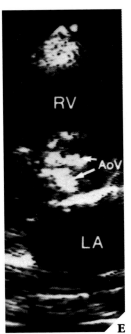

FIG. 4.8 *Cross-sectional echocardiograms were obtained from two patients with severe aortic stenosis, one with bicuspid valve (A–C) and the other with a calcified trileaflet valve (D,E). (A) Parasternal long-axis view shows systolic doming of the anterior and the posterior cusps of the aortic valve (AoV). During diastole (not shown) the aortic cusps prolapse into the left ventricular outflow tract. Left ventricular hypertrophy is present, and the left atrium (LA) is dilated. (B) Parasternal short-axis view at the level of the aortic valve in systole shows only two aortic cusps that are parallel to the anterior (AAW) and the posterior (PAW) aortic walls. (C) In the parasternal short-axis view at the level of the aortic valve in diastole the closure of the aortic valve is represented by an abnormal, dominant, single echo, which appears S-shaped. (D) Parasternal long-axis view in systole shows a dense mass of calcium totally obscuring the leaflets and the orifice of the aortic valve. (E) Parasternal short-axis view at the level of the aorta in systole shows a heavily calcified trileaflet* aortic valve with markedly reduced opening (VST, *ventricular septal thickness;* PWT, *posterior wall thickness;* Ao, *aorta;* LV, *left ventricle;* RV, *right ventricle;* MV, *mitral valve). (Fig. 120-31,* The Heart, *6th ed; see Figure Credits)*

catheterization, when it is used to determine the mean systolic gradient across the aortic valve rather than the peak-to-peak systolic gradient across the valve.

CARDIAC CATHETERIZATION. The purpose of cardiac catheterization is to confirm the presence of aortic valve stenosis, measure its severity, and exclude or identify the presence of other cardiac disease, especially coronary disease.

The normal valve area is 2–3 cm². A reduction of 75% or more resulting in an orifice size less than 0.8 cm² is necessary to produce significant impairment of flow and cardiac output (Hancock and Fleming, 1960). This degree of stenosis is usually accompanied by a left ventricular–aortic systolic pressure gradient exceeding 50 mmHg (Fig. 4.10). A gradient must always be assessed in relationship to the cardiac

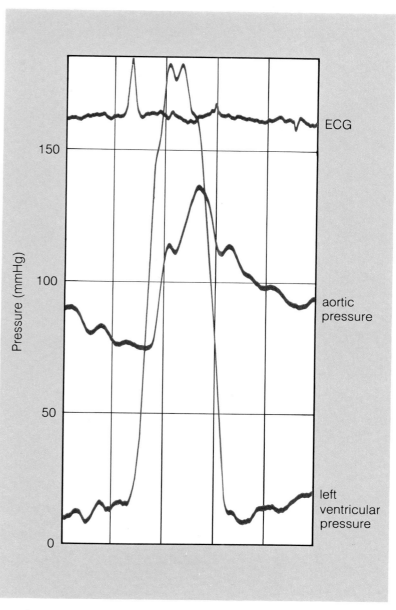

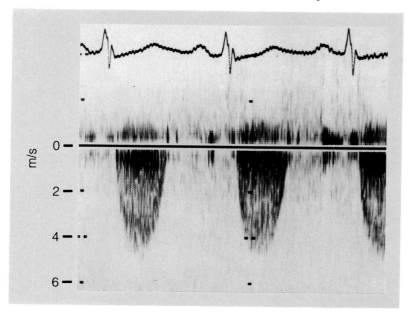

FIG. 4.9 *Severe aortic stenosis is evaluated from the apical approach using a nonimaging, continuous-wave Doppler device. The waveform shows flow away from the transducer with a peak velocity of approximately 4.6 m/s, predicting a peak pressure gradient of 86 mmHg. (Fig. 122-6,* The Heart, *6th ed; see Figure Credits)*

FIG. 4.10 *Left ventricular and aortic pressures were recorded in a patient with aortic valve stenosis. This figure illustrates a peak-to-peak pressure gradient of about 48 mmHg between the left ventricular systolic pressure and the aortic pressure. (Redrawn; courtesy of Robert H. Franch, MD, Atlanta, Georgia)*

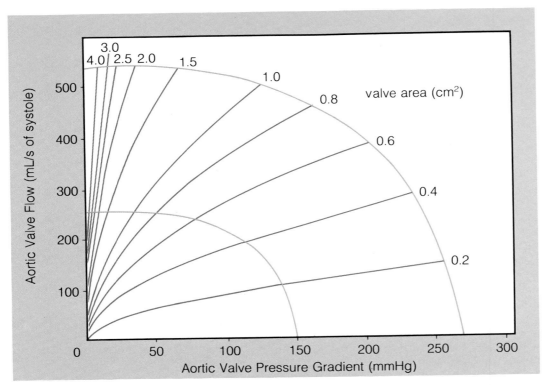

FIG. 4.11 *This diagram illustrates the relationship of cardiac output to the pressure gradient across the aortic valve in patients with aortic stenosis. When the valve area remains the same, the transaortic valve gradient increases as the cardiac output increases. (Redrawn; reproduced with permission of the author and publisher; see Figure Credits)*

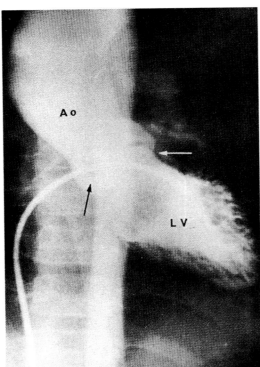

FIG. 4.12 *In this frontal-view angiogram of a patient with valvar aortic stenosis the catheter is passed from the right atrium to the left atrium by transseptal puncture, and then advanced into the left ventricle. Selective left ventricular injection reveals a dome-shaped defect of the aortic valve with bulging of the leaflets into the dilated ascending aorta (arrows) (Ao, aorta; LV, left ventricle). (Fig. 9-13, The Heart, 1st ed; see Figure Credits)*

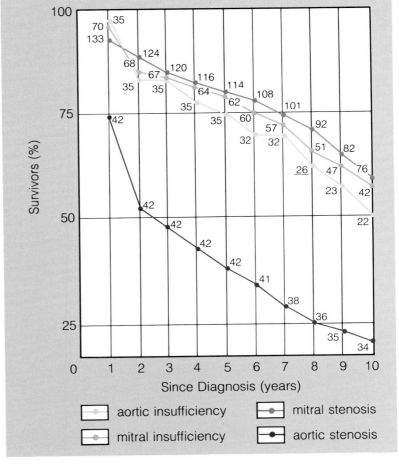

FIG. 4.13 *The actuarial survival of patients with valvar heart disease treated medically is graphed from the time of diagnosis. (The numbers at each of the circles indicate the number of patients known to be dead or alive at a point in time. The percentage survival figures have been corrected accordingly to reflect the actual number of patients in the series at that time.) (Redrawn; reproduced with permission of the author and publisher; see Figure Credits. Also, Fig. 38-7,* The Heart, *6th ed, p 761)*

PART II: DISEASES OF THE HEART

output (Fig. 4.11); for example a gradient of 30 mmHg may be very significant if the cardiac output is low.

Quantitative angiography provides measurements of end-diastolic and systolic volumes, the ejection fraction, and left ventricular mass (Fig. 4.12) (Rackley, 1976).

Coronary arteriography in adults reveals a 50% prevalence of coronary atherosclerosis regardless of reported angina. If obstructive coronary disease is present, coronary bypass surgery may be needed; it should be performed at the time of valve surgery.

RADIONUCLIDE STUDIES. Radionuclide ventriculography using technetium-99m (^{99m}Tc) can be employed to determine the resting and the exercise ejection fractions. ^{201}Thallium (^{201}Tl) scanning at rest and with exercise may identify areas of myocardial scarring or ischemia. Exercise testing in patients with severe aortic valvar stenosis may be dangerous; accordingly these tests are usually performed at rest.

NATURAL HISTORY

Adults with aortic stenosis have an average mortality of 9% per year (Dexter, 1969). The survival time is often less than five years once symptoms develop; then the incidence of sudden death is 15%–20% (Frank et al, 1973). Angina is associated with an average life expectancy of five years; less than 5% of patients with this symptom survive for 10–20 years (Wood, 1958). The survival time after syncope is three to four years, and the survival after the development of left ventricular failure is about two years (Baker and Sommerville, 1959). The actuarial survival of patients with aortic stenosis treated medically is depicted from the time of diagnosis in Figure 4.13.

In a subset of adult patients with accelerated aortic stenosis a rather rapid acceleration of the narrowing of the valve may occur. The aortic valve gradient in such cases may increase from 40 mmHg to 75 mmHg within two years.

TREATMENT

Patients with aortic valve stenosis should be treated prophylactically for bacterial endocarditis; heart failure is treated with digitalis and diuretics. Measures to decrease preload and afterload should be used with great discretion, if at all. Angina should be treated cautiously with nitrates. It is obvious that patients with symptoms caused by aortic valve stenosis need surgical intervention. Patients without symptoms require very careful assessment and follow-up to determine when surgery should be performed.

Treatment of stenosis by balloon dilation of the aortic valve is currently under investigation. Patients chosen for this investigation are not eligible for valve replacement because they are elderly, have serious concomitant disease, and have severe symptoms. Preliminary results are encouraging in these carefully selected patients, but more research and experience is needed before this procedure is used routinely (Cribier et al, 1986).

INDICATIONS FOR SURGERY

Symptomatic patients and asymptomatic patients with a systolic gradient of 75 mmHg across the aortic valve should have surgery. Patients who are asymptomatic but have a systolic gradient of less than 75 mmHg across the aortic valve should be followed every six months. Surgery should then be performed if the patient has symptoms, an increase in heart size, an increase in aortic valve systolic pressure gradient as measured by the Doppler technique, or a decline in the resting ejection fraction as determined by ^{99m}Tc ventriculography.

SURGICAL PROCEDURE

The young patient may have an aortic valvotomy (Fig. 4.14), but the older patient requires valve replacement. The operative risk is very small with aortic valvotomy and about 2% with aortic valve replacement. When coronary bypass surgery is also needed, the surgical risk

FIG. 4.14 *In this operative view of aortic valve stenosis in an infant (A) the fused commissure is opened (B). Care is taken not to extend the incision all the way to the aortic wall.*

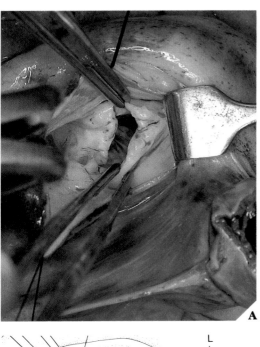
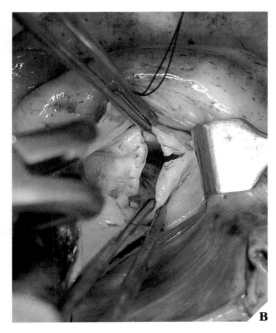

A

B

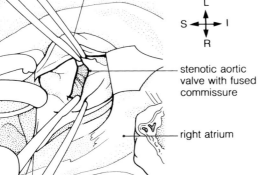

stenotic aortic valve with fused commissure

right atrium

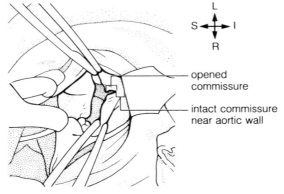

opened commissure

intact commissure near aortic wall

rises to about 4%. The operative risk is 4%–8% when the heart is large and heart failure is present.

When a valvotomy cannot be performed in young patients, valve replacement is necessary, using a synthetic valve (Fig. 4.15). The surgeon may use a tissue valve (porcine or pericardial) in older patients (Fig. 4.16). The advantages of the tissue valve are that episodes of thromboembolism are rare, anticoagulants are not needed, and de-

terioration is usually slow compared with some of the acute problems that arise when synthetic valves are used.

The surgical approach to the diseased aortic valve is invariably through the aortic root. This does not present a problem except under unusual circumstances, as in an abnormal origin of one or more of the coronary arteries. These vessels usually arise from within the appropriate sinus of Valsalva; however, they may arise virtually anywhere in the aortic

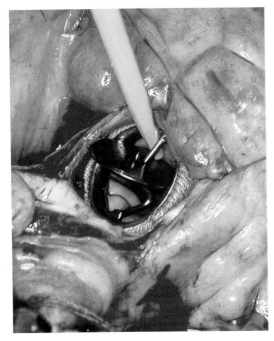

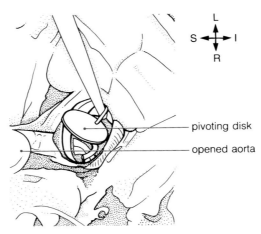

FIG. 4.15 A Medtronic–Hall synthetic prosthesis is seen in this operative view, already sewn in place. The wide opening angle (80°) and sturdy Pyrolyte block construction make this a particularly satisfactory prosthesis to replace the aortic valve. Pledgeted sutures must be placed on the aortic side of the native valve remnant, and the suture ends must be controlled to avoid interference with the pivoting disk.

pivoting disk
opened aorta

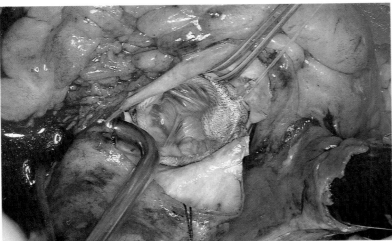

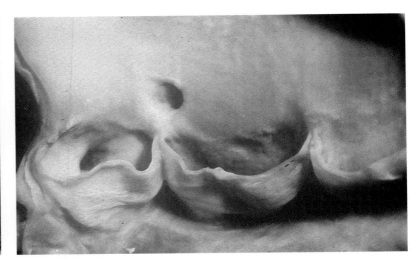

FIG. 4.16 In this operative view a Carpentier–Edwards stent-mounted, glutaraldehyde-preserved porcine bioprosthesis is seen sewn in place. This valve is quite satisfactory in older individuals whose aortic orifice will accept a 23 mm or larger prosthesis. Pledgeted sutures may be placed on the ventricular side of the native valve remnant if the coronary orifices are not obstructed with the stent.

FIG. 4.17 The right coronary orifice lies above the aortic bar. The left coronary artery can be seen arising in its more usual location. (Reproduced with permission of the authors and publisher; see Figure Credits)

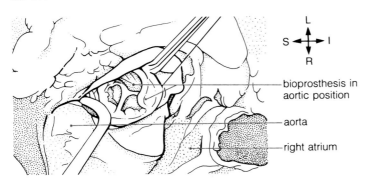

bioprosthesis in aortic position

aorta

right atrium

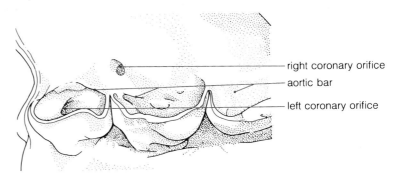

right coronary orifice
aortic bar
left coronary orifice

root. When the ostium of a coronary artery lies above the aortic bar (Fig. 4.17), it may well pose a problem at the time of aortotomy and an alternate site must be chosen (Fig. 4.18).

Occasionally the heart is so malformed or displaced that access from the usual approach is impaired. The heart, for example, may be rotated and displaced into the right chest because of a pulmonary abnormality, and consequently it is easier to approach the valve from the patient's left side (Fig. 4.19). Malrotation does not usually affect

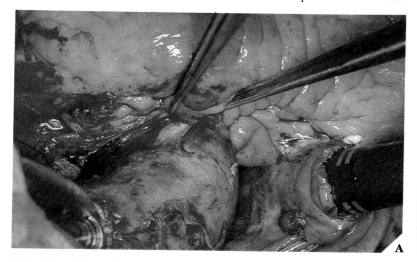
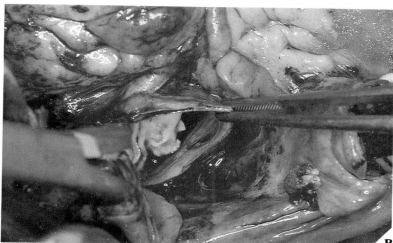

FIG. 4.18   (A) *In this operative view a right coronary artery arises high on the aortic root.* (B) *The aortotomy must then be more distal than usual to avoid injury to this artery.*

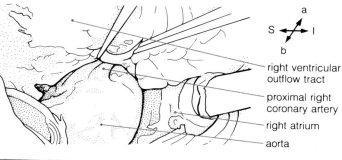

right ventricular outflow tract
proximal right coronary artery
right atrium
aorta

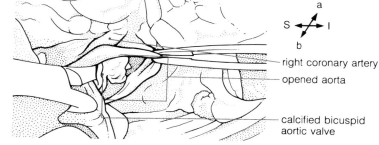

right coronary artery
opened aorta
calcified bicuspid aortic valve

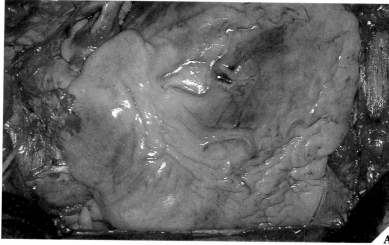
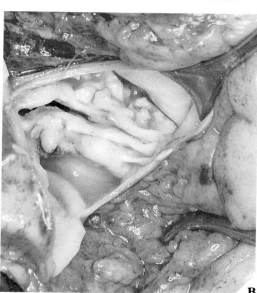

FIG. 4.19   (A) *Rightward rotation of the heart in an elderly patient with right lung hypoplasia and calcific aortic stenosis causes the aorta to take an almost transverse course across the base of the heart.* (B) *Aortotomy in this patient reveals the densely calcified bicuspid valve.*

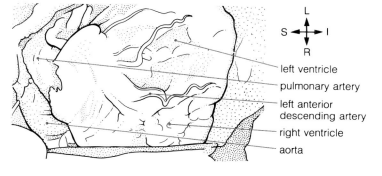

left ventricle
pulmonary artery
left anterior descending artery
right ventricle
aorta

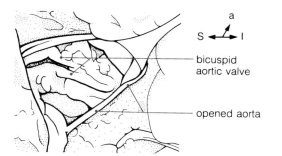

bicuspid aortic valve
opened aorta

the critical anatomic relationships of the aortic valve that are so important for the surgeon to keep in mind when performing aortic valve surgery. The fundamental feature of this anatomy is the pivotal position of the valve in relation to other vital structures within the heart (Figs. 4.20, 4.21).

In heavily calcified aortic valves calcium deposits do not usually extend beyond the confines of the cusps, but they may involve the anterior leaflet of the mitral valve (Fig. 4.22). Overzealous pursuit of such lesions can easily lead to detachment of that leaflet with resultant mitral incompetence, necessitating a difficult repair or replacement of the mitral apparatus. Such calcification may also cause problems

when it extends toward the central fibrous body and the adjacent conduction tissue (Fig. 4.23). Here again a vigorous attempt at decalcification to facilitate placement of an aortic prosthesis can lead to complications, including fistula formation through the central fibrous body to right-sided chambers of the heart, complete heart block, and/or detachment of the aortic root. The commissure between the right and the noncoronary cusps serves as an excellent guidepost in trying to avoid these complications (Fig. 4.24).

On occasion the surgeon is required to enlarge the aortic root to accommodate a prosthetic valve. Such an undertaking cannot be safely effected without a clear understanding of the anatomic relationships

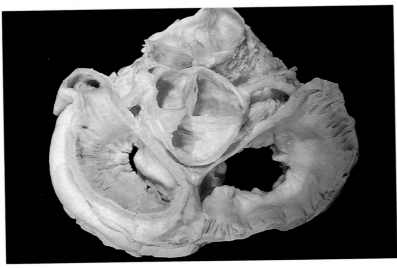

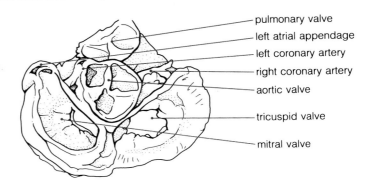

FIG. 4.20 *The wedged position of the aortic valve can easily be appreciated in this short-axis view of the heart.*

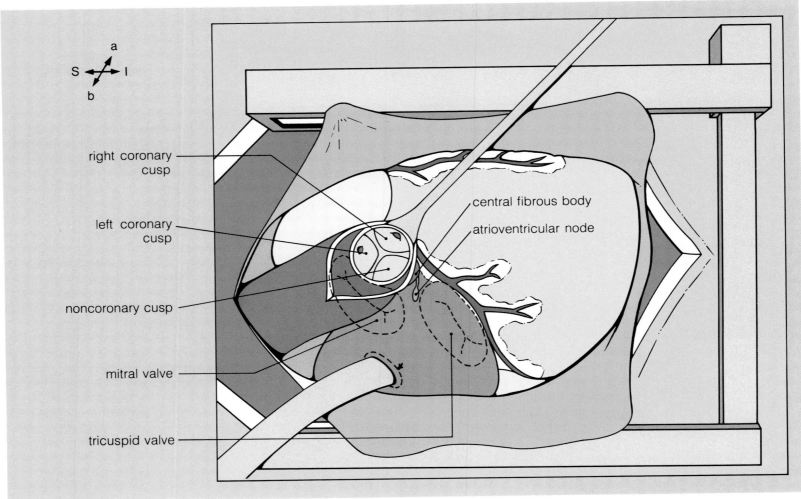

FIG. 4.21 *This diagram of the heart in surgical orientation shows the important relationships of the aortic valve. (Redrawn; reproduced with permission of the authors and publisher; see Figure Credits)*

PART II: DISEASES OF THE HEART

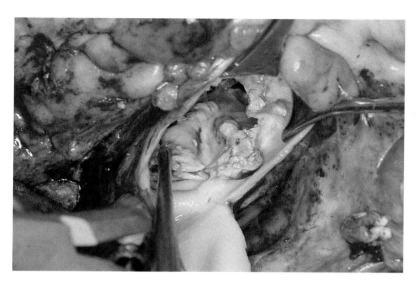

FIG. 4.22 *In this operative view of the area of aortic–mitral continuity after resection of the densely calcified aortic cusps, a prominent ridge of calcium can be seen extending onto the anterior mitral leaflet.*

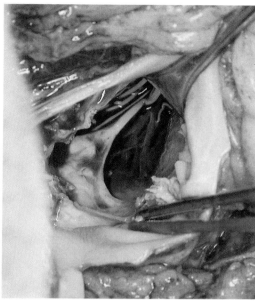

FIG. 4.23 *The edge of the anterior mitral leaflet is shown as it leads into the septal area just beneath the commissure of the excised aortic cusps. At this point beneath the central fibrous body, the left bundle sends its branches down the muscular septum.*

FIG. 4.23 *The edge of the anterior mitral leaflet is shown as it leads into the septal area just beneath the commissure of the excised aortic cusps. At this point beneath the central fibrous body, the left bundle sends its branches down the muscular septum.*

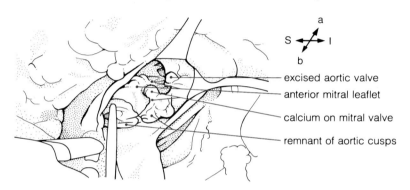

a
S ← → I
b

— excised aortic valve
— anterior mitral leaflet
— calcium on mitral valve
— remnant of aortic cusps

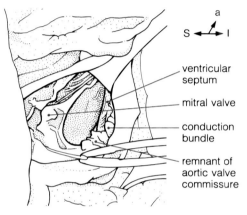

a
S ← → I

ventricular septum
mitral valve
conduction bundle
remnant of aortic valve commissure

FIG. 4.24 *The important relationships of the aortic valve are depicted as seen through an aortotomy. (Adapted; see Figure Credits)*

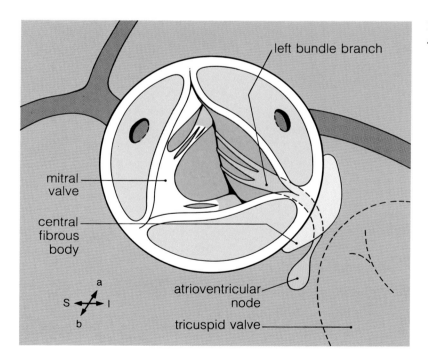

left bundle branch

mitral valve

central fibrous body

atrioventricular node

tricuspid valve

a
S ← → I
b

of the surrounding structures. Enlargement can only be accomplished in either of two directions. In the anterior alternative the left ventricular outflow tract and the aortic root are enlarged (Fig. 4.25). This technique has been particularly effective in children requiring valve replacement (Misbach et al, 1982). The longitudinal aortic incision is extended slightly to the left of the right coronary artery into the right ventricular outflow tract just inferior to the pulmonary valve. By continuing in this same plane, the subsequent incision into the outlet septum avoids the left bundle branches as they descend on the inter-

ventricular septum (Konno et al, 1975). Although this procedure is possible in adults as well as children, the extensive surgery and the complex reconstruction make this technique less appealing when dealing with the fragile tissues of a septuagenarian with calcific aortic valve disease and a narrow aortic orifice. Under these and other circumstances the less difficult posterior alternative is advocated by various investigators (Blank et al, 1976; Manouguian and Seybold–Epting, 1979; Nicks et al, 1970). This approach takes advantage of the anatomic arrangement of the adjacent parts of the left and the noncoronary

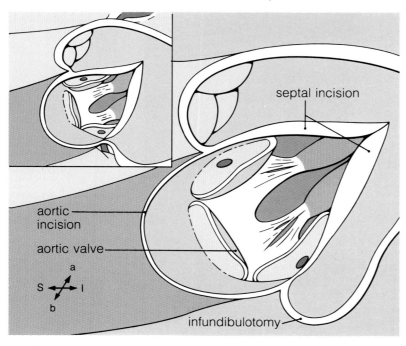

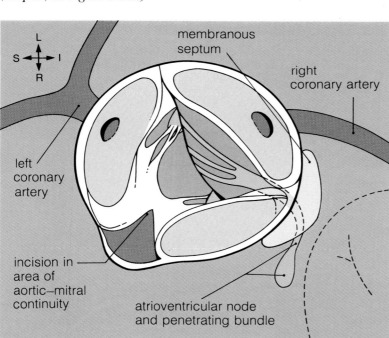

FIG. 4.25   *The anterior approach for enlargement of the left ventricular outflow tract and the aortic orifice is illustrated in surgical orientation. (Adapted; see Figure Credits)*

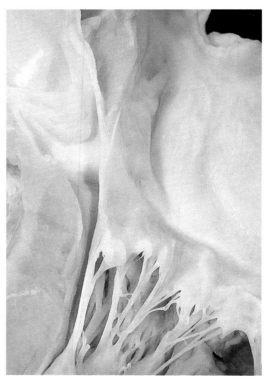

FIG. 4.26   *An anatomically oriented section has been taken through the noncoronary–left coronary commissure of the aortic valve. Note that the aortic–mitral curtain is directly related to the transverse sinus of the pericardial sac.*

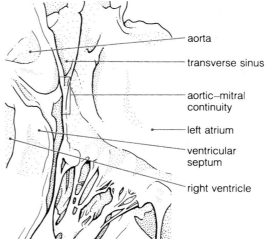

FIG. 4.27   *The posterior approach for enlargement of the aortic orifice is represented diagrammatically in surgical orientation.*

cusps of the aortic valve. Part of the free aortic wall forms the anterior aspect of the transverse sinus of the pericardial sac; at this point the attachments of the noncoronary cusps rise to their common commissure (Fig. 4.26). Thus this area may be safely incised; the incision may even be extended into the anterior leaflet of the mitral valve (Fig.

4.27). Autologous pericardium or other patch material may then be inserted into the resultant defect in the aorta, the mitral valve, and/or the left atrium to enlarge the diameter of the aortic orifice by as much as 5–15 mm (Fig. 4.28).

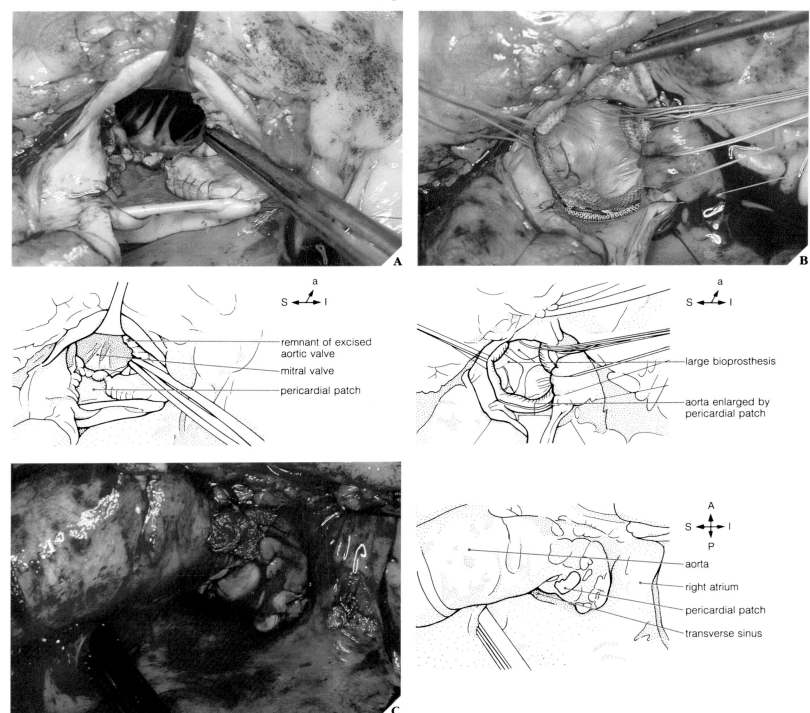

FIG. 4.28 (A) *In this operative view the aortic orifice has been enlarged by incising the aortic–mitral curtain and inserting a pericardial patch.* (B) *With the new valve in place the increased circumference is approximately* *equivalent to one third of that of the bioprosthesis.* (C) *The external appearance of the enlarged aorta is shown.*

The survival curve of patients who have had aortic valve replacement is shown in Figure 4.29; left ventricular dysfunction is a significant determinant of late results (Fig. 4.30). Late complications are determined by the type of artificial valve that is used. Mechanical prostheses are associated with a 2%–3% per year incidence of thromboembolic complications. Tissue prostheses are associated with valve failure re-quiring reoperation within eight years in about 20% of patients (Gallo et al, 1983).

Patients should take antibiotics prophylactically for bacterial endo-carditis after valve replacement. Patients with mechanical valves should have long-term anticoagulation therapy. Patients should be followed about twice a year in order to detect deterioration of the valve.

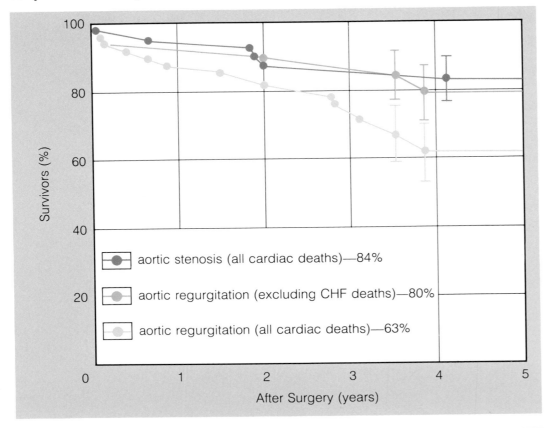

FIG. 4.29 *Actuarial survival times following aortic valve replacement are compared for aortic stenosis and aortic regurgitation. (Redrawn; reproduced with permission of the authors and publisher; see Figure Credits. Also, Fig. 37-35, The Heart, 6th ed, p 750)*

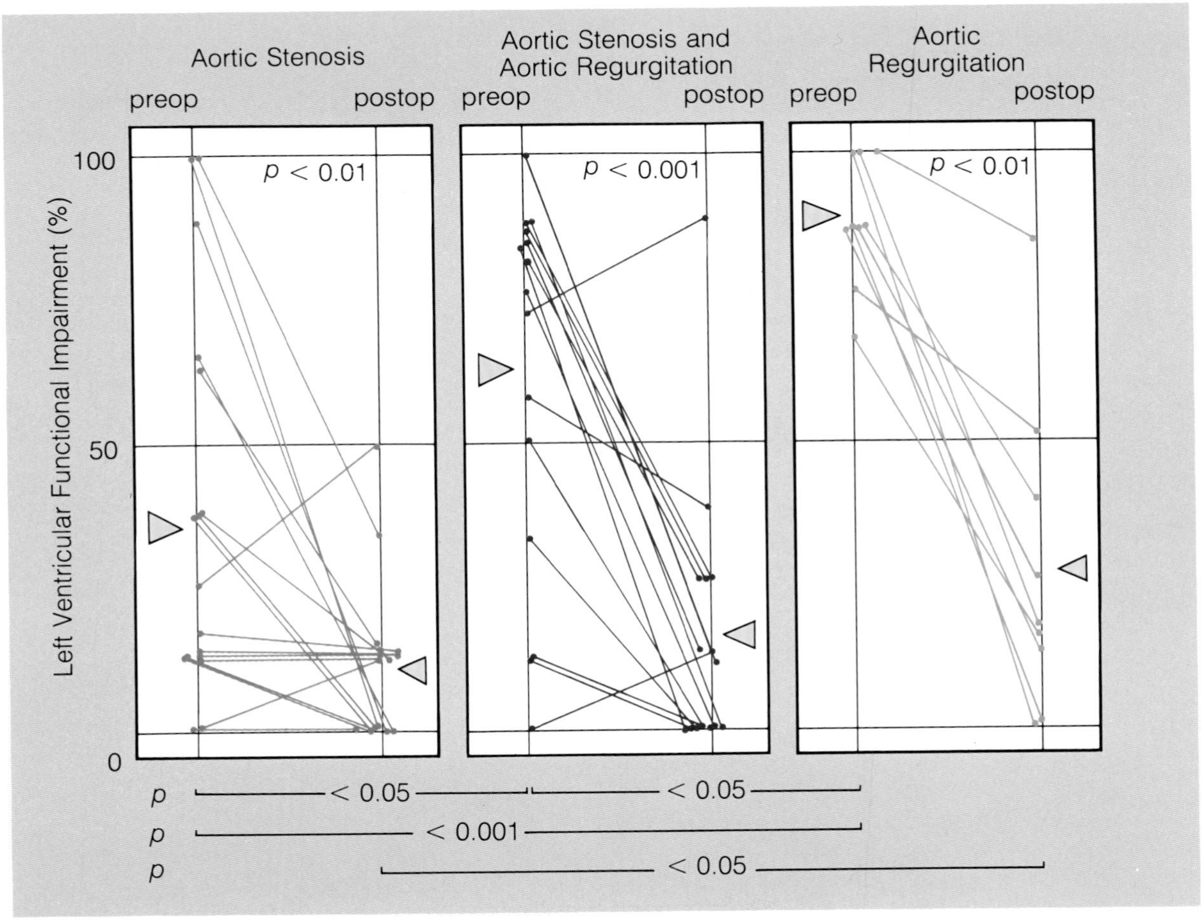

- aortic stenosis (all cardiac deaths)—84%
- aortic regurgitation (excluding CHF deaths)—80%
- aortic regurgitation (all cardiac deaths)—63%

Survivors (%)

After Surgery (years)

FIG. 4.30 *Change in multiple parameters of left ventricular impairment after aortic valve replacement is graphed for patients with aortic stenosis, mixed lesion, and aortic regurgitation. (Redrawn; reproduced with permission of the authors and publisher; see Figure Credits. Also, Fig. 37-12, The Heart, 6th ed, p 739)*

Aortic Stenosis

Aortic Stenosis and Aortic Regurgitation

Aortic Regurgitation

preop   postop   preop   postop   preop   postop

Left Ventricular Functional Impairment (%)

$p < 0.01$

$p < 0.001$

$p < 0.01$

p < 0.05 < 0.05
p < 0.001
p < 0.05

AORTIC VALVE REGURGITATION*
ETIOLOGY AND PATHOLOGY

In past decades rheumatic fever and syphilis were the major causes of aortic valve regurgitation; however, with the decline in incidence and prevalence of these diseases other etiologies should be considered (Table 4.1). The pathology of this condition is diverse; acute or chronic pathological processes may be responsible. Basically abnormalities of the valve leaflets and/or the aortic root may result in aortic regurgitation.

In chronic regurgitation the valve may show fibrosis of the leaflets with retraction and immobilization with or without accompanying calcification. The sequelae of rheumatic fever are a good example of the chronic condition (Fig. 4.31), but most other types of abnormalities that affect the connective tissue core of the leaflets can also produce these changes (see Table 4.1). Congenitally bicuspid aortic valve is an important condition, particularly in the setting of a large conjoined cusp; prolapse toward the left ventricular cavity may occur with or without dystrophic calcification (Fig. 4.32). Conditions affecting the aortic root are manifold; Marfan's syndrome may be the best example (Fig. 4.33). An important abnormality of uncertain origin is aorticoan-

---

*Abstracted with permission of the authors and publisher from Rackley CE, Edwards JE, Wallace RB, Katz NM: Aortic valve disease, Chapter 37, pp 729–754, in Hurst JW (ed): *The Heart*, 6th ed. New York, McGraw-Hill, 1986. Figures and tables above reproduced in this section from the chapter or other sources are also reprinted with permission of the authors and publishers. For the full bibliographic citations of the sources of figures and tables other than the above chapter, see Figure Credits at the end of this chapter.

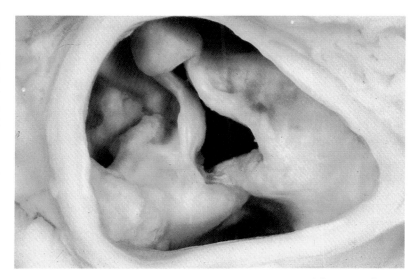

FIG. 4.31   *This rheumatic aortic valve shows commissural fusion and leaflet fibrosis. The pathology suggests stenosis and regurgitation as a functional consequence. (Reproduced with permission of the authors and publisher; see Figure Credits)*

Table 4.1 Etiology of Chronic and Acute Aortic Regurgitation*

CHRONIC AORTIC REGURGITATION

Rheumatic fever	Aortic root disease
Syphilis	Aorticoannuloectasia
Aortitis (Takayasu)	Cystic medial necrosis of
Heritable disorders of	aorta
connective tissue	Hypertension
Marfan's syndrome	Arteriosclerosis
Ehlers–Danlos syndrome	Myxomatous degeneration
Osteogenesis imperfecta	of valve
Congenital heart disease	Infective endocarditis
Bicuspid aortic valve	Following prosthetic valve
Interventricular septal	surgery
defect	Associated with aortic
Sinus of Valsalva	stenosis
aneurysm	
Arthritic diseases	
Ankylosing spondylitis	
Reiter's syndrome	
Rheumatoid arthritis	
Lupus erythematosus	

ACUTE AORTIC REGURGITATION

Rheumatic fever	Acute aortic dissection
Infective endocarditis	Following prosthetic valve
Congenital (rupture of sinus	surgery
of Valsalva)	Trauma

(Table 37-1, *The Heart*, 6th ed, p 740)
*Please note that certain disorders are capable of producing both acute and chronic regurgitation.

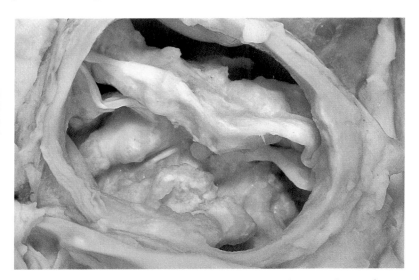

FIG. 4.32   *This bicuspid aortic valve from an adult shows evidence of fibrosis and calcification; prolapse of the conjoined leaflet results in aortic valve regurgitation.*

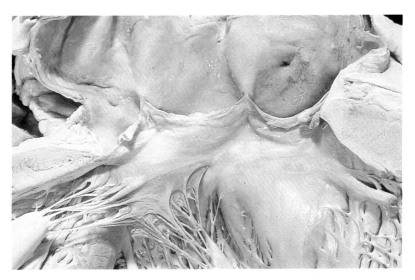

FIG. 4.33   *Aortic root dilation in a patient with Marfan's disease causes aortic regurgitation. (Reproduced with permission of the authors and publisher; see Figure Credits)*

nuloectasia (Fig. 4.34). Acute regurgitation is generally due to sudden disruption of the integrity of the aortic valve; infective endocarditis is by far the most common cause (Fig. 4.35).

ABNORMAL PHYSIOLOGY

Chronic aortic valve regurgitation causes a gradual increase in end-diastolic volume of the left ventricle. As a result of this volume load the heart remodels itself by left ventricular dilation and an increase in left ventricular wall thickness. The left ventricular stroke volume is also increased. The increase in end-diastolic volume may be associated with a minimal increase in pressure in the early stages of the condition. The diastolic compliance of the left ventricle is increased, and compensatory left ventricular hypertrophy normalizes systolic wall stress or afterload. Forward cardiac output remains normal during rest and exercise.

In the late stages of chronic aortic valve regurgitation primary myocardial factors or secondary lesions, such as coronary disease, may depress the contractile state of the left ventricular myocardium, producing an increase in end-systolic volume and a decrease in the ejection fraction. This is associated with an increase in end-diastolic pressure due to a decrease in compliance, leading to elevation of left atrial pressure and, hence, to pulmonary venous hypertension.

The hemodynamic changes of acute aortic valve regurgitation differ from the chronic condition if the acute damage occurs in a patient with no previous regurgitation. The left ventricle does not have sufficient time to adapt to considerable aortic regurgitation. Accordingly an abrupt rise in left ventricular end-diastolic pressure may occur with little ventricular dilation. The left ventricular end-diastolic pressure may rise and approach, or even exceed, left atrial pressure, prematurely closing the mitral valve. These sudden changes may produce pulmonary venous hypertension and pulmonary edema.

If acute regurgitation is superimposed on chronic aortic valve regurgitation, the hemodynamic and clinical consequences depend on the summation of the chronic and the acute hemodynamic changes.

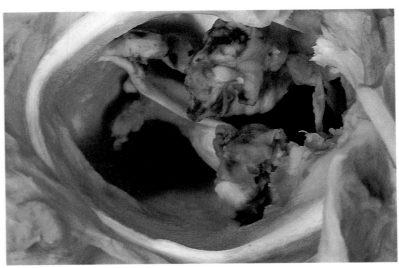

FIG. 4.34 *Aorticoannuloectasia with a markedly dilated ascending aorta results in chronic aortic regurgitation.*

FIG. 4.35 *Infective endocarditis of the aortic valve with extensive destruction of leaflet tissue leads to acute regurgitation.*

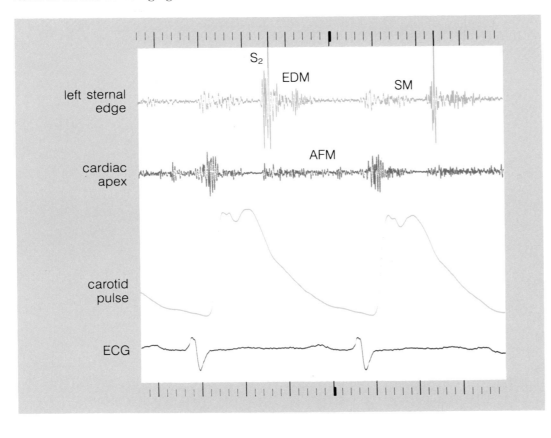

FIG. 4.36 *These phonocardiograms and carotid pulse recording were obtained from a patient with aortic regurgitation. At the left sternal edge a decrescendo diastolic murmur (EDM) following the second sound (S₂) is recorded. At the cardiac apex a low-frequency mid-diastolic and a presystolic (Austin Flint) murmur (AFM) culminate at the time of the first heart sound. The carotid arterial tracing shows a bisferious pattern in the absence of the dicrotic notch. (Redrawn; Fig. 37-21, The Heart, 6th ed, p 745. Courtesy of Ernest Craige, MD)*

CLINICAL MANIFESTATIONS
SYMPTOMS

The patient may notice prominent pulsations in the carotid artery and at the apex of the heart when he or she lies on the left side. The patient may be aware of premature heart beats, since the stroke volume is quite large after the long diastole.

SYMPTOMS DUE TO HEART FAILURE. Patients with long-standing chronic aortic valve regurgitation develop symptoms of heart failure, including dyspnea with effort, orthopnea, paroxysmal nocturnal dyspnea, pulmonary edema, and fatigue.

ANGINA PECTORIS. The angina associated with aortic valve regurgitation tends to occur at rest when bradycardia is present and lasts longer than angina due to coronary disease alone. The exact cause of the angina, however, cannot be determined by an analysis of the symptoms.

OTHER SYMPTOMS. Patients with severe aortic valve regurgitation may have carotid sheath pain, abdominal pain, postural dizziness, and excessive sweating (Harvey et al, 1957). Patients with acute aortic valve regurgitation may develop abrupt pulmonary edema, hypotension, and even shock.

PHYSICAL EXAMINATION

The etiology of aortic valve regurgitation may be immediately evident upon physical examination if it is associated with Marfan's syndrome, osteogenesis imperfecta, or ankylosing spondylitis.

A rapid carotid upstroke and a wide pulse pressure may result in a hyperdynamic state with a pulsus bisferiens (Fig. 4.36). When the regurgitation is severe, it produces a profound effect on the peripheral arterial pulsation. When heart failure is severe, however, the systemic diastolic blood pressure may be normal because of the elevation of the diastolic pressure in the left ventricle.

The heart may be normal in size when chronic aortic valve regurgitation is slight or when the regurgitation is acute. Patients with moderately severe chronic regurgitation have enlarged hearts; the apex impulse is displaced inferolaterally, and is hyperdynamic and larger than normal.

The first heart sound at the apex may be diminished in intensity especially if the P-R interval is long. A systolic ejection sound may be heard along the left sternal border due to abrupt distention of the aorta. Secondary to aortic valve regurgitation there may be a systolic aortic murmur in the second left intercostal space, a systolic murmur at the apex, a diastolic rumble (Austin Flint murmur) at the apex, and a systolic tricuspid murmur.

The characteristic diastolic murmur of aortic valve regurgitation is high-pitched. It is best heard along the left sternal border, using the diaphragm of the stethoscope with firm pressure; the patient should be leaning forward after exhaling. When there is aortic root disease, the murmur may be best heard to the right of the sternum. A high-pitched, cooing, diastolic murmur may be heard when an aortic leaflet is lacerated, retroverted, or when a hole develops because of endocarditis (Fig. 4.37). This type of murmur is often heard with acute aortic regurgitation. The first sound is usually faint in such cases be-

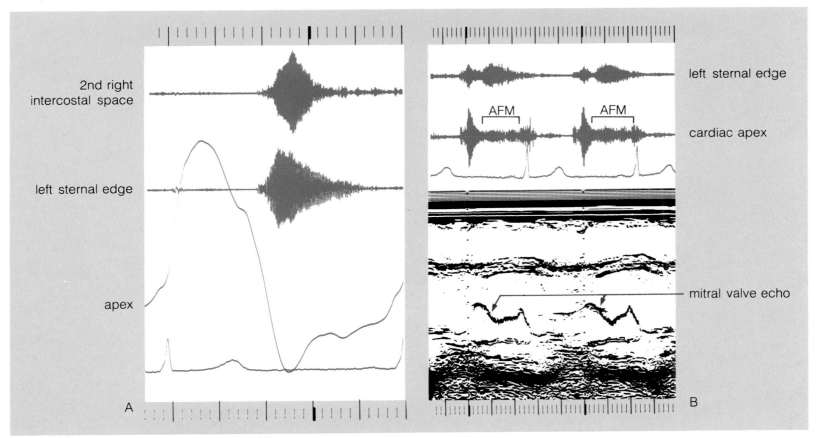

FIG. 4.37 *These phonocardiograms and M-mode echocardiogram were obtained from a patient with aortic regurgitation.* (**A**) *The murmur is loudest at the left sternal edge with a high-frequency and diminuendo configuration. The musical quality of the murmur is indicated by the pattern of the vibrations, which suggests an everted cusp as the cause of the valvar incompetence.* (**B**) *At a slower paper speed the contrast in the phonocardiographic appearance of the murmur at different precordial locations is evident. At the left sternal edge the early diastolic murmur has a diminuendo silhouette. At the apex the murmur is of lower frequency; it becomes accentuated prior to the next systole owing to the addition of an Austin Flint murmur (AFM). The vibrations of the anterior leaflet of the mitral valve, seen in the M-mode echocardiogram, coincide with the early diastolic murmur and not the Austin Flint murmur. (Fig. 37-22, The Heart, 6th ed, p 746. Courtesy of Ernest Craige, MD)*

cause of premature closure of the mitral valve. A ventricular gallop sound heard at the apex is usually a sign of left ventricular dysfunction.

The Austin Flint diastolic rumble heard at the apex is due to the impingement of aortic regurgitant flow on the anterior leaflet of the mitral valve, which produces functional mitral stenosis.

LABORATORY STUDIES

CHEST RADIOGRAPHY. Chronic aortic valve regurgitation produces a dilated left ventricle, an enlarged left atrium, and a dilated aortic root (Fig. 4.38). The heart size or shape may not be altered in acute regurgitation, but pulmonary edema may be present.

ELECTROCARDIOGRAPHY. The ECG shows left ventricular hypertrophy (Selzer et al, 1962). The QRS voltage is increased, and the ST-T wave may be of the diastolic overload type; that is, the mean vector representing the large ST and T waves is parallel to the mean QRS vector. The pattern of left ventricular strain may also be present when the mean ST-T vector is pointed in a direction that is opposite to the mean QRS vector (Fig. 4.39). The P-R interval may be prolonged.

ECHOCARDIOGRAPHY. The echocardiogram can provide anatomic information about the aortic root and the aortic valve, including vegetations. It can also give measurements of ventricular function. An

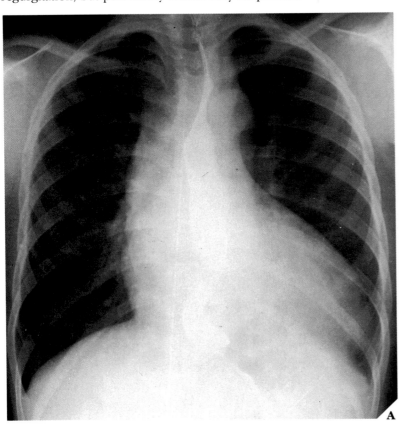
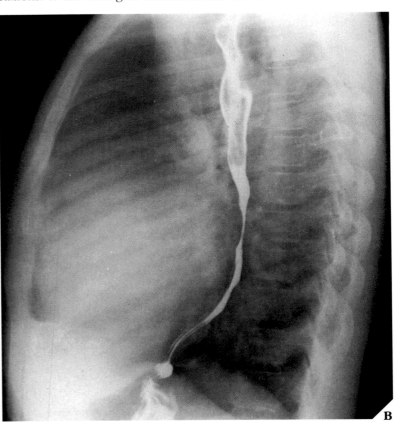

FIG. 4.38 *Barium opacifies the esophagus on the chest films of a patient with aortic regurgitation.* (**A**) *Posteroanterior view reveals marked enlargement of the left ventricle with dilation of the aorta beginning in the root and extending through the distal arch. The lung fields are normal.*

(**B**) *Lateral projection demonstrates posterior displacement of the esophagus by an enlarged left atrium. (Courtesy of Wade H. Shuford, MD, Atlanta, Georgia)*

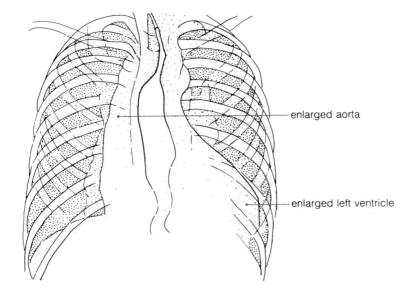
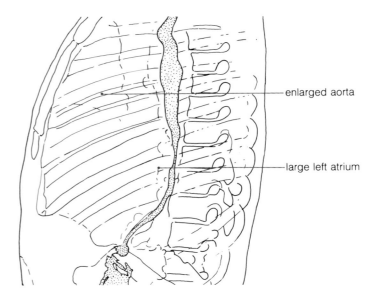

enlarged aorta

enlarged left ventricle

enlarged aorta

large left atrium

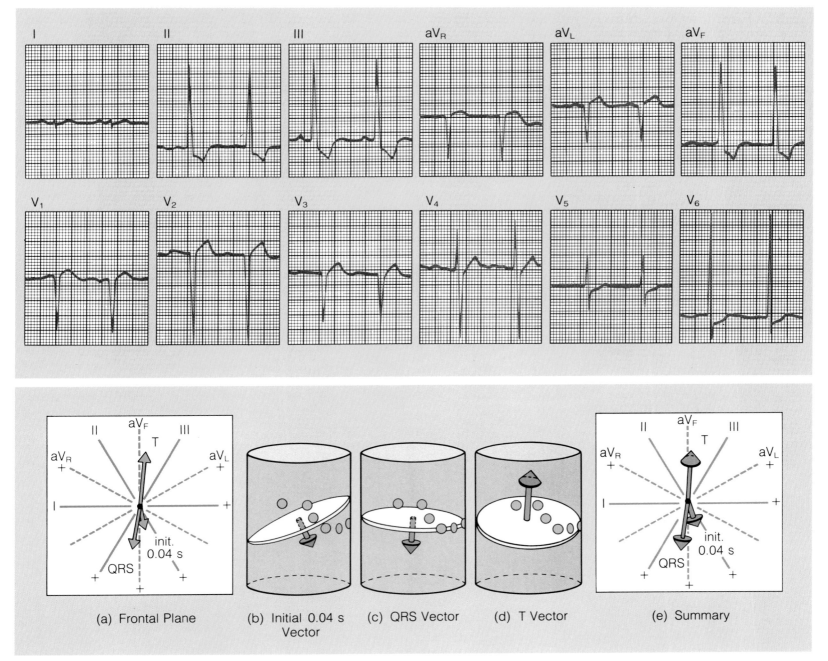

I   II   III   aV_R   aV_L   aV_F

V₁   V₂   V₃   V₄   V₅   V₆

(a) Frontal Plane (b) Initial 0.04 s Vector (c) QRS Vector (d) T Vector (e) Summary

FIG. 4.39 *This ECG was obtained from a 16-year-old girl with Marfan's syndrome and severe aortic regurgitation.* (**a**) *Frontal plane projection shows the mean QRS, initial 0.04 second, and T vectors.* (**b**) *The initial 0.04 second vector is slightly positive in lead I and negative in aV_R and aV_L; therefore it is just to the left of aV_F. There are Q waves in leads V₁–V₃ and R waves in leads V₄–V₆.* (**c**) *The mean QRS vector is resultantly negative in lead I and slightly more positive in lead III compared with lead II. The vector must be just to the right of aV_F. The mean QRS vector is transitional between V₄ and V₅.* (**d**) *The mean T vector is opposite the mean QRS vector; and since it is positive in lead I, it is drawn slightly to the left of the perpendicular to lead I.* (**e**) *Final summary figure shows the spatial arrangement of the vectors. The striking ventricular forces and the vertical mean QRS axis are common in young people with left ventricular hypertrophy. Decreased anterior forces and ST-segment elevation in V₁ and V₂ are common findings with severe left ventricular hypertrophy. (Redrawn; reproduced with permission of the authors and publisher; see Figure Credits)*

increase in aortic dimension suggests chronic regurgitation. Left ventricular stroke volume and the ejection fraction can be calculated at rest and during supine exercise.

Mitral valve abnormalities recognized on the echocardiogram include diastolic fluttering of the anterior mitral valve leaflet and rapid early closure of a thickened mitral valve (Fig. 4.40) (Pridie et al, 1971). In acute aortic regurgitation a flail aortic leaflet may be seen, and aortic dissection can often be recognized (Whipple et al, 1977).

Pre- and postoperative studies suggest that a left ventricular end-systolic dimension greater than 55 mm may identify a group of patients at high risk for the development of heart failure (Henry et al, 1973). The aortic valve should be replaced before irreversible left ventricular damage has occurred. The echocardiogram is useful in identifying such patients.

The diastolic flow across the aortic valve can be determined by the Doppler technique (Fig. 4.41).

CARDIAC CATHETERIZATION. Cardiac catheterization is indicated to assess the severity of aortic regurgitation in patients thought to have moderately severe to severe regurgitation (Fig. 4.42), to determine left ventricular function, and to identify other cardiac abnormalities, such as mitral valve disease or coronary artery disease.

Cardiac catheterization results may easily be misinterpreted. A dilated left ventricular chamber may dilute the contrast medium, giving

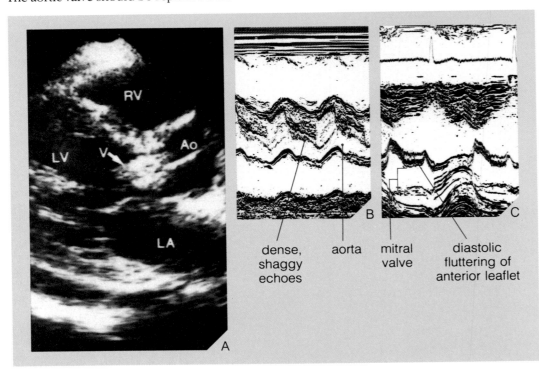

dense, shaggy echoes   aorta   mitral valve   diastolic fluttering of anterior leaflet

FIG. 4.40 *These cross-sectional and M-mode echocardiograms were obtained from a patient with aortic regurgitation due to infective endocarditis. (A) Cross-sectional echocardiogram in the long-axis parasternal view reveals a large aortic vegetation (V) (Ao, aortic valve; LA, left atrium; LV, left ventricle; RV, right ventricle). (B) M-mode echocardiogram of the aortic valve shows dense, shaggy echoes visible on the aortic leaflets during diastole consistent with an aortic valve vegetation. (C) M-mode echocardiogram of the mitral valve shows high-frequency diastolic fluttering of the anterior leaflet of the mitral valve consistent with aortic regurgitation. (Courtesy of Joel M. Felner, MD, Atlanta, Georgia)*

FIG. 4.41 *Continuous-wave Doppler recording from the apex toward the aortic valve shows the high velocity diastolic flow jet due to aortic regurgitation. (Courtesy of Joel M. Felner, MD, Atlanta, Georgia)*

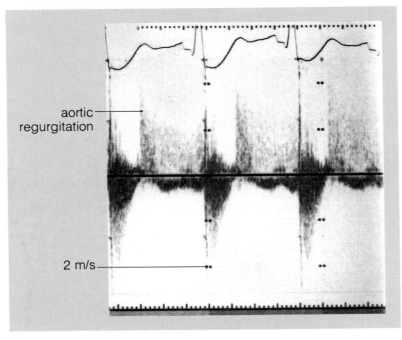

aortic regurgitation

2 m/s

the impression of minimal regurgitation, whereas regurgitation into a normal-sized left ventricular chamber may create an impression of severe aortic regurgitation (Hunt et al, 1973). Left ventricular end-diastolic pressure cannot be used as an index of left ventricular function in patients with chronic aortic regurgitation, because there may be an increase in the diastolic compliance and the end-diastolic wall stress with a normal preload. This measurement is more useful in patients with acute aortic regurgitation. The ejection fraction is useful, but this value is artificially preserved in the volume overload of chronic aortic regurgitation, since systolic ejection begins at a lower than normal level of left ventricular pressure.

Contractility can be studied in patients with chronic aortic regurgitation. It is more depressed in patients with heart failure than in asymptomatic patients (Osbakken et al, 1981).

Coronary arteriography should be performed in adults who are undergoing cardiac catheterization for aortic regurgitation, since coronary disease may produce angina and left ventricular dysfunction. Bypass surgery may be required when the aortic valve is replaced.

RADIONUCLIDE STUDIES. ^{99m}Tc ventriculograms at rest and during exercise can be used to quantify the amount of regurgitant flow and to determine the ejection fraction (Borer et al, 1978). With normal

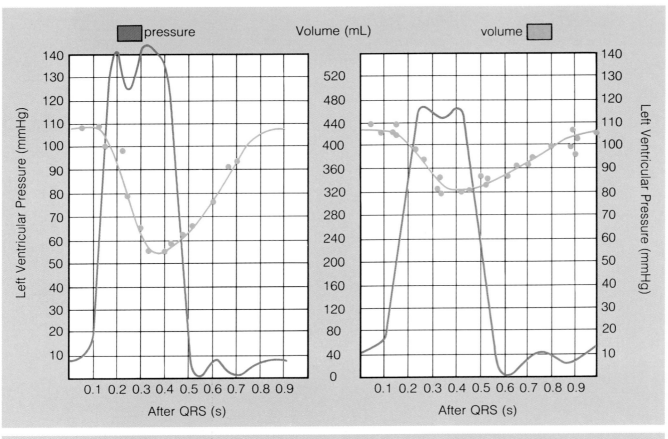

FIG. 4.42 *Left ventricular pressure and volume was recorded in two patients with aortic regurgitation. The patient on the left enjoyed unrestricted activity without symptoms, whereas the patient on the right was extremely limited by left ventricular failure. (Redrawn; reproduced with permission of the authors and publisher; see Figure Credits. Also, Fig. 37-23, The Heart, 6th ed, p 748)*

Unrestricted Activity		Restricted Activity
436	end-diastolic volume (mL)	430
219	end-systolic volume (mL)	329
217	left ventricular stroke volume (mL)	101
97	forward stroke volume (mL)	67
120	aortic regurgitation (mL)	34
217/436 = 50	ejection fraction (%)	101/430 = 23
474	left ventricular weight (g)	561
8	left ventricular end-diastolic pressure (mmHg)	13

cardiac function the ejection fraction should be in the normal range, increasing with exercise. A fall in ejection fraction with exercise indicates poor myocardial contractility, which can occur before the patient becomes symptomatic (Fig. 4.43). The test is often used in following patients to establish the optimum time for aortic valve replacement.

[201]Tl scintigraphy can identify perfusion defects in the myocardium that suggest the presence of associated coronary disease.

NATURAL HISTORY

Seventy-five percent of patients with significant chronic aortic valve regurgitation survive five years, and 50% survive for ten years after the diagnosis has been made. Patients with mild-to-moderate aortic regurgitation are likely to survive ten years (Rapaport, 1975). Many patients with trivial aortic regurgitation live a normal life span, but they are predisposed to infective endocarditis. Patients who develop heart failure often expire within two years; the average survival after the onset of angina is five years.

Patients with a preoperative ejection fraction of 45% and cardiac indices greater than 2.5 liters/min/m² have a greater long-term survival after surgery than do patients with less than 45% ejection fractions and cardiac indices of less than 2.5 liters/min/m² (Greves et al, 1981).

The actuarial survival of patients with chronic aortic regurgitation treated medically from the time of diagnosis is shown in Figure 4.13. Patients with acute aortic regurgitation and pulmonary edema have a very poor prognosis; surgical intervention is usually necessary.

TREATMENT

Patients with aortic regurgitation should be treated prophylactically for bacterial endocarditis. Heart failure is treated with digitalis, diuretics, and vasodilating drugs, such as hydralazine and nitrates, to reduce afterload.

INDICATIONS FOR SURGERY

Symptomatic patients with severe chronic regurgitation are advised to have surgery. Asymptomatic patients who have evidence of left ventricular dysfunction at rest determined by the identification of a decreased ejection fraction using ^{99m}Tc ventriculography, echocardiography, or angiography should be advised to have surgery. Those patients who do not increase their ejection fractions with exercise are probably in the same category, and it is highly likely that they will need surgery even if it is delayed for a period of time.

Acute aortic regurgitation is often due to bacterial endocarditis, aortic dissection, or rupture of a myxomatous valve. Prompt surgical intervention is usually required to prevent death due to pulmonary edema. Although destruction of the valve cusps (Fig. 4.44A) is usually the principal problem when infective endocarditis is the cause of acute aortic regurgitation, fistula formation may also result from infections in the aortic root (Fig. 4.44B). Sometimes, with dissection, a prosthetic valve is not needed when the aorta can be repaired (Croft et al, 1983).

SURGICAL PROCEDURE

Anatomic considerations in the replacement of regurgitant valves are identical to those for stenotic valves (see above).

The choice of a prosthetic valve is determined by the patient's age, need, contraindications for anticoagulants, and the durability of valves. Patients with tissue valves, either porcine or pericardial, may not require the long-term use of anticoagulants. However, the durability of these valves is probably less than it is for synthetic valves.

The operative risk is about 2% in patients with moderate chronic regurgitation and normal coronary arteries. The operative risk in patients with more severe regurgitation with heart failure and in patients with associated coronary disease is much higher, ranging from 4%–10% or more depending on the clinical state of the patient.

Survival following valve replacement for aortic regurgitation is shown in Figure 4.29. Late results are best in patients who had good left ventricular function at the time of surgery, but the etiology of the condition also influences long-term survival.

Patients should be instructed about antibiotic prophylaxis for endocarditis following surgery; those patients with mechanical valves should receive long-term anticoagulation therapy. Patients should be followed semi-annually to detect deterioration of the valve.

MITRAL VALVE STENOSIS*
ETIOLOGY AND PATHOLOGY

Mitral valve stenosis is usually caused by scarring of the valve following rheumatic fever. Fibrosis affects the valve leaflets and the commissures, restricting valve mobility. Retraction may eventually lead to a funnel-type valve (Fig. 4.45), cordal fibrosis, and obliteration of the intercordal spaces (Fig. 4.46), thus contributing markedly to the inflow obstruction. Congenital mitral valve stenosis is almost always part of a more complex cardiac malformation; usually the patient becomes symptomatic at an early age.

---

*Abstracted with permission of the authors and publisher from Rackley CE, Edwards JE, Karp, RB: Mitral valve disease, Chapter 38, pp 754–784, in Hurst JW (ed): *The Heart,* 6th ed. New York, McGraw-Hill, 1986. Figures and tables reproduced in this section from the above chapter, other chapters in *The Heart,* or other sources are also reprinted with permission of the authors and publishers. For the full bibliographic citations of the sources of figures other than the above chapter, see Figure Credits at the end of this chapter.

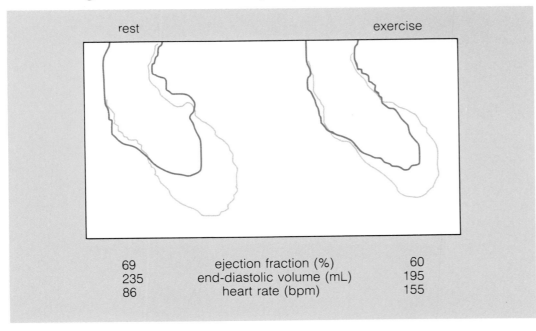

FIG. 4.43 *The results of rest and exercise radionuclide angiograms in a patient with aortic regurgitation show a decrease in the ejection fraction and the end-diastolic volume with peak exercise. (Redrawn; reproduced with permission of the author and publisher; see Figure Credits)*

rest		exercise
69	ejection fraction (%)	60
235	end-diastolic volume (mL)	195
86	heart rate (bpm)	155

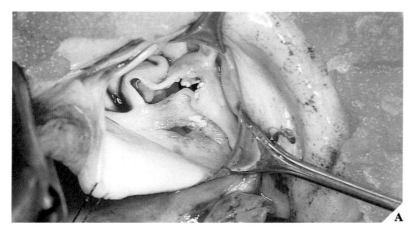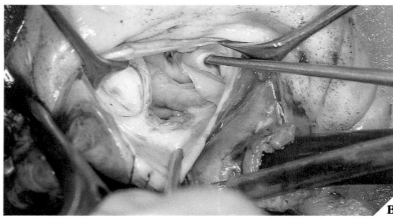

FIG. 4.44 (A) *This operative view shows a severely damaged aortic valve secondary to bacterial endocarditis. Urgent surgical intervention was required due to intractable heart failure, which was aggravated by the* presence of an aortic–right atrial fistula, shown here with a probe inserted through the aortic aspect of the fistula (B).

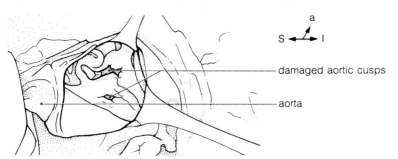

a

S ← → I

— damaged aortic cusps

— aorta

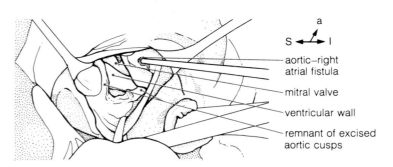

a

S ← → I

— aortic–right atrial fistula

— mitral valve

— ventricular wall

— remnant of excised aortic cusps

FIG. 4.45 *Long-axis cross-section through a heart with a rheumatic mitral valve shows funnel-like stenosis. (Reproduced with permission of the authors and publisher; see Figure Credits)*

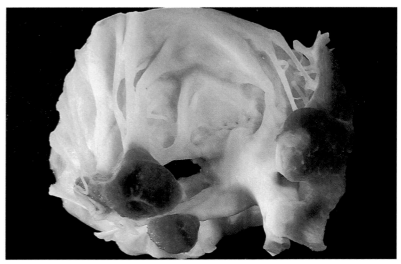

FIG. 4.46 *A resected rheumatic mitral valve shows extensive obliteration of intercordal spaces and leaflet fibrosis—features underlying mitral stenosis.*

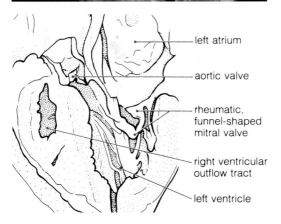

— left atrium

— aortic valve

— rheumatic, funnel-shaped mitral valve

— right ventricular outflow tract

— left ventricle

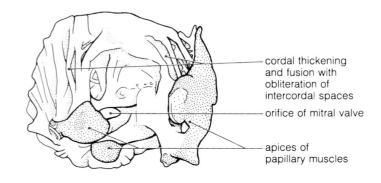

— cordal thickening and fusion with obliteration of intercordal spaces

— orifice of mitral valve

— apices of papillary muscles

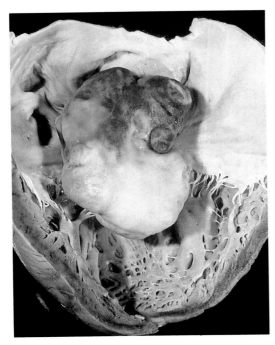

FIG. 4.47 *A left atrial myxoma obstructs the mitral orifice. (Reproduced with permission of the authors and publisher; see Figure Credits)*

Other conditions, such as methysergide maleate (Sansert) toxicity, causing mitral stenosis are rare. Left atrial myxoma may obstruct the orifice (Fig. 4.47). Occasionally endocarditis may present with signs of mitral stenosis due to excessive thrombotic vegetations occluding the orifice. A malfunctioning mitral prothesis may also produce stenosis of the mitral orifice (Fig. 4.48), and the large papillary muscles of idiopathic cardiac hypertrophy may impede the flow of blood into the left ventricle. A calcified mitral ring usually produces regurgitation rather than stenosis.

ABNORMAL PHYSIOLOGY

Significant mitral valve blockade produces a decrease in diastolic blood flow through the valve, resulting in a pressure gradient between the left atrium and the left ventricle. The relationship of the mean diastolic pressure gradient and flow across the mitral valve is shown in Figure 4.49. The mean diastolic gradient is determined by the cardiac output and the time required for diastole. As the left atrial pressure rises, it produces an elevation of pulmonary venous pressure. This leads to compensatory dilation of the lymphatics (Fig. 4.50) and the bronchial veins due to pulmonary bronchial venous shunting (Fig. 4.51); soon medial hypertrophy and arterialization of the pulmonary veins occur (Fig. 4.52). The muscular pulmonary arteries and arterioles hypertrophy, and intimal fibrosis develops (Fig. 4.53); the resulting pulmonary

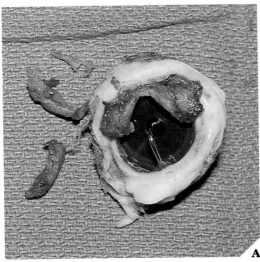

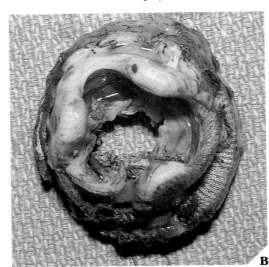

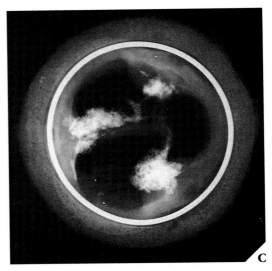

A   B   C

FIG. 4.48 *Examples of malfunctioning mitral prostheses.* (A) *A pivoting disk valve with pannus formation results in mitral stenosis.* (B) *A bioprosthesis with calcified leaflets may cause mitral stenosis and regurgita-* tion. (C) *Radiograph of a bioprosthesis four years after implantation in a 50-year-old female shows marked calcification.*

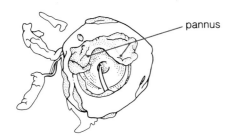

pannus

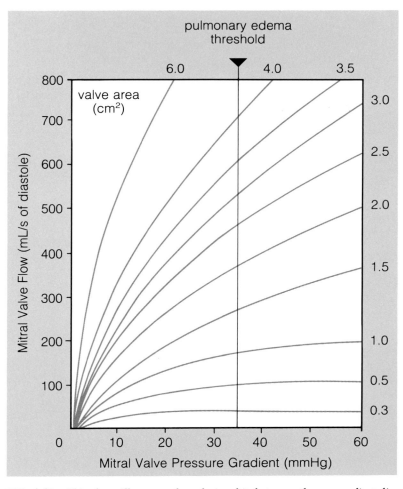

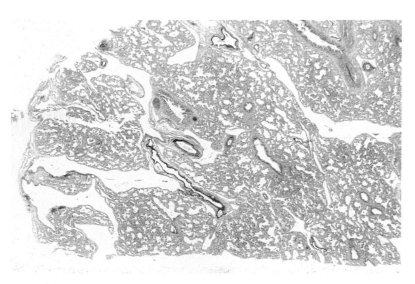

FIG. 4.50 *Histologic section of lung tissue shows dilation of lymphatics consequent to chronic pulmonary venous hypertension. (Reproduced with permission of the authors and publisher; see Figure Credits)*

FIG. 4.49 *This chart illustrates the relationship between the mean diastolic gradient across the mitral valve and the rate of flow across the mitral valve per second of diastole, as predicted by the Gorlin and Gorlin formula. When the mitral valve area is 1.0 cm² or less, very little additional flow can be achieved by an increased pressure gradient. Transudation of fluid from the pulmonary capillaries and the development of pulmonary edema begin when pulmonary capillary pressure exceeds the oncotic pressure of plasma, which is about 25–35 mmHg. It is also apparent that severe mitral regurgitation is incompatible with very tight mitral stenosis. (Redrawn; Fig. 44-2, The Heart, 2nd ed; see Figure Credits. Courtesy of Robert C. Schlant, MD, Atlanta, Georgia)*

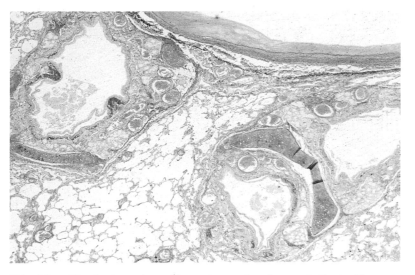

FIG. 4.51 *Histologic section of lung tissue taken from a patient with chronic pulmonary venous hypertension shows a dilated bronchial venous plexus.*

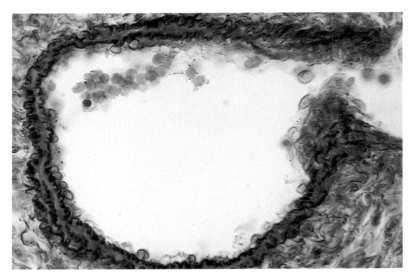

FIG. 4.52 *Arterialization of the pulmonary vein may occur in a patient with congenital mitral valve stenosis. A distinct muscular media is formed, sandwiched between an inner and an outer elastic lamina.*

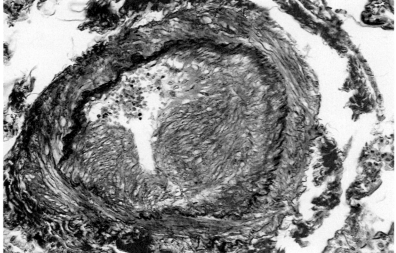

FIG. 4.53 *Histologic section of lung tissue taken from a patient with chronic pulmonary venous hypertension shows a muscular pulmonary artery with medial hypertrophy and cushion-like intimal fibrosis.*

hypertension causes right ventricular hypertrophy (Fig. 4.54) (Kennedy et al, 1970).

CLINICAL MANIFESTATIONS

About 50% of patients with mitral stenosis due to rheumatic fever give a history of rheumatic fever (Rowe et al, 1960). This condition occurs more often in women; symptoms begin to appear in the early 30s or older, although mitral stenosis due to rheumatic fever may occur at a younger age in certain countries. Congenital mitral stenosis may produce symptoms at an early age (see Chapter 3).

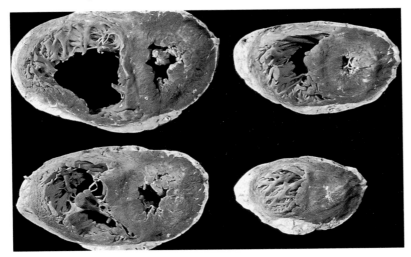

FIG. 4.54 *Right ventricular wall hypertrophy and chamber dilation are the results of long-standing pulmonary hypertension. (Reproduced with permission of the authors and publisher; see Figure Credits)*

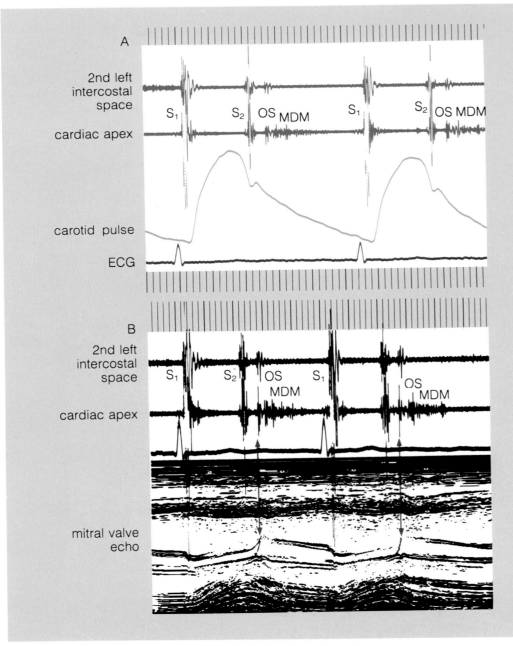

FIG. 4.55 *These phonocardiographic tracings, obtained at the second left intercostal space and cardiac apex, and carotid pulse tracing were recorded in a patient with mitral stenosis and atrial fibrillation. (A) A loud first sound (S$_1$) and the opening snap (OS) of the mitral valve occurs 0.11 second after the second heart sound (S$_2$), which is in turn followed by a low-frequency mid-diastolic murmur (MDM) at the cardiac apex. (B) A phonocardiogram, obtained at a slower paper speed (50 mm/s), and an M-mode echocardiogram show a relation between the first heart sound and the completion of the closing movement of the mitral valve and, similarly, the opening snap accompanying the termination of the opening movement of the valve. (Fig. 38-3,* The Heart, *6th ed, p 757. Courtesy of Ernest Craige, MD)*

SYMPTOMS

Patients complain of dyspnea on effort, fatigue, palpitation, hemoptysis, and hoarseness. The symptoms that result from embolic events and the symptoms that accompany infective endocarditis are also noted (Selzer and Cohn, 1972).

DYSPNEA. Patients may be asymptomatic for many years, and then gradually develop dyspnea on effort. They may walk less rapidly and, by limiting their activity, avoid dyspnea. Such patients may then deny dyspnea, although the mitral valve obstruction may be gradually increasing.

Patients with slight or no dyspnea may develop severe dyspnea and pulmonary edema when atrial fibrillation develops. Left ventricular filling is compromised by the rapid rate and the short diastoles in such patients. Pulmonary edema may develop during pregnancy (Szekely et al, 1973).

FATIGUE. Fatigue usually accompanies dyspnea in patients with mitral stenosis, but occasionally it dominates the clinical picture.

PALPITATION. Atrial fibrillation, either paroxysmal or persistent, is a common complication of mitral stenosis. The patient usually detects the tumultuous heart action and develops dyspnea and weakness.

HEMOPTYSIS. Hemoptysis may occur as a result of an increase in pulmonary venous pressure, pulmonary emboli, or recurrent bronchitis. At times hemoptysis may be severe enough to require emergency valve surgery (Schwartz et al, 1966).

HOARSENESS. Hoarseness occasionally occurs when the enlarged left atrium compresses the recurrent laryngeal nerve.

PERIPHERAL EMBOLI. Emboli to the brain may produce strokes and seizures; peripheral emboli to the arms and legs may also occur (Baker and Finnegan, 1957).

PHYSICAL EXAMINATION

The patient may exhibit a malar flush, and the internal jugular veins may pulsate abnormally due to tricuspid regurgitation.

The heart rhythm may be normal, or it may reveal the signs of atrial fibrillation. The apex impulse is normal or diminished in patients with isolated mitral stenosis. There may be a sustained anterior lift of the precordium, signifying right ventricular hypertrophy. A diastolic rumble may be palpated at the apex, and the first heart sound may be easily palpated. The second heart sound may be felt when there is pulmonary hypertension.

The auscultatory features of mitral stenosis are a loud first heart sound, the opening snap of the mitral valve, a diastolic rumble with presystolic accentuation, and a loud pulmonary valve closure (Fig. 4.55) (Dack et al, 1960; Wood, 1954). The pulmonary component of the second sound may increase in intensity due to pulmonary hypertension; it is heard best in the second and the third left intercostal spaces. The murmur of pulmonary regurgitation may be present with advanced disease.

The examiner must listen for the murmur of mitral stenosis with the patient in the left lateral recumbent position after exercise. The opening snap, the loud first sound, and the loud pulmonary component of the second sound are heard best by using the diaphragm of the stethoscope applied with firm pressure. These abnormalities are distributed over a wide area on the chest. The diastolic rumble, which is heard in a localized area at the apex, is best heard with the bell of the stethoscope applied with light pressure.

Other conditions may produce a diastolic rumble at the apex, including mitral regurgitation, aortic regurgitation causing an Austin Flint rumble, patent arterial duct, interventricular septal defect, left atrial myxoma, the Carey–Coombs murmur of acute rheumatic fever, and, rarely, calcification of the mitral valve annulus. A tricuspid valve rumble secondary to atrial septal defect may be mistaken for a mitral valve rumble.

LABORATORY STUDIES

CHEST RADIOGRAPHY. On the chest films of a patient with mitral stenosis the pulmonary arterial trunk, the left atrial appendage, the large left atrium, and Kerley B lines are all prominent (Fig. 4.56) (Felson, 1973). Calcification of the mitral valve leaflets is often seen.

ELECTROCARDIOGRAPHY. The ECG of a patient with mitral stenosis reveals broad and notched P waves when there is normal rhythm

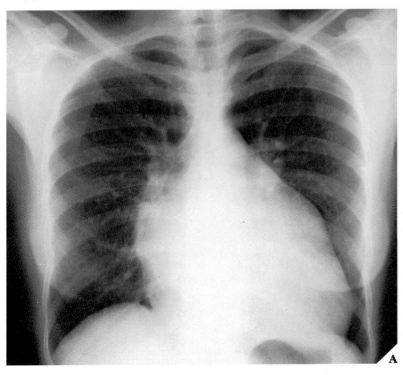

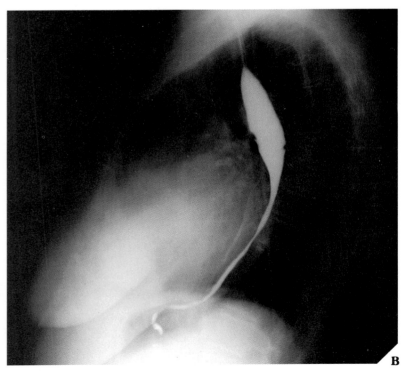

FIG. 4.56 **(A)** *Posteroanterior view of the chest in a patient with rheumatic mitral stenosis shows an enlarged left atrium that can be seen as a double density through the heart shadow. The superior pulmonary veins are distended, while the inferior pulmonary veins are not prominent.* **(B)** *Lateral view of a barium-filled esophagus shows posterior displacement due to an enlarged left atrium. (Courtesy of Robert G. Sybers, MD, Atlanta, Georgia)*

(Fig. 4.57). The mean QRS vector may be normal or directed to the right; it may show right ventricular hypertrophy. Atrial fibrillation is frequently present (Lee et al, 1965).

ECHOCARDIOGRAPHY. The M-mode echocardiogram of a patient with mitral stenosis shows a decrease in the E-F slope of the anterior leaflet of the mitral valve, and failure of the posterior leaflet to move downward (Fig. 4.58). Doppler recordings may also be used to evaluate mitral stenosis (Fig. 4.59).

CARDIAC CATHETERIZATION. The mitral valve pressure gradient, the mitral valve area, and the pulmonary artery pressure can be cal-culated from data acquired at cardiac catheterization (Gorlin and Gorlin, 1951). The normal mitral valve area is 4–6 cm². Hemodynamic abnormalities develop when the valve area is reduced to 1.5–2.5 cm²; pulmonary congestion develops when the valve area is 1.1–1.5 cm². Symptoms such as dyspnea usually indicate a valve area of 1.0 cm² or less.

Patients with dyspnea due to mitral stenosis usually exhibit a pulmonary arterial wedge pressure greater than 15–20 mmHg (Hungenholtz et al, 1962). The pulmonary arterial pressure and the pulmonary arteriolar resistance become elevated in patients with mitral stenosis. The pressure may almost reach systemic levels in some patients. In some symptomatic patients with normal pulmonary wedge

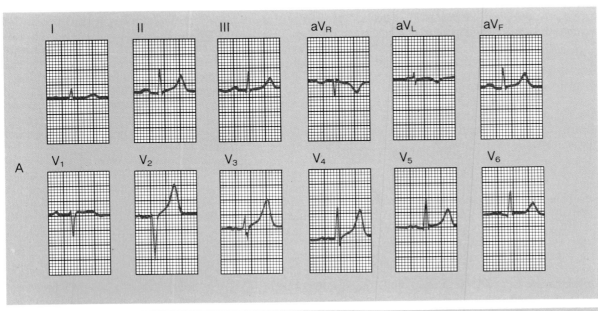

FIG. 4.57 *ECG recordings from a patient with mitral stenosis were made seven years apart, during which time the patient's symptoms and hemodynamic findings had progressed.* (**A**) *The first ECG shows a left atrial abnormality and a +60° frontal mean QRS vector.* (**B**) *The recording obtained seven years later shows atrial fibrillation with coarse fibrillatory waves and a +85° mean QRS vector. (Redrawn; Fig. 38-5,* The Heart, *6th ed, p 759. Courtesy of I. Sylvia Crawley, MD, Atlanta, Georgia)*

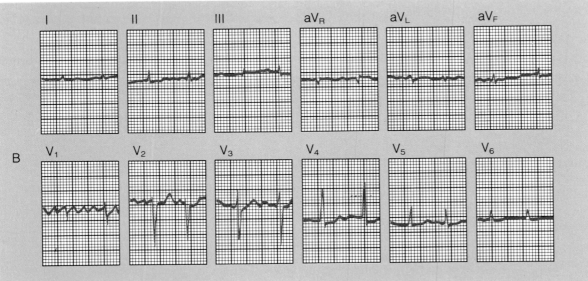

FIG. 4.58 *These M-mode echocardiograms were recorded from a patient with moderately severe mitral stenosis.* (**A**) *At the level of the papillary muscles the left ventricle (LV) is reduced in size, and the right ventricle (RV) is dilated. Ventricular septal (VS) motion is reduced.* (**B**) *Moderately thickened mitral valve shows reduced diastolic slope of the anterior mitral leaflet (AML) and paradoxical motion of the posterior leaflet (PML).* (**C**) *The anterior tricuspid leaflet (ATL) shows evidence of atrial fibrillation with a long diastole, but is otherwise normal.* (**D**) *The aorta (Ao) is normal in size, but the aortic valve is thickened with reduced excursion suggestive of aortic stenosis. The left atrium (LA) is dilated.* (**E**) *The pulmonary valve shows evidence of pulmonary hypertension with a flat diastolic slope and midsystolic closure (arrow). (Fig. 120-29,* The Heart, *6th ed; see Figure Credits)*

pressures it is necessary to measure the pulmonary arterial pressure after exercise.

Segmental and global wall abnormalities may be detected by left ventriculography (Hildner et al, 1972). Angiography is also used to detect mitral regurgitation and left atrial tumor (Fig. 4.60). Coronary arteriography is used to detect coronary atherosclerosis in all adult patients undergoing cardiac catheterization for mitral stenosis (Chun et al, 1982).

RADIONUCLIDE STUDIES. The ^{99m}Tc ventriculogram can be used to determine left ventricular function. It is possible to measure the

left ventricular ejection fraction, the end-diastolic volume, the cardiac output, and the stroke volume at rest and after exercise. Right ventricular function can also be assessed (Newman et al, 1979).

NATURAL HISTORY

While rheumatic fever usually occurs at ages 8–12 years, mitral stenosis is usually detected about 20 years later. Symptoms usually occurring by ages 40–50 years include dyspnea, fatigue, and palpitation (atrial fibrillation). Atrial fibrillation occurs in about 50%, and systemic emboli occur in about 10%–20% of patients with mitral stenosis (Abernathy and Willis, 1973).

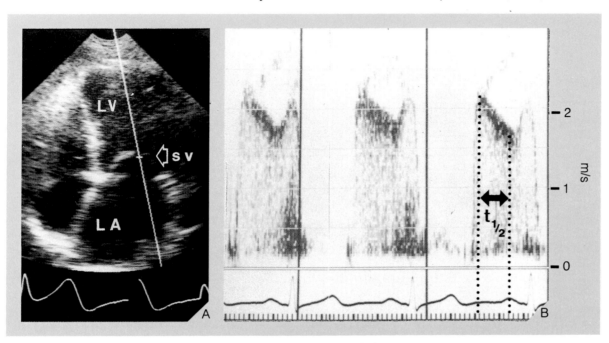

FIG. 4.59 *Doppler recording from a patient with mitral stenosis is taken from the apical approach.* (**A**) *The Doppler sample volume (SV, open arrow) is positioned in the stenotic mitral valve orifice (LA, left atrium; LV, left ventricle).* (**B**) *The flow velocity curve shows an increased peak of approximately 2.2 m/s, predicting a peak early diastolic gradient of 19 mmHg. The pressure half-time (t$_{\frac{1}{2}}$, double-headed arrow) is 260 ms, predicting a mitral valve area of 220/260 = 0.8 cm^2. (Fig. 122-7, The Heart, 6th ed; see Figure Credits)*

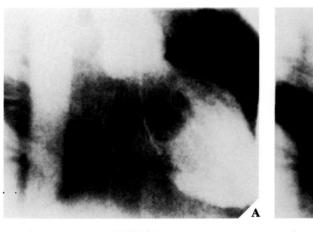
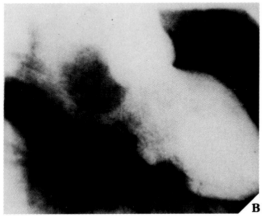

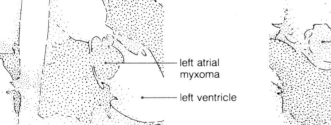
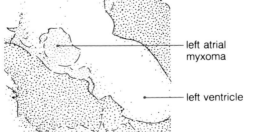

left atrial myxoma

left ventricle

left atrial myxoma

left ventricle

FIG. 4.60 (**A**) *In this left ventriculogram in the right anterior oblique projection a mobile left atrial myxoma is seen as a space-filling defect within the mitral valve in diastole.* (**B**) *Sufficient mitral regurgitation is present to delineate the myxoma in the left atrium in systole. (Fig. 61-4, The Heart, 6th ed; see Figure Credits)*

Bacterial endocarditis may develop in patients with mitral stenosis. It is less frequent in patients with isolated severe stenosis than it is in those with milder degrees of stenosis associated with mitral regurgitation.

The average age of patients who are treated medically is 48 years. The survival curve of patients with mitral stenosis is shown in Figure 4.13.

TREATMENT

Digitalis helps very little in patients with normal rhythm. Patients with atrial fibrillation should receive digoxin in sufficient dosage to control the ventricular rate; propranolol and verapamil can be used additionally to achieve a desired rate.

Quinidine or direct-current cardioversion may be used to revert atrial fibrillation to normal rhythm when it is associated with no symptoms or little hemodynamic deterioration. Direct-current cardioversion should be used when atrial fibrillation is associated with dyspnea and altered hemodynamics. To prevent emboli it is wise to give an anticoagulant for two weeks prior to an attempt at reverting the rhythm to normal and for several weeks afterwards, when there is no contraindication to its use. When atrial fibrillation is recent in onset and is associated with pulmonary edema and hypotension, it may be necessary to use direct-current cardioversion as an emergency form of treatment without the prior administration of anticoagulant. Quinidine may be used to prevent atrial fibrillation after the rhythm is restored to normal. Patients with chronic atrial fibrillation who have a large left atrium may not remain in normal rhythm; one must be satisfied with the control of ventricular rate. Patients with mitral stenosis and chronic atrial fibrillation should receive an anticoagulant, such as Coumadin, if there is no contraindication to its use.

Patients who experience systemic emboli should be placed on anticoagulant therapy, and surgical intervention for mitral stenosis should be considered. The patient with mitral stenosis must be instructed in antibiotic prophylaxis of bacterial endocarditis.

Balloon dilation of the mitral valve is currently under investigation (Lock et al, 1985); the exact place of this procedure must be determined after further research and experience.

INDICATIONS FOR SURGERY

Surgery should be performed in patients who have increasing dyspnea with effort. A casual history may be misleading, because patients walk slower and exert less to avoid dyspnea; accordingly they may deny dyspnea. In fact some patients knowing that cardiac surgery is being considered deny all symptoms. Because of this it is wise to observe some patients perform on the treadmill. Certain patients have more fatigue than dyspnea; this may be an indication for surgery.

Patients who have mitral stenosis with few symptoms but have evidence of pulmonary hypertension on physical examination and cardiac catheterization should have surgery. This is also true for patients with systemic emboli.

SURGICAL PROCEDURE

There is some disagreement as to whether cardiac catheterization should be performed on all patients. Some physicians believe that catheterization is not necessary in young patients, especially females, in whom coronary disease is uncommon, and when estimates of valve disease can be determined by noninvasive methods.

The pliability of the mitral valve should be determined prior to anticipated surgery. Pliability is believed to be present if the patient is young, an opening snap is heard, and no calcium is detected in the echocardiogram or with fluoroscopy. Rarely when such conditions do exist, closed mitral commissurotomy may be performed; however, in general open commissurotomy is the surgical procedure of choice (Fig. 4.61). The open approach is considered to be safer and more

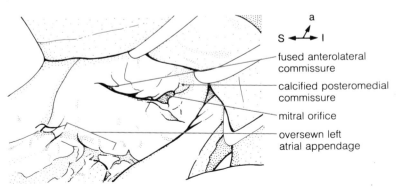
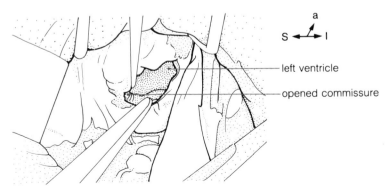

FIG. 4.61 (**A**) *Operative view of a stenotic mitral valve shows a small eccentric orifice.* (**B**) *After open commissurotomy the valve orifice has been greatly enlarged.*

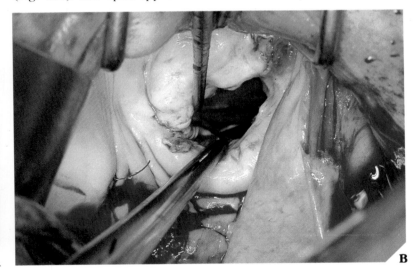

PART II: DISEASES OF THE HEART

effective; it allows the surgeon to perform a more precise valvoplasty, and it lessens the risk of embolization from an unsuspected left atrial clot (Fig. 4.62).

Patients with severely diseased and calcified valves require valve replacement with a tissue or a synthetic valve. The type of valve is dictated by the same conditions that pertain in regard to the choice of aortic valve prosthesis. Emboli occur less often with bioprostheses, and unless the left atrium is large or atrial fibrillation persists, it is usually not necessary to use long-term anticoagulant therapy after a tissue valve has been inserted. Many surgeons do, however, prescribe anticoagulants during the initial three-month postoperative period un-

til the valve strut is endothelialized. An anticoagulant, such as Coumadin, is always prescribed after insertion of a synthetic valve.

The operative risk varies according to the procedure used and the condition of the patient. The risk associated with mitral valvotomy may be as low as 2%. The operative risk of a patient with advanced heart failure who has mitral valve replacement may be as high as 8%.

The standard surgical approach to the mitral valve is through a median sternotomy, although on occasion access through the right hemithorax or, exceedingly rarely, the left chest may be advantageous. Waterston's groove serves as an excellent guidepost to the right lateral aspect of the left atrium (Fig. 4.63). Usually a simple vertical incision

FIG. 4.62 *An unsuspected thrombus was encountered at operation in the patient shown in Figure 4.61. The clot originated in the left atrial appendage; it was found loosely attached to the atrial wall.*

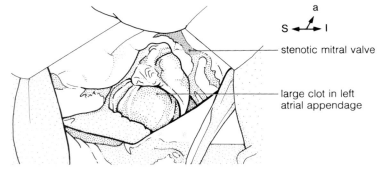

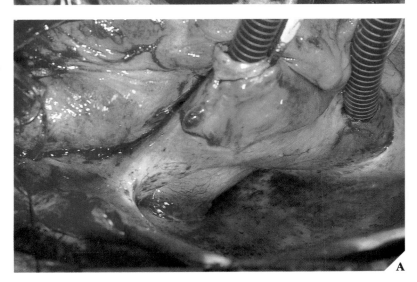

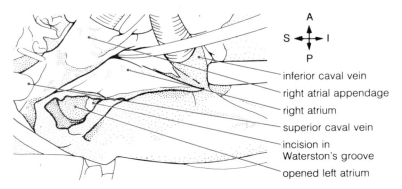

FIG. 4.63 (A) *Waterston's groove is viewed through a median sternotomy.* (B) *Incision into the left atrium is made just lateral to Waterston's groove.*

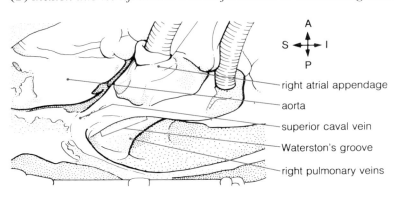

into the anterior aspect of the atrial wall affords adequate access, particularly if the left atrium is dilated. However, if the atrium is small, one may need to extend the incision behind either or both of the caval veins. The pericardial curtain suspending the caval veins is especially well seen in Figure 4.64. Division of these pericardial reflections allows extension of the incision into the inferior wall or superiorly into the so-called roof of the left atrium. Such extensions are quite safe; the only risk is damaging the sinus node artery when it originates from the left coronary artery. In approximately 50% of patients the artery runs over the left atrial roof (Fig. 4.65), passing in front of or behind the superior caval vein to supply the sinus node. The mitral valve may also be exposed by using a transverse incision, opening both atria and cutting into the oval fossa. This transseptal

approach may be useful if one anticipates the need for tricuspid repair or replacement at the time of mitral valve surgery.

Having gained access to the mitral valve, the surgeon must be aware of the important "invisible anatomy" associated with the valve annulus (Fig. 4.66). The posterior medial commissure indicates the area where the atrioventricular node and the penetrating bundle lie in close proximity to the central fibrous body. The coronary sinus is another rather constant relationship that must be kept in mind during mitral valve surgery (Fig. 4.67). Depending on whether the coronary artery dominance is right (see Fig. 4.67) or left (Fig. 4.68), the circumflex branch of the left coronary artery is less or more critically related to the valve annulus. In either instance the artery to the atrioventricular node lies close to the valve in its course to the apex of the triangle of Koch. All

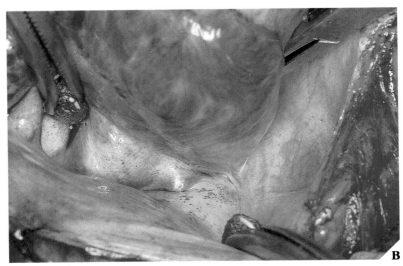

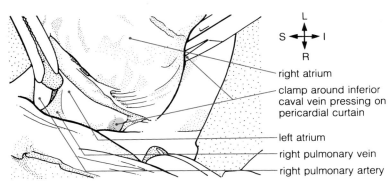

FIG. 4.64 (A) The right lateral aspect of the heart is viewed through a median sternotomy. The thin pericardial curtain suspending the superior caval vein is unusually well seen. (B) In a different patient the inferior pericardial curtain is demonstrated with a right-angle clamp passed behind the inferior caval vein.

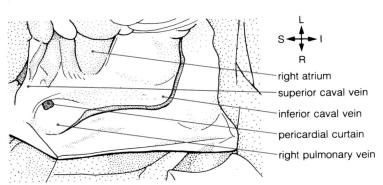

right atrium
superior caval vein
inferior caval vein
pericardial curtain
right pulmonary vein

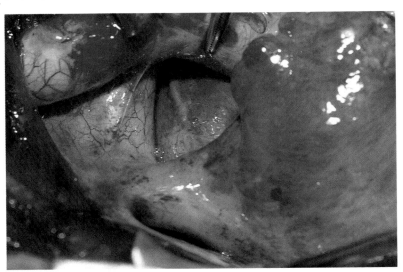

right atrium
clamp around inferior caval vein pressing on pericardial curtain
left atrium
right pulmonary vein
right pulmonary artery

FIG. 4.65 The sinus node artery courses across the roof of the left atrium in this operative view.

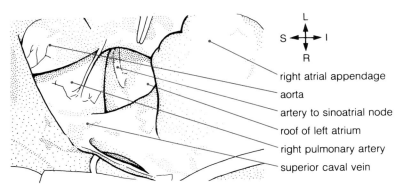

right atrial appendage
aorta
artery to sinoatrial node
roof of left atrium
right pulmonary artery
superior caval vein

PART II: DISEASES OF THE HEART

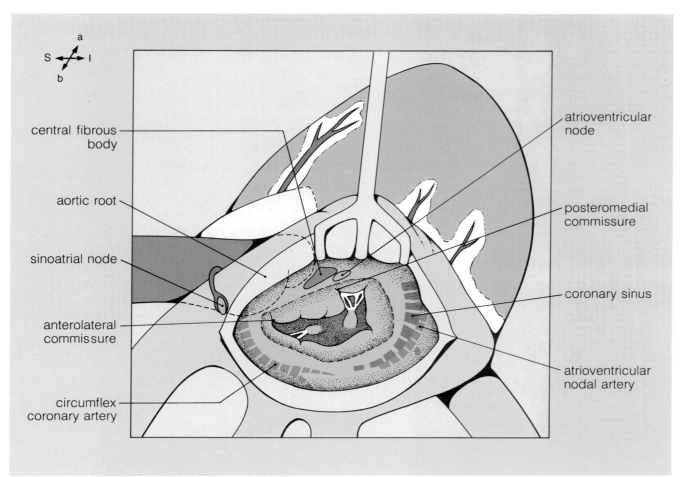

central fibrous body

aortic root

sinoatrial node

anterolateral commissure

circumflex coronary artery

atrioventricular node

posteromedial commissure

coronary sinus

atrioventricular nodal artery

FIG. 4.66 *This diagram represents the left atrium opened through an incision parallel to Waterston's groove. The important relationships of the mitral valve are superimposed. (Adapted; see Figure Credits)*

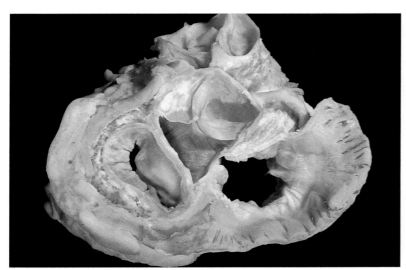

FIG. 4.67 *A short-axis view of the heart shows the close relationship of the coronary sinus and the conduction system to the mitral valve.*

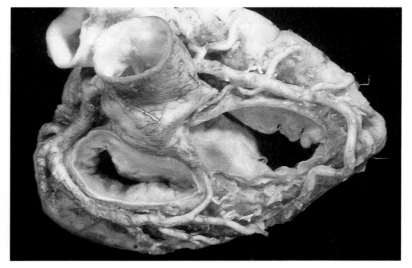

FIG. 4.68 *Dissection of a heart with a left dominant coronary system demonstrates the intimate relationship of the circumflex coronary artery to the mitral valve.*

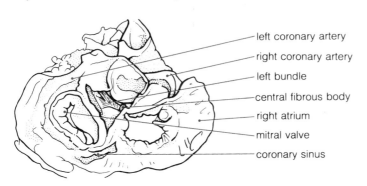

left coronary artery

right coronary artery

left bundle

central fibrous body

right atrium

mitral valve

coronary sinus

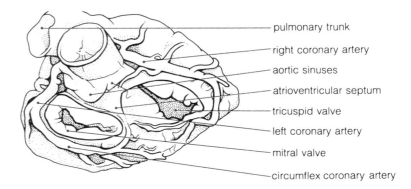

pulmonary trunk

right coronary artery

aortic sinuses

atrioventricular septum

tricuspid valve

left coronary artery

mitral valve

circumflex coronary artery

VALVAR HEART DISEASE

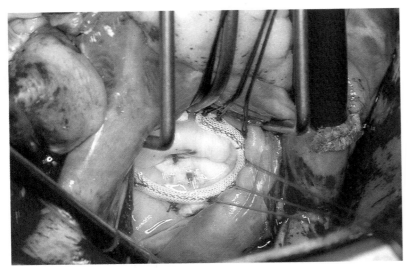

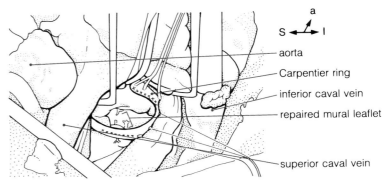

FIG. 4.69 *In this operative view of a mitral valvoplasty and annuloplasty in a patient with ruptured tendinous cords, the Carpentier ring is seen sewn in place. The mural leaflet of the mitral valve has also been repaired.*

aorta

Carpentier ring

inferior caval vein

repaired mural leaflet

superior caval vein

FIG. 4.70 *A Medtronic–Hall pivoting disk valve is sewn in place using interrupted pledgeted mattress sutures. The valve is oriented so that the major disk excursion extends into the left ventricular outflow tract.*

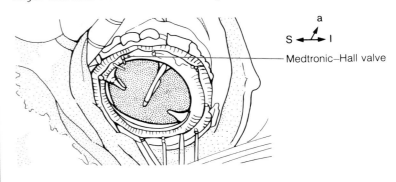

Medtronic–Hall valve

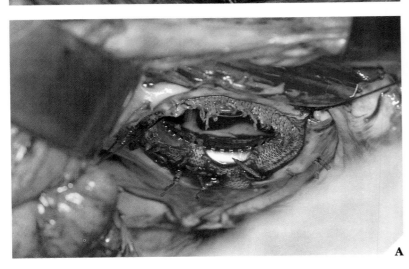

FIG. 4.71 (**A**) *Starr–Edwards mitral prosthesis has been in place in this patient for 15 years.* (**B**) *The mitral annulus is shown after the prosthesis has been enucleated.*

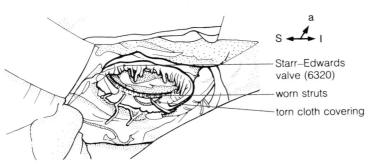

Starr–Edwards valve (6320)

worn struts

torn cloth covering

left ventricle

suture from previous valve

seat of previous valve

PART II: DISEASES OF THE HEART

of these structures are vulnerable to injury by the injudicious placement of annular sutures during valve repair (Fig. 4.69) or replacement (Fig. 4.70). A particular problem exists for the patient requiring removal of a malfunctioning mitral prosthesis. Because the annulus is distorted and sometimes deficient, in such cases it is advisable to enucleate the device without excising any adjacent tissue (Fig. 4.71). This avoids the risk of cutting into the surrounding structures, and leaves a cuff of tissue through which the new sutures may be placed safely.

Long-term anticoagulant therapy is indicated in patients who have a synthetic valve and in patients with a tissue valve in whom the left atrium is large and atrial fibrillation is present. As mentioned earlier, anticoagulant therapy is used for three months after insertion of a tissue valve in patients with normal rhythm and normal-sized left atrium.

The patient's symptoms should be greatly improved after surgery, but detailed instructions regarding the prevention of bacterial endocarditis must be given repeatedly.

The patient with a valvotomy must be followed to determine if re-stenosis occurs, since the re-stenosis rate is about 10% per year. The patient who has had valve replacement must be followed to determine if the valve remains competent.

The long-term survival of patients who have had mitral valve surgery is far better than in patients without valve surgery.

MITRAL VALVE REGURGITATION*
ETIOLOGY AND PATHOLOGY

The causes of chronic and acute mitral regurgitation are listed in Table 4.2. Rheumatic fever is the most common cause of chronic mitral valve regurgitation; in these cases leaflet retraction usually dominates the pathologic state (Fig. 4.72). In the Western world mitral valve prolapse has become an important cause of regurgitation. The underlying pathology is a floppy valve characterized by myxomatous degeneration of the leaflets and tendinous cords, and accompanied by dilation of the valve annulus (Fig. 4.73). Cordal rupture is a frequent complication, leading

---

*Abstracted with permission of the authors and publisher from Rackley CE, Edwards JE, Karp RB: Mitral valve disease, Chapter 38, pp 754–784, in Hurst JW (ed): *The Heart,* 6th ed. New York, McGraw-Hill, 1986. Figures and tables reproduced in this section from the above chapter, other chapters in *The Heart,* or other sources are also reprinted with permission of the authors and publishers. For the full bibliographic citations of the sources of figures other than the above chapter, see Figure Credits at the end of this chapter.

Table 4.2 Etiology of Chronic and Acute Mitral Regurgitation

CHRONIC REGURGITATION

Mitral leaflet prolapse (congenital, myxomatous degeneration)
Coronary artery disease
Left ventricular dilation (numerous causes)
Rheumatic fever
Calcified mitral annulus
Heritable disorders of connective tissue (Marfan's syndrome, Ehlers–Danlos syndrome, osteogenesis imperfecta)
Papillary muscle dysfunction (infarction)
Lupus erythematosus

ACUTE REGURGITATION

Rupture of tendinous cords (myxoma, endocarditis, trauma)
Rupture of papillary muscle (infarction, trauma)
Perforation of leaflet (endocarditis)

(Table 38-1, *The Heart,* 6th ed, p 764)

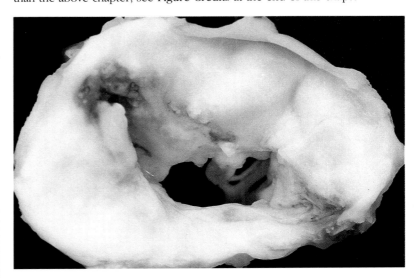

FIG. 4.72 *This resected mitral valve shows leaflet retraction due to scarring secondary to rheumatic fever. Leaflet retraction is the dominant clinical feature in mitral valve regurgitation.*

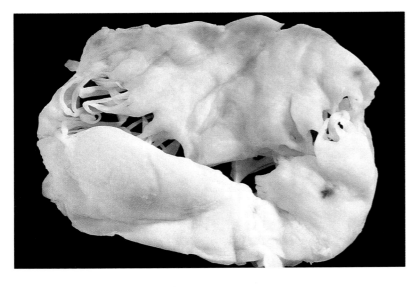

FIG. 4.73 *A resected mitral valve shows prolapse of the middle scallop of the posterior leaflet due to myxomatous degeneration of the mitral valve and tendinous cords.*

to abrupt onset of signs of left heart failure (Fig. 4.74). Patients with coronary disease and its complications may have mitral regurgitation because of papillary muscle dysfunction (Fig. 4.75). Patients with cardiomyopathy may also develop mitral regurgitation. Acute mitral regurgitation may be due to infarction of the papillary muscle due to coronary disease, particularly when this is complicated by partial or complete rupture of the muscle (Fig. 4.76). Mitral regurgitation may also be caused by infective endocarditis (Fig. 4.77) or ruptured tendinous cords in the setting of trauma.

ABNORMAL PHYSIOLOGY

The amount of the left ventricular stroke volume that is ejected into the left atrium determines the extent of left atrial and left ventricular dilation (Braunwald, 1969). Chronic mitral regurgitation produces a volume overload on the left ventricle and the left atrium; the pressure also gradually rises in the left atrium, the pulmonary veins, and the pulmonary capillaries (Fig. 4.78).

The left ventricle dilates to accommodate the increase in diastolic volume that occurs as a result of regurgitation (Rackley, 1975). In addition the left ventricle remodels itself by increasing its wall thickness (see Fig. 2.6A). During the remodeling the alignment of the tendinous cords and the papillary muscles becomes deranged, which may increase the mitral regurgitation. The left ventricular compliance increases, and the left ventricular end-diastolic pressure remains normal or slightly elevated for a long period of time.

Mitral valve prolapse is associated with large, thin leaflets, elongated cords, dilation of the valve annulus, and abnormal systolic contraction patterns of the left ventricle ranging from hyperkinesis to akinesis (Nutter et al, 1975). Regurgitation may be slight, moderate, or severe.

The magnitude of chronic regurgitation is related predominantly to the position of the valve leaflets during systole.

Patients with coronary disease may have chronic mitral regurgitation, usually due to a combination of papillary muscle dysfunction, dilation of the left ventricle, and dyskinetic motion of the posterior myocardial wall (Rackley et al, 1970).

Mitral regurgitation occurs in patients with dilated cardiomyopathy; the left ventricle dilates, and the tendinous cords and the papillary muscles have a new physical relationship to the valve leaflets (Boltwood et al, 1983). The dilation of the left ventricle seems to have more influence on the amount of regurgitation than the degree of dilation of the valve annulus.

The altered physiology that results from acute mitral valve regurgitation is quite different from that produced by chronic incompetence of the valve. The abrupt development of mitral regurgitation is not associated with abrupt dilation of the atrium or the left ventricle (Klughaupt et al, 1969). These structures have inadequate time to adjust to the increased volume; because of this, the end-diastolic pressure of the left ventricle, the left atrial pressure, and the pulmonary artery pressure become markedly elevated. A severe pressure load is created, which is in marked contrast to the volume overload that is secondary to chronic mitral regurgitation. As stated earlier, the causes of acute mitral regurgitation are rupture of the tendinous cords due to myxomatous degeneration, infective endocarditis, trauma, and papillary muscle rupture due to myocardial infarction.

CLINICAL MANIFESTATIONS

The clinical picture that results from mitral regurgitation is determined by the amount of regurgitation, whether it is chronic, acute or a com-

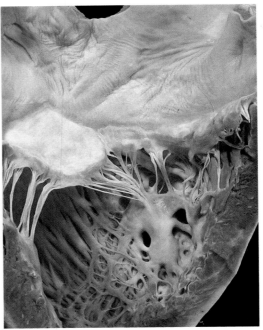

FIG. 4.75 *In this heart specimen scarred myocardium in the area of the posteromedial papillary muscle due to obstructive coronary heart disease underlies papillary muscle dysfunction as the cause of mitral regurgitation.*

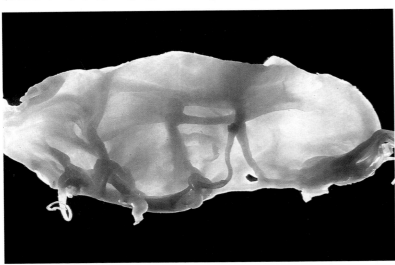

FIG. 4.74 *The undersurface of a prolapsing mitral valve leaflet shows the middle scallop with ruptured cords.*

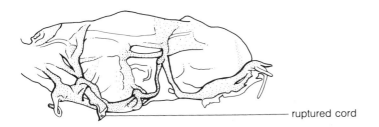

ruptured cord

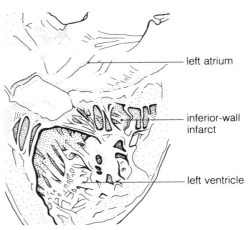

left atrium

inferior-wall infarct

left ventricle

bination of the two, and other abnormalities that may be present in the heart.

SYMPTOMS

Patients with chronic but mild mitral valve regurgitations have no symptoms (Selzer and Katayama, 1972). Severe chronic regurgitation produces symptoms associated with heart failure, such as fatigue and dyspnea on effort (Jeresaty, 1973). Palpitation may be related to atrial fibrillation. Some patients with mitral valve prolapse have atrial and ventricular arrhythmias, chest pain of uncertain etiology, and anxiety (Winkle et al, 1975).

Patients with acute mitral regurgitation may experience the symptoms associated with abrupt and severe pulmonary edema and shock.

PHYSICAL EXAMINATION

Palpation of the precordium may be normal in patients with mild chronic regurgitation. More severe regurgitation may produce a pal-

pable thrill at the apex, a hyperdynamic apical impulse that is displaced leftward, and a hyperdynamic anterior lift of the precordium located to the left of the sternum, secondary to abrupt dilation of the left atrium.

The murmur secondary to rheumatic mitral regurgitation is usually holosystolic; it begins with the first sound, which may be diminished in intensity because the valve leaflets may not coapt properly. The increased volume of blood entering the left ventricle during diastole produces a ventricular gallop sound. When the volume of blood is large, it causes a low-pitched, diastolic rumbling murmur at the apex. The second sound may be split abnormally, because ventricular systole is shortened and aortic valve closure occurs earlier than usual.

Patients with mitral valve prolapse have additional anomalies. Abnormalities of the chest wall may be apparent; the anteroposterior diameter of the chest may be narrow, or pectus excavatum or scoliosis may be present. Evidence of Marfan's syndrome may be obvious. The murmur may appear after an early systolic click. A change in the size

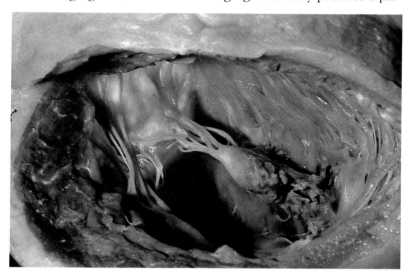

FIG. 4.76 *Acute mitral regurgitation may result from a ruptured anterolateral papillary muscle as a complication of acute myocardial infarction. (Reproduced with permission of the authors and publisher; see Figure Credits)*

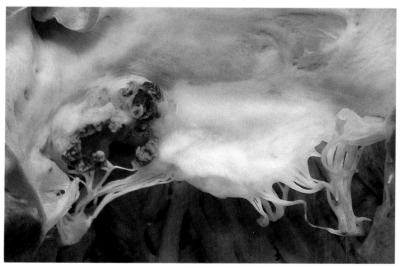

FIG. 4.77 *Infective endocarditis of the mitral valve, localized in this specimen in the area of the anterolateral commissure, may result in mitral regurgitation.*

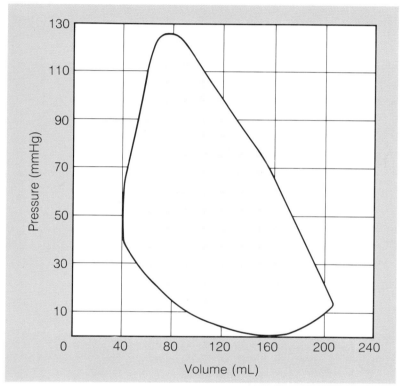

FIG. 4.78 *This pressure–volume diagram was recorded from a patient with mitral regurgitation. There is a loss of the isovolumic contraction phase on the right side of the pressure–volume loop due to the mitral valve regurgitation. The early diastolic filling is initiated by the 40 mmHg V wave in the left atrium. (Redrawn; reproduced with permission of the authors and publisher; see Figure Credits. Also, Fig. 38-17, The Heart, 6th ed, p 769)*

of the left ventricular cavity produced by standing causes the click and the murmur to occur earlier in systole (Fig. 4.79).

The systolic murmur produced by chronic regurgitation secondary to coronary disease may begin in early, mid- or late systole, and is often associated with atrial and ventricular gallop sounds (Holmes et al, 1968).

Patients with acute regurgitation due to rupture of the tendinous cords or the papillary muscle usually exhibit signs of pulmonary edema

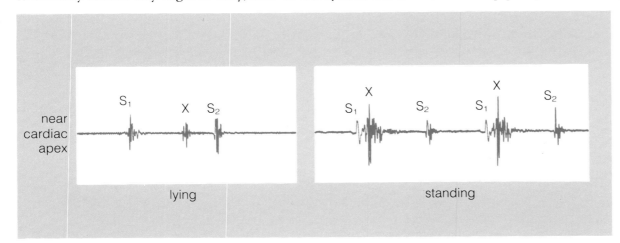

FIG. 4.79 *These phonocardio-grams recorded near the apex in a patient with mitral valve prolapse show that a late systolic click* (x) *moves to a position early in systole when the patient is standing. (Re-drawn; Fig. 38-19,* The Heart, *6th ed, p 771. Courtesy of Ernest Craige, MD)*

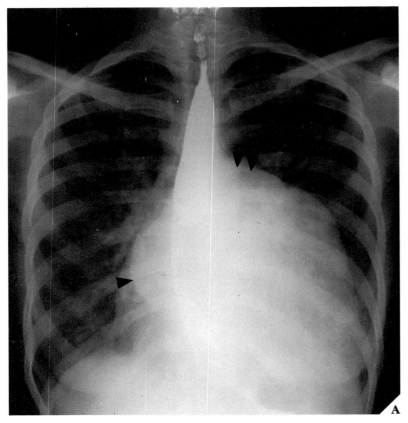

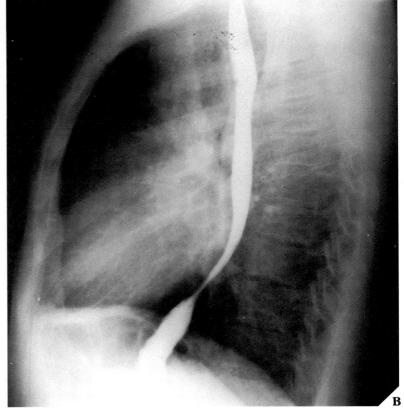

FIG. 4.80 **(A)** *Posteroanterior chest radiograph shows the barium-filled esophagus of a patient with rheumatic mitral regurgitation. Cardiomegaly is present, with the left ventricle extending toward the lateral chest wall. The enlarged left atrium can be seen as a double density* (single arrow), *and the pulmonary artery segment* (double arrows) *is prominent.* **(B)** *Lateral view reveals the large left atrium. (Courtesy of Robert G. Sybers, MD, Atlanta, Georgia)*

(Ronan et al, 1971). The heart is not large, unless it was large before the cordal rupture. The apical systolic murmur of ruptured tendinous cords is usually loud, radiating laterally or toward the base of the heart. It is often heard over the cervical and the thoracic areas of the spine, and it may even be heard on the top of the head and over the sacrum. An atrial gallop is usually heard.

Papillary muscle rupture due to myocardial infarction may not produce a murmur, because the infarcted ventricular muscle may not be capable of vigorous contraction (Shelburne et al, 1969). A systolic murmur is usually heard as well as an atrial gallop sound. The patient may display signs of shock and pulmonary edema.

LABORATORY STUDIES
CHEST RADIOGRAPHY. The chest film may show no abnormality when mitral regurgitation is slight. Moderate and severe mitral regurgitation may produce evidence of left atrial enlargement, left ven-

tricular enlargement, calcification of the mitral annulus or the leaflets, and signs of heart failure (Fig. 4.80).

ELECTROCARDIOGRAPHY. The ECG may be normal. When mitral regurgitation is moderately severe, the ECG usually reveals left ventricular hypertrophy, left atrial abnormality when normal rhythm is present, or atrial fibrillation.

ECHOCARDIOGRAPHY. The echocardiogram may show evidence of mitral valve prolapse (Fig. 4.81), calcification, increased diastolic dimensions of the left ventricle, systolic wall-motion abnormalities, and an increase in size of the left atrium. Acute mitral regurgitation may be associated with echocardiographic abnormalities that can be attributed to ruptured tendinous cords, papillary muscle rupture, or a perforated valve leaflet. The cross-sectional echocardiogram of a patient with mitral regurgitation may reveal a prolapsing anterior mi-

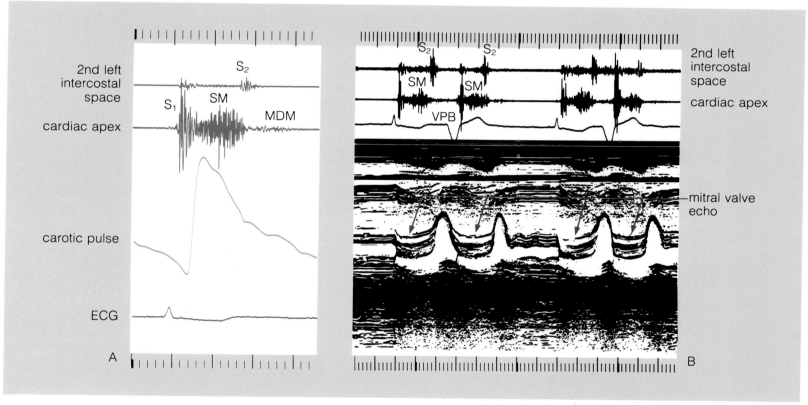

FIG. 4.81 *These phono- and echocardiograms were obtained in a patient with mitral valve prolapse. (A) The phonocardiograms, obtained at the second left intercostal space and the cardiac apex, demonstrate an intense high-frequency pansystolic murmur (SM) with accentuation in late systole. There is also a minimal mid-diastolic murmur (MDM). (B) The echo-* *cardiogram demonstrates the hammock-shaped appearance of the valve leaflets, which coincides with the pansystolic murmur. The rhythm is atrial fibrillation with bigeminy. (Redrawn; Fig. 38-18,* The Heart, *p 771. Courtesy of Ernest Craige, MD)*

tral leaflet (Fig. 4.82). Mitral regurgitation can also be detected by the Doppler technique (Fig. 4.83).

CARDIAC CATHETERIZATION. Cardiac catheterization is used to assess ventricular function, to identify other cardiac abnormalities, and to determine the presence or absence of coronary disease.

An abnormal V wave may be seen in the pulmonary wedge pressure tracing. Left ventricular function can be determined by measuring the end-diastolic pressure and the ejection fraction and estimating the amount of blood that is regurgitated (Fig. 4.84). Quantitative angiography may be used to measure left ventricular stroke volume, which is identified as the difference between end-diastolic and end-systolic volumes. The end-diastolic volume may be increased, but the ejection

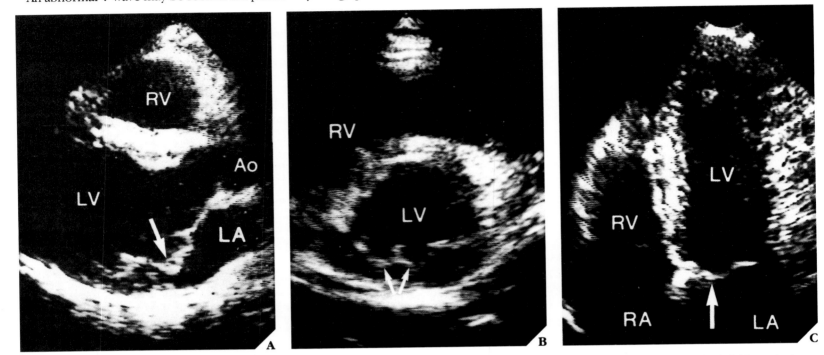

FIG. 4.82 **(A)** *Cross-sectional echocardiogram obtained from a patient with severe mitral valve prolapse shows, on the parasternal long-axis view in systole, the anterior and posterior leaflets arching posteriorly* (arrow), *above the level of the atrioventricular groove and behind the normal coaptation point into the left atrium.* **(B)** *Parasternal short-axis view at the level of the mitral valve and the left ventricular outflow tract in systole shows the anterior leaflet buckling posteriorly* (arrows). **(C)** *The apical four-chamber view in systole shows the classic image of a prolapsing anterior mitral leaflet* (arrow) (RV, *right ventricle;* LV, *left ventricle;* Ao, *aorta;* RA, *right atrium;* LA, *left atrium*). *As stated, this example represents severe prolapse; most cases are mild.* (Fig. 120-30, The Heart, 6th ed; see Figure Credits)

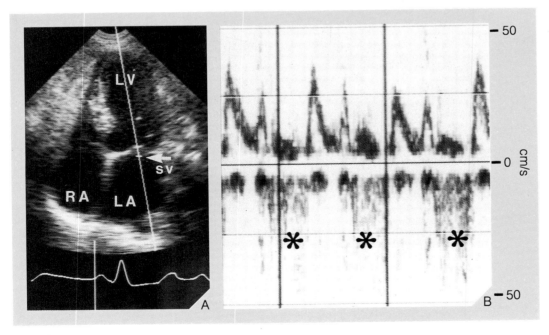

FIG. 4.83 *Mitral regurgitation is examined from the apical approach in this Doppler recording.* **(A)** *The sample volume* (SV, arrow) *is positioned just to the left of the left atrial* (LA) *side of the closed mitral leaflets in systole* (LV, *left ventricle;* RA, *right atrium*). **(B)** *The flow waveform shows the laminar diastolic emptying of the left atrium; a systolic flow disturbance* (asterisks) *is diagnostic of mitral regurgitation.* (Fig. 122-9, The Heart, 6th ed; see Figure Credits)

PART II: DISEASES OF THE HEART

fraction may be normal until left ventricular dysfunction occurs. Eventually the pressure in the left atrium, the pulmonary veins, and the capillaries becomes elevated. The ratio of end-systolic wall stress to end-systolic volume index can be computed; this measure of left ventricular function can be used to determine the likelihood of postoperative improvement.

Left ventriculography also enables one to detect mitral valve prolapse and associated anomalies, such as wall-motion abnormalities. It must be emphasized that minor degrees of mitral valve prolapse are not detected with this technique.

Mitral regurgitation secondary to coronary artery disease is usually associated with left ventricular dilation and abnormal posterior wall

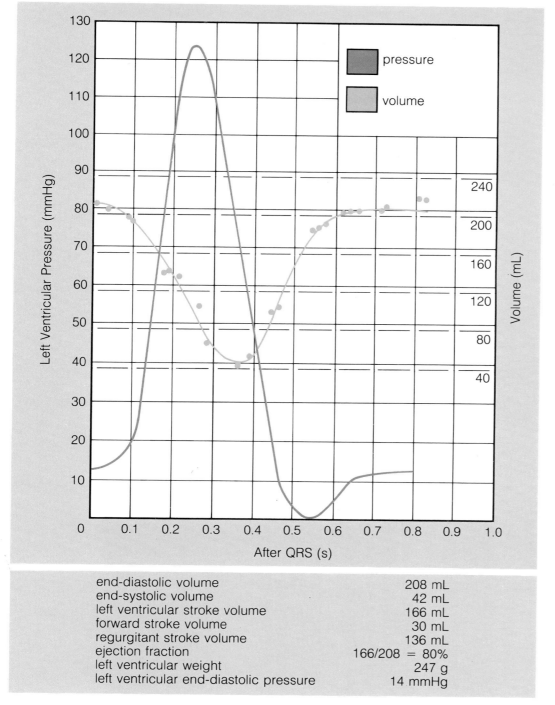

FIG. 4.84 *Left ventricular pressure and volume were recorded in a patient with mitral regurgitation. (Redrawn; Fig. 38-21, The Heart, 6th ed, p 773)*

end-diastolic volume	208 mL
end-systolic volume	42 mL
left ventricular stroke volume	166 mL
forward stroke volume	30 mL
regurgitant stroke volume	136 mL
ejection fraction	166/208 = 80%
left ventricular weight	247 g
left ventricular end-diastolic pressure	14 mmHg

motion, usually located at the base of the papillary muscle (Fig. 4.85).

The left atrial V wave may be huge; it is often identified during the insertion of a Swan–Ganz catheter to the wedge position in patients with acute mitral regurgitation (Klughaupt et al, 1969). The left ventricular angiogram reveals a large amount of regurgitation into the left atrium and the pulmonary veins when there is severe mitral valve regurgitation (Fig. 4.86).

RADIONUCLIDE STUDIES. Radionuclide ventriculography can be used to identify the resting (Fig. 4.87) and exercise ejection fractions.

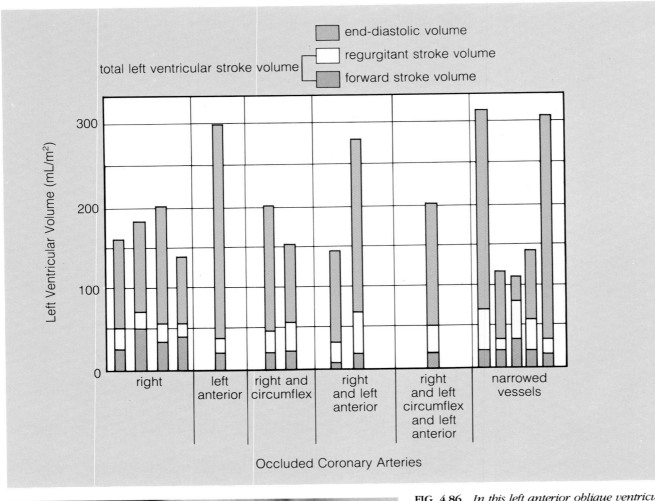

FIG. 4.85 *Left ventricular volume is compared in patients with mitral regurgitation due to various coronary lesions. The total height of each bar is the end-diastolic volume. (Redrawn; reproduced with permission of the authors and publisher; see Figure Credits. Also, Fig. 38-23,* The Heart, *6th ed, p 775)*

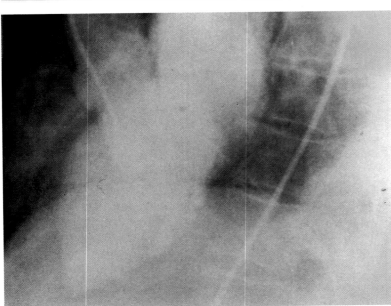

FIG. 4.86 *In this left anterior oblique ventriculogram in a patient with mitral regurgitation the contrast medium opacifies the left atrium as a result of severe mitral regurgitation. (Courtesy of Henry W. Smith, MD, Atlanta, Georgia)*

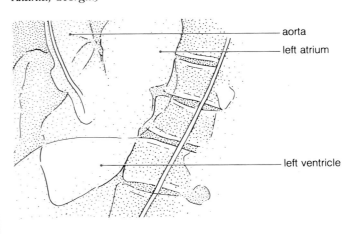

Thallium scans can be used to exclude myocardial ischemia in patients with mitral valve prolapse, since stress exercise ECGs often yield false-positive results for ischemia (Fig. 4.88) (Slutsky et al, 1979).

NATURAL HISTORY

The natural history and prognosis depend on the etiology of the condition. Patients with chronic mitral regurgitation may have no symptoms for many years. The pressure in the pulmonary veins may not rise and the ejection fraction may be normal, because left atrial compliance remains normal, protecting the lungs. The left atrium may actually become "giant-sized" and the patient may not be severely disabled. Atrial fibrillation may develop and systemic emboli may occur, although not as often as with mitral stenosis. Endocarditis may occur, producing further valve damage. The survival curve of patients with chronic mitral regurgitation is shown in Figure 4.13.

Patients with mitral valve prolapse may have atrial and ventricular arrhythmias that do not correlate with the severity of the anatomic abnormality. The prognosis is excellent in most patients with prolapse; a small percentage have sudden death, ruptured tendinous cords, endocarditis, and heart failure.

The prognosis of patients with mitral valve regurgitation due to coronary disease depends on the state of the myocardium, the degree of coronary disease, and the amount of regurgitation (Selzer and Katayama, 1972).

Acute mitral valve regurgitation is serious and may lead to shock, pulmonary edema, and death. Although the majority of patients die, an increasing number are saved by modern surgery.

TREATMENT

The patient with chronic mitral regurgitation must be advised regarding the prevention of bacterial endocarditis. Atrial fibrillation is treated with digitalis; propranolol and verapamil may also be needed. At least in the beginning the rhythm may revert to normal with quinidine or cardioversion. Anticoagulant therapy should be given for two weeks before and several weeks after reversion of the rhythm. Anticoagulants should also be administered to the patient with chronic atrial fibrillation. Drugs that alter the preload and the afterload may be given in addition to digitalis and diuretics to relieve symptoms of heart failure. When the condition warrants the use of such drugs, the hemodynamic problem should be corrected with mitral valve surgery. It is wise to anticipate the need for surgery before myocardial contractility is impaired.

Patients with mitral valve prolapse and cardiac arrhythmias may profit from the administration of propranolol.

INDICATIONS FOR SURGERY

Surgery should be performed before there is clinical evidence of heart failure or impaired contractility of the left ventricle. The ejection fraction remains deceptively high because of the low impedance of the left atrium. Surgery should be considered when the patient begins to limit activity to avoid symptoms, and as the left ventricle becomes larger and the ejection fraction decreases with exercise. The ratio of the end-systolic wall stress to the end-systolic volume index is believed by some to indicate that the patient will have a good result from surgery (Carabello and Spann, 1984).

Patients with pulmonary congestion as a result of acute mitral regurgitation due to any cause usually require surgical treatment.

SURGICAL PROCEDURE

The surgeon may replace the valve with either a tissue or a synthetic valve, or reconstruct the valve (valvoplasty). The operative risk ranges from 4%–15%, depending on the cause and the severity of the regurgitation. (See the surgical procedure section under "Mitral Valve Stenosis" for a discussion of the surgical anatomy.)

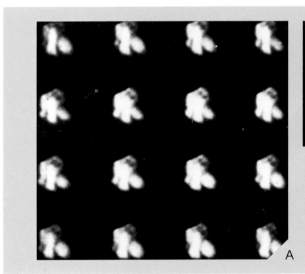
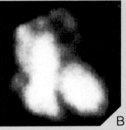
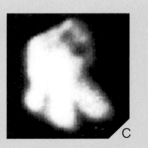

left ventricular ejection fraction 29%
right ventricular ejection fraction 7%

FIG. 4.87 (A) *These sixteen frames of a gated equilibrium radionuclide angiogram were obtained in a patient with severe mitral regurgitation. The end-diastolic (B) and end-systolic (C) images show left ventricular and right ventricular dysfunction. The pulmonary artery wedge pressure in the patient was 29 mmHg, and the pulmonary artery pressure was 60/30 mmHg. The pulmonary artery, the right atrium, and the left atrium are prominent. (Reproduced with permission of the author and publisher; see Figure Credits)*

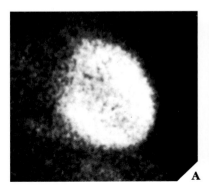
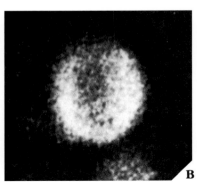
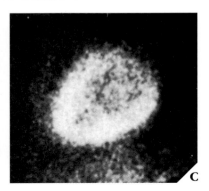

FIG. 4.88 *These normal* ^{201}Tl *scans in the anterior (A) and 30° (B) and 65° (C) left anterior oblique projections were obtained in a patient with mitral valve prolapse and a normal coronary arteriogram. (Reproduced with permission of the author and publisher; see Figure Credits)*

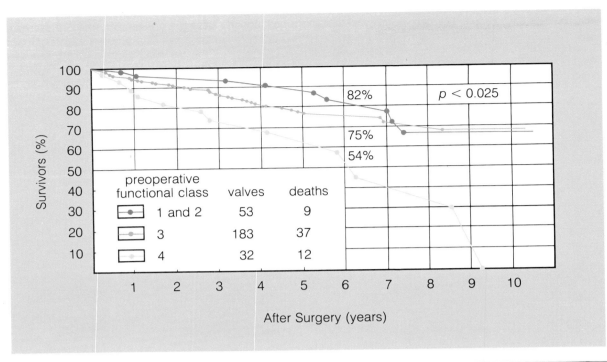

FIG. 4.89 *Actuarial survival over a ten-year period for patients having Starr–Edwards mitral valve replacement varies according to preoperative functional class. Only operative survivors are included. (Redrawn; reproduced with permission of the authors and publisher; see Figure Credits. Also, Fig. 38-28, The Heart, 6th ed, p 780)*

Survivors (%)

After Surgery (years)

preoperative functional class	valves	deaths
1 and 2	53	9
3	183	37
4	32	12

82%

75%

54%

$p < 0.025$

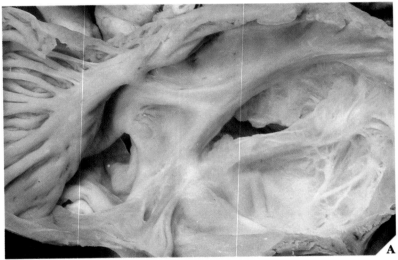

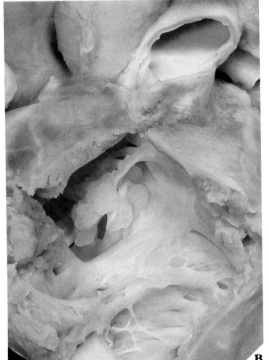

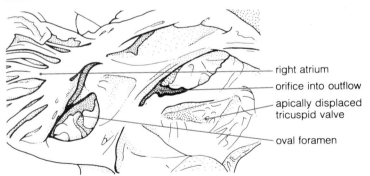

right atrium
orifice into outflow
apically displaced tricuspid valve
oval foramen

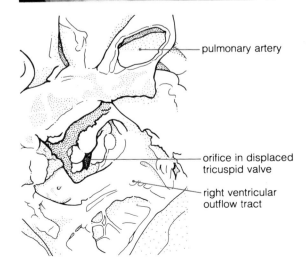

pulmonary artery

orifice in displaced tricuspid valve

right ventricular outflow tract

FIG. 4.90 **(A)** *Right-atrial view of a heart specimen with Ebstein's disease of the tricuspid valve shows extreme apical displacement, which causes extensive atrialization of part of the right ventricle. Valve dysplasia leads to a small outlet from the atrialized part into the remaining right ventricular pumping chamber.* **(B)** *The outlet view shows the restricted tricuspid valve orifice close to the pulmonary artery.*

The ten-year actuarial survival curve for patients with the Starr–Edwards valve is shown in Figure 4.89. The survival curves vary considerably with the functional classification assigned to the patient at the time of surgery.

Tissue valves are preferred in older adults because long-term anticoagulation is not usually needed. Anticoagulation is always necessary in patients who have a Bjork–Shiley or a Starr–Edwards valve. Prophylaxis against bacterial endocarditis must be emphasized to patients with either a tissue or a synthetic valve prosthesis.

TRICUSPID VALVE STENOSIS*
ETIOLOGY AND PATHOLOGY

Tricuspid valve stenosis may be congenital in origin. Usually it is part of a more complex cardiac malformation, leading to symptoms early in life (see Chapter 3). An exception is Ebstein's malformation, which

*Abstracted with permission of the authors and publisher from Rackley CE, Edwards JE, Wallace RB, Katz NM: Tricuspid and pulmonary valve disease, Chapter 40, pp 792–800, in Hurst JW (ed): *The Heart,* 6th ed. New York, McGraw-Hill, 1986. Figures reproduced in this section from the above chapter or other sources are also reprinted with permission of the authors and publishers. For the full bibliographic citations of the sources of figures other than the above chapter, see Figure Credits at the end of this chapter.

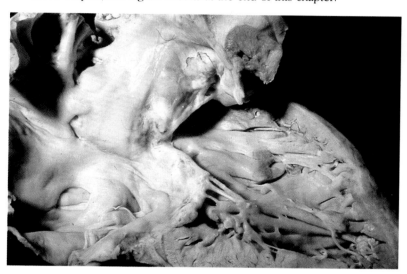

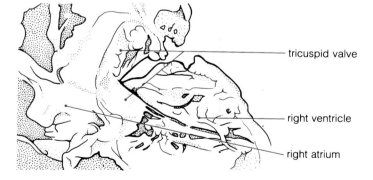

— tricuspid valve

— right ventricle

— right atrium

FIG. 4.91 *The carcinoid syndrome may affect the tricuspid valve; valve thickening and partial immobilization may cause regurgitation and often stenosis. (Reproduced with permission of the authors and publisher; see Figure Credits)*

can occasionally produce tricuspid stenosis (Fig. 4.90), although regurgitation more commonly dominates. While rheumatic fever may affect the tricuspid valve, it is extremely uncommon that this progresses to valve stenosis (Clawson, 1940). Other rare conditions, such as the carcinoid syndrome, may affect the tricuspid valve to such an extent that stenosis occurs (Fig. 4.91). Blockade of the tricuspid valve may be due to right atrial mxyoma (Fig. 4.92), other neoplasms, or thrombi. Tricuspid valve stenosis may be the result of the thrombotic obstruction of a tricuspid valve prosthesis.

(For a discussion of congenital tricuspid atresia, see Chapter 3.)

ABNORMAL PHYSIOLOGY

The normal area of the tricuspid valve is 7 cm². The flow of blood from the right atrium into the right ventricle is impeded when the valve area is reduced to 1.5 cm². An elevation of the right atrial pressure to 10 mmHg is usually associated with peripheral edema. The cardiac output falls with significant tricuspid stenosis (El–Sherif, 1971). When the condition is due to rheumatic fever, it is usually associated with mitral valve disease, which may also play a role in the altered hemodynamics.

CLINICAL MANIFESTATIONS
SYMPTOMS

Patients with significant tricuspid stenosis experience fatigue and dyspnea. Tricuspid stenosis may, to some degree, protect the lungs in

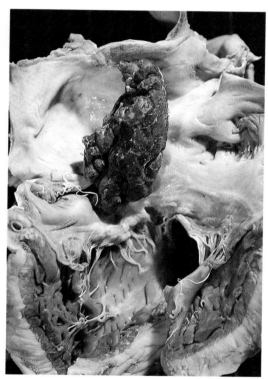

FIG. 4.92 *A right atrial myxoma obstructs the tricuspid orifice.*

patients with mitral stenosis (Kitchin and Turner, 1964). The patient may notice large a waves in the internal jugular venous pulse.

PHYSICAL EXAMINATION

A large a wave may be detected by the examiner in the internal jugular venous pulse. The right ventricle is not palpable. Respiratory variation in splitting of the second heart sound may be absent, since right ventricular filling remains fairly constant throughout the respiratory cycle.

The tricuspid component of the first sound may be louder than normal. A diastolic rumble that becomes louder with inspiration may be heard at the end of the left sternal border (Fig. 4.93). An opening snap may also be heard.

The physical signs of aortic and/or mitral valve disease are often present and may in fact mask the physical signs of tricuspid stenosis.

LABORATORY STUDIES

CHEST RADIOGRAPHY. The right atrium may be large, and calcium may be seen in the tricuspid valve leaflets or annulus (Perloff and Harvey, 1960).

ELECTROCARDIOGRAPHY. The P waves may become large, or atrial fibrillation may be present. Congenital tricuspid atresia may produce left ventricular hypertrophy in the ECG, but acquired isolated tricuspid stenosis is not associated with right or left ventricular hypertrophy.

ECHOCARDIOGRAPHY. The echocardiogram (Fig. 4.94) and the Doppler technique (Fig. 4.95) may be used to identify tricuspid stenosis.

CARDIAC CATHETERIZATION. The pressure gradient between the right ventricle and the right atrium is normally less than 1 mmHg (Killip and Lukas, 1957). The gradient is elevated in patients with tricuspid stenosis; however, small gradients may not be detected. The tricuspid valve area in patients with tricuspid stenosis is less than 1.5 cm^2.

(Congenital tricuspid atresia is discussed in Chapter 3. An atrial septal defect is always present in such patients.)

NATURAL HISTORY

The natural history depends on the etiology of the tricuspid valve blockade. Rheumatic tricuspid valve disease is usually associated with mitral stenosis, and the natural history depends more on the severity of the mitral valve disease. Some observers believe that pulmonary congestion is less and that peripheral edema dominates the clinical picture when both mitral and tricuspid stenosis are present. The presence of tricuspid stenosis may lead one to underestimate the degree of mitral stenosis.

The natural history of tricuspid stenosis in patients with carcinoid syndrome is determined by the other aspects of the syndrome and the degree of stenosis of the valve, which, in general, progresses slowly.

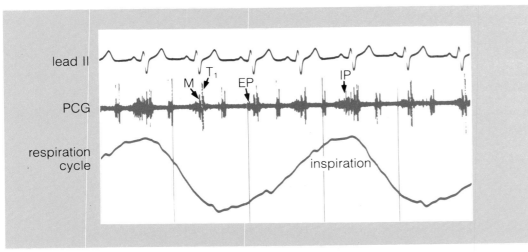

FIG. 4.93 *The striking features of a phonocardiogram obtained in a patient with tricuspid stenosis are the prominent tricuspid component of the first sound* (T$_1$) *in comparison with the mitral component* (M), *and the late diastolic murmur, which increases during the inspiratory phase* (IP) *of respiration. (Redrawn; Fig. 40-3,* The Heart, *6th ed, p 795. Courtesy of I. Sylvia Crawley, MD, Atlanta, Georgia)*

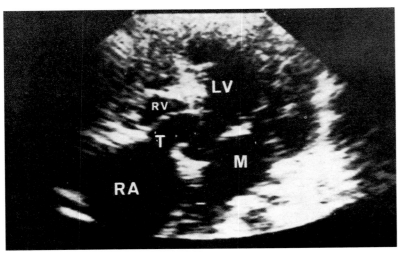

FIG. 4.94 *Cross-sectional echocardiogram in the apical four-chamber view was obtained in a child with a severely stenotic tricuspid valve. The tricuspid annulus* (T) *is smaller than the mitral annulus* (M). *The right ventricle* (RV) *is diminutive; the tricuspid leaflets open dome-wise. The right atrium* (RA) *is enlarged* (LV, *left ventricle). (Reproduced with permission of the author and publisher; see Figure Credits)*

(The natural history of congenital tricuspid atresia is discussed in Chapter 3.)

TREATMENT

The patient must be advised regarding the prevention of bacterial endocarditis. Patients with heart failure must be treated with diuretics and digitalis, but results are poor.

Balloon dilation of the tricuspid valve is currently under investigation; the indications for the use of this technique cannot be stated without further research and experience (Feit et al, 1986).

INDICATIONS FOR SURGERY

Surgery is indicated for patients with evidence of severe tricuspid stenosis. It is important to assess the other valves carefully prior to surgery, since they too may need to be replaced at the same operation.

SURGICAL PROCEDURE

Operations on the tricuspid valve are performed through some type of right atriotomy. As in any operation requiring a right atriotomy the sinus node and its blood supply are at risk (Fig. 4.96). When the nodal artery lies in its usual location in relation to the superior cavoatrial

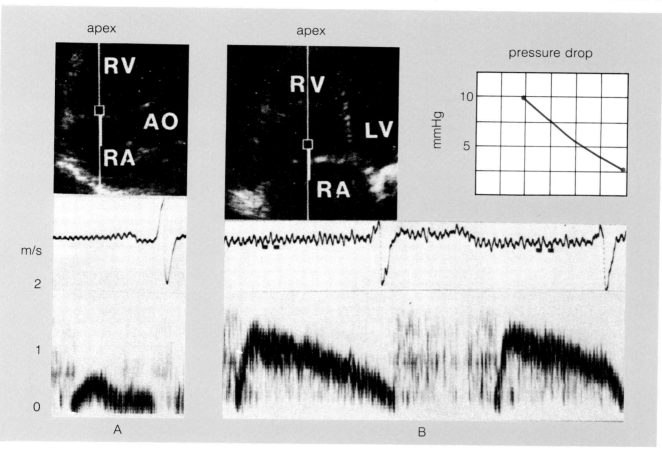

FIG. 4.95 *Tricuspid flow velocity is recorded from the apex in a normal subject (A) and in a patient with tricuspid stenosis and atrial fibrillation (B). The calculated pressure drop for the last beat is shown; the mean pressure drop is 6 mmHg (RV, right ventricle; RA, right atrium; LV, left ventricle, AO, aorta). (Partially redrawn; reproduced with permission of the author and publisher; see Figure Credits)*

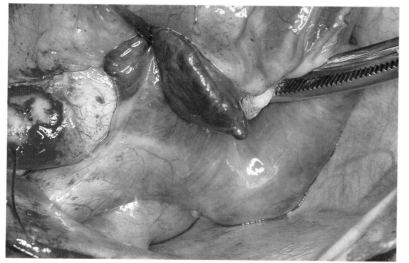

FIG. 4.96 *Operative view through a median sternotomy shows the superior cavoatrial junction; the location of the sinoatrial node is clearly apparent.*

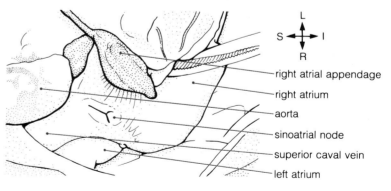

- right atrial appendage
- right atrium
- aorta
- sinoatrial node
- superior caval vein
- left atrium

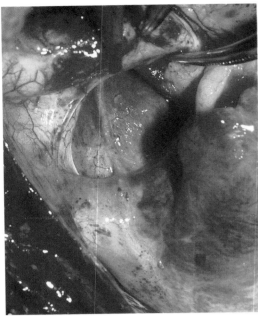

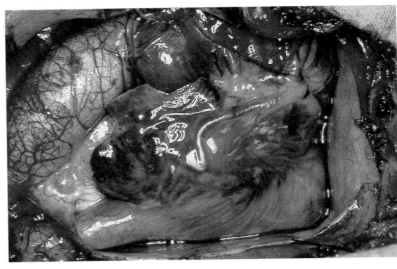

FIG. 4.97 *The artery to the sinus node courses across the roof of the left atrium, over the superior cavoatrial junction, to the terminal sulcus. (Reproduced with permission of the authors and publisher; see Figure Credits)*

FIG. 4.98 *The anomalous course of a sinus node artery runs across the lateral wall of the left atrium. (Reproduced with permission of the authors and publisher; see Figure Credits)*

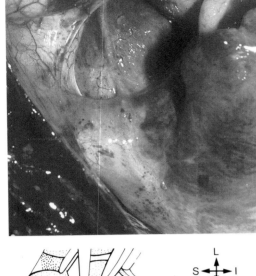

L
S ← → I
R

aorta

roof of
left atrium

right atrial
appendage

artery to
sinoatrial node

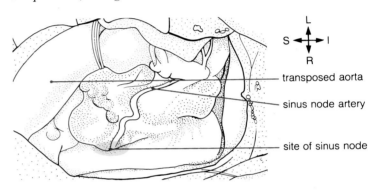

L
S ← → I
R

transposed aorta

sinus node artery

site of sinus node

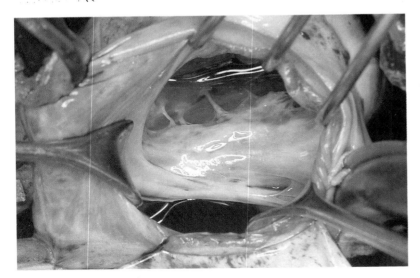

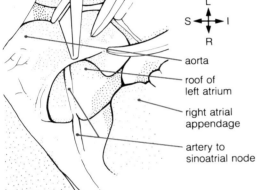

FIG. 4.99 *In this operative view of the triangle of Koch the atrial portion of the membranous septum is particularly well seen. The oval fossa is absent in this patient with a secundum atrial septal defect.*

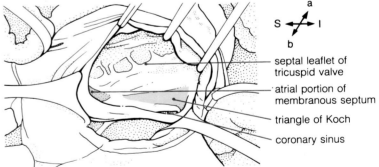

a
S ← → I
b

septal leaflet of
tricuspid valve

atrial portion of
membranous septum

triangle of Koch

coronary sinus

junction, both the node and the artery are relatively safe (Fig. 4.97). However, one may occasionally encounter cases in which the artery originates quite distally from the right coronary artery and traverses the midportion of the right atrial wall (Fig. 4.98).

Operations on the tricuspid valve usually accompany operative repair of lesions elsewhere in the heart. The most frequent operation is tricuspid valvoplasty for primary or secondary tricuspid insuffi-

ciency. Valve replacement may be necessary when the valve is stenosed or damaged to the degree that repair is not possible. In either instance the important anatomic considerations are concentrated at the apex of the triangle of Koch (Fig. 4.99). Figure 4.100 illustrates the position of the tricuspid valve in relation to other critical structures within the heart. The right coronary artery, lying in the right atrioventricular groove, may be intimately related to the tricuspid annulus (Fig. 4.101),

FIG. 4.100 *Anatomic relations of the tricuspid valve to other critical structures are illustrated in operative orientation. The structures at risk are superimposed. (Adapted; see Figure Credits)*

tricuspid valve

central fibrous body

atrioventricular node

aorta

triangle of Koch

superior caval vein

oval fossa

coronary sinus

FIG. 4.101 *A dissected specimen shows the tricuspid valve orifice and its intimate relationship to the right coronary artery. (Reproduced with permission of the authors and publisher; see Figure Credits)*

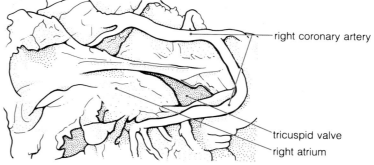

right coronary artery

tricuspid valve

right atrium

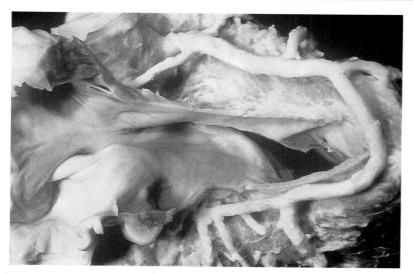

placing this vessel at risk during operative repair of the valve (Fig. 4.102).

The risk of surgery is about 5%–15%, depending on the number of valves replaced and the severity of the condition at the time of surgery.

After surgery the patient must continue to use prophylaxis against bacterial endocarditis. Therapy with anticoagulants and dipyridamole is usually indicated; dipyridamole may be especially useful in patients with tricuspid and pulmonary prosthetic valves (Chesebro et al, 1983).

TRICUSPID VALVE REGURGITATION*
ETIOLOGY AND PATHOLOGY

Tricuspid valve regurgitation is usually secondary to right ventricular dilation and heart failure caused by disease of the left side of the heart.

---

*Abstracted with permission of the authors and publisher from Rackley CE, Edwards JE, Wallace RB, Katz NM: Tricuspid and pulmonary valve disease, Chapter 40, pp 792–800, in Hurst JW (ed): *The Heart,* 6th ed. New York, McGraw-Hill, 1986. Figures reproduced in this section from other sources are also reprinted with permission of the authors and publishers. For the full bibliographic citations of the sources of figures, see Figure Credits at the end of this chapter.

Bacterial endocarditis, particularly in drug addicts, is the most common cause of isolated regurgitation of the tricuspid valve (Fig. 4.103). Other causes include myocardial infarction, which may cause right ventricular overload leading to regurgitation or, rarely, rupture of the septal papillary muscles to the tricuspid valve (Fig. 4.104), carcinoid syndrome (see Fig. 4.91), prolapse of the tricuspid valve particularly in patients with Marfan's syndrome, and congenital heart disease, such as ostium primum atrioventricular septal defect or Ebstein's malformation. Trauma with laceration of the tricuspid valve apparatus or a faulty prosthetic tricuspid valve may also cause tricuspid valve regurgitation.

ABNORMAL PHYSIOLOGY

Tricuspid valve regurgitation during systole produces an increase in the right atrial pressure and a large V wave in the right atrial pressure curve and in the internal jugular vein (Hansing and Rowe, 1972).

CLINICAL MANIFESTATIONS
SYMPTOMS

Tricuspid regurgitation that is secondary to right ventricular dilation related to left-sided heart disease is associated with dyspnea and fatigue (Salazar and Levine, 1962). Paroxysmal nocturnal dyspnea and pulmonary edema may be diminished in such patients because of the

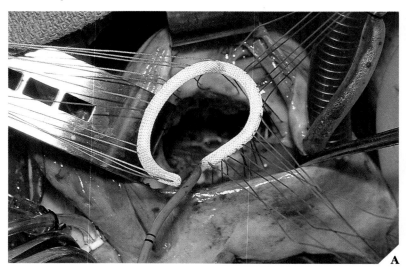
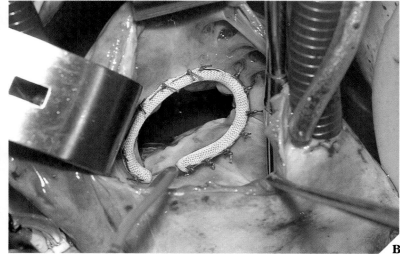

A

B

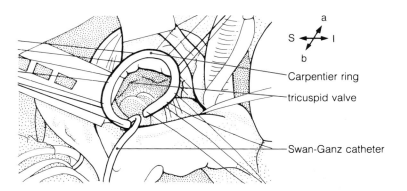
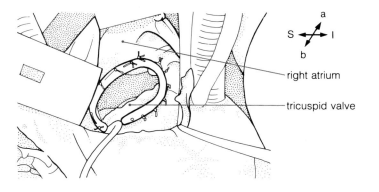

FIG. 4.102 (A,B) *In these operative views of a tricuspid valvoplasty utilizing a Carpentier ring the blue Swan-Ganz catheter identifies the gap* *in the ring where sutures are omitted to avoid damage to the atrioventricular node.*

PART II: DISEASES OF THE HEART

tricuspid regurgitation, but the decrease in symptoms is more likely to be due to an increase in pulmonary arteriolar resistance. Patients who have bacterial endocarditis may have fever and fatigue. Patients with the carcinoid syndrome have flushing and other features of this unusual disease.

PHYSICAL EXAMINATION

Atrial fibrillation is often present. Tricuspid regurgitation produces a large V wave in the internal jugular venous pulse. The liver may be large and pulsate with each systole.

A holosystolic murmur may be heard at the lower end of the sternum; it may increase in intensity with inspiration. An opening snap of the tricuspid valve may be heard on rare occasion. The pulmonary component of the second sound may be louder than normal, and the murmur of pulmonary regurgitation may be heard in patients with tricuspid regurgitation associated with pulmonary hypertension. The signs of additional valve disease or myocardial disease are usually evident in patients with tricuspid valve regurgitation.

The abnormalities noted in patients with tricuspid regurgitation due to bacterial endocarditis are usually isolated to the tricuspid valve, although other signs of endocarditis may be present.

LABORATORY STUDIES

CHEST RADIOGRAPHY. Chest films of patients with secondary tricuspid regurgitation reveal the abnormalities of the primary heart disease, including right atrial enlargement. The chest film of a patient with tricuspid regurgitation due to endocarditis may show right atrial enlargement.

ELECTROCARDIOGRAPHY. The ECG of a patient with secondary tricuspid regurgitation may reveal abnormal P waves and right, left, and combined ventricular hypertrophy that reflects the primary heart disease. Right or left bundle branch block may be present in patients with severe heart disease. Atrial fibrillation may be detected.

The ECG of a patient with primary tricuspid regurgitation may show right atrial abnormality.

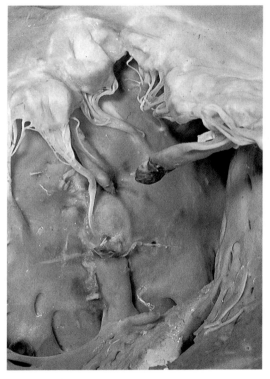

FIG. 4.104 *Papillary muscle rupture due to myocardial infarction leads to severe regurgitation of the tricuspid valve.*

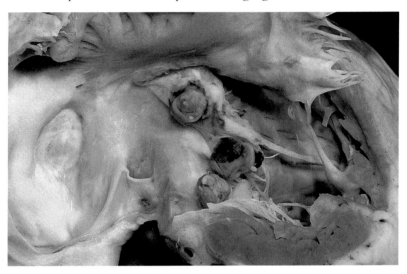

FIG. 4.103 *Infective endocarditis in a drug addict led to isolated tricuspid valve regurgitation. (Reproduced with permission of the authors and publisher; see Figure Credits)*

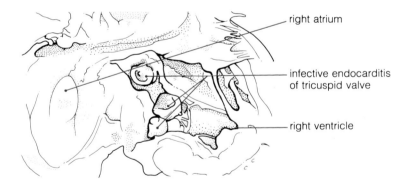

right atrium

infective endocarditis of tricuspid valve

right ventricle

ECHOCARDIOGRAPHY. Systolic prolapse of the tricuspid valve may be detected on the echocardiogram. Valvar calcification and an increase in the left and right ventricular dimensions may be noted. Vegetations on the tricuspid valve may also be identified by echocardiography in patients with endocarditis (Fig. 4.105).

CARDIAC CATHETERIZATION. A prominent V wave in the right atrial pressure curve indicates tricuspid regurgitation. Catheterization may reveal abnormalities of the aortic and the mitral valves, evidence of dilated cardiomyopathy including ischemic cardiomyopathy, and coronary disease.

Angiographic evidence of tricuspid regurgitation is difficult to demonstrate, since the catheter itself may produce an incompetent tricuspid valve.

NATURAL HISTORY

Secondary tricuspid regurgitation is a marker of severe, advanced heart disease; the natural history is that of the causative disease of the left side of the heart.

The natural history of primary tricuspid regurgitation due to endocarditis is that of endocarditis plus the associated hemodynamic alteration. The condition is lethal unless antibiotic and surgical therapy is implemented in a timely fashion.

TREATMENT

Heart failure is treated with digitalis, diuretics, and drugs that alter preload and afterload. Endocarditis must be treated with appropriate antibiotics.

INDICATIONS FOR SURGERY

When surgery is planned for aortic and mitral valve disease, one must consider surgery for secondary tricuspid regurgitation, if it is present. Surgery should be performed on the tricuspid valve in such patients if the regurgitation is severe and long-standing, and there is chronic pulmonary hypertension. At times the decision to repair or replace the tricuspid valve is made at surgery.

The need for tricuspid valve surgery for endocarditis is determined by the severity of the regurgitation and the presence of septic pulmonary emboli.

SURGICAL PROCEDURE

The tricuspid valve may be repaired (valvoplasty) or replaced with a tissue or a synthetic valve (Carpentier et al, 1974). The same anatomic conditions pertain in replacement of a regurgitant tricuspid valve as described in relation to tricuspid valve stenosis (see above).

The operative risk is high and may reach 25% in patients who have severe multivalvar disease and heart failure. Medical treatment must

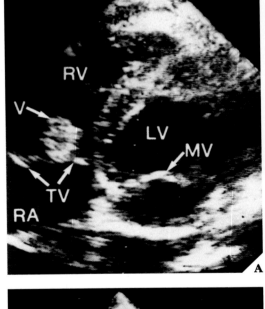

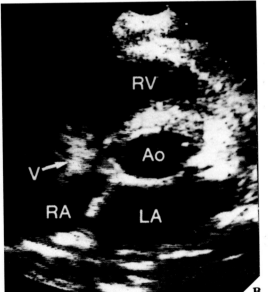

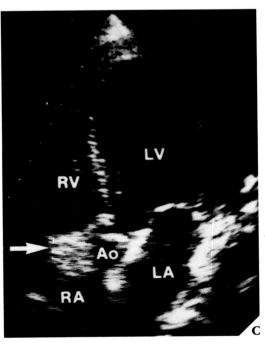

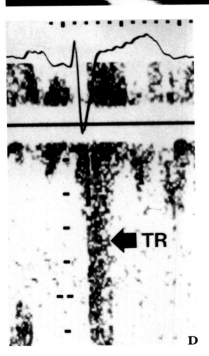

FIG. 4.105 *Cross-sectional echocardiograms and a Doppler recording were obtained in a patient with tricuspid valve endocarditis.* (**A**) *On the parasternal short-axis view of the tricuspid valve a large vegetation* (V) *is seen on the tricuspid valve* (TV). (**B**) *On the parasternal short-axis view of the tricuspid valve at the level of the aortic valve* (Ao), *the vegetation can be seen prolapsing into the right ventricle* (RV). (**C**) *The apical five-chamber view reveals the vegetation* (arrow) *prolapsing into the right atrium* (RA) (LA, *left atrium;* LV, *left ventricle;* RV, *right ventricle;* MV, *mitral valve*). (**D**) *A continuous-wave Doppler recording was obtained with the transducer placed to show the apical four-chamber view. Systolic flow* (TR) *away from the transducer is seen.* (*Courtesy of Joel M. Felner, MD, Atlanta, Georgia*)

be continued after surgery, including digitalis, diuretics, anticoagulants, and prophylaxis against endocarditis.

The information on long-range follow-up is inadequate. Since the procedure is often performed to save lives and decrease severe symptoms, the survivors fare better than patients who are not treated surgically.

PULMONARY VALVE STENOSIS*
ETIOLOGY AND PATHOLOGY

Pulmonary valve stenosis is almost always due to congenital heart disease (see Chapter 3), although it may be related to the carcinoid

---

*Abstracted with permission of the authors and publisher from Rackley CE, Edwards JE, Wallace RB, Katz NM: Tricuspid and pulmonary valve disease, Chapter 40, pp 792–800, in Hurst JW (ed): *The Heart,* 6th ed. New York, McGraw-Hill, 1986. Figures reproduced in this section from other sources are also reprinted with permission of the authors and publishers. For the full bibliographic citations of the sources of figures, see Figure Credits at the end of this chapter.

syndrome (Hurst et al, 1985). When due to carcinoid, the leaflets become immobilized due to a proliferation of connective tissue on the arterial side of the cusps (Fig. 4.106).

ABNORMAL PHYSIOLOGY

For a discussion of the abnormal physiology of pulmonary valve stenosis the reader is referred to the relevant section under "Pulmonary Stenosis with Intact Ventricular Septum" in Chapter 3.

CLINICAL MANIFESTATIONS
SYMPTOMS

Patients with the carcinoid syndrome and pulmonary valve stenosis exhibit episodes of flushing, and less commonly diarrhea and asthma. (The symptoms associated with congenital pulmonary valve stenosis is discussed in Chapter 3.)

PHYSICAL EXAMINATION

The patient with carcinoid syndrome may have telangiectasia, an enlarged liver, flushing, wheezing, and a systolic murmur heard in the second intercostal space to the left of the sternum. The pulmonary

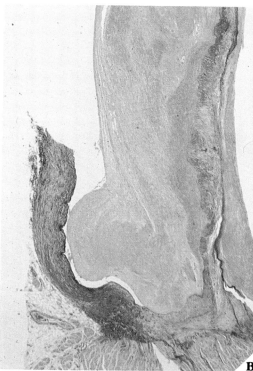
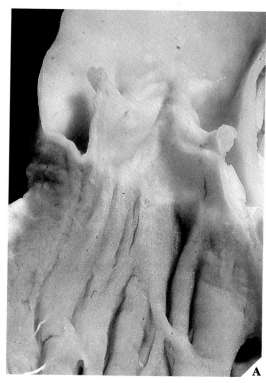
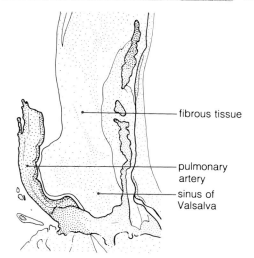
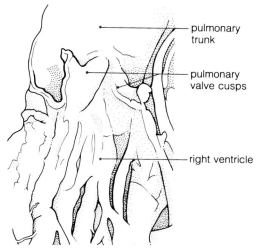

FIG. 4.106 (A) *In pulmonary valve stenosis in carcinoid syndrome the pulmonary valve shows marked thickening.* (B) *Histologic section shows the deposition of collagenous material on the arterial side of the valve cusp, underlying immobilization and stenosis (elastic tissue stain, counterstained with van Gieson's stain).*
(B: *Reproduced with permission of the authors and publisher; see Figure Credits*)

component of the second sound may be delayed and decreased in intensity.

(The abnormalities associated with congenital pulmonary valve stenosis are discussed in Chapter 3.)

LABORATORY STUDIES

CHEST RADIOGRAPHY. The pulmonary trunk may be prominent on chest radiographs of patients with pulmonary valve stenosis due to the carcinoid syndrome. (For the chest film in patients with congenital pulmonary valve stenosis see Figure 3.96.)

ELECTROCARDIOGRAPHY. The ECG of a patient with pulmonary valve stenosis associated with the carcinoid syndrome may show prominent right atrial P waves and right axis deviation of the mean QRS vector. (For the ECG of patients with congenital pulmonary stenosis, see Figure 3.97.)

ECHOCARDIOGRAPHY. The echocardiogram may reveal pulmonary valve stenosis in patients with the carcinoid syndrome.

(For the echocardiogram of a patient with congenital pulmonary valve stenosis, see Figure 3.98.)

CARDIAC CATHETERIZATION Pulmonary valve stenosis is identified when there is a pressure gradient across the pulmonary valve. Angiographic studies on patients with the carcinoid syndrome may reveal decreased contractility of the right ventricle.

SPECIAL LABORATORY TESTS. When the carcinoid syndrome is suspected, the urine should be examined for the presence of 5-hydroxyindoleacetic acid.

NATURAL HISTORY

The natural history of the patient with the carcinoid syndrome depends on the site of the tumor, the extent of metastases, and the degree of heart damage. (The natural history of a patient with congenital pulmonary valve stenosis is discussed in Chapter 3.)

TREATMENT

The patient with pulmonary valve stenosis must be advised regarding the prevention of bacterial endocarditis.

Several drugs are purported to decrease the symptoms associated with the carcinoid syndrome, but none are entirely satisfactory.

The surgical treatment of pulmonary valve stenosis associated with the carcinoid syndrome usually entails replacement with a tissue rather than a synthetic valve. The bioprosthesis is used in an effort to minimize thrombosis, which is more likely to occur with the synthetic valves.

The surgical treatment of congenital pulmonary valve stenosis is discussed in Chapter 3. Balloon dilation of the pulmonary valve has been used successfully but the indications for the use of this technique cannot be determined without further research and experience.

PULMONARY VALVE REGURGITATION*
ETIOLOGY AND PATHOLOGY

The absent pulmonary valve syndrome is discussed in Chapter 3. Pulmonary valve regurgitation may be associated with congenital pulmonary valve stenosis (see Chapter 3) or pulmonary hypertension. Primary pulmonary hypertension occurs without an obvious cause. Pulmonary hypertension may be due to congenital heart disease, including ventricular or atrial septal defect, or a patent arterial duct. Acquired causes of pulmonary hypertension include rheumatic mitral stenosis (in which the murmur of pulmonary regurgitation is referred to as a Graham Steele murmur), severe chronic lung disease, pulmonary emboli, and primary pulmonary hypertension. Pulmonary valve

---

*Abstracted with permission of the authors and publisher from Rackley CE, Edwards JE, Wallace RB, Katz NM: Tricuspid and pulmonary valve disease, Chapter 40, pp 792–800, in Hurst JW (ed): *The Heart,* 6th ed. New York, McGraw-Hill, 1986. Figures reproduced in this section from other sources are also reprinted with permission of the authors and publishers. For the full bibliographic citations of the sources of figures, see Figure Credits at the end of this chapter.

FIG. 4.107 *Cross-sectional* (**A**) *and M-mode* (**B**) *echocardiograms were obtained in a patient with pulmonary valve regurgitation due to primary pulmonary hypertension.* (**A**) *The parasternal short-axis view of the pulmonary valve* (PV) *shows a dilated main pulmonary artery* (PA) (Ao, *aorta*). (**B**) *An M-mode tracing of the pulmonary valve demonstrates the absence of the* a *wave and premature closing of the pulmonary valve referred to as a "notch"* (arrow). (*Courtesy of Joel M. Felner, MD, Atlanta, Georgia*)

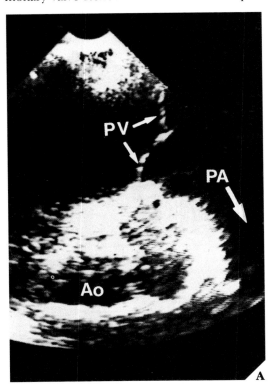
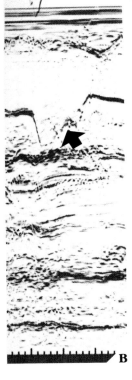

regurgitation may be associated with an atrial septal defect when the pulmonary flow is large and the pulmonary pressure is only slightly elevated. The murmur of pulmonary valve regurgitation may be heard in patients who undergo chronic renal dialysis. Pulmonary valve regurgitation may be caused by carcinoid involvement of the pulmonary valve or by previous surgery on the valve. Bacterial endocarditis may involve the pulmonary valve, producing incompetence.

ABNORMAL PHYSIOLOGY
Pulmonary valve regurgitation produces a volume overload on the right ventricle; this alone can usually be tolerated without producing heart failure (Holmes et al, 1968). Since most of the causes of pulmonary valve regurgitation are associated with right ventricular hypertension, the volume load is superimposed on the pressure load, which is the cause of right ventricular hypertrophy.

CLINICAL MANIFESTATIONS
SYMPTOMS
Pulmonary valve regurgitation itself rarely causes any symptoms. When present, symptoms are usually related to the causative disease and to pulmonary arteriolar disease. Patients with pulmonary hypertension may experience dyspnea, syncope, and even sudden death.

PHYSICAL EXAMINATION
When pulmonary valve regurgitation is secondary to some other type of heart disease, the abnormalities found on physical examination are those of the primary disease.

When pulmonary valve regurgitation is caused by pulmonary hypertension, the second component of the second heart sound is louder than normal. A high-pitched, decrescendo, diastolic murmur may be heard along the left sternal border. The murmur immediately follows the second heart sound. It is difficult to differentiate this murmur from the murmur of aortic valve regurgitation.

When pulmonary valve regurgitation is due to heart disease that is associated with normal or low pulmonary arterial pressure, it produces a low-pitched, decrescendo, diastolic murmur, which is heard along the left sternal border. The pulmonary component of the second sound may be normal or decreased in intensity. The murmur may not immediately follow the second heart sound.

LABORATORY STUDIES
CHEST RADIOGRAPHY. The chest films of patients with secondary pulmonary valve regurgitation reveal the characteristics of the primary disease. The chest films of patients with primary pulmonary valve regurgitation may be normal, or they may reveal a large pulmonary trunk with or without enlargement of the right ventricle and right atrium.

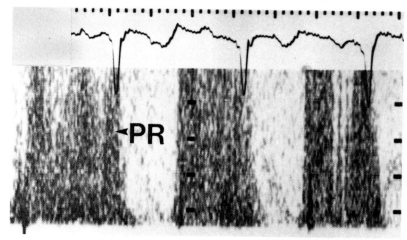

ELECTROCARDIOGRAPHY. The ECG reveals the abnormalities associated with the heart disease responsible for secondary pulmonary regurgitation. The ECG of a patient with pulmonary regurgitation due to primary pulmonary hypertension may show right atrial abnormality and other features signifying right ventricular hypertrophy.

ECHOCARDIOGRAPHY. M-mode and cross-sectional echocardiograms of a patient with pulmonary hypertension and valve regurgitation are shown in Figure 4.107. The Doppler technique is an excellent method of identifying pulmonary regurgitation (Fig. 4.108); however, regurgitant turbulent flow may be recorded in normal subjects (Kostucki et al, 1986).

CARDIAC CATHETERIZATION. Pulmonary valve regurgitation cannot be detected by pressure measurements, but the features of the heart disease that is responsible for pulmonary valve regurgitation may be detected. It is also difficult to demonstrate pulmonary valve regurgitation by angiography.

NATURAL HISTORY
The natural history of patients with secondary pulmonary valve regurgitation is that of the heart disease responsible for it. The natural history of patients with primary pulmonary valve regurgitation due to endocarditis or carcinoid is also that of the primary disease.

TREATMENT
The treatment of secondary pulmonary valve regurgitation is limited to the treatment used for the heart disease that produced it. There is no satisfactory treatment for primary pulmonary hypertension. The treatment of pulmonary valve regurgitation due to endocarditis includes antibiotic therapy and surgical replacement with a tissue valve. The surgical treatment of patients with pulmonary valve regurgitation due to carcinoid disease may require replacement with a tissue valve, but isolated pulmonary valve regurgitation may be present for years without causing difficulty.

Pulmonary valve surgery may be needed in patients with pulmonary valve regurgitation that is secondary to prior surgery performed on the pulmonary valve.

REFERENCES
Abernathy WS, Willis PW III (1973) Thromboembolic complications of rheumatic heart disease. *Cardiovasc Clin* 5:131
Baker C, Sommerville J (1959) Clinical features and surgical treatment of fifty patients with severe aortic stenosis. *Guys Hosp Rep* 108:101
Baker CG, Finnegan TRL (1957) Epilepsy and mitral stenosis. *Br Heart J* 19:159
Blank RH, Pupello DF, Besone LN, et al (1976) Method of managing a small aortic root annulus during valve replacement. *Ann Thorac Surg* 22:356

FIG. 4.108 *In this continuous-wave Doppler recording obtained from the parasternal short-axis view in a patient with pulmonary regurgitation, diastolic flow (PR) is recorded flowing toward the transducer. (Courtesy of Joel M. Felner, MD, Atlanta, Georgia)*

Boltwood CM, Tei C, Wong M, Shah PM (1983) Quantitative echocardiography of the mitral complex in dilated cardiomyopathy: The mechanism of functional mitral regurgitation. *Circulation* 68:498

Borer JS, Bacharach SL, Greene MV, et al (1978) Exercise-induced left ventricular dysfunction in symptomatic and asymptomatic patients with aortic regurgitation: Assessment with radionuclide cineangiography. *Am J Cardiol* 42:351

Braunwald E (1969) Mitral regurgitation: Physiologic, clinical and surgical considerations. *N Engl J Med* 281:425

Carabello BA, Spann JF (1984) The uses and limitations of end-systolic indexes of left ventricular function. *Circulation* 69:1058

Carpentier A, Deloche A, Hanania G, et al (1974) Surgical management of acquired tricuspid valve disease. *J Thorac Cardiovasc Surg* 67:53

Chesebro JH, Fuster V, Elveback LR, et al (1983) Trial of combined Warfarin plus dipyridamole or aspirin therapy in prosthetic heart valve replacement: Danger of aspirin compared with dipyridamole. *Am J Cardiol* 51:1537

Chun PK, Gertz E, Davisa JE, Cheitlin MD (1982) Coronary atherosclerosis in mitral stenosis. *Chest* 81:36

Clawson BJ (1940) Rheumatic heart disease. An analysis of 796 cases. *Am Heart J* 20:454

Crawley IS, Morris DC, Silverman BD: Valvular heart disease, in Hurst JW (ed): *The Heart* 4th ed. New York, McGraw-Hill, 1978, p 992

Cribier A, Saoudi N, Berland J, Savin T, Rocha P, Letac B (1986) Percutaneous transluminal valvoplasty of acquired aortic stenosis in elderly patients: An alternative to valve replacement? *Lancet* 1:63

Croft CH, Woodward W, Elliott A, et al (1983) Analysis of surgical versus medical therapy in active complicated native valve infective endocarditis. *Am J Cardiol* 51:1650

Dack S, Bleifer S, Grishman A, Donoso E (1960) Mitral stenosis: Auscultatory and phonocardiographic findings. *Am J Cardiol* 5:815

Dexter L (1969): Evaluation of the results of cardiac surgery, in Jones AM (ed): *Modern Trends in Cardiology*, vol. 2. New York, Appleton-Century-Crofts, p 311

Dodge HT, Baxley WA (1969) Left ventricular volume and mass and their significance in heart disease. *Am J Cardiol* 23:528

Edwards JE (1979) On the etiology of acquired valvular disease of the heart. *Semin Roentgenol* 14:96

El–Sherif N (1971) Rheumatic tricuspid stenosis: A haemodynamic correlation. *Br Heart J* 33:16

Feit F, Stecy PJ, Nachamie MS (1986) Percutaneous balloon valvoplasty for stenosis of a porcine bioprosthesis in the tricuspid valve position. *Am J Cardiol* 58:363

Felson B (1973) *Chest Roentgenology*. Philadelphia, WB Saunders Co., 1973

Flamm MD, Braiff BA, Kimball R, Hancock EW (1967) Mechanism of effort syncope in aortic stenosis. *Circulation* 36(suppl 2):II-109

Frank S, Johnson A, Ross J Jr (1973) Natural history of valvular aortic stenosis. *Br Heart J* 35:41

Gallo I, Ruiz B, Duran CMG (1983) Five to eight year follow-up of patients with the Hancock cardiac prosthesis. *J Thorac Cardiovasc Surg* 86:897

Gorlin R, Gorlin SG (1951) Hydraulic formula for calculation of the area of the stenotic mitral valve, other cardiac valves and central circulatory shunts. *Am Heart J* 41:1

Greves J, Rahimtoola SH, McAnulty JH, et al (1981) Preoperative criteria predictive of late survival following valve replacement for severe aortic regurgitation. *Am Heart J* 101:300

Hancock EW (1966) The ejection sound in aortic stenosis. *Am J Med* 40:569

Hancock EW, Fleming PR (1960) Aortic stenosis. *Q J Med* 29:209

Hansing CE, Rowe GG (1972) Tricuspid insufficiency: A study of hemodynamics and pathogenesis. *Circulation* 45:793

Harvey WP, Segal JP, Hufnagel CA (1957) Unusual clinical features associated with severe aortic insufficiency. *Ann Intern Med* 47:27

Henry WL, Bonow RO, Borer JS, et al (1973) Observations on the optimum time for operative intervention for aortic regurgitation. I. Evaluation of the results of aortic valve replacement in symptomatic patients. *Circulation* 31:696

Hildner FJ, Javier RP, Cohen LS, et al (1972) Myocardial dysfunction associated with valvular heart disease. *Am J Cardiol* 30:319

Holmes AM, Logan WF, Winterbottom T (1968) Transient systolic murmurs in angina pectoris. *Am Heart J* 76:680

Holmes JC, Fowler NO, Kaplan S (1968) Pulmonary valvular insufficiency. *Am J Med* 44:851

Hood WP Jr, Thompson WJ, Rackley CE, Rolett EL (1969) Comparison of calculations of left ventricular wall stress in man from thin-walled and thick-walled ellipsoidal models. *Circ Res* 24:575

Hungenholtz PG, Ryan TJ, Stein SW, Abelmann WH (1962) The spectrum of pure mitral stenosis: Hemodynamic studies in relation to clinical disability. *Am J Cardiol* 10:773

Hunt D, Baxley WA, Kennedy JW, et al (1973) Quantitative evaluation of cineaortography in the assessment of aortic regurgitation. *Am J Cardiol* 31:696

Hurst JW, Whitworth HB, O'Donoghue S, et al (1985): Heart disease due to ovarian carcinoid: Successful replacement of the pulmonary and tricuspid valves with porcine heterografts and removal of the tumor, in Hurst JW (ed): *Clinical Essays on The Heart*, vol. 5. New York, McGraw-Hill

Jeresaty RM (1973) Mitral valve prolapse–click syndrome. *Prog Cardiovasc Dis* 15:623

Kennedy JW, Twiss RD, Blackmon JR, Dodge HT (1968) Quantitative angiocardiography. III. Relationships of left ventricular pressure, volume and mass in aortic valve disease. *Circulation* 38:838

Kennedy JW, Yarnall SR, Murray JA, Figley MM (1970) Quantitative angiocardiography. IV. Relationships of left atrial and ventricular pressure and volume in mitral valve disease. *Circulation* 41:817

Killip T, Lukas DS (1957) Tricuspid stenosis: Physiologic criteria for diagnosis and hemodynamic abnormalities. *Circulation* 16:3

Kitchin A, Turner R (1964) Diagnosis and treatment of tricuspid stenosis. *Br Heart J* 26:354

Klatte EC, Tampas JP, Campbell JA, Lurie PR (1962) The roentgenographic manifestations of aortic stenosis and aortic valvular insufficiency. *Am J Roentgenol Radium Ther Nucl Med* 87:57

Klughaupt M, Flamm MD, Hancock EW, Harrison DC (1969) Nonrheumatic mitral insufficiency: Determination of operability and prognosis. *Circulation* 39:307

Konno S, Imai Y, Iida Y, et al (1975) A new method for prosthetic valve replacement in congenital aortic stenosis associated with hypoplasia of the aortic valve ring. *J Thorac Cardiovasc Surg* 70:909

Kostucki W, Vandenbossche JL, Friart A, Englert M (1986) Pulsed Doppler regurgitant flow patterns of normal valves. *Am J Cardiol* 58:309

Lee YC, Scherlis L, Singleton RT (1965) Mitral stenosis: Hemodynamic, electrocardiographic and vector cardiographic studies. *Am Heart J* 69:559

Lock JE, Khalilullah M, Shrivastavas S, Bahl V, Keane JF (1985) Percutaneous catheter commissurotomy in rheumatic mitral stenosis. *N Engl J Med* 313:1515

Manouguian S, Seybold–Epting W (1979) Patched enlargement of the aortic valve ring by extending the aortic incision into the anterior mitral leaflet: New operative techniques. *J Thorac Cardiovasc Surg* 78:402

Misbach GA, Turley K, Ullyot DJ, Ebert PA (1982) Left ventricular outflow enlargement by the Konno procedure. *J Thorac Cardiovasc Surg* 84:696

Newman GE, Bounous PW, Jones RH, Saliston DC (1979) Noninvasive assessment of hemodynamic effects of mitral valve commissurotomy during rest and exercise in patients with mitral stenosis. *J Thorac Cardiovasc Surg* 78:750

Nicks R, Cartmill T, Bernstein L (1970) Hypoplasia of the aortic root: The problem of aortic valve replacement. *Thorax* 25:339

Nutter DO, Wickliffe C, Gilbert CA, et al (1975) The pathophysiology of idiopathic mitral valve prolapse. *Circulation* 52:297

Osbakken M, Bove AA, Spann JF (1981) Left ventricular function in chronic aortic regurgitation with reference to end-systolic pressure, volume and stress relations. *Am J Cardiol* 47:193

Perloff JK, Harvey WP (1960) Clinical recognition of tricuspid stenosis. *Circulation* 22:346

Pomerance A (1972) Pathogenesis of aortic stenosis and its relation to age. *Br Heart J* 34:569

Pridie RB, Benham MB, Oakley CM (1971) Echocardiography of the mitral valve in aortic valve disease. *Br Heart J* 33:296

Rackley CE (1976) Quantitative evaluation of left ventricular function by radiographic techniques. *Circulation* 54:862

Rackley CE (1975) Value of ventriculography in cardiac function and diagnosis. *Cardiovasc Clin* 6:283

Rackley CE, Dear HD, Baxley WA, et al (1970) Left ventricular chamber volume, mass and function in severe coronary artery disease. *Circulation* 41:605

Rackley CE, Hood WP Jr (1976): Aortic valve disease, in Levine HJ (ed): *Clinical Cardiovascular Physiology*. New York, Grune & Stratton, p 493

Rackley CE, Hood WP Jr (1976): Quantitative angiographic evaluation and pathophysiologic mechanisms in valvular heart disease, in Sonnenblick EJ and Lesch M (eds): *Valvular Heart Disease*. New York, Grune & Stratton, Inc., p 109

Rackley CE, Russell RO Jr, Mantle JA, Rogers WJ (1979): Recognition of acute myocardial infarction, in Rackley CE and Russell RO Jr (eds): *Coronary Artery Disease: Recognition and Management*. Mount Kisco, N.Y., Futura Publishing Company, p 315

Radford DJ, Bloom KR, Izukawa T, et al (1976) Echocardiographic assessment of bicuspid aortic valves: Angiographic and pathological correlates. *Circulation* 53:80

Rapaport E (1975) Natural history of aortic and mitral valve disease. *Am J Cardiol* 35:221

Reigenbaum H (1976) *Echocardiography.* Philadelphia, Lea & Febiger

Ronan JA Jr, Steelman RB, de Leon AC Jr, et al (1971) The clinical diagnosis of acute severe mitral insufficiency. *Am J Cardiol* 27:284

Rotman M, Morris JJ, Behar VW, et al (1971) Aortic valve disease: Comparison of types and their medical and surgical management. *Am J Med* 51:241

Rowe JC, Bland EF, Spague HB, White PD (1960) The course of mitral stenosis without surgery: Ten and twenty year perspectives. *Ann Intern Med* 52:741

Salazar E, Levine HD (1962) Rheumatic tricuspid regurgitation: The clinical spectrum. *Am J Med* 33:111

Sandler H, Dodge HT, Hay RE, Rackley CE (1963) Quantitation of valvular insufficiency in man by angiocardiography. *Am Heart J* 65:501

Schwartz R, Meyerson RM, Lawrence LT, Nichols HT (1966) Mitral stenosis, massive pulmonary hemorrhage and emergency valve replacement. *N Engl J Med* 272:755

Selzer A, Cohn KE (1972) Natural history of mitral stenosis: A review. *Circulation* 45:878

Selzer A, Katayama F (1972) Mitral regurgitation: Clinical patterns, pathophysiology and natural history. *Medicine* 51:337

Selzer A, Naruse DY, York E, Kahn KA, Matthew HB (1962) Electrocardiographic findings in concentric and eccentric left ventricular hypertrophy. *Am Heart J* 63:320

Shelburne JC, Rubenstein D, Gorlin R (1969) A reappraisal of papillary muscle dysfunction. *Am J Med* 46:862

Slutsky R, Karliner J, Ricci D, et al (1979) Left ventricular volumes by gated equilibrium radionuclide angiography: A new method. *Circulation* 60:556

Stott DK, Marpole DG, Bristow JD, et al (1970) The role of left atrial transport in aortic and mitral stenosis. *Circulation* 41:1031

Szekely P, Turner R, Snaith L (1973) Pregnancy and the changing pattern of rheumatic heart disease. *Br Heart J* 35:1293

Whipple RL, Morris DC, Felner JM, Merrill AJ, Miller JI (1977) Echocardiographic manifestations of the flail aortic valve leaflet syndrome. *J Clin Ultrasound* 5:417

Winkle RA, Lopes MG, Fitzgerald JW, et al (1975) Arrhythmias in patients with mitral valve prolapse. *Circulation* 52:73

Wood P (1958) Aortic stenosis. *Am J Cardiol* 1:553

Wood P (1954) An appreciation of mitral stenosis. *Br Heart J* 1:1051

FIGURE CREDITS

FIG. 4.4 From Becker AE, Anderson RH: *Cardiac Pathology.* New York, Raven Press, 1983, p 4.18.

FIG. 4.7 Redrawn from Hurst JW, Goodson GC Jr: *Atlas of Spatial Vector Electrocardiography.* New York, The Blakiston Company, 1952, pp 88,89.

FIG. 4.8 From Felner JM: Echocardiography, Chapter 120 in Hurst JW (ed): *The Heart,* 6th ed. New York, McGraw-Hill, 1986, p 1960.

FIG. 4.9 From Pearlman AS: The use of Doppler in the evaluation of cardiac disorders and function, Chapter 122 in Hurst JW (ed): *The Heart,* 6th ed. New York, McGraw-Hil, 1986, p 1982.

FIG. 4.11 Redrawn from Grossman W: *Cardiac Catheterization and Angiography.* Philadelphia, Lea & Febiger, 1980, p 129.

FIG. 4.12 From Franch RH, Shuford WH: Selective angiocardiography, negative-contrast roentgenography, and radioisotope photoscanning, Chapter 9 in Hurst JW, Logue RB (eds): *The Heart,* 1st ed. New York, McGraw-Hill, 1964, p 202.

FIG. 4.13 From Rapaport E: Natural history of aortic and mitral valve disease. *Am J Cardiol* 35:221, 1975.

FIG. 4.17 From Wilcox BR, Anderson RH: *Surgical Anatomy of the Heart.* New York, Raven Press, 1985, p 3.2.

FIG. 4.21 Redrawn from Wilcox BR, Anderson RH: *Surgical Anatomy of the Heart.* New York, Raven Press, 1985, p 2.18.

FIG. 4.24 Adapted from Wilcox BR, Anderson RH: *Surgical Anatomy of the Heart.* New York, Raven Press, 1985, p 2.19.

FIG. 4.25 Adapted from Wilcox BR, Anderson RH: *Surgical Anatomy of the Heart.* New York, Raven Press, 1985, p 2.19.

FIG. 4.29 Redrawn from Henry WL, Bonow RO, Borer JS, et al: Evaluation of aortic valve replacement in patients with valvular aortic stenosis. *Circulation* 61:823, 1980; with permission of the American Heart Association, Inc.

FIG. 4.30 Redrawn from Krayenbuehl HP, Lurina M, Hess O, Rothlin M, Senning A: Pre- and postoperative left ventricular contractile function in patients with aortic valve disease. *Br Heart J* 41:204, 1979.

FIG. 4.31 From Becker AE, Anderson RH: *Cardiac Pathology.* New York, Raven Press, 1983, p 4.7.

FIG. 4.33 From Becker AE, Anderson RH: *Cardiac Pathology.* New York, Raven Press, 1983, p. 4.20.

FIG. 4.39 Redrawn from Silverman ME, Myerburg RJ, Hurst JW: *Electrocardiography: Basic Concepts and Clinical Application.* New York, McGraw-Hill, 1983, pp 202, 203.

FIG. 4.42 Redrawn from Rackley CE, Hood WP Jr, Wilcox BR, Peters RM: Quantitation of myocardial function in valvular heart disease, in Brewer III LA (ed): *Prosthetic Heart Valves.* Springfield, IL, Charles C Thomas, 1969.

FIG. 4.43 Redrawn from Iskandrian AS: *Nuclear Cardiac Imaging: Principles and Applications.* Philadelphia, FA Davis Company, 1987, p 433.

FIG. 4.45 From Becker AE, Anderson RH: *Cardiac Pathology.* New York, Raven Press, 1983, p 4.3.

FIG. 4.47 From Becker AE, Anderson RH: *Cardiac Pathology.* New York, Raven Press, 1983, p 8.2.

FIG. 4.49 Redrawn from Schlant RC: Altered cardiovascular function of rheumatic heart disease and other acquired valvular disease, Chapter 44 in Hurst JW (ed): *The Heart,* 2nd ed. New York, McGraw-Hill, 1970, p 754.

FIG. 4.50 From Becker AE, Anderson RH: *Cardiac Pathology.* New York, Raven Press, 1983, p 2.9.

FIG. 4.54 From Becker AE, Anderson RH: *Cardiac Pathology.* New York, Raven Press, 1983, p 2.11.

FIG. 4.58 From Felner JM: Echocardiography, Chapter 120 in Hurst JW (ed): *The Heart,* 6th ed. New York, McGraw-Hill, 1986, p 1959.

FIG. 4.59 From Pearlman AS: The use of Doppler in the evaluation of cardiac disorders and function, Chapter 122 in Hurst JW (ed): *The Heart,* 6th ed. New York, McGraw-Hill, 1986, p 1983.

FIG. 4.60 From Hall RJ, Cooley DA: Neoplastic heart disease, Chapter 61 in Hurst JW (ed): *The Heart,* 6th ed. New York, McGraw-Hill, 1986, p 1290.

FIG. 4.66 Adapted from Wilcox BR, Anderson RH: *Surgical Anatomy of the Heart.* New York, Raven Press, 1985, p 2.12.

FIG. 4.76 From Becker AE, Anderson RH: *Cardiac Pathology.* New York, Raven Press, 1983, p 3.26.

FIG. 4.78 Redrawn from Rackley CE: Value of ventriculography in cardiac function and diagnosis, in Fowler NO (ed): *Diagnostic Methods in Cardiology.* Philadelphia, FA Davis Company, 1975, p 283.

FIG. 4.82 From Felner JM: (1986) Echocardiography, Chapter 120 in Hurst JW (ed): *The Heart,* 6th ed. New York, McGraw-Hill, 1986, p 1959.

FIG. 4.83 From Pearlman AS: The use of Doppler in the evaluation of cardiac disorders and function, Chapter 122 in Hurst JW (ed): *The Heart,* 6th ed. New York, McGraw-Hill, 1986, p 1984.

FIG. 4.85 Redrawn from Rackley CE, Dear HD, Baxley WA, Jones WB, Dodge HT: Left ventricular chamber volume, mass and function in severe coronary artery disease. *Circulation* 41:605, 1970; with permission of the American Heart Association, Inc.

FIG. 4.87 From Iskandrian AS: *Nuclear Cardiac Imaging: Principles and Applications.* Philadelphia, FA Davis Company, 1987, p 453.

FIG. 4.88 From Iskandrian AS: *Nuclear Cardiac Imaging: Principles and Applications.* Philadelphia, FA Davis Company, 1987, p 459.

FIG. 4.89 Redrawn from Starr A, Grunkemeier G, Lambert L, Okies JE, Thomas D: Mitral valve replacement: a 10-year followup of non-cloth vs. cloth-covered caged-ball prostheses. *Circulation* 54:111–147, 1976; with permission of the American Heart Association, Inc.

FIG. 4.91 From Becker AE, Anderson RH: *Cardiac Pathology.* New York, Raven Press, 1983, p 4.23.

FIG. 4.94 From Lintermans JP: *Two-Dimensional Echocardiography in Infants and Children.* Dordrecht, The Netherlands, Martinus Nijhoff, 1986, p 103.

FIG. 4.95 From Iskandrian AS: *Nuclear Cardiac Imaging: Principles and Applications.* Philadelphia, FA Davis Company, 1987, p 152.

FIG. 4.97 From Wilcox BR, Anderson RH: *Surgical Anatomy of the Heart.* New York, Raven Press, 1985, p 3.6.

FIG. 4.98 From Wilcox BR, Anderson RH: *Surgical Anatomy of the Heart.* New York, Raven Press, 1985, p 2.5.

FIG. 4.100 Adapted from Wilcox BR, Anderson RH: *Surgical Anatomy of the Heart.* New York, Raven Press, 1985, p 2.10.

FIG. 4.101 From Wilcox BR, Anderson RH: *Surgical Anatomy of the Heart.* New York, Raven Press, 1985, p 3.3.

FIG. 4.103 From Becker AE, Anderson RH: *Cardiac Pathology.* New York, Raven Press, 1983, p 4.16.

FIG. 4.106B From Becker AE, Anderson RH: *Cardiac Pathology.* New York, Raven Press, 1983, p 4.7.

5
MYOCARDIAL DISEASE

MYOCARDITIS

J. Willis Hurst, MD
Nanette K. Wenger, MD
Walter H. Abelmann, MD
Anton E. Becker, MD

CARDIOMYOPATHY

J. Willis Hurst, MD
Nanette K. Wenger, MD
John F. Goodwin, MD
Anton E. Becker, MD
Benson R. Wilcox, MD

MYOCARDITIS*
ETIOLOGY AND PATHOLOGY

Myocarditis is an inflammatory response within the myocardium due to a variety of causes. Among the most common are infectious diseases caused by viral, bacterial, mycotic, rickettsial, or parasitic organisms (Lansdown, 1978; Walsh et al, 1980; Kean and Breslau, 1964). Infectious myocarditis is a common complication in patients who are immunocompromised due to disease or immunosuppressive drugs.

---

*Abstracted with permission of the authors and publisher from Wenger NK, Abelmann WH, Roberts WC: Myocarditis, Chapter 57, pp 1158–1180, in Hurst JW (ed): *The Heart*, 6th ed. New York, McGraw-Hill, 1986. Figures and tables reproduced in this section from the above chapter or other sources are also reprinted with permission of the authors and publishers. For the full bibliographic citations of the sources of figures and tables other than the above chapter, see Figure Credits at the end of this chapter.

In the United States and Europe virus infections, such as coxsackievirus type B (especially strains B1–5 and A4), are responsible for most cases of myocarditis (Fig. 5.1) (Bell and Grist, 1971). In South America the most common cause of myocarditis is *Trypanosoma cruzi*, which is responsible for Chagas' disease (Puigbo et al, 1966). In New Zealand, Australia, and Uruguay, where sheep are raised in abundance, echinococcosis is often seen (Murphy et al, 1971). Trichinosis caused by eating uncooked pork is a serious but rare cause of myocarditis.

Bacterial myocarditis is most often due to staphylococci, streptococci, pneumococci, or meningococci. A suppurative response prevails, and microabscesses are common (Fig. 5.2). Tuberculosis in some parts of the world is still a common cause of myocarditis (Fig. 5.3), often complicated further by hemorrhagic pericarditis. Other causes of bacterial myocarditis, such as syphilis, are rare (Table 5.1).

Drug-induced myocarditis may result from direct toxic effect on the myocardium or from an immune reaction, termed allergic or hyper-

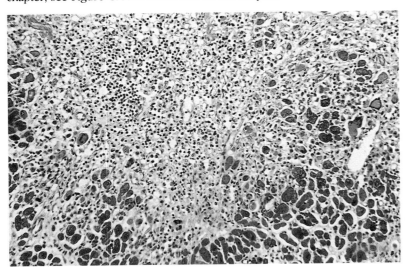

FIG. 5.1 *In this histologic section of the myocardium in a case of viral myocarditis extensive loss of myocytes is accompanied by massive infiltration of inflammatory cells, mainly lymphocytes. (Reproduced with permission of the authors and publisher; see Figure Credits)*

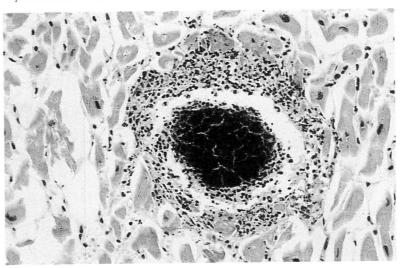

FIG. 5.2 *Histologic section of myocardium shows a microabscess containing a colony of staphylococci due to sepsis. (Reproduced with permission of the authors and publisher; see Figure Credits)*

FIG. 5.3 *Histologic section of myocardium shows a granulomatous inflammation with multinucleated giant cells in a case of tuberculous myocarditis. (Reproduced with permission of the authors and publisher; see Figure Credits)*

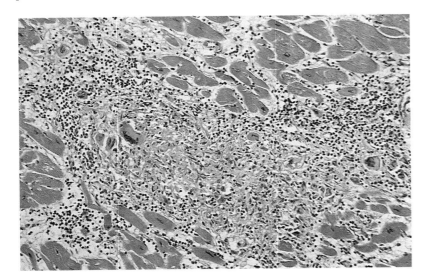

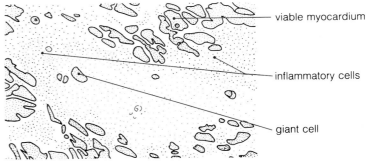

viable myocardium

inflammatory cells

giant cell

Table 5.1 Rarer Forms of Myocarditis

| ETIOLOGY | DISTINCTIVE FEATURES | | | | |
	PHYSICAL EXAMINATION	LABORATORY	MORPHOLOGIC MANIFESTATIONS	SPECIFIC THERAPY*	REFERENCE
BACTERIAL					
Diphtheria	(see discussion in *The Heart*, 6th ed, p 1168)				
Tuberculosis	Arrhythmias	Arrhythmias	Tubercles with caseation	Isoniazid, plus rifampin, plus ethambutol or streptomycin	Claiborne, *Am J Cardiol* 33:920, 1974
Typhoid fever (*Salmonella*)	Early: peripheral circulatory collapse; ? endotoxin effect Late: congestive heart failure	—	Coronary arteritis Abscesses	Chloramphenicol Vasopressor drugs	Diem, *Am J Trop Med Hyg* 23:218 1974
Scarlet fever Rheumatic fever	—	—	Valve lesions Aschoff bodies	Penicillin G Salicylates Corticosteroid hormones	Ewy, *Am Heart J* 78:259, 1969
Meningococcemia	Circulatory collapse	Disseminated intravascular coagulation	Petechiae	Penicillin Isoproterenol	Denmark, *Arch Intern Med* 127:238, 1971
Infective endocarditis	—	—	Valve vegetations Microabscesses	Depends on specific etiology	Roberts, *Cardiovasc Med* 3:699, 1978
Staphylococcal Pneumococcal Gonococcal infection	—	—	Abscesses Valve vegetations	Antistaphylococcal penicillin (staph) Penicillin G (pneumo) Penicillin G (gono)	—
Clostridial infection	—	—	Air cysts with organisms in wall	Penicillin G	Roberts, *Am Heart J* 74:482, 1967
Psittacosis (*Chlamydia psittaci*)	—	—	Psittacosis inclusion bodies in plasma cells	Tetracycline	Sutton, *Am Heart J* 81:597, 1971
Chlamydia trachomatis	Heart failure	—	—	Tetracycline, erythromycin	Grayston, *JAMA* 246:2823, 1981
Brucellosis	—	—	—	Tetracycline plus streptomycin	Buczynska-Hencner, *Pol Tyg Lek* 20:761, 1966
Actinomycosis	—	—	Abscesses with actinomycotic granules	Penicillin G or tetracycline	Edwards, *Am J Dis Child* 41:1419, 1931
Tetanus	—	—	Nerve cell degeneration	Penicillin G Tetanus antitoxin Propranolol	Murphy, *Med J Aust* 2:542, 1970
Tularemia	—	—	—	Streptomycin	—
Melioidosis	Mimic AMI	Mimic AMI	Abscesses	Tetracycline plus streptomycin	Baumann, *Ann Intern Med* 67:836, 1967
Legionnaires' disease	Heart failure	—	—	Erythromycin	Gross, *Chest* 79:232, 1981
SPIROCHETAL					
Syphilis	Arrhythmias, heart block Conduction abnormalities		Gumma	Penicillin G	Boss, *Ann Intern Med* 55:824, 1961
Leptospirosis	Valve "pseudostenosis" Arrhythmias	Arrhythmias	Focal hemorrhage Edema Necrosis	Penicillin G Tetracycline	Nusynowitz, *Hawaii Med J* 23:41, 1963

Table 5.1 Rarer Forms of Myocarditis

ETIOLOGY	DISTINCTIVE FEATURES			SPECIFIC THERAPY*	REFERENCE
	PHYSICAL EXAMINATION	LABORATORY	MORPHOLOGIC MANIFESTATIONS		
Relapsing fever	Vasoconstriction Hypotension Heart failure Conduction abnormalities, arrhythmias	Conduction abnormalities, arrhythmias	—	Tetracycline Penicillin	Judge, *Arch Pathol* 97:136, 1974
Lyme disease	—	Conduction abnormalities Complete heart block	—	Penicillin Tetracycline ± Prednisone	Steere, *Ann Intern Med* 93:8, 1980

RICKETTSIAL

ETIOLOGY	PHYSICAL EXAMINATION	LABORATORY	MORPHOLOGIC MANIFESTATIONS	SPECIFIC THERAPY*	REFERENCE
Typhus	—	—	Vasculitis	Tetracycline or chloramphenicol	Woodward, *Ann Intern Med* 53:1130, 1960
Rocky Mountain spotted fever	Hypovolemia, hypotension Peripheral vascular collapse	—	Vasculitis	Colloid Tetracycline or chloramphenicol	Walker, *Arch Pathol Lab Med* 104:171, 1980
Q fever	—	—	—	Tetracycline	Barraclough, *Br Med J* 2:423, 1975

VIRAL

ETIOLOGY	PHYSICAL EXAMINATION	LABORATORY	MORPHOLOGIC MANIFESTATIONS	SPECIFIC THERAPY*	REFERENCE
Coxsackie B	(see discussion in *The Heart*, 6th ed, p 1169)				—
Echovirus	(see discussion in *The Heart*, 6th ed, p 1169)				
Poliomyelitis	Pulmonary edema Vascular collapse	—	—	Tracheostomy Oxygen Vasopressor drugs Pacemaker ? Amantadine for influenza A	Trimbos, *Folia Med Neerl* 1963, p. 49
Influenza	Peripheral circulatory failure Arrhythmias, complete heart block	Arrythmias, complete heart block	Myofiber necrosis		Verel, *Am Heart J* 92:290, 1976
Mumps	—	Complete heart block	—	—	Arita, *Br Heart J* 46:342, 1981
Infectious mononucleosis (virus Epstein-Barr)	—	—	Abnormal perivascular lymphocytes	Corticosteroid hormones	Hudgins, *JAMA* 235:2626, 1976
Viral hepatitis	—	—	—	—	Bell, *JAMA* 218:387, 1971
Rubella	Congestive heart failure	ECG: mimic AMI	Extensive myocardial vacuolation necrosis	—	Ainger, *Cardiol Dig* 2:21, 1967
Rubeola	Pericarditis Arrhythmias	—	—	—	Guistra, *AMA J Dis Child* 79:487, 1950
Rabies	—	—	—	Vaccine	Roux, *Coeur Med Intern* 15:37, 1976
Varicella	—	Bundle branch block Arrhythmia	Eosinophilic intranuclear inclusion bodies	—	Fiddler, *Br Heart J* 39:1150, 1977
Mycoplasma pneumoniae	Myalgia	ECG: mimic AMI Arrhythmias	—	Erythromycin	Ponka, *Acta Med Scand* 206:77, 1979
Lymphocytic choriomeningitis	—	—	—	—	Thiede, *Arch Intern Med* 109:104, 1962
Viral encephalitis	—	—	—	—	Ungar, *Am J Clin Pathol* 18:48, 1948

Table 5.1 Rarer Forms of Myocarditis

ETIOLOGY	DISTINCTIVE FEATURES			SPECIFIC THERAPY*	REFERENCE
	PHYSICAL EXAMINATION	LABORATORY	MORPHOLOGIC MANIFESTATIONS		
Herpes simplex	—	—	—	? Adenine arabinoside	Bell, *Am Heart J* 74:309, 1967
Cytomegalovirus	—	—	Intranuclear inclusion bodies	—	Wilson, *Br Heart J* 34:865, 1972
Variola	—	—	—	—	
Herpes zoster	—	—	—	? Acyclovir	—
Adenovirus infection	—	—	—	—	Henson, *Am J Dis Child* 121:334, 1971
Arbovirus infection	Arrhythmias Heart failure	Arrhythmias	—	—	Obeyesekere, *Am Heart J* 85:186, 1973
Respiratory syncytial virus	—	—	—	—	Giles, *JAMA* 236:1128, 1976
Viral hemorrhagic fever	Shock	—	Myocardial hemorrhage	—	Milei, *Am Heart J* 104:1385, 1982

MYCOTIC

ETIOLOGY	PHYSICAL EXAMINATION	LABORATORY	MORPHOLOGIC MANIFESTATIONS	SPECIFIC THERAPY*	REFERENCE
Blastomycosis	—	—	Tubercle with caseation and giant cells	Amphotericin B	Baker, *Am J Pathol* 13:139, 1937
Candidiasis	Debilitated or immunosuppressed host	ECG: Bundle branch block, AV block, mimic AMI	Multiple abscesses with pseudohyphae, yeast forms	Amphotericin B	Franklin, *Am J Cardiol* 38:924, 1976
Aspergillosis	Debilitated or immunosuppressed host	—	Granulomas or microabscesses; mycelial and filamentous forms	Amphotericin B	Williams, *Am J Clin Pathol* 61:247, 1974
Histoplasmosis	—	—	Granulomas *H. capsulatum* in phagocytes	Amphotericin B	Owen, *Am J Med* 32:552, 1962
Sporotrichosis	—	—		Amphotericin B Potassium iodide	Collins, *Arch Dermatol* 56:523, 1947
Coccidioidomycosis	—	—	Miliary granulomas with *C. immitis* spherules	Amphotericin B	Reingold, *Am J Clin Pathol* 20:1044, 1950
Cryptococcosis	—	—	*C. neoformans* in granulomas	Amphotericin B plus 5-fluoro-cytosine	Jones, *Br Heart J* 27:462, 1965
Mucormycosis	Debilitated or immunosuppressed host	—	Septic thromboses	Amphotericin B	Virmani, *Am J Clin Path* 78:42, 1982

PROTOZOAL

ETIOLOGY	PHYSICAL EXAMINATION	LABORATORY	MORPHOLOGIC MANIFESTATIONS	SPECIFIC THERAPY*	REFERENCE
Chagas' disease	(see discussion in *The Heart*, 6th ed, pp 1169–1170)				
Sleeping sickness (trypanosomiasis)	—	Frequent ECG abnormalities and arrhythmias	—	Early infection: *T. gambiense*– Pentamidine *T. rhodesiense*– Suramin Late infection: Melarsoprol	Poltera, *Br Heart J* 38:827, 1976
Toxoplasmosis	—	Arrhythmias	Parasitized myofiber→ rupture	Pyrimethamine plus trisulfa-pyrimidines	Leak, *Am J Cardiol* 43:841, 1979

Table 5.1 Rarer Forms of Myocarditis

ETIOLOGY	DISTINCTIVE FEATURES				REFERENCE
	PHYSICAL EXAMINATION	LABORATORY	MORPHOLOGIC MANIFESTATIONS	SPECIFIC THERAPY*	
Malaria	Peripheral circulatory collapse Angina	—	Parasitized RBC Myocardial vascular occlusion	Chloroquine unless resistant falciparum–then quinine, pyrimethamine and sulfonamides	Herrera, *Arch Inst Cardiol Mex* 30:26, 1960
Leishmaniasis	—	—	Clasmatocytes with Leishman-Donovan bodies	Stibogluconate	Benhamou, *Arch Mal Coeur* 31:81, 1938
Balantidiasis	—	—	—	Tetracycline	Sidorov, *Ann Anat Pathol* 12:711, 1935
Sarcosporidiosis	—	—	Sarcocysts in myofiber with basophilic bodies	—	Aral, *J Mt Sinai Hosp* 15:367, 1949
Amebiasis	—	—	Microabscesses	Metronidazole	Markowitz, *Am J Clin Pathol* 62:619, 1974
HELMINTHIC					
Trichinosis	(see discussion in *The Heart*, 6th ed, pp 1170, 1172)				—
Echinococcosis	(see discussion in *The Heart*, 6th ed, p 1172)				—
Schistosomiasis	Cor pulmonale	—	Microscopic pseudotubercle or granuloma	*S. japonicum:* praziquantel *S. haematobium* and *S. mansoni:* niridazole, praziquantel	Lima, *Rev Inst Med Trop São Paulo*, 11:290, 1969
Ascariasis	—	—	—	Mebendazole Pyrantel pamoate	Ferreira, *Rev Med Aeroaut* 15:35, 1963
Heterophydiasis	—	—	—	Tetrachloro-ethylene	Africa, *Acta Med Philippina*, Monograph Series, no. 1, 118, 1940
Filariasis	Congestive heart failure	Eosinophilia	Pericardial effusion Restrictive endocarditis	Corticosteroid hormones Diethylcarbamazine	Tatibouet, *Semaine Hop Paris* 37:3418, 1961
Paragonimiasis	—	—	—	Bithional Praziquantel	Kean, *Parasites of the Human Heart*. New York, Grune & Stratton, 1964, p 104
Strongyloidiasis	—	—	—	Thiabendazole	Kyle, *Ann Intern Med* 29:1014, 1948
Cysticercosis	—	—	Myocardial scolex-containing cysts	—	Ibarra-Perez, *South Med J* 65:484, 1972
Visceral larva migrans	—	—	Allergic granulomatosis	Corticosteroid hormones Thiabendazole	Becroft, *NZ Med J* 63:729, 1964

(Table 57-2, *The Heart*, 6th ed, pp. 1173–1176)

*With appreciation to Jonas A Shulman, MD, Professor of Medicine (Infectious Diseases), Emory University School of Medicine, for review of drug therapy.

Notes: (—) indicates no distinctive physical findings, laboratory data, or morphological manifestations other than heart failure and nonspecific cardiac enlargement; or no specific therapy.

PART II: DISEASES OF THE HEART

sensitivity myocarditis (Fig. 5.4). Drug-induced toxic myocarditis is usually dose-dependent and cumulative. Drugs that cause myocarditis are manifold; well-known examples are emetine, barbiturates, theophylline, the herbicide paraquat, amphetamines, and a number of immunosuppressive agents. Allergic or hypersensitivity myocarditis is not dose-dependent; it usually regresses when administration of the drug is stopped. Sulfonamides are the best-known drugs in this category, but others, such as penicillin, streptomycin, tetracycline, and phenylbutazone, have been reported to cause myocarditis.

Autoimmune myocarditis is also reported in patients with rheumatic fever, systemic lupus erythematosus, and rheumatoid arthritis. Active myocarditis under these circumstances is usually of a temporary nature, but occasionally it may have a profound effect on the clinical profile of the autoimmune disease. In years past it was not uncommon for children to die as a result of rheumatic myocarditis. Necrotizing arteritis of coronary arteries in infancy, known as Kawasaki's disease (mucocutaneous lymph node syndrome), may belong to this category; in the acute stage of the disease it is often accompanied by myocarditis (Fig. 5.5).

Finally, particular types of myocarditis occur that cannot be related to a known etiology. These include granulomatous myocarditis, giant cell myocarditis (Fig. 5.6), and Fiedler's myocarditis. Myocarditis may also coexist with pericarditis (Bell and Grist, 1971).

ABNORMAL PHYSIOLOGY

Myocardial cells are damaged by the invading organisms. In addition evidence suggests that certain organisms activate the autoimmune system; this in turn damages the heart muscle. Myocarditis due to rheumatic fever is an example of this type of myocardial damage. Infections such as diphtheria have a special affinity for the conduction system (Lerner et al, 1975; Burch and Giles, 1972).

Both ventricles are usually involved. The right and the left ventricular diastolic volumes and pressures may increase; myocardial contractility may diminish. Atrial and ventricular tachycardia may occur, further compromising cardiac function. Complete heart block and shock may occur with diphtheria; right bundle branch block is common in patients with Chagas' disease.

CLINICAL MANIFESTATIONS

No effort is made here to characterize the unique features of all causes of myocarditis. As indicated earlier, specific causes are common to certain geographic areas. In addition myocarditis due to rheumatic fever and myocarditis due to diphtheria have different clinical manifestations. These examples indicate that the clinical setting and the systemic manifestations of a large number of clinical conditions due to infectious agents vary considerably. The purpose of this discussion is to emphasize the damage that is done to the heart muscle rather

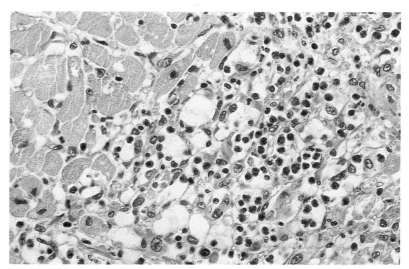

FIG. 5.4 *Histologic section of myocardium reveals a dense infiltration of inflammatory cells, predominately eosinophilic cells, suggesting hypersensitivity myocarditis. (Reproduced with permission of the authors and publisher; see Figure Credits).*

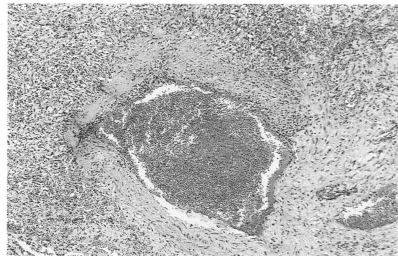

FIG. 5.5 *Histologic section of a coronary artery from a patient with Kawasaki's disease demonstrates an extensive inflammatory cellular infiltrate affecting the arterial wall and spreading onto adjacent tissues.*

FIG. 5.6 *Histologic section of myocardium from a patient with idiopathic giant cell myocarditis shows inflammatory foci containing giant cells.*

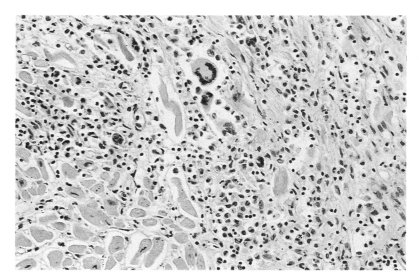

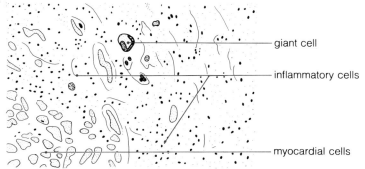

than to describe the entire clinical picture related to specific etiologies. The clinical clues used to recognize myocarditis are similar regardless of the etiology.

SYMPTOMS

The individual may have no complaints relative to the heart if there is minimal involvement of the heart in the overall process of infection. Severe involvement of the heart may produce cardiac failure, which in turn may lead to fatigue, dyspnea, and palpitations. The chest pain of pericarditis may be associated with myocarditis. Syncope and sudden death may occur (Wentworth et al, 1979).

PHYSICAL EXAMINATION

Fever and tachycardia are usually present; the latter is often out of proportion to the fever. Bradycardia may be present, usually due to an atrioventricular conduction disturbance.

The heart may be enlarged, and hypotension may be present. Neck vein abnormalities and pulsus alternans are often detected. The apex impulse may be diffuse; atrial and ventricular gallop sounds are commonly heard. The first heart sound may be faint, and new murmurs of mitral and tricuspid regurgitation are sometimes present (Woodward et al, 1967). A pericardial rub may be heard, and the liver may be enlarged.

Atrial and ventricular arrhythmias and conduction abnormalities may account for the abnormal rhythm found in patients on physical examination.

LABORATORY STUDIES

CHEST RADIOGRAPHY. The chest film may show enlargement of the left and the right ventricles and evidence of heart failure.

ELECTROCARDIOGRAPHY. The electrocardiogram (ECG) may show low voltage of the QRS complexes, nonspecific ST-T wave abnormalities, sinus and atrial tachycardia, conduction defects including right or left bundle branch block, atrioventricular block of varying degrees, and, on rare occasion, signs of acute infarction.

ECHOCARDIOGRAPHY. This technique is used to identify ventricular chamber size, wall-motion abnormalities, and pericardial effusion. It is especially useful in following the progress of patients with myocarditis (Fig. 5.7) (Nieminen et al, 1984).

CARDIAC CATHETERIZATION. Cardiac catheterization is not performed in patients who have diagnostic evidence of myocarditis. On rare occasion it may be needed to exclude certain other diseases, such as coronary artery disease or valvar heart disease.

RADIONUCLIDE STUDIES. Ventricular function and wall-motion abnormalities can be identified with radionuclide ventriculography. Patients with myocarditis may show global myocardial dysfunction or regional wall-motion abnormalities. A gallium scan showing considerable uptake in the myocardium is believed to indicate an active inflammatory process; in certain cases it suggests that therapy with corticosteroids may be helpful (O'Connell et al, 1984).

ENDOMYOCARDIAL BIOPSY. Endomyocardial biopsy of the right or the left ventricle can be safely performed (Fig. 5.8); at times a specific etiology may be discovered. When the biopsy reveals considerable inflammation, the condition may respond more readily to corticosteroid medication (Edwards et al, 1982; Kereiakes and Parmley, 1984).

ROUTINE AND SPECIAL LABORATORY TESTS. Routine laboratory tests may reveal eosinophilia, elevated sedimentation rates, and elevated creatine kinase levels. Tests for specific infectious agents, such as acute and convalescent antibody titers, are useful, but the results are often negative.

NATURAL HISTORY

Many patients with mild myocarditis recover completely. However, myocarditis is a serious condition, and, depending on its etiology, the recovery rate is variable. Many patients either die from heart failure or cardiac arrhythmia, or develop chronic dilated cardiomyopathy. A few patients with severe myocarditis recover and exhibit no cardiac dysfunction. One problem in establishing the natural history of myocarditis is the inability to determine the cause of dilated cardiomyopathy.

TREATMENT

The patient with myocarditis should be placed at rest, restricted to a bed or a chair, with minimal activity. Heart failure should be treated with diuretics and digitalis, although the latter is not obviously beneficial. Some patients with sinus or atrial tachycardia may profit from

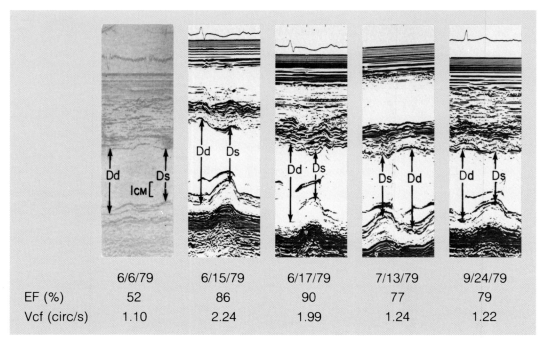

	6/6/79	6/15/79	6/17/79	7/13/79	9/24/79
EF (%)	52	86	90	77	79
Vcf (circ/s)	1.10	2.24	1.99	1.24	1.22

FIG. 5.7 *Serial M-mode echocardiograms were obtained from a 34-year-old male with acute viral myocarditis who presented with cardiogenic shock. The first study shows hypokinesis of the posterior wall of the left ventricle. Nine days later movement of the posterior wall is normal [Dd, left ventricular end-diastolic diameter; Ds, left ventricular end-systolic diameter; EF (%), ejection fraction percentage (normal, 55 %); Vcf, mean velocity of circumferential fiber shortening (normal, 1.29 ± 0.23 circ/s)]. (Fig. 57-9, The Heart, 6th ed, p 1167)*

the use of beta-blockers, such as propranolol, when the beneficial effect on heart rhythm outweighs the harmful effect on contractility.

Corticosteroid therapy is contraindicated in the early phase of viral myocarditis, but it may be beneficial in patients who show considerable myocardial inflammation on endomyocardial biopsy. Rheumatic myocarditis is often treated with corticosteroids; myocardial biopsy is not indicated. Therapy for specific types of myocarditis is listed in Table 5.1.

CARDIOMYOPATHY*
DILATED CARDIOMYOPATHY
Etiology and Pathology

Dilated cardiomyopathy is the most common type of myocardial disease. This condition is seen in patients who abuse alcohol over long periods of time (see Chapter 18). It may also be seen in hypertensive

---

*Abstracted with permission of the authors and publisher from Wenger NK, Goodwin JF, Roberts WC: Cardiomyopathy and myocardial involvement in systemic disease, Chapter 58, pp 1181–1248, in Hurst JW (ed): *The Heart*, 6th ed. New York, McGraw-Hill, 1986. Figures in this section from the above chapter or other sources are also reprinted with permission of the authors and publishers. For the full bibliographic citations of the sources of figures other than the above chapter, see Figure Credits at the end of this chapter.

patients, during the latter part of pregnancy or in the pueperium, and following viral myocarditis. It may be caused by toxic effects of drugs, such as daunorubicin and cobalt, or by selenium deficiency. The cause of dilated cardiomyopathy is usually difficult or impossible to establish in an individual patient. It is likely that many different causes are responsible, eventually leading to irreversible myocardial damage and, as a final common pathway, becoming clinically manifest as *idiopathic* (or more accurately identified as *cryptogenic) dilated cardiomyopathy*.

Ischemic cardiomyopathy due to atherosclerotic coronary artery disease may simulate other types of cardiomyopathy. Some physicians object to this term since the primary problem is coronary disease. This is true because all types of dilated cardiomyopathy may have angina and electrocardiographic abnormalities simulating infarction of the myocardium and because ischemic cardiomyopathy due to coronary atherosclerosis may not be associated with angina or other signs of infarction.

The pathology of dilated cardiomyopathy is characterized by gross dilation of the chambers of the heart, accompanied by marked hypertrophy (Fig. 5.9). Interstitial myocardial fibrosis is usually present (Fig. 5.10). In a number of cases the endocardium is thickened and often shows hyperplasia of smooth muscle cells; lymphocytes may be recognized. This finding is often interpreted as an indication that the disease is initiated by myocarditis, which in its end stage results in dilated cardiomyopathy.

FIG. 5.8. *This endomyocardial biopsy contains a lymphocytic inflammatory infiltrate indicative of active myocarditis.*

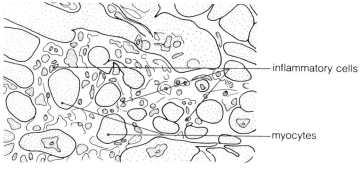

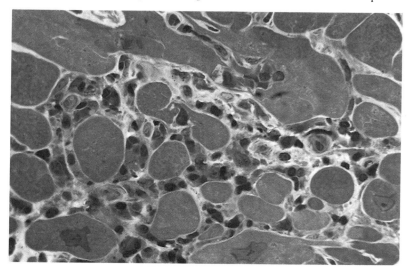

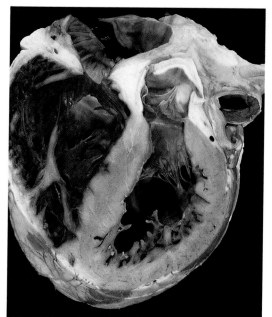

FIG. 5.9 *Cross-section through a heart shows biventricular chamber dilation with wall hypertrophy in dilated congestive cardiomyopathy.*

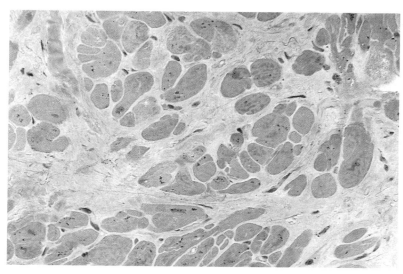

FIG. 5.10 *In a case of dilated congestive cardiomyopathy a histologic section shows hypertrophied myocytes amid dense fibrosis. There is no evidence of inflammatory infiltrate.*

Abnormal Physiology

During the early stages of the condition, stroke volume is reduced. Cardiac output is maintained at a normal level by an increase in heart rate. While this type of compensation is adequate at rest, it may not be adequate with exercise, when there may be an increase in left ventricular end-diastolic pressure.

Later in the course of the disease the stroke output and the minute output become decreased. Eventually, as dictated by Laplace's law (see Fig. 2.7), dilation becomes increasingly harmful. Myocardial wall tension and pressure increase, as do the oxygen demand and the metabolic needs of the myocardium. There is also a decreased rate of myocardial fiber shortening and a decrease in the maximal rate of rise of pressure (max dP/dT) and in the velocity of ejection. The systolic and the diastolic volumes of the ventricles are increased and the ejection fraction is decreased, while the left ventricular end-diastolic pressure is increased (Kristinsson, 1969). The pulmonary venous pressure rises, producing dyspnea. The pulmonary arterial pressure and the pulmonary vascular resistance are often slightly increased. The decrease in cardiac output sets in motion the compensatory mechanisms that, in an effort to correct the fault, produce congestive heart failure. Angina pectoris due to myocardial ischemia may occur; it is thought to be due to an increase in coronary arterial resistance together with the exercise-precipitated elevation in left ventricular end-diastolic volume and pressure (Opherk et al, 1983).

Clinical Manifestations
SYMPTOMS

The condition is more commonly seen in adult males. The patient may be asymptomatic when first seen. Eventually dyspnea on effort becomes apparent, and the symptoms of advanced heart failure with paroxysmal nocturnal dyspnea and pulmonary edema may develop. The patient may have arrhythmias and chest pain consistent with angina pectoris. Serious arrhythmias are commonly linked to the severity of hemodynamic disturbance.

PHYSICAL EXAMINATION

There may be signs of heart failure, but the systemic blood pressure is usually normal or elevated. Pulsus alternans may be present, and the neck veins are usually distended. A systolic jugular pulsation may be detected in the internal jugular veins, signifying tricuspid regurgitation. The apex impulse is usually larger than normal. Atrial and ventricular diastolic gallop sounds are usually heard; the systolic murmurs of mitral and tricuspid regurgitation may be detected. There may be reversed splitting of the second sound when left bundle branch block is present.

LABORATORY STUDIES

CHEST RADIOGRAPHY. The chest film reveals cardiac enlargement due to dilation of the ventricles and the atria. Signs of heart failure are frequently present.

ELECTROCARDIOGRAPHY. The ECG may show nonspecific ST-T wave changes, left ventricular hypertrophy, low voltage, left bundle branch block (common), atrial abnormalities, atrial arrhythmias, ventricular arrhythmias, atrioventricular conduction defects, and abnormal Q waves suggesting myocardial infarction (Gau et al, 1972).

Ambulatory Electrocardiography. Patients with rhythm disturbances may be studied with ambulatory electrocardiography (Holter monitoring).

ECHOCARDIOGRAPHY. The echocardiogram reveals dilation of both ventricles and decreased contractility of the myocardium, especially the posterior free wall of the left ventricle, with paradoxical movement of the septum (Fig. 5.11). The free wall and septal thickness are usually normal. Left ventricular thrombi may be seen in the cross-sectional echocardiogram (DeMaria et al, 1980). Echocardiography cannot be used reliably to separate nonischemic cardiomyopathy from ischemic cardiomyopathy.

CARDIAC CATHETERIZATION. Cardiac catheterization reveals an elevated left ventricular diastolic pressure. Angiography shows dilation of the left and the right ventricles, decreased myocardial contractility, decreased ejection fraction, slight mitral regurgitation, and either normal coronary arteries, nonobstructive coronary artery disease, or severe obstructive coronary disease. The latter finding usually signifies the presence of ischemic cardiomyopathy, although dilated

FIG. 5.11 *A cross-sectional echocardiogram in the long-axis view was recorded during systole in a 35-year-old male with dilated cardiomyopathy. The systolic dimension of the left ventricle was 7.4 cm, and the diastolic dimension was 8.6 cm. (Courtesy of Stephen D. Clements, Jr, MD, Atlanta, Georgia)*

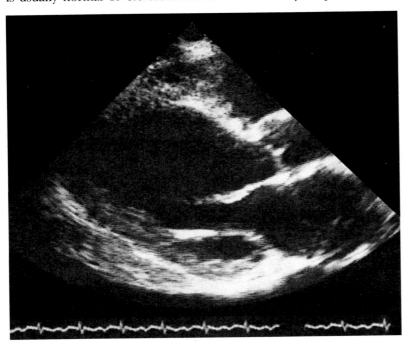

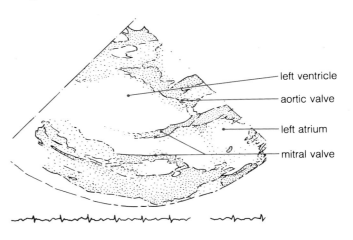

left ventricle
aortic valve
left atrium
mitral valve

cardiomyopathy may be accompanied by unrelated coronary atherosclerosis.

RADIONUCLIDE STUDIES. Nuclear ventriculography reveals enlargement of both ventricles and global hypokinesis. The ejection fraction may be as low as 10%–15%. This test may be useful in following the progress of a patient with cardiomyopathy (Goldman et al, 1980). However, this procedure cannot reliably separate coronary disease from cardiomyopathy (Dunn et al, 1982).

Thallium scanning may reveal areas of poor perfusion. This test does not always separate nonischemic from ischemic cardiomyopathy.

ENDOMYOCARDIAL BIOPSY. Whereas endomyocardial biopsy was formerly used only for research purposes, it is now commonly used in patients who may be candidates for transplantation. Myocarditis may be found, which may dictate certain treatment, or the biopsy may give evidence of a systemic disease that would make cardiac transplantation inadvisable. The procedure is also used to detect the early signs of cardiac rejection in patients who have had a heart transplant.

Treatment

The treatment of dilated cardiomyopathy is unsatisfactory. Medical treatment consists of the management of heart failure with diuretics, digitalis, and drugs that alter the preload and the afterload. Cardiac arrhythmias are commonly present and they are often resistant to

therapy (Chatterjee, 1982). The activity of the patient should be curtailed.

INDICATIONS FOR SURGERY

Cardiac transplantation is indicated in patients with terminal heart failure who are under 60 years of age, do not respond to medical therapy, and have no other organ pathology.

SURGICAL PROCEDURE: CARDIAC TRANSPLANT

The surgical preparation for cardiac transplantation is much the same as for any other open heart procedure. The heart is approached through a standard median sternotomy, and bypass is established using a distally placed aortic cannula and individual caval cannulas (Fig. 5.12). Extracorporeal perfusion and excision of the heart are not initiated until the donor organ is immediately available to the transplant surgeon. The aorta is clamped, and the cardiectomy is begun by incising the lateral wall of the right atrium. This incision is extended medially toward the atrioventricular groove and superiorly to the roof of the left atrium. At this point the left atrium may be entered through a separate incision to facilitate optimal exposure of the interatrial septum. Inferiorly the left atrium is entered adjacent to the coronary sinus and the septal incision is completed, leaving the heart attached posteriorly by only the lateral left atrial wall. The great arteries are transected, and the last atrial connections are divided to remove the heart. Figure 5.13 illustrates the nearly empty pericardial cavity with the

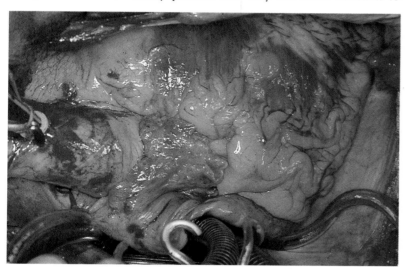

FIG. 5.12 *This operative view shows a heart with severe idiopathic cardiomyopathy cannulated in the standard fashion prior to excision in preparation for transplantation.*

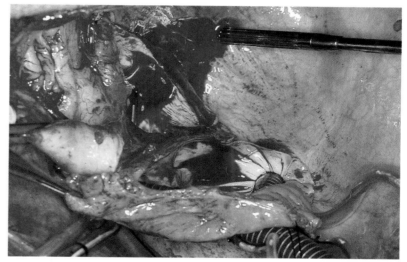

FIG. 5.13 *After excision the depth of the pericardium, the right and the left atrial walls, and the interatrial septum are clearly seen. The pulmonary venous drainage and the oval fossa are visible in the left and the right atria; the ascending aorta and pulmonary trunk are also visible* (continued—Fig. 5.14).

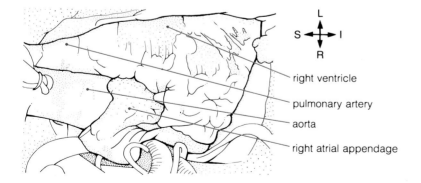

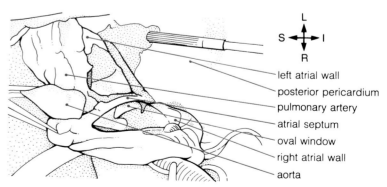

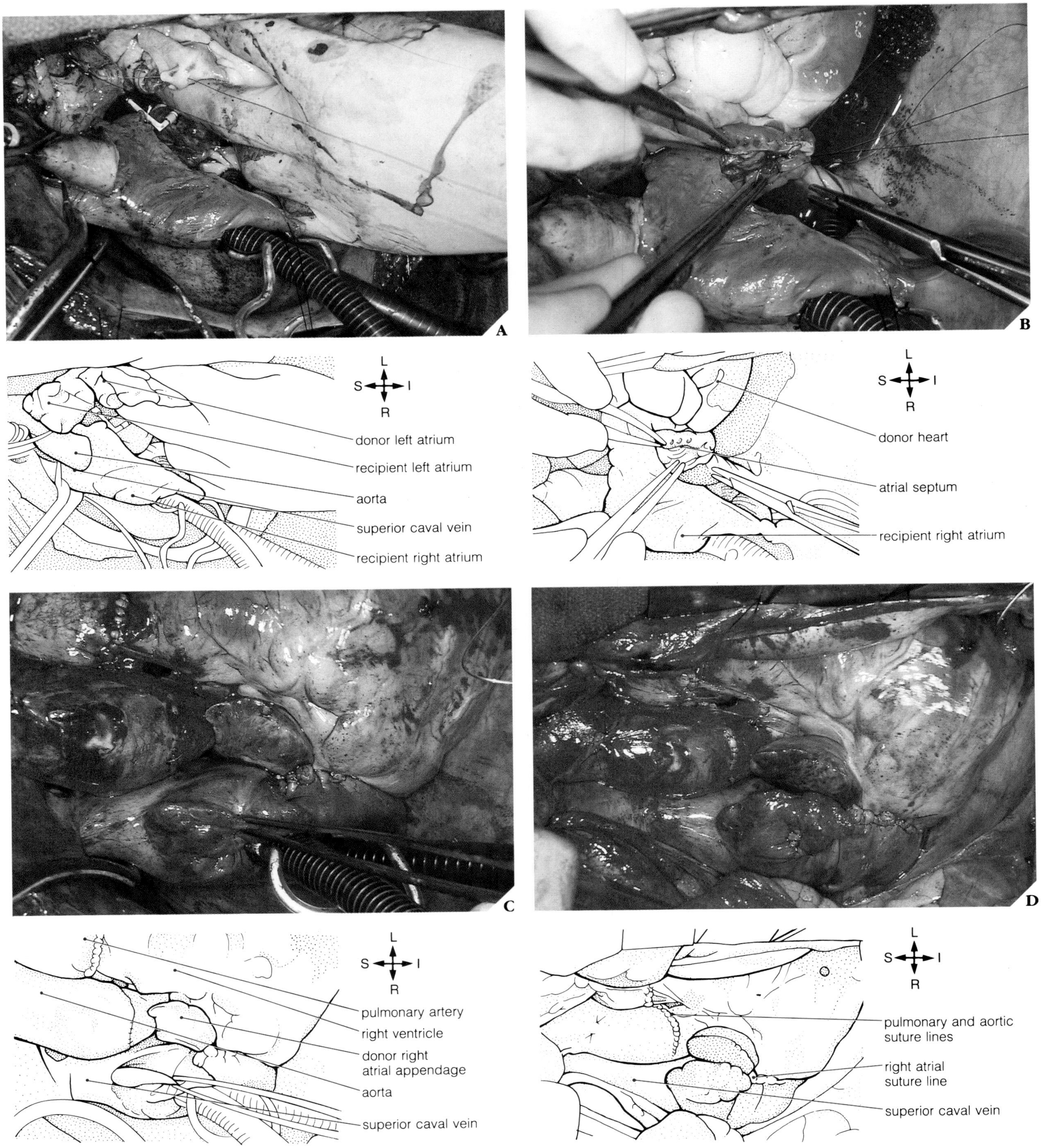
A
B
C
D
L
S
I
R
donor left atrium
recipient left atrium
aorta
superior caval vein
recipient right atrium
donor heart
atrial septum
recipient right atrium
pulmonary artery
right ventricle
donor right
atrial appendage
aorta
superior caval vein
pulmonary and aortic
suture lines
right atrial
suture line
superior caval vein

FIG. 5.14 *Cardiac transplantation* (continued). (A) *Implantation of a donor heart begins by suturing the left atrial walls in a continuous fashion.* (B) *The suture line is carried onto the atrial septum and then to the right atrial wall.* (C) *All anastomoses are completed. The heart is rewarmed, and air is evacuated.* (D) *The operation is completed and the patient is taken off bypass. Both right atrial appendages can be seen to contract independently.*

remaining atrial walls and aortic cuff ready to receive the new heart.

The donor heart is sewn in place using continuous sutures. Beginning on the left superior aspect of the atrial cuff (Fig. 5.14A) and sewing within the heart, the left atrial wall and the septum are attached. Attention is then directed to the right atrial suture line (Fig. 5.14B), taking care not to injure the sinus node and its blood supply. Next the aortic and the pulmonary trunk anastomoses are completed (Fig. 5.14C). After an adequate period of reperfusion and warming, the donor heart begins to contract, often spontaneously, with a normal sinus rhythm. Meticulous attention must be given to assure that all air has been evacuated and that the extensive suture lines are completely hemostatic. Discontinuation of bypass and decannulation can then be effected in the usual manner. Except for the iatrogenically imposed "juxtaposition" of the right atrial appendages, the donor heart looks remarkably natural in its new setting (Fig. 5.14D).

CARDIAC REJECTION. Today, with modern techniques, the one-year survival of patients who have had cardiac transplantation is in the range of 60%–75%. Rejection of the donor heart, however, is one of the major problems that blunts the success of this phenomenal surgical feat. The clinical signs of rejection include fever, atrial fibrillation, and heart failure. Endomyocardial biopsy is considered to be the best method of detecting the early signs of cardiac rejection.

HYPERTROPHIC CARDIOMYOPATHY
Etiology and Pathology

Hypertrophic cardiomyopathy is a disease of unknown origin characterized by massive myocardial hypertrophy. It usually involves the mid- and upper parts of the ventricular septum and the adjacent anterior wall of the left ventricle, producing asymmetric hypertrophy (Fig. 5.15). However, concentric hypertrophy affecting all of the left ventricle or predominately the apex also occurs. The left ventricular cavity is usually small, and the mitral valve may be thickened. The corresponding septal surface on the left ventricle may show fibroelastosis as a secondary effect of mitral valve impact during systole. Hypertrophic cardiomyopathy restricted to the right ventricle may also occur.

Microscopically the disease is characterized by extensive myocardial fiber disarray throughout the grossly affected areas (Fig. 5.16). The myocardial cells are markedly hypertrophic, often with a perinuclear halo. The texture is distorted in the sense that bundles may cross each other in different directions, often exhibiting whorls or cartwheel configurations. Perpendicular branchings and intercellular junctions are often seen.

The abnormal architecture of the myocardium is generally considered to underlie the abnormal compliance of the ventricles, which leads to the restricted inflow of blood during diastole.

Abnormal Physiology

Overemptying of the left ventricle with an ejection fraction of 80%–90% or more is an important feature of hypertrophic cardiomyopathy. Authorities have argued about the importance of *obstruction* versus *elimination* of the left ventricular cavity. Hypertrophic cardiomyopathy produces a decrease in ventricular compliance, impedance to diastolic filling of the ventricle, and abnormal ventricular contraction. The filling of the ventricle takes a longer time than normal, and there is a greatly prolonged isovolumic relaxation period (Sanderson et al, 1977).

While these diastolic abnormalities are well documented, further study is needed to understand fully the entire diastolic abnormality associated with this disorder.

The obstructive type of the disease is characterized by a peak systolic pressure gradient below the aortic valve between the body of the left ventricle and the aorta. The magnitude of the gradient varies from time to time; it is increased by an ectopic beat, increased myocardial contractility, hypovolemia, or decreased systemic blood pressure. The outflow tract of such patients becomes muscle-bound; the anterior leaflet of the mitral valve is entrapped in the obstructing process. The early phase of ventricular contraction is rapid; the subsequent ventricular contraction pattern produces a pulsus bisferiens–type contour in the carotid artery pulsation. Whereas the gradient does not directly correlate with symptoms or prognosis in all patients, it is important in some patients. Accordingly some patients profit from muscle resection to remove the obstructing area (Braunwald et al, 1964).

Myocardial ischemia occurs because the thickened myocardium needs more blood than normal. Additional causes of myocardial ischemia in such patients are myocardial bridging of the coronary arteries, abnormal diastolic function of the ventricles, and unrelated atherosclerotic coronary disease.

Clinical Manifestations
SYMPTOMS

The patient, who is usually male, may be asymptomatic or may complain of angina or syncope. Late in the course of the condition the patient may complain of dyspnea and palpitation. Sudden death is the mode of death in 50% of those who die of this disease.

PHYSICAL EXAMINATION

The general appearance of the patient is usually normal, although the skeletal muscles may be prominent.

Patients with a left ventricular outflow tract pressure gradient may have a diamond-shaped, systolic murmur that is heard to the left of the midsternal area, at the apex, and less well in the aortic area. The murmur becomes louder when the patient stands or performs a Valsalva maneuver, but it becomes fainter with squatting and handgrip.

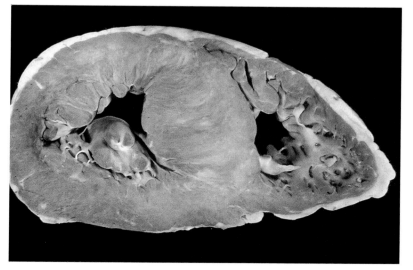

FIG. 5.15 *Cross-section through a heart reveals hypertrophic cardiomyopathy and asymmetry of the affected interventricular septum. (Reproduced with permission of the authors and publisher; see Figure Credits)*

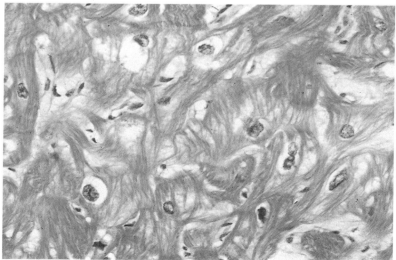

FIG. 5.16 *Histologic section of the myocardium in hypertrophic cardiomyopathy demonstrates marked hypertrophy of individual myocytes and an abnormal texture known as myocardial disarray.*

The murmur may not become louder during the systole that follows an ectopic beat, as it does with aortic valve stenosis. The murmur of mitral regurgitation may be heard. On rare occasion a low-pitched, diastolic rumble may be heard at the apex. Slight aortic regurgitation has also been noted.

A pulsus bisferiens may be detected in the carotid artery pulsation. An atrial gallop may be heard and felt at the cardiac apex. During systole the apex impulse may be bifid.

A prominent a wave may be seen in the jugular venous pulse when there is involvement of the right ventricle with obstruction of its outflow tract (Goodwin, 1982).

LABORATORY STUDIES

CHEST RADIOGRAPHY. The heart may appear normal on the chest radiograph. Alternately there may be slight-to-moderate cardiac enlargement. The left atrium may be large and, late in the course of the disease, pulmonary congestion may be evident. Valvar calcification is not seen.

ELECTROCARDIOGRAPHY. The ECG usually shows left ventricular hypertrophy with increased amplitude of the QRS complexes. The ST-T wave abnormality may simulate myocardial infarction with elevated ST segments and inverted T waves in some leads. Abnormal Q waves may also suggest myocardial infarction (Fig. 5.17). The T waves may be deeply inverted and large in apical hypertrophic cardiomyopathy. The P-R interval may be short and a delta wave may be noted in the QRS complex, signifying that an atrioventricular bypass tract is present (Wolff-Parkinson-White syndrome) (Vacek et al, 1984). Ventricular arrhythmias may be seen on the routine ECG, but they are more often detected by ambulatory monitoring (Frank et al, 1984).

ECHOCARDIOGRAPHY. The M-mode echocardiogram shows increased thickness of the ventricular wall (Fig. 5.18). The septum is often thicker than the posterior left ventricular wall, and it may contract less than the free wall of the left ventricle. The left ventricular cavity size may be decreased. There is abnormal anterior motion of the mitral valve during systole, and its rate of closure is slowed (Gilbert et al,

FIG. 5.17 *The ECG of a 77-year-old woman with apical hypertrophic cardiomyopathy shows normal sinus rhythm, a tall R wave in lead V_1, and very unusual ST and T waves. The ST and T wave abnormalities persisted for years; they simulate the ST and T wave abnormalities of myocardial infarction.*

| I | II | III | aV$_R$ | aV$_L$ | aV$_F$ |

| V$_1$ | V$_2$ | V$_3$ | V$_4$ | V$_5$ | V$_6$ |

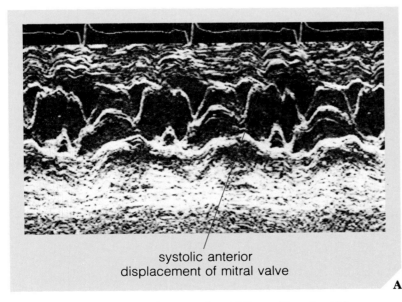

systolic anterior
displacement of mitral valve

A

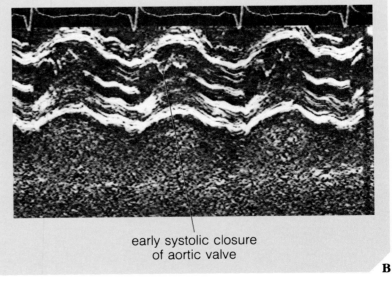

early systolic closure
of aortic valve

B

FIG. 5.18 *M-mode echocardiogram of a middle-aged female with hypertrophic cardiomyopathy and left ventricular outflow tract obstruction demonstrates (A) abnormal systolic anterior motion of the mitral valve and (B) early* systolic closure of the aortic valve. (Courtesy of Stephen D. Clements, Jr, MD, Atlanta, Georgia)

1980). The aortic valve tends to close in mid-systole. The left atrial size may be increased.

Cross-sectional echocardiography is superior to the M-mode technique in detecting hypertrophy of the septum and studying the mitral apparatus (Fig. 5.19) (DeMaria et al, 1980).

CARDIAC CATHETERIZATION. A systolic pressure gradient between the left ventricle and the aorta may be identified when the patient is at rest (Fig. 5.20). The gradient may be provoked with amyl nitrate, a Valsalva maneuver, or isoproterenol; it may also be detected following a ventricular ectopic beat. Catheter entrapment must be avoided to prevent the spurious recording of an elevated left ventricular pressure (Braunwald et al, 1960).

Left ventriculography, performed at the time of cardiac catheterization, may reveal the thick ventricular muscle in the region of the apex, mid-left ventricle, or subaortic area. Coronary arteriography is useful to identify coronary atherosclerosis, which may occasionally coexist with hypertrophic cardiomyopathy.

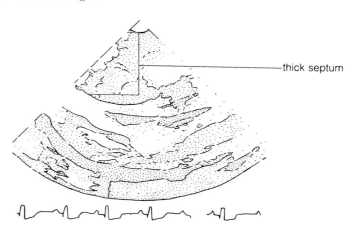

FIG. 5.19 *A diastolic frame of a cross-sectional echocardiogram of a young man who has hypertrophic cardiomyopathy with obstruction indicates severe hypertrophy of the septum. (Courtesy of Stephen D. Clements, Jr, MD, Atlanta, Georgia)*

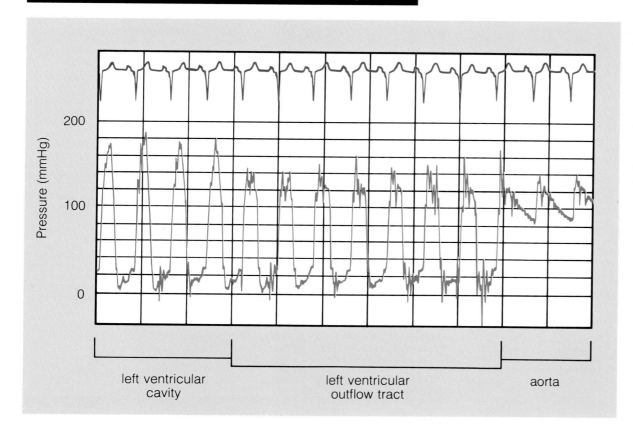

FIG. 5.20 *Obstruction in the outflow tract of the right ventricle in this case of idiopathic hypertrophic subaortic stenosis is demonstrated when the catheter is pulled from the interventricular cavity through the outflow tract into the aorta. Pressure recordings are shown from the left ventricular cavity, the outflow tract of the left ventricle, and the aorta. (Courtesy of Jerre F. Lutz, MD, Atlanta, Georgia)*

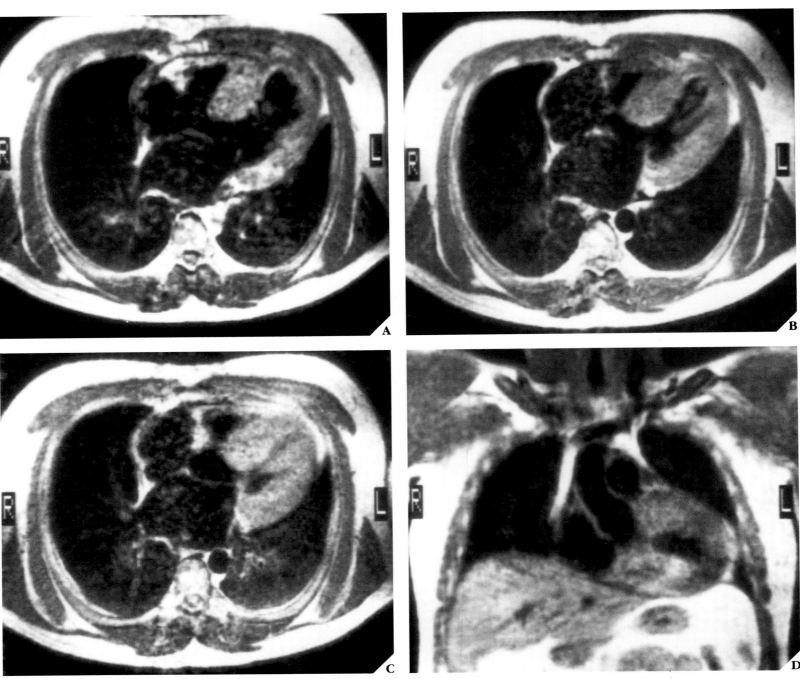

FIG. 5.21 *These MRI sections were recorded in a 31-year-old male with hypertrophic cardiomyopathy who had had two episodes of syncope. The transverse sections were made during end-diastole (A), mid-diastole (B), and end-systole (C). An image in the coronal plane was also made during mid-systole (D). Left ventricular hypertrophy is evident, and systolic anterior motion of the mitral valve is seen in all of the systolic images. (Courtesy of Roderic I. Pettigrew, PhD, MD, Atlanta, Georgia)*

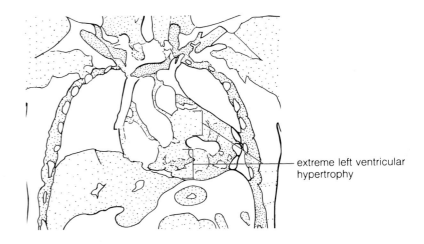

extreme left ventricular hypertrophy

MAGNETIC RESONANCE IMAGING. Magnetic resonance imaging (MRI) may reveal the thick myocardium of hypertrophic cardiomyopathy (Fig. 5.21).

Natural History

The survival period for patients with hypertrophic cardiomyopathy varies from a short period to a long life. About half of patients die suddenly due to an arrhythmia or severe left ventricular outflow tract obstruction (Shah et al, 1973). Syncope may occur, and it is considered to be a serious and dangerous event. Both supraventricular and ventricular arrhythmias are common. Some patients have preexcitation due to atrioventricular bypass tracts. When atrial fibrillation develops in this setting, the ventricular rate is very rapid. Congestive heart failure occurs late in the natural course of the condition, often precipitated by atrial fibrillation.

Episodes of myocardial ischemia produce angina pectoris in many patients. A few patients experience prolonged chest pain due to myocardial ischemia. This, in addition to the electrocardiographic abnormalities that may simulate myocardial infarction, may lead the physician to erroneously diagnose atherosclerotic coronary heart disease (Ouzts et al, 1980).

Infective endocarditis may occur in patients with obstruction of the outflow tract. Peripheral emboli, which are usually related to atrial fibrillation, occur in about 10% of patients. Severe mitral regurgitation may develop, and this contributes to the development of heart failure.

Treatment

There is no satisfactory treatment at present. Arrhythmias are treated according to their type. Digitalis produces an increase in contractility, but this may increase the outflow tract obstruction. Beta-blockers are used in an effort to decrease the resistance to the inflow of blood and, by improved filling, to increase cardiac output. It now appears that verapamil may not be as useful in the treatment of this condition as was originally thought (Webb–Peploe et al, 1971; Alvares and Goodwin, 1982; Epstein and Rosing, 1981). Amiodarone may improve survival of patients with hypertrophic cardiomyopathy and ventricular tachycardia (McKenna et al, 1985).

INDICATIONS FOR SURGERY

No surgery can be performed when there is diffuse cardiac hypertrophy without outflow tract, apical, or mid-ventricular obstruction. Surgical removal of a portion of the septum is indicated when the patient has syncope or angina despite medical treatment, a proven outflow tract pressure gradient of 50 mmHg at rest, and a thick ventricular septum (Maron et al, 1980). The procedure can be done with an operative risk of about 2%–8%. Survival is improved; about three-fourths of patients live longer than ten years after surgery. Mitral valve replacement is not indicated unless the regurgitation is moderately severe.

SURGICAL PROCEDURE

The surgical anatomy in an operation to relieve the left ventricular outflow obstruction is shown in Figure 5.22.

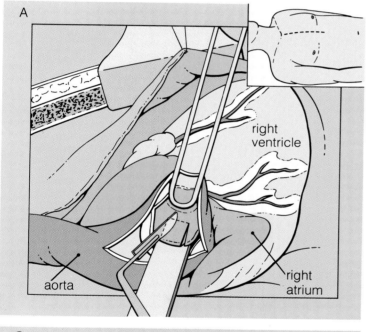

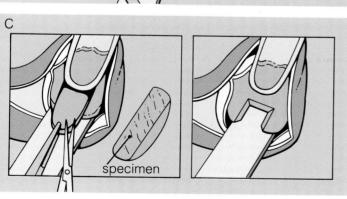

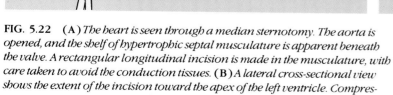

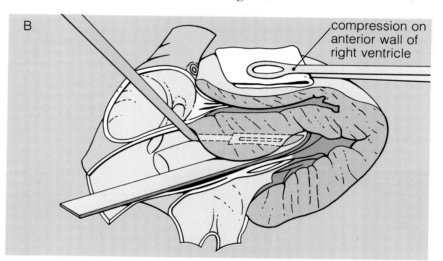

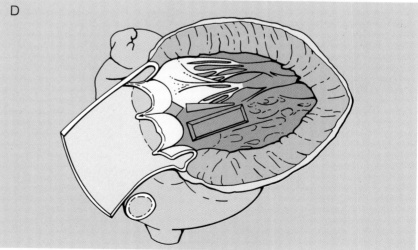

FIG. 5.22 (A) *The heart is seen through a median sternotomy. The aorta is opened, and the shelf of hypertrophic septal musculature is apparent beneath the valve. A rectangular longitudinal incision is made in the musculature, with care taken to avoid the conduction tissues. (B) A lateral cross-sectional view shows the extent of the incision toward the apex of the left ventricle. Compression on the anterior wall of the right ventricle facilitates this maneuver. A "plug" of myocardium is removed. (C) The resultant defect is illustrated from the anterior viewpoint of the septum. (D) A view of the septum shows the long segment removed. (Redrawn; reproduced with permission of the publisher; see Figure Credits)*

RESTRICTIVE CARDIOMYOPATHY
Etiology and Pathology

Restrictive cardiomyopathy, the least common type of cardiomyopathy, is caused by conditions such as endomyocardial fibrosis (with or without eosinophilia), amyloid disease (Fig. 5.23), and hemochromatosis (Roberts et al, 1970). The decreased diastolic volume and the diminished ability of the ventricle to stretch in response to a volume load causes a decrease in cardiac output. Myocardial contraction is usually normal until late in the course of the disease (Chew et al, 1977). The ventricular cavity may become small during the late phase of the disease, at which time the condition is described as *obliterative cardiomyopathy* (Goodwin, 1979).

Abnormal Physiology

During the early phase of the condition restricted ventricular filling is caused by endomyocardial fibrosis; later there is progressive obliteration of the ventricular cavity with thrombus and fibrous tissue. This process involves the papillary muscles and the tendinous cords, producing mitral and tricuspid regurgitation.

Early diastolic filling of the ventricles may be normal, but the condition limits diastolic filling during the later part of diastole. Systolic function is preserved until late in the course of the disease. The physiologic picture is similar to that found in constrictive pericarditis. Accordingly the pressure curve in the right ventricle shows the *dip-and-plateau* waveform during diastole, while elevation of peak pressure in the right atrium and the right ventricle may be the same. A small paradoxical pulse may be present. The stroke output is decreased, and tachycardia may be present. Pulmonary hypertension may be present when the left ventricle is severely damaged and mitral regurgitation is present. The right atrium may become enlarged.

The physiologic derangement of Loeffler's endomyocardial fibrosis with eosinophilia and tropical endomyocardial fibrosis without eosinophilia is similar.

The ventricular filling is slow throughout diastole in patients with amyloid infiltration of the heart. Early in the course of the disease the contractility is normal, but it decreases later. The ventricular distortion does not occur as it does in endomyocardial fibrosis.

Hemochromatosis decreases the compliance of the ventricles; this limits diastolic filling.

Clinical Manifestations
SYMPTOMS

The patient with acute eosinophilic endomyocardial disease (Loeffler's disease) may experience fever, dyspnea, and edema. These abnormalities may disappear for a while or continue as fatigue and fever. Gradually the patient develops a syndrome not unlike constrictive pericarditis, with dyspnea, cough, ascites, and edema.

Tropical endomyocardial fibrosis may involve the left, the right, or both ventricles. Dyspnea and cough dominate the clinical picture when the left ventricle is predominantly involved. Ascites and edema dominate the clinical picture when the right ventricle is primarily involved. However, usually the clinical picture is a mixture of the left and the right ventricular forms of the disease. Both ventricles are usually involved in the pathologic process.

Primary amyloid involvement of the heart produces a similar clinical picture. Angina pectoris may be present when the coronary arteries themselves are involved.

Hemochromatosis of the heart also gives a similar clinical picture. The patient's skin may be bronze in color, and symptoms of diabetes may be present.

PHYSICAL EXAMINATION

The physical findings may suggest constrictive pericarditis. The cardiac rhythm is usually normal, but atrial fibrillation may be present. The neck veins are distended, and the deep jugular venous pulsation may show a prominent a wave and rapid descent of the x and y waves. Inspiration produces a marked increase in the abnormalities of the neck vein.

Amyloid disease may be characterized by isolated heart disease, but systemic features may include the presence of a large tongue, petechiae, purpura, peripheral neuropathy, and downward displacement of the submaxillary glands due to involvement of the base of the tongue. Postural hypotension may be present, and the sick sinus node syndrome may occur.

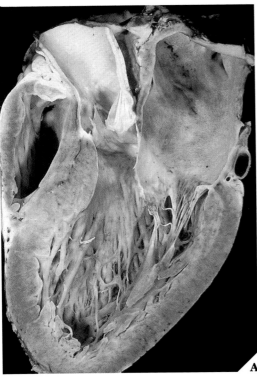
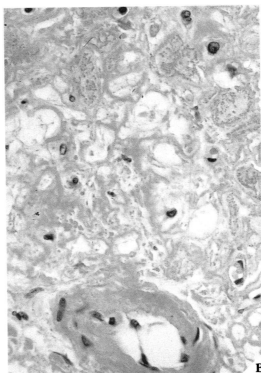
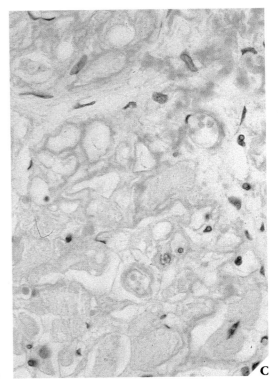

FIG. 5.23 (A) *Long-axis section through a heart with amyloid disease demonstrates the sandy appearance of the left atrial endocardium.* (B) *Histologic section shows myocardial cell degeneration and extensive extracellular deposition of amorphous eosinophilic material enclosing the cells.* (C) *The amyloid stains positive with a Congo red stain. (Reproduced with permission of the authors and publisher; see Figure Credits)*

LABORATORY STUDIES

CHEST RADIOGRAPHY. The chest film shows moderate cardiomegaly, an enlarged left atrium, and prominent pulmonary veins. Calcium may be seen as a linear streak in the endocardial area of the left ventricular apex in patients with endomyocardial fibrosis.

ELECTROCARDIOGRAPHY. The ECG of patients with endomyocardial fibrosis of the left ventricle may show left ventricular hypertrophy and a left atrial abnormality. Patients with right ventricular endomyocardial fibrosis may exhibit low voltage of the QRS complexes and large P waves due to a right atrial abnormality. The ECG associated with amyloid heart disease may show low voltage of the QRS complexes and evidence of a sick sinus node and atrioventricular conduction block. Abnormal Q waves suggesting infarction may be present (Fig. 5.24) (Carroll et al, 1982).

ECHOCARDIOGRAPHY. The M-mode echocardiogram of patients with endomyocardial fibrosis may not be helpful. The cross-sectional echocardiogram may show the obliteration of the ventricular cavities, an increase in left ventricular mass, thrombi in the ventricular cavity, normal ventricular contractility, and a large left atrium.

The cross-sectional echocardiogram in patients with amyloid heart disease may show brilliant echoes involving the myocardium; this abnormality is almost diagnostic when it is present (Fig. 5.25) (DeMaria et al, 1980).

CARDIAC CATHETERIZATION. The pressure curves may simulate those found in constrictive pericarditis with the dip-and-plateau waveform recorded during diastole in the right ventricle (see Fig. 7.19).

There may be evidence of tricuspid and mitral valve regurgitation.

Angiography reveals obliterated areas in the apices of the ventricles. The ventricular cavity size may be decreased, and the myocardial wall may be thicker than normal. Contractility is usually normal during the early stages of the disease, while relaxation of the myocardial wall is abnormal.

RADIONUCLIDE STUDIES. Radionuclide ventriculography reveals a normal or a decreased ventricular cavity size; this assists in the differentiation from dilated cardiomyopathy. The relaxation abnormality of the myocardial wall may be identified. Cardiac amyloidosis is less likely to show a distorted ventricular cavity.

COMPUTED TOMOGRAPHY AND MAGNETIC RESONANCE IMAGING. These modalities may help differentiate several conditions that produce somewhat similar clinical pictures. They may show the thick ventricular muscle and distorted cavity in patients with endomyocardial fibrosis or may reveal a thick pericardium and normal cardiac muscle thickness in patients with constrictive pericarditis.

ENDOMYOCARDIAL BIOPSY. Endomyocardial biopsy may be diagnostic of endomyocardial fibrosis, amyloid involvement of the heart, or hemochromatosis.

OTHER STUDIES. The hypereosinophilic syndrome is associated with eosinophilic infiltration of tissues, including the heart. The eosinophils may constitute 75% of the total white blood cell count, which may be as high as 100,000/mm³. There may be no recognizable cause of the eosinophilia, but the abnormality may be an immunologic response

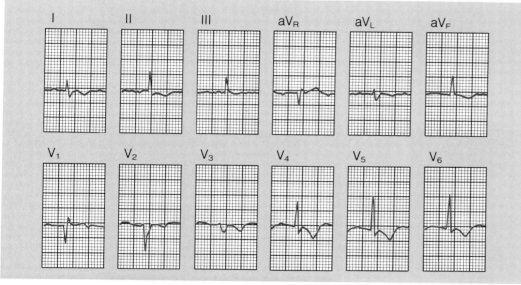

FIG. 5.24 *The ECG of a 65-year-old woman with amyloid of the heart shows normal sinus rhythm. The P waves are just barely visible in lead aV$_R$, and the P-R interval is 0.24 s. Large abnormal Q waves are seen in leads V$_1$–V$_3$. The T waves are deeply inverted in leads I, II, aV$_F$, and V$_2$–V$_6$. Initially the condition was diagnosed as myocardial infarction with normal coronary arteries.*

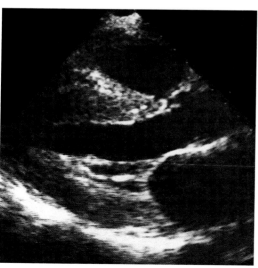

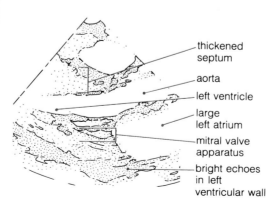

thickened septum
aorta
left ventricle
large left atrium
mitral valve apparatus
bright echoes in left ventricular wall

FIG. 5.25 *A cross-sectional echocardiogram in the long-axis view was obtained during systole in a 66-year-old male with amyloid involving the heart. Sparkling echoes involving the myocardium are evident. Both the interventricular septum and the posterior wall are thickened. (Courtesy of Stephen D. Clements, Jr, MD, Atlanta, Georgia)*

of some sort. The response may be associated with parasitic infections, or it may be of unknown origin, as in Loeffler's disease.

Biopsy of the rectal mucosa, gums, skin lesions, and other sites may be performed if one suspects amyloid heart disease, but endomyocardial biopsy is more diagnostic.

Natural History

Patients with restrictive myocardial disease may survive only a few months or a few years, because treatment is unsatisfactory.

Treatment

The medical treatment for restrictive myocardial disease is unsatisfactory. Digitalis is used but helps very little. Diuretics are necessary, but to diurese the patient to the point that the filling pressures of the heart are diminished is detrimental. Corticosteroid therapy may be used when eosinophilia is present; ascites may be removed for comfort.

Resection of the endocardium has been performed in patients with endomyocardial fibrosis, but this technique is in the developmental stage. Mitral and tricuspid valves have been replaced with prosthetic valves and the Glenn procedure has been used, but these operations do not save the patient (Cherian et al, 1983; Davies et al, 1983). Cardiac transplantation is the surgical treatment of choice and should be performed when conditions are proper (see Figs. 5.12–5.14).

MYOCARDIAL INVOLVEMENT IN SYSTEMIC DISEASE

There are many causes of myocardial disease; some are limited to the heart, while others represent the heart's participation in systemic disease, as in Pompe's disease (Fig. 5.26) or tumor metastases to the heart (Fig. 5.27). For systemic diseases involving the heart, see Table 5.2.

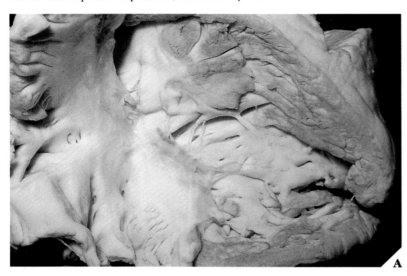

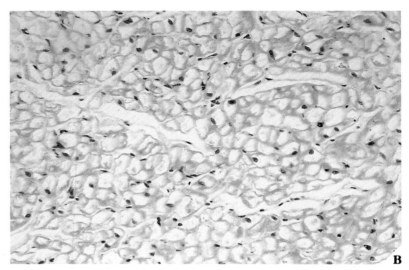

FIG. 5.26 (**A**) *Right ventricular view of the heart in a case of Pompe's disease shows the pale-staining myocardial wall.* (**B**) *Histologic section shows vacuolated cells where the glycogen has been washed out.*

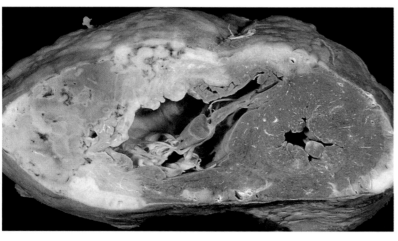

FIG. 5.27 *Extensive tumor involvement of the heart is consequent to spread from a primary bronchial carcinoma.*

Table 5.2 Myocardial Involvement in Systemic Disease

Infectious disease
Sarcoidosis
Nutritional disorders
Metabolic disorders
Endocrine disorders
Hematologic diseases
Neurologic and neuromuscular diseases
Collagen vascular diseases
Neoplastic diseases
Chemical and drug effects
Physical causes
Miscellaneous systemic syndromes

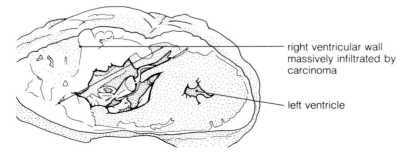

right ventricular wall
massively infiltrated by
carcinoma

left ventricle

REFERENCES

Alvares RF, Goodwin JF (1982) Non-invasive assessment of diastolic function in hypertrophic cardiomyopathy on and off beta-adrenergic blocking drugs. *Br Heart J* 48:204

Bell GJ, Grist NR (1971) Echoviruses, carditis, and acute pleurodynia. *Am Heart J* 82:133

Braunwald E, Lambrew CT, Morrow AG, et al (1964) Idiopathic hypertrophic subaortic stenosis. *Circulation* 29/30(suppl IV):1

Braunwald E, Morrow AG, Cornell WP, Aygen MM, Hilbish TF (1960) Idiopathic hypertrophic subaortic stenosis: Clinical, hemodynamic and angiographic manifestations. *Am J Med* 29:24

Burch GE, Giles TD (1972) The role of viruses in the production of heart disease. *Am J Cardiol* 29:231

Carroll JD, Gaasch WH, McAdam KPWJ (1982) Amyloid cardiomyopathy: Characterization by a distinctive voltage/mass relation. *Am J Cardiol* 49:9

Chatterjee K (1982) Digitalis versus newer inotropic agents: Which to use. *Drug Therapy* 12:834

Cherian G, Vijayaraghavan G, Krishnaswami S, et al (1983) Endomyocardial fibrosis: Report on the hemodynamic data in 29 patients and review of the results of surgery. *Am Heart J* 105:659

Chew CYC, Ziady GM, Raphael JM, et al (1977) Primary restrictive cardiomyopathy: Non-tropical endomyocardial fibrosis and hypereosinophilic heart disease. *Br Heart J* 39:399

Davies J, Spry CJF, Sapsford R, et al (1983) Cardiovascular features of 11 patients with eosinophilic endomyocardial disease. *Q J Med* 52:23

DeMaria AN, Bommer W, Lee G, Mason DT (1980) Value and limitations of two-dimensional echocardiography in assessment of cardiomyopathy. *Am J Cardiol* 46:1224

Dunn RF, Uren RF, Sadick N, et al (1982) Comparison of thallium-201 scanning in idiopathic dilated cardiomyopathy and severe coronary artery disease. *Circulation* 66:804

Edwards WD, Holmes DR Jr, Reeder GS (1982) Diagnosis of active lymphocytic myocarditis by endomyocardial biopsy: Quantitative criteria for light microscopy. *Mayo Clin Proc* 57:419

Epstein SE, Rosing DR (1981) Verapamil: Its potential for causing serious complications in patients with hypertrophic cardiomyopathy. *Circulation* 64:437

Frank MJ, Watkins LO, Prisant M, et al (1984) Potentially lethal arrhythmias and their management in hypertrophic cardiomyopathy. *Am J Cardiol* 53:1608

Gau GT, Goodwin JF, Oakley CM, et al (1972) Q waves and coronary arteriography in cardiomyopathy. *Br Heart J* 34:1034

Gilbert BW, Pollick C, Adelman AG, Wigle ED (1980) Hypertrophic cardiomyopathy: Subclassification by M-mode echocardiography. *Am J Cardiol* 45:861

Goldman MR, Boucher CA (1980) Value of radionuclide imaging techniques in assessing cardiomyopathy. *Am J Cardiol* 46:1232

Goodwin JF (1982) The frontiers of cardiomyopathy. *Br Heart J* 48:1

Goodwin JF: Cardiomyopathy: An interface between fundamental and clinical cardiology, in Hayase S, Murao S (eds): *Cardiology* (Proceedings VIII World Congress of Cardiology, Tokyo, 1978). Amsterdam, Excerpta Medica, 1979, p 103

Kean BH, Breslau RC (1964) *Parasites of the Human Heart.* New York, Grune & Stratton

Kereiakes DJ, Parmley WW (1984) Myocarditis and cardiomyopathy. *Am Heart J* 108:1318

Kristinsson A (1969) Diagnosis, natural history and treatment of congestive cardiomyopathy. PhD thesis, University of London, Royal Postgraduate Medical School of London

Lansdown ABG (1978) Viral infections and diseases of the heart. *Prog Med Virol* 24:70

Lerner AM, Wilson FM, Reyes MP (1975) Enteroviruses and the heart (with special emphasis on the probable role of coxsackie viruses, group B, types 1–5). I. Epidemiological and experimental studies. II. Observations in humans. *Mod Concepts Cardiovasc Dis* 44:7, 11

Maron BJ, Koch J–P, Kent KM, et al (1980) Results of surgery for idiopathic hypertrophic subaortic stenosis. *J Cardiovasc Med* 5:145

McKenna WJ, Oakley CM, Krikler DM, Goodwin JF (1985) Improved survival with amiodarone in patients with hypertrophic cardiomyopathy and ventricular tachycardia. *Br Heart J* 53:412–416

Murphy TE, Kean BH, Venturini A, Lillehei CW (1971) Echinococcus cyst of the left ventricle: Report of a case with review of the pertinent literature. *J Thorac Cardiovasc Surg* 61:443

Nieminen MS, Heikkila J, Karjalainene J (1984) Echocardiography in acute infectious myocarditis: Relation to clinical and electrocardiographic findings. *Am J Cardiol* 53:1331

O'Connell JB, Henkin RE, Robinson JA, Subramanian R, Scanlon PJ, Gunnar RM (1984) Gallium-67 imaging in patients with dilated cardiomyopathy and biopsy proven myocarditis. *Circulation* 70:58

Opherk D, Schwarz F, Mall G, et al (1983) Coronary dilatory capacity in idiopathic dilated cardiomyopathy: Analysis of 16 patients. *Am J Cardiol* 51:1657

Ouzts HG, Turner JL, Douglas JS Jr, Hurst JW: Prolonged chest pain suggesting myocardial infarction in patients with hypertrophic cardiomyopathy, in Hurst JW (ed): *Update III: The Heart.* New York, McGraw-Hill, 1980, p 139

Puigbo JJ, Rhode JRN, Barrios HG, Suarez JA, Yepez CG (1966) Clinical and epidemiological study of chronic heart involvement in Chagas' disease. *Bull WHO* 34:655

Roberts WC, Bjua LM, Ferrans VJ (1970) Loeffler's fibroplastic parietal endocarditis, eosinophilic leukemia, and Davies' endomyocardial fibrosis: The same disease at different stages? *Pathol Microbiol* 35:90

Sanderson JE, Gibson DG, Brown DJ, Goodwin JF (1977) Left ventricular filling in hypertrophic cardiomyopathy: An angiographic study. *Br Heart J* 39:661

Shah PM, Adelman AG, Wigle ED, et al (1973) The natural (and unnatural) course of hypertrophic obstructive cardiomyopathy—a multicenter study. *Circulation* 47/48 (suppl 4):IV-5

Vacek JL, Davis WR, Bellinger RL, et al (1984) Apical hypertrophic cardiomyopathy in American patients. *Am Heart J* 108:1501

Walsh TJ, Hutchins GM, Bulkley BH, Mendelsohn G (1980) Fungal infections of the heart: Analysis of 51 autopsy cases. *Am J Cardiol* 45:357

Webb–Peploe MM, Croxson RS, Oakley CM, Goodwin JF (1971) Cardioselective beta-adrenergic blockade in hypertrophic obstructive cardiomyopathy. *Postgrad Med J* 47(suppl):93

Wentworth P, Jentz LA, Croal EA (1979) Analysis of sudden unexpected death in southern Ontario, with emphasis on myocarditis. *Can Med Assoc J* 120:676

Woodward TE, Togo Y, Lee Y–C, Hornick RB (1967) Special microbial infections of the myocardium and pericardium. A study of 82 patients. *Arch Intern Med* 120:270

FIGURE CREDITS

FIG. 5.1 From Becker AE, Anderson RH: *Cardiac Pathology.* New York, Raven Press, 1983, p 3.37.

FIG. 5.2 From Becker AE, Anderson RH: *Cardiac Pathology.* New York, Raven Press, 1983, p 3.37.

FIG. 5.3 From Becker AE, Anderson RH: *Cardiac Pathology.* New York, Raven Press, 1983, p 3.37.

FIG. 5.4 From Becker AE, Anderson RH: *Cardiac Pathology.* New York, Raven Press, 1983, p 3.36.

FIG. 5.15 From Becker AE, Anderson RH: *Cardiac Pathology.* New York, Raven Press, 1983, p 3.51.

FIG. 5.22 A–D: Redrawn from Morrow AG: Hypertrophic subaortic stenosis: Operative methods utilized to relieve left ventricular outflow obstruction. *J Thorac Cardiovasc Surg* 76:423, 1978.

FIG. 5.23 (A,B) From Becker AE, Anderson RH: *Cardiac Pathology.* New York, Raven Press, 1983, p 3.46.

6
CORONARY HEART DISEASE

J. Willis Hurst, MD
Anton E. Becker, MD
Benson R. Wilcox, MD

Abstracted with permission of the authors and publisher from Hurst JW, King SB III, Friesinger GC, Walter PF, Morris DC: Atherosclerotic coronary heart disease: recognition, prognosis, and treatment, Chapter 45, pp 882–1008, in Hurst JW (ed): *The Heart,* 6th ed. New York, McGraw-Hill, 1986. Additional contributions were made by Theodore Hersh MD, Robert B. Smith MD, George Beller MD, and Burton Sobel MD. Figures, tables, or extracts of text reproduced from the above chapter, other chapters in *The Heart,* or other sources are also reprinted with permission of the authors and publishers. For the full bibliographic citations of the sources of figures and tables other than the above chapter, see Figure Credits at the end of this chapter.

Myocardial ischemia is usually due to an imbalance between myocardial oxygen consumption and oxygen supply. The most common condition underlying myocardial ischemia is obstructive coronary artery disease, which may be aggravated by additional cardiac abnormalities such as hypertrophy and dilation. Myocardial ischemia and infarction may also complicate various types of cardiac disease, such as valve abnormalities, cardiomyopathies, and congenital heart malformations.

Coronary atherosclerosis is the most common condition underlying obstructive coronary artery disease. However, other abnormalities may occur, including coronary artery spasm, coronary artery embolism, coronary ostial stenosis, coronary arteritis, coronary artery dissection, and congenital artery anomaly.

PATHOLOGY

Coronary atherosclerosis is the most common cause of coronary disease (Fig. 6.1). The abnormality, which is confined mainly to the intima, consists of a fibrocellular proliferation with an accumulation of lipids. The latter may form a distinct mass, and this particular lesion is designated as an atheroma. Usually the atheroma is delineated from the

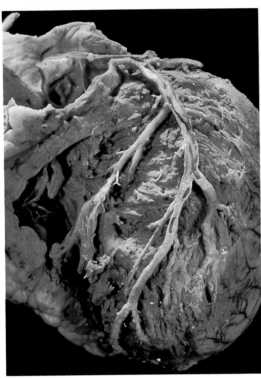

FIG. 6.1 *The anterior descending coronary artery and major branches in this specimen show multiple obstructive lesions due to atherosclerosis.*

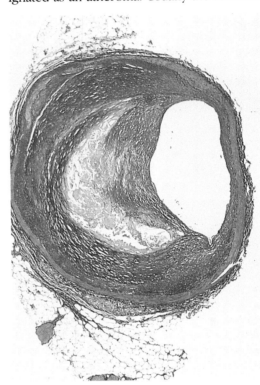

FIG. 6.2. *Histologic cross-section through a coronary artery shows an eccentric atherosclerotic lesion. The atheroma is separated from the lumen by a fibrous cap. The medial layer is intact.*

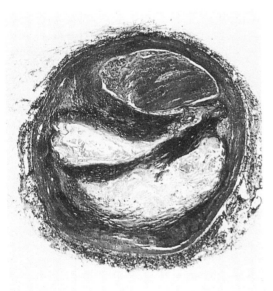

FIG. 6.3 *Histologic cross-section through a coronary artery showing two distinct layers of atherosclerotic lesions suggests different episodes of growth. The lumen is obliterated by a recent thrombosis.*

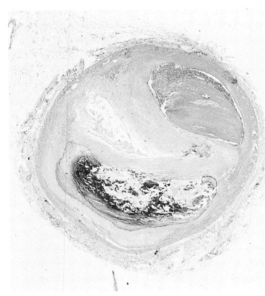

FIG. 6.4 *In this particular stain of the same artery shown in Figure 6.3 the calcified atheroma is clearly recognized by its distinct purple color. Calcification is a common phenomenon in advanced atherosclerotic lesions.*

lumen by a fibrous cap (Fig. 6.2). Macrophages are dispersed throughout the lesion.

The extent and severity of the obstructive atherosclerotic lesion may vary considerably. In the majority of patients the atherosclerotic lesion is in an eccentric position, but concentric lesions do occur. In advanced lesions one may often observe a layering suggesting different episodes of growth of the plaque (Fig. 6.3). Calcification of advanced lesions is a common feature (Fig. 6.4).

The composition of atherosclerotic lesions may also differ. Occasionally the lesion is dominated by a fibrocellular proliferation (Fig.

6.5). In other instances the lesion may be composed almost totally of atheroma (Fig. 6.6), or it may be almost totally fibrosed (Fig. 6.7). Coronary thrombosis is an important complication, which may be initiated by plaque fissure (Fig. 6.8).

The muscular media of the affected coronary artery is usually intact, providing a morphologic substrate for vasospasm. Thus, in the majority of cases, the fixed stenosis caused by the atherosclerotic lesion can be aggravated by contraction of the intact muscular wall. Coronary arteries with early atherosclerotic lesions appear to be particularly sensitive in this phenomenon.

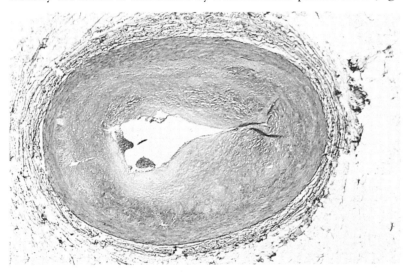

FIG. 6.5 *Concentric lesion of a coronary artery is dominated by a fibrocellular proliferation. (Reproduced with permission of the authors and publisher; see Figure Credits)*

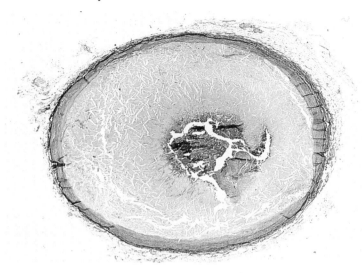

FIG. 6.6 *Cross-section through a coronary artery shows an extensive atherosclerotic lesion almost totally composed of atheroma. There is hemorrhage in a crack of the atheromatous plaque.*

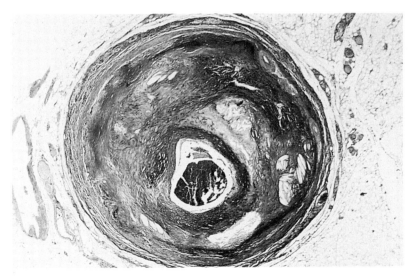

FIG. 6.7 *Cross-section through a coronary artery shows an atherosclerotic lesion almost totally composed of fibrosed tissue.*

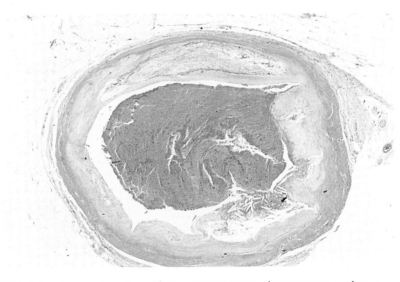

FIG. 6.8 *Cross-section through a coronary artery demonstrates a plaque fissure and adherent thrombus occluding the lumen. (Reproduced with permission of the authors and publisher; see Figure Credits)*

ETIOLOGY

The etiology of atherosclerosis is not known. The condition is more common in males, in individuals who smoke tobacco, have hypertension, are obese, have elevated serum cholesterol, eat a high-fat diet, have diabetes, or are inactive. These risk factors or markers seem to regulate the acceleration rate of the disease in individuals who have a genetically determined tendency toward the disease. The response-to-injury theory is considered one of the best hypotheses to explain how the lesion develops in patients with or without risk factors (Fig. 6.9).

ABNORMAL PHYSIOLOGY

An adequate amount of blood carrying a proper amount of oxygen must reach the myocardial cells so that they can contract and relax 60–90 times each minute for as long as one lives. Blood flow is de-termined by pressure gradients. The left ventricular myocardium in the normal heart is perfused during diastole when the pressure in the coronary arteries is about 80 mmHg and the pressure within the left ventricle is 0–5 mmHg. There is less myocardial perfusion during systole because the systolic pressure in the coronary epicardial arteries is about equal to the systolic pressure within the left ventricle. The myocardial perfusion of the right ventricle is different from that of the left ventricle and septum. It occurs during diastole and systole, because the pressure in the coronary arteries during diastole and systole is always higher than that within the right ventricle. It is easy to understand why tachycardia, with consequent short diastoles, influences myocardial perfusion of the left ventricle and septum. Furthermore the amount of blood delivered to the myocardium must be regulated so that more blood can be delivered during exercise than during rest. Although the epicardial coronary arteries can change their

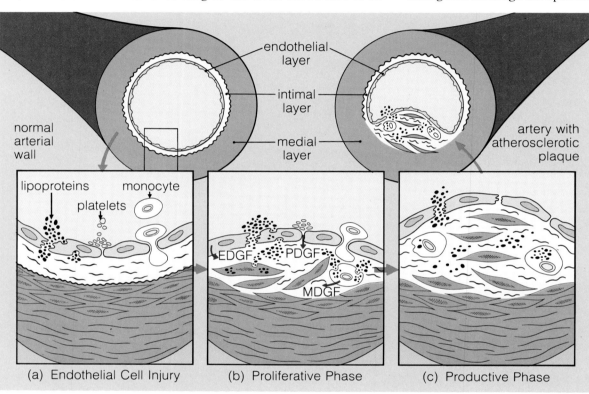

FIG. 6.9 *In the genesis of an atherosclerotic plaque, endothelial cell injury* (a) *leads to excessive influx of lipoproteins, invasion of monocytes/macrophages, and adherence of platelets. This leads to a proliferative phase* (b) *in which a macrophage reaction and release of growth factors (EDGF, MDGF, PDGF) set in motion a process of smooth muscle proliferation, eventually resulting in a productive phase* (c) *in which connective tissue elements are formed leading to distinct plaque formation. (Adapted; see Figure Credits)*

(a) Endothelial Cell Injury   (b) Proliferative Phase   (c) Productive Phase

---

Table 6.1 Clinical Spectrum of Atherosclerotic Coronary Heart Disease*

Coronary atherosclerosis without angina or other evidence of ischemia
Coronary atherosclerosis with reversible myocardial ischemia
  Stable subsets
    Stable angina pectoris
    Positive exercise test
    Angina equivalents
  Unstable subsets
    Unstable angina pectoris and equivalents
    Postinfarction angina pectoris
    Prinzmetal's angina pectoris
    Prolonged myocardial ischemia without objective evidence of infarction

Coronary atherosclerosis with irreversible myocardial ischemia and necrosis
  Very early profound ischemia
  Early evolving infarction
  Uncomplicated completed infarction
  Complicated infarction
Sudden death†
Syncope†
Cardiac arrhythmias†
Ischemic cardiomyopathy‡
Atherosclerotic coronary heart disease in combination with other conditions

(Table 45-1, *The Heart,* 6th ed, p 888)

*This classification of atherosclerotic coronary heart disease permits the linkage of pathophysiology, clinical syndromes, prognosis, and specific treatment. Clear definitions of the syndromes and their treatment are discussed in the text.

†Sudden death may occur in patients with reversible myocardial ischemia. It may also occur in patients who have had infarction due to irreversible myocardial ischemia. The mechanism for syncope may be similar to the mechanism for sudden death. Cardiac arrhythmias occurring in patients with coronary atherosclerotic heart disease may be, but are not always, due to myocardial ischemia.

‡The hearts of patients with ischemic cardiomyopathy have areas of infarction due to irreversible ischemia. The same patients may also experience episodes of reversible ischemia.

size, they do not control coronary flow as much as the small intra-myocardial coronary branches, which are called *resistance arterioles*. Considerable research is now designed in an effort to understand the factors that control the resistance vessels. One of these factors is the effect of end-diastolic ventricular pressure on myocardial perfusion (see Fig. 2.11).

Coronary blood flow is not impeded until an obstructing lesion occludes about 50% of the luminal diameter of the artery, which is equivalent to 75% cross-sectional obstruction. This degree of stenosis may permit adequate myocardial perfusion when the individual is at rest but not during exercise. This leads to consideration of the supply–demand concept of myocardial perfusion. The supply end of the system includes the coronary artery pressure, size of the coronary artery lumen, and oxygen content of the blood, while the demand end of the system includes the work of the myocardium and myocardial cellular metabolism. Certain clinical syndromes, which are discussed later, can be analyzed in terms of this concept: Is the myocardial ischemia due to a problem in the supply end of the myocardial perfusion system, in the demand end of the myocardial perfusion system, or in both ends of the system? At times specific therapy can be linked to the pathophysiologic fault that is deduced to be present. The condition is then designated by a certain carefully chosen term. This approach has ushered in a new era in which it is possible to think in pathophysiologic terms about the basic mechanisms responsible for clinical syndromes.

CLINICAL MANIFESTATIONS

The clinical syndromes associated with atherosclerotic coronary disease are listed in Table 6.1. These syndromes and subsets are defined later and, when possible, the pathophysiology responsible for each subset is stated along with the prognosis and treatment. Initially it is necessary to discuss the methods of identifying the various syndromes.

Table 6.2 Grading of Effort Required to Produce Angina By The Canadian Cardiovascular Society

Class 1: Ordinary physical activity does not cause . . . angina, such as walking and climbing stairs. Angina with strenuous or rapid or prolonged exertion at work or recreation.

Class 2: Slight limitations of ordinary activity. Walking or climbing stairs rapidly, walking uphill, walking or stair climbing after meals, or in cold, or in wind, or under emotional stress, or only during the few hours after awakening. Walking more than two blocks on the level and climbing more than one flight of ordinary stairs at a normal pace and in normal conditions.

Class 3: Marked limitation of ordinary physical activity. Walking one to two blocks on the level and climbing one flight of stairs in normal conditions and at normal pace.

Class 4: Inability to carry on any physical activity without discomfort. Anginal syndrome *may* be present at rest.

(Reproduced with permission of the author and publisher; see Figure Credits. Also, Table 6-1, *The Heart*, 6th ed, p 108)

CLINICAL SETTING

Coronary atherosclerosis is more common in males than in females, but in either sex it occurs more frequently in individuals who are in a certain age range (30–70 years); smoke tobacco; are hypertensive; have hyperlipidemia; are obese; have a carotid artery bruit, abdominal aneurysm, or peripheral arterial disease; have diabetes; are inactive; have hyperuricemia; have certain electrocardiographic abnormalities; have a type A personality; have a family history of premature atherosclerotic coronary disease; have xanthoma; have had mediastinal irradiation; are undergoing renal dialysis; or have had a cardiac transplant. In females the use of contraceptive pills is an additional risk factor.

Coronary atherosclerosis is common even when the factors listed above are absent. Conversely the disease may not be present even when several of the risk factors are present. However, the disease is more common in a population of subjects when risk factors are present, as compared with a population of subjects when risk factors are absent. Data other than risk factors are required to diagnose the presence of the disease in an individual patient.

HISTORY

The patient may have serious and advanced coronary atherosclerosis without symptoms. Sudden death from the disease may occur without preceding symptoms. The patient may even have objective evidence of repeated bouts of myocardial ischemia with no symptoms; this is called *silent ischemia*.

In patients who experience *angina pectoris* due to myocardial ischemia the discomfort is usually located in the retrosternal area. They may use a variety of adjectives to describe the discomfort: tightness, indigestion, burning, aching, pain, or simply a "bad" feeling in the chest. Angina pectoris is classified as any unpleasant feeling in the retrosternal area that has not been noted previously. The discomfort may radiate into the left arm, right arm, throat, mandible, or upper back. It is occasionally located in the precordial area. The duration of the discomfort is usually one to three minutes and rarely lasts longer than ten minutes. The discomfort is usually precipitated by effort, emotional distress, exposure to cold, or eating. Angina pectoris is usually relieved by nitroglycerin.

The chest discomfort thought to be angina pectoris due to atherosclerotic heart disease must be differentiated from discomfort associated with other diseases, such as emotional disturbances, esophageal reflux, esophageal spasm, esophageal rupture, peptic ulcer, gallbladder disease, herpes zoster, Tietze's syndrome, chest wall syndromes, thoracic outlet syndrome, pneumothorax, mediastinal emphysema, pulmonary emboli, pericarditis, other causes of myocardial ischemia such as aortic valve disease and cardiomyopathy, and other causes of coronary disease such as coronary spasm, dissecting aneurysm, and pulmonary hypertensive pain (see Chapter 45, *The Heart*, 6th ed). It is important to remember that angina pectoris due to coronary atherosclerosis is common as are many of the other causes of chest discomfort. Accordingly the coexistence of two conditions, each causing chest discomfort, is also common. The identification of one cause of chest discomfort does not exclude another cause.

There are several different types of angina pectoris (see Table 6.1). The effort necessary to product angina can be graded according to the guidelines established by The Canadian Cardiovascular Society (Table 6.2). The predictive value of the history of angina pectoris depends upon the type of history obtained (Table 6.3).

Table 6.3 Predictive Value of the History Indicating Atherosclerotic Heart Disease

TYPE 1	TYPE 2	TYPE 3
Male, aged 45 and over; retrosternal chest discomfort produced by effort; history easily obtained. —predictive value >90%.	Male, aged 45 and over; retrosternal chest discomfort not always produced by effort and often occurring at rest; history difficult to obtain. —predictive value 75%.	Female, aged 45–50; retrosternal chest discomfort produced by effort or occurring at rest; history easily obtained or obtained with difficulty. —predictive value 50%.

Patients may experience chest discomfort that lasts longer than angina pectoris. This symptom is designated as *prolonged chest discomfort due to myocardial ischemia*. The discomfort is similar to angina pectoris but lasts from 10–20 minutes to several hours, usually occurring while the patient is at rest. Cardiac muscle may or may not be permanently damaged; when it is, *myocardial infarction* is diagnosed. The condition must be differentiated from many of the same conditions listed under angina pectoris.

There are several subsets of both angina pectoris and prolonged myocardial ischemia (see Table 6.1). These are discussed later (see below, "Definition and Treatment of Various Subsets of Coronary Atherosclerotic Heart Disease").

Angina equivalents are due to ischemia but are not associated with chest pain (see Table 6.1). The patient may have palpitation, dyspnea on effort, or exhaustion. *Palpitation* may occur at rest or with effort. Palpitation due to a cardiac arrhythmia is usually not caused by ischemia

except under certain circumstances. *Dyspnea* on effort or at rest as a new symptom in a patient without lung disease may be due to transient global myocardial ischemia, which results in an elevation of left ventricular diastolic pressure, left atrial pressure, and pulmonary venous pressure. *Exhaustion* on effort or at rest in a middle-aged person who has no other cause for the symptom may be due to global ischemia secondary to coronary atherosclerosis, which results in decreased cardiac output during exercise. Angina equivalents have less predictive value than angina, but they provide important clues to pursue.

PHYSICAL EXAMINATION

The physical examination of a patient with coronary atherosclerosis is usually normal. Carotid artery bruit, abdominal aneurysm, or peripheral arterial disease in a man indicates that the patient is more likely to have coronary atherosclerosis. Examination during an attack of angina pectoris may reveal pallor and an atrial or ventricular gallop sound.

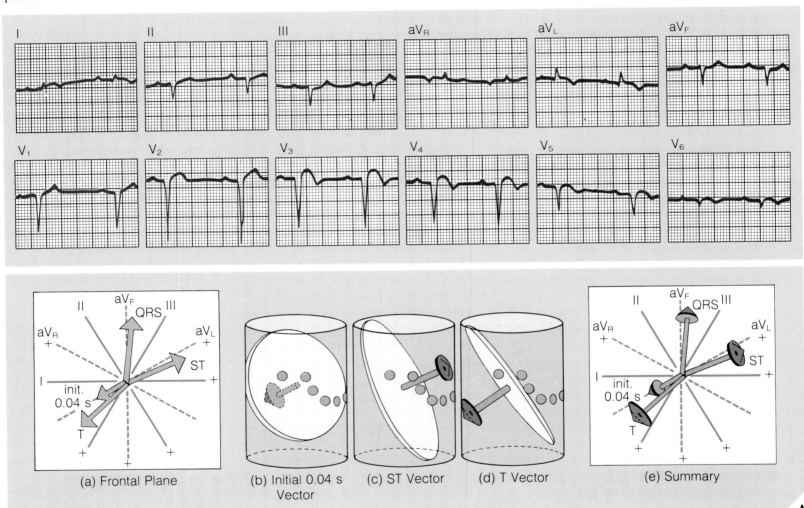

A

FIG. 6.10 (A) *ECG of a 48-year-old patient shows an extensive anterior myocardial infarction. (a) The QRS complexes are resultantly negative in leads II and III and slightly positive in lead I; this can be represented by a mean vector directed relatively parallel with the negative limb of lead aV_F but directed so that a small positive quantity will be projected on lead I. The initial 0.04 second portion of the QRS cycle is negative in leads I and aV_L and positive in lead III and can be represented by a small mean vector directed perpendicular to lead II. The T wave is large and positive in lead III and slightly positive in lead aV_R and can be represented by a mean vector directed just to the right of the positive limb of lead III. The ST segment is elevated in leads I, II, and aV_L and slightly depressed in leads III, aV_R, and aV_F. Accordingly the mean ST vector is directed relatively parallel with the positive limb of aV_L but directed so that a small positive quantity will be projected on lead II. (b,c,d) The mean initial 0.04 second vector is rotated markedly posteriorly and deviated from the frontal plane approximately*

80° because the initial 0.04 second is negative in all the precordial leads. The mean ST vector is rotated at least 45° anteriorly because the ST segment is elevated in all the precordial leads but is less elevated in V_1 and V_6. The mean T vector is approximately flush with the frontal plane because the T wave is upright in lead V_1 and inverted in leads V_2–V_6. (e) Final summary figure illustrates the spatial arrangement of the vectors. The mean spatial initial 0.04 second vector is located abnormally to the right and is posteriorly directed. This vector is directed away from a large area of anterior dead zone. The mean ST vector is directed toward an area of epicardial injury located in the anterolateral portion of the left ventricle. The mean T vector is rotated away from an area of anterolateral epicardial ischemia. It is interesting that the tracing was made three months after the acute infarction and that the abnormal ST vector is still present, suggesting the possibility of ventricular aneurysm at the site of infarction. (Redrawn; reproduced with permission of the authors and publisher; see Figure Credits)

The patient with septal rupture due to infarction may have a systolic murmur that is heard to the left of the midsternal area or occasionally at the apex. Rupture of a papillary muscle due to infarction may produce a systolic murmur at the apex. Such a murmur may not be present when the systolic pressure is low.

The patient with ischemic cardiomyopathy may exhibit an abnormally prolonged apex impulse and atrial and ventricular gallop sounds, as well as other physical signs of heart failure. A myocardial aneurysm may produce an abnormal pulsation of the precordium; such a pulsation may be seen and felt.

LABORATORY STUDIES
CHEST RADIOGRAPHY

The chest film of a patient with coronary atherosclerosis is usually normal. The heart may be large when there is ischemic cardiomyopathy or when multiple myocardial infarcts have occurred; evidence of heart failure may be found in such patients. A ventricular aneurysm may be noted. On rare occasion calcification of the coronary arteries or of the myocardium due to an old infarction may be seen.

ELECTROCARDIOGRAPHY

The resting electrocardiogram (ECG) is usually normal in patients with angina pectoris due to coronary atherosclerosis. A small percentage of patients show ST-segment displacement (mean ST vector directed away from the cardiac apex) or T-wave abnormalities.

The ECG may be normal or nondiagnostic in about 20% of patients with other evidence of myocardial infarction. The abnormalities, when present, include the following: the mean vector for the initial 0.04 second of the QRS complexes points away from the infarction; the mean ST vector points toward the area of infarction; the mean T vector points away from the area of infarction. ECGs showing anterior and inferior myocardial infarctions are shown in Figure 6.10A,B.

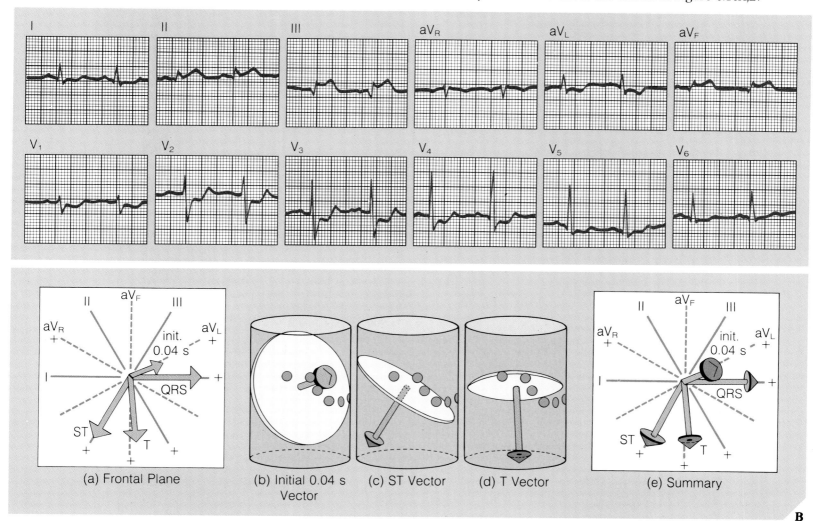

B

FIG. 6.10 (B) *ECG of a 62-year-old patient shows an acute posterior myocardial infarction. (a) The frontal plane projection shows the mean QRS, ST, T, and initial 0.04 second vectors. The mean QRS vector is directed perpendicular to lead aV_F because the QRS complex is resultantly zero in lead aV_F. The ST-segment displacement is greatest in lead III and least in lead aV_R and can be represented by a mean vector directed parallel with the positive limb of lead III. The mean T vector is directed just to the left of the positive limb of lead aV_F because the T wave is slightly positive in lead I and large and positive in lead aV_F. The initial 0.04 second of the QRS complex is negative in lead III and aV_F and is resultantly slightly positive in lead II. The initial 0.04 second of the QRS cycle can be represented by a mean vector directed relatively perpendicular to lead II, but it is located so that a small positive quantity will be projected on lead II. (b,c,d) The mean spatial initial 0.04 second vector is rotated approximately 80° anteriorly because the initial 0.04 second of the QRS complex is resultantly*

positive in leads V_1–V_4. (The Q wave in V_5 is 0.02 second in duration and the transitional pathway for the mean initial 0.04 second vector lies near V_6.) The mean spatial ST vector is rotated posteriorly since the ST segment is depressed in all the precordial leads. The mean spatial T vector is tilted at least 15° anteriorly since all the precordial leads record upright T waves. (e) The mean spatial initial 0.04 second vector is abnormal in position because it is located too far to the left of the horizontally directed mean spatial QRS vector. The mean spatial ST vector is directed toward the area of inferoposterior epicardial injury and the mean spatial initial 0.04 second vector is directed away from the area of posterior myocardial necrosis. The infarction is clinically only three hours old and the mean T vector has not yet assumed the position of being directed away from the ischemia surrounding an area of necrosis. (Redrawn; reproduced with permission of the authors and publisher; see Figure Credits)

When the method of vector electrocardiography is understood, it is easy to predict the electrocardiographic signs of infarction of different areas of the left ventricle and septum (Fig. 6.11A–I). All three abnormalities may not be present in every patient. There may be only T wave abnormalities, ST-T abnormalities, or there may be abnormalities of the initial 0.04 second of the QRS complex, T waves, and ST segments.

There are several conditions that may be mistaken for myocardial

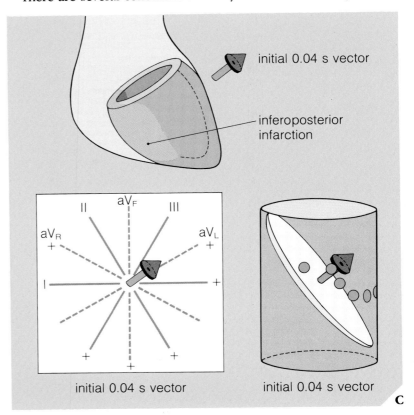

FIG. 6.11 (A) *In this frontal view of the left ventricle as seen within the cardiac silhouette, the dashed lines indicate the endocardial surface. Various regions of the left ventricle are identified. (Redrawn; reproduced with permission of the authors and publisher; see Figure Credits)*

FIG. 6.11 (C) Top, *The myocardial infarction is located on the inferoposterior surface of the left ventricle. The electrical forces generated by the diametrically opposite part of the heart dominate the electrical field during the initial 0.04 second of the QRS cycle and the mean initial 0.04 second vector is directed away from the area of infarction.* **Left,** *The mean initial 0.04 second vector is treated as though it originates in the center of the chest and the hexaxial reference system has been superimposed. This enables one to study the projection of the mean initial 0.04 second vector on the frontal lead axes. In this case a Q wave will be recorded in leads II, III, aV$_F$, and aV$_R$, and an R wave will be recorded in leads I and aV$_L$.* **Right,** *This figure illustrates how the mean initial 0.04 second vector will influence the precordial leads. In this case initial R waves will be recorded in all the precordial leads. (Redrawn; reproduced with permission of the authors and publisher; see Figure Credits)*

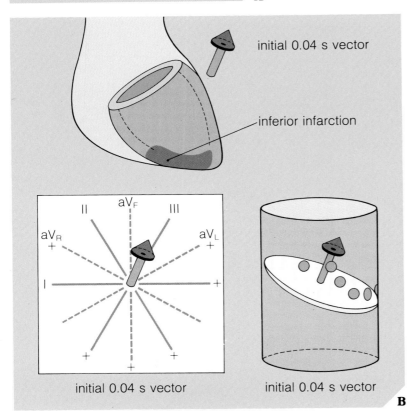

FIG. 6.11 (B) Top, *In myocardial infarction located in the inferior wall of the left ventricle, the electrical forces generated by the muscle of the diametrically opposite wall dominate the electrical field during the initial 0.04 second of the QRS cycle and the mean initial 0.04 second vector is directed away from the area of infarction.* **Left,** *The mean initial 0.04 second vector is treated as though it originates in the center of the chest and the hexaxial reference system has been superimposed. This enables one to study the projection of the mean initial 0.04 second vector on the frontal lead axes. In this case a Q wave will be written in leads II, III, and aV$_F$ and an R wave will be written in leads I, aV$_R$, and aV$_L$. This type of myocardial infarction is usually called an inferior infarction.* **Right,** *This figure illustrates how the mean initial 0.04 second vector will influence the precordial leads. In this case there will be initial R waves in all the precordial leads. (Redrawn; reproduced with permission of the authors and publisher; see Figure Credits)*

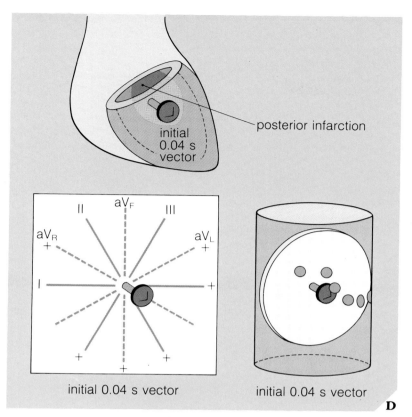

initial 0.04 s vector

initial 0.04 s vector

D

FIG. 6.11 (D) Top, *The myocardial infarction is located on the posterior wall of the left ventricle—a true posterior infarct. The electrical forces generated by the anterior surface of the heart dominate the electrical field during the initial 0.04 second of the QRS cycle.* **Left,** *The mean initial 0.04 second vector is treated as though it originates in the center of the chest and the hexaxial reference system has been superimposed. This enables one to study the projection of the mean spatial 0.04 second vector on the frontal lead axes. In this case the frontal plane projection of the vector is quite small, producing an R wave in leads I, II, aV_F, and aV_L, and a Q wave in lead aV_R. The mean 0.04 second vector is perpendicular to lead III, and therefore the initial 0.04 second of the QRS complex in lead II will be resultantly zero.* **Right,** *This figure illustrates how the mean initial 0.04 second vector will influence the precordial leads. In this cases initial R waves will be recorded in all the precordial leads and the R wave in the right precordial leads will be quite large. (Redrawn; reproduced with permission of the authors and publisher; see Figure Credits)*

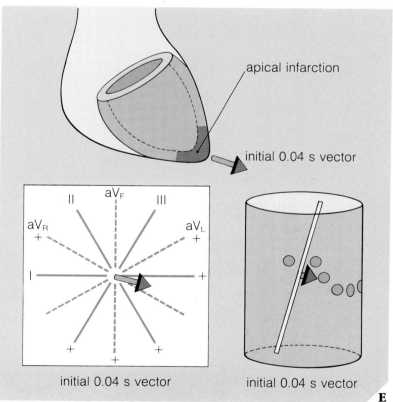

apical infarction

initial 0.04 s vector

initial 0.04 s vector

initial 0.04 s vector

E

FIG. 6.11 (E) Top, *The myocardial infarction is located in the apical portion of the left ventricle. If the infarcted area is relatively small, there may be little change in the QRS contour other than reduced magnitude. This is because a large number of normal initial QRS forces can still be generated by the intact muscle. In addition there may be little ventricular muscle opposite the area of infarction located at the apex and therefore few opposing forces are generated.* **Left,** *The mean initial 0.04 second vector is treated as though it originates in the center of the chest, and the hexaxial reference system is superimposed. This enables one to study the projection of the mean initial 0.04 second vector on the frontal lead axes. In this case the initial 0.04 second vector is quite small and is directed in a normal manner. A small Q wave will be recorded in lead III, but leads I, II, aV_L, and aV_F will record a resultantly positive deflection for the first 0.04 second of the QRS cycle.* **Right,** *This figure illustrates how the mean 0.04 second vector will influence the precordial leads. In this case an initial Q wave will be recorded in lead I and positive R waves will be recorded in leads V_2–V_6. (Redrawn; reproduced with permission of the authors and publisher; see Figure Credits)*

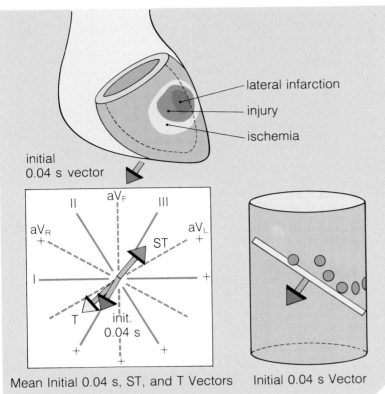

Mean Initial 0.04 s, ST, and T Vectors   **Initial 0.04 s Vector**

F

FIG. 6.11 (F) Top, *The myocardial infarction is located in the lateral portion of the left ventricle. The electrical forces generated in the opposite portion of the heart dominate the electrical field during the initial 0.04 second of the QRS cycle, and the mean initial 0.04 second vector is directed away from the infarction. The area of infarcted tissue is surrounded by an area of myocardial injury located predominantly in the epicardial region of the left ventricle. The mean ST vector will be directed toward the area of epicardial injury. The area of dead and injured tissue is surrounded by an area of epicardial ischemia. The mean T vector will be directed away from the area of epicardial ischemia.* **Left,** *The mean initial 0.04 second, ST, and T vectors are treated as though they originate in the center of the chest and the hexaxial reference system has been superimposed. This enables one to study the projection of the vectors on the lead axes. In this case a Q wave will be recorded in leads I and aV_L and an R wave will be recorded in leads, II, III, and aV_F. The mean initial 0.04 second vector is perpendicular to lead aV_R, and therefore the initial 0.04 second of the QRS complex in lead aV_R will be resultantly zero. The ST segment will be elevated in leads I and aV_L and depressed in leads II, III, aV_F, and aV_R. The T wave will be inverted in leads I and aV_L and upright in leads II, III, aV_F, and aV_R.* **Right,** *This figure illustrates how the mean initial 0.04 second vector will influence the precordial leads. In this case a Q wave will be recorded in leads V_2–V_6. Although it is not illustrated, the ST segment would be elevated in leads V_2–V_6 and depressed in lead V_1. The T wave would be inverted in V_2–V_6, and upright in lead V_1. (Redrawn; reproduced with permission of the authors and publisher; see Figure Credits)*

Mean Initial 0.04 s, ST, and T Vectors   **Initial 0.04 s Vector**

G

FIG. 6.11 (G) Top, *The myocardial infarction is located in the anterior and septal region of the left ventricle. The electrical forces generated in the opposite portion of the ventricular muscle dominate the electrical field during the initial 0.04 second of the QRS cycle, and the mean initial 0.04 second vector is directed away from the infarcted area. The area of infarction is surrounded by an area of epicardial myocardial injury. The mean ST vector will be directed toward the area of epicardial injury. The area of dead and injured tissue is surrounded by a zone of epicardial ischemia. The mean T vector will be directed away from the area of epicardial ischemia.* **Left,** *The mean initial 0.04 second, ST, and T vectors are treated as though they originate in the center of the chest, and the hexaxial reference system has been superimposed. This enables one to study the projection of the vectors on the frontal lead axes. In this case the frontal plane projection of the mean initial 0.04 second vector is quite small, producing a Q wave in leads I and aV_L and and an R wave in leads III, aV_F, and aV_R. The mean 0.04 second vector is perpendicular to lead II, and therefore the initial 0.04 second of the QRS complex in lead II will be resultantly zero. The ST segment will be elevated in leads I and aV_L and will be depressed in leads III, aV_F, and aV_R. There will be no ST-segment displacement in lead II. The T wave will be inverted in leads I and aV_L and will be upright in leads II, III, aV_F, and aV_R.* **Right,** *This figure illustrates how the mean initial 0.04 second vector will influence the precordial leads. In this case a Q wave will be recorded in all the precordial leads. Although it is not illustrated, the ST segment would be elevated and the T waves would be inverted in all the precordial leads. (Redrawn; reproduced with permission of the authors and publisher; see Figure Credits)*

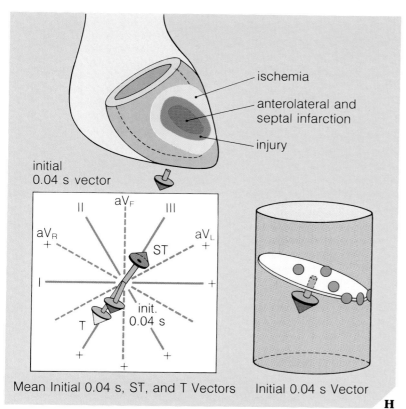

initial
0.04 s vector

Mean Initial 0.04 s, ST, and T Vectors

Initial 0.04 s Vector

H

FIG. 6.11 (H) Top, *The myocardial infarction is located in the anterolateral and septal portion of the left ventricle. The electrical forces generated in the opposite portion of the heart dominate the electrical field during the initial 0.04 second of the QRS cycle, and the mean initial 0.04 second vector is directed away from the infarcted area. The area of dead tissue is surrounded by an area of epicardial myocardial injury, and the ST vector will be directed toward the area of epicardial injury. Surrounding the latter area is an area of epicardial myocardial ischemia. The mean T vector will be directed away from the area of epicardial ischemia.* Left, *The mean initial 0.04 second, ST, and T vectors are treated as though they originate in the center of the chest, and the hexaxial reference system has been superimposed. This enables one to study the projection of the vectors on the frontal lead axes. In this case a Q wave will be recorded in leads I, aV_L, and aV_R and an R wave will be recorded in leads II, III, and aV_F. The ST segment will be elevated in leads I and aV_L and depressed in leads II, III, aV_F, and aV_R. The T wave will be inverted in leads I and aV_L, resultantly zero in lead aV_R, and upright in leads II, III, and aV_F.* Right, *This figure illustrates how the mean initial 0.04 second vector will influence the precordial leads. In this case a Q wave will be recorded in leads V_1–V_3, and the initial 0.04 second of the QRS cycle will be resultantly zero in leads V_4–V_6. Although it is not illustrated, the ST segment would be elevated in leads V_1–V_3, and isoelectric in leads V_4–V_6. The T waves would be inverted in leads V_1–V_3 and flat in leads V_4–V_6. (Redrawn; reproduced with permission of the authors and publisher; see Figure Credits)*

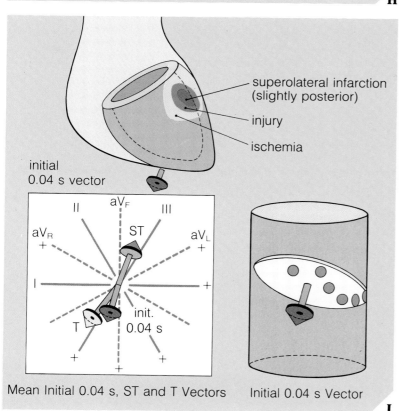

initial
0.04 s vector

Mean Initial 0.04 s, ST and T Vectors

Initial 0.04 s Vector

I

FIG. 6.11 (I) Top, *The myocardial infarction is located in the superolateral wall of the left ventricle and slightly posteriorly. The electrical forces generated in the opposite portion of the ventricular muscle dominate the electrical field during the initial 0.04 second of the QRS cycle and the mean initial 0.04 second vector is directed away from the infarcted area. The area is surrounded by a zone of epicardial injury, and the mean ST vector will be directed toward the area of epicardial injury. The zone of injury is surrounded by a zone of epicardial ischemia, and the mean T vector will be directed away from the zone.* Left, *The mean initial 0.04 second, ST, and T vectors are treated as though they originate in the center of the chest, and the hexaxial reference system has been superimposed. This enables one to study the projection of the vectors on the frontal lead axes. In this case a Q wave will be recorded in leads I, aV_L, and aV_R and an R wave will be recorded in leads II, III, and aV_F. R waves will be written in the precordial leads because the infarct is located in a slightly posterior position. The ST segment will be elevated in leads I, aV_L, and aV_R and depressed in leads II, III, and aV_F. The T wave will be inverted in leads I and aV_L and upright in leads II, III, aV_F, and aV_R.* Right, *This figure illustrates how the mean initial 0.04 second vector would influence the precordial leads in this particular case. Initial R waves will be recorded in all the precordial leads. Although it is not illustrated, the ST segment would be slightly depressed and the T waves would be upright in all the precordial leads. (Redrawn; reproduced with permission of the authors and publisher; see Figure Credits)*

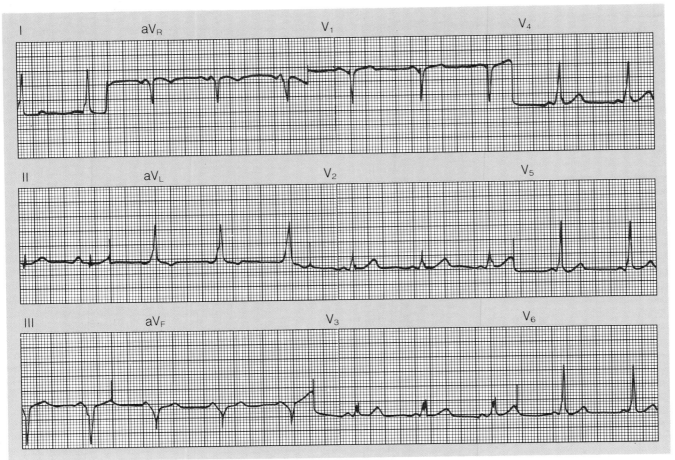

FIG. 6.12 This figure demonstrates the electrocardiographic features of the WPW syndrome (type B). Note the short PR interval and delta waves. There are deep Q waves in leads III and aV_F. Such Q waves may at times be misinterpreted as being due to myocardial infarction. (Redrawn; Fig. 14-22, The Heart, 6th ed; see Figure Credits)

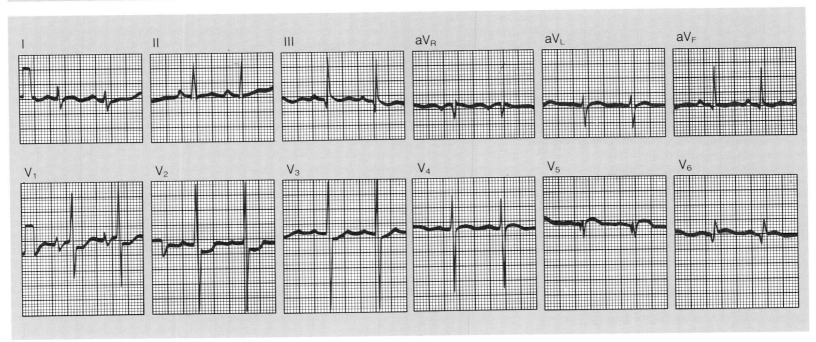

FIG. 6.13 A ten-year-old boy with muscular dystrophy was on digitalis, sodium restriction, and diuretics for heart failure. The abnormal Q waves and ST segment in V_5 and V_6 could be mistaken for myocardial infarction.

(Redrawn; reproduced with permission of the authors and publisher; see Figure Credits)

infarction. The ECG of a patient with the Wolff-Parkinson-White (WPW) syndrome may simulate infarction (Fig. 6.12). The ECGs of patients with hypertrophic cardiomyopathy or dilated cardiomyopathy (including neuromuscular disorders) may mimic infarction (Fig. 6.13).

The ECGs of patients with acute pulmonary embolism may suggest myocardial infarction (Fig. 6.14). Patients with complex congenital lesions, myocardial abnormalities due to sarcoid, amyloid, or neoplastic disease, and acute myocarditis may all exhibit ECGs that re-

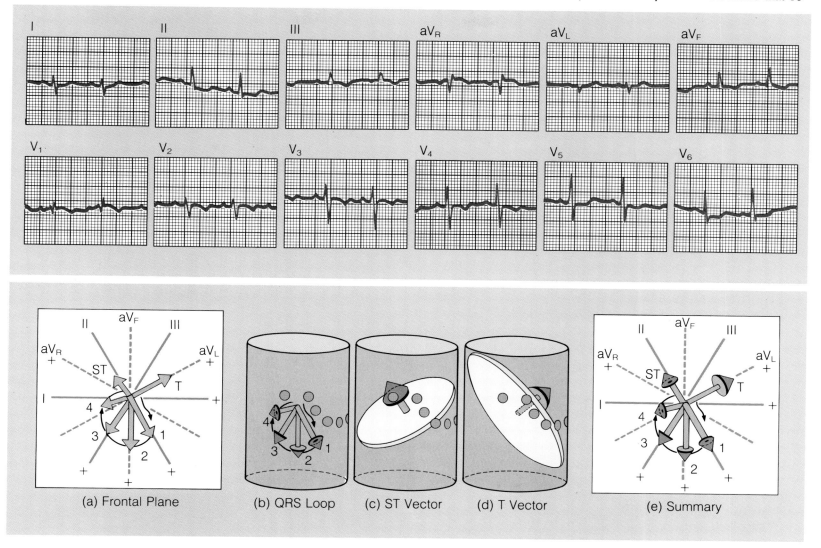

(a) Frontal Plane   (b) QRS Loop   (c) ST Vector   (d) T Vector   (e) Summary

FIG. 6.14 *This ECG of a 54-year-old patient was made shortly after pulmonary embolism. (a) The frontal plane projection shows the mean spatial QRS loop and ST and T vectors. (b) The QRS loop is broken down into four successive spatial instantaneous vectors. Each of these instantaneous vectors is oriented in space producing a rough outline of the mean spatial QRS loop. (c) The mean ST vector is rotated 40° anteriorly because the ST segment is elevated in V_1–V_3 and depressed in V_5 and V_6. (d) The mean T vector is rotated approximately 20° posteriorly because the T wave is inverted in V_1–V_4 and upright in V_5 and V_6. Note that when the mean T vector, or any vector, is in this position, only a small amount of posterior rotation is necessary to produce inverted T waves in several of the precordial leads. (e) Final summary figure illustrates the spatial arrangement of the vectors. The QRS loop is rotund and is inscribed in a clockwise manner.*

The initial forces are to the left and are rotated anteriorly, producing an initial R wave in lead V_1. Vector 4, illustrating the terminal QRS vectors, is directed to the right and anteriorly, producing an S wave in leads I and V_2–V_6, and an R wave in V_1. The mean ST vector is directed toward the right shoulder and indicates subendocardial injury, while the mean T vector is directed to the left and posteriorly, indicating right ventricular ischemia. These findings are typical of acute cor pulmonale secondary to pulmonary embolism. At times only right ventricular ischemia may be present. The inverted T waves in leads V_1–V_4 may stimulate the physician to believe they are due to the ischemic effects of myocardial infarction due to coronary atherosclerotic heart disease, whereas they are actually due to acute pulmonary embolism. (Redrawn; reproduced with permission of the authors and publisher; see Figure Credits)

semble the tracing of myocardial infarction due to coronary atherosclerosis (Figs. 6.15, 6.16).

Right or left bundle branch block may occur, but these abnormalities are also seen with many other forms of heart disease. This is also true for atrial fibrillation, ventricular rhythm disturbances, and atrioventricular block.

The ECG obtained during an exercise stress test may reveal abnormalities not seen in the tracing made while the patient is at rest

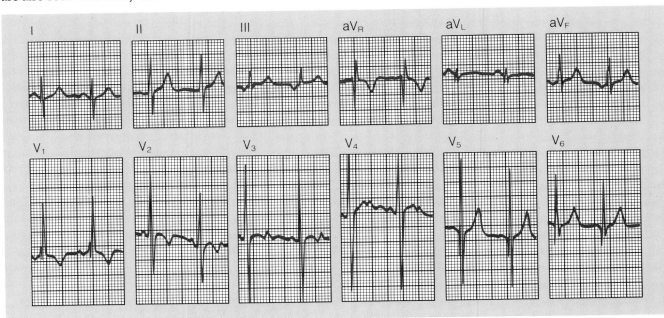

FIG. 6.15 *In a seven-year-old male with aortic septal defect, the large Q waves in leads aV$_L$, V$_5$ and V$_6$ could be misinterpreted as myocardial infarction. They are probably related to septal hypertrophy in this patient with congenital heart disease. (Redrawn; reproduced with permission of the authors and publisher; see Figure Credits)*

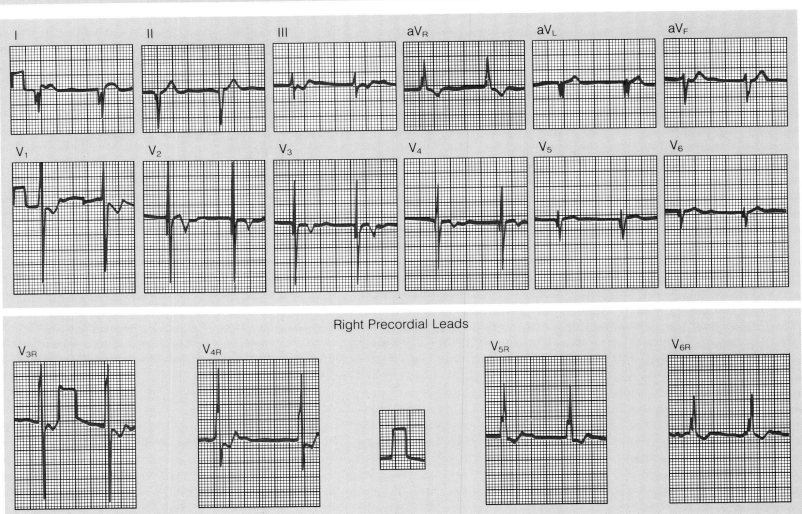

FIG. 6.16 *In a nine-year-old boy with congenital heart disease the diagnostic studies were compatible with isolated dextrocardia, transposition of the great vessels, and intracardiac shunt. The Q wave in leads I, II, aV$_L$, and V$_2$–V$_6$ could be misinterpreted as being due to myocardial infarction. (Redrawn; reproduced with permission of the authors and publisher; see Figure Credits)*

PART II: DISEASES OF THE HEART

(Fig. 6.17). The Bruce protocol is commonly used as the standard test. One millimeter or more of downward displacement of the ST segment at the J point that continues for 0.08 second is considered to be a positive response. The predictive value of a positive response in a middle-aged male is about 80%. Therefore a false-positive response occurs in 10%–20% of male patients. The predictive value of a negative response in a middle-aged male excluding coronary disease is about 90%. The predictive value of a positive response in a female 40–50 years of age is about 50%. Therefore a false-positive response is com-

mon in females. The predictive value of a negative response excluding coronary disease in a woman 40–50 years of age is 90% or more.

The exercise ECG is not indicated for diagnostic reasons when the history of stable angina pectoris has a predictive value of 90% (see Table 6.3). An exercise test should not be done routinely in patients thought to have unstable angina. The exercise test rarely clarifies the diagnosis of chest pain in women who are 40–50 years of age. A negative test in such patients is helpful but in practice the number of false-positives makes the test less useful. Other information is obtained

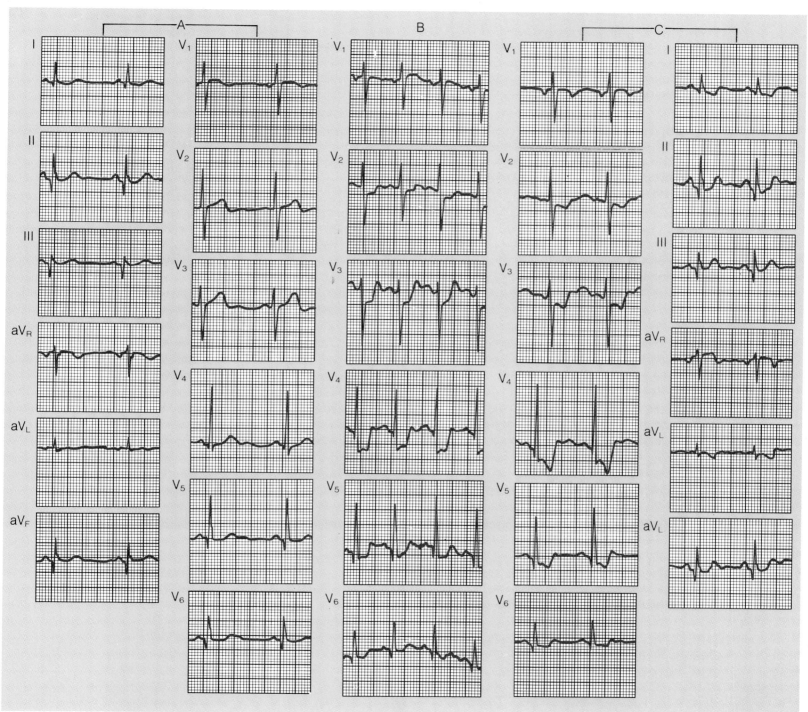

FIG. 6.17 *Rest* (**A**), *exercise* (**B**), *and recovery* (**C**) *ECGs were recorded on a 59-year-old man who underwent treadmill testing to evaluate increasingly severe angina pectoris in the previous six months. Inferior myocardial infarction had occurred six years previously. The resting ECG demonstrates old inferolateral infarction and left atrial abnormality. Exercise was terminated by exertional angina pectoris at a peak heart rate of 110 beats per minute (bpm) and peak workload of 6 METs. Ischemic ST-segment depression is noted during exercise in leads V_2–V_5, maximally (0.5 mV) in lead V_4. Post-* *exertional T-wave inversion is noted in V_2–V_5 accompanied by ischemic ST depression maximally (0.4 mV) in lead V_4. Major lesions in the three major coronary arteries were bypassed surgically. The patient had been largely asymptomatic and without recurrent infarction during the six years following initial infarction; an exercise test performed six months previously demonstrated similar ST-segment abnormalities at a peak heart rate of 145 bpm and peak workload of 9 METs. Beta blockers were withdrawn 72 hours prior to testing. (Redrawn; Fig. 98-4, The Heart, 6th ed; see Figure Credits)*

from an exercise test, including angina or a fall in blood pressure during the test, and the degree of exercise tolerance.

Long-term monitoring of the ECG is indicated when the physician suspects cardiac arrhythmia after myocardial infarction. Artifacts may occur in such recordings and the physician must be aware of their appearance.

ECHOCARDIOGRAPHY

Most patients with coronary atherosclerosis have normal echocardiograms prior to the development of cardiac muscle damage. The echocardiogram (Fig. 6.18) can be used to detect left ventricular thrombi, right ventricular thrombi, or wall-motion abnormalities including a left ventricular aneurysm; it is also used to calculate the ejection fraction and to show pericardial effusion. Other conditions may also be identified. This is important because coronary disease may coexist with many other conditions or other diseases may mimic coronary disease.

CARDIAC CATHETERIZATION

Coronary arteriography and left ventriculography are now commonplace since it became obvious that both types of studies are necessary in the majority of patients in whom coronary atherosclerosis is suspected. The risk of the procedure is about 0.01% or less. Coronary arteriography and left ventriculography are used for diagnostic purposes and to determine if coronary bypass surgery or coronary angioplasty are needed for proper treatment (Fig. 6.19).

Coronary arteriography and left ventriculography are indicated in the following cases:

in patients with a positive exercise ECG or thallium stress test;
in young patients with stable angina pectoris;
in elderly patients with disabling stable angina pectoris;
in patients with unstable angina (unless they are elderly and have other reasons why angioplasty or surgery should not be employed);
early in infarction when thrombolytic therapy is used or when emergency angioplasty or surgery is to be used in therapy;
following infarction when angina continues or occurs for the first time;
following infarction when the submaximal ECG stress test or the thallium stress test is positive;
in patients in whom surgery is planned for abdominal aneurysm or peripheral arterial disease and the dipyridamole [201]thallium (^{201}Tl) test is abnormal;
and in patients undergoing cardiac catheterization for valve disease.

NUCLEAR STUDIES

The technetium-99m (^{99m}Tc) ventriculogram, including the first pass, can be used to measure the ejection fraction at rest and with exercise (Fig. 6.20). The normal resting ejection fraction is 50%–70% and normally should increase with exercise. Patients with myocardial ischemia

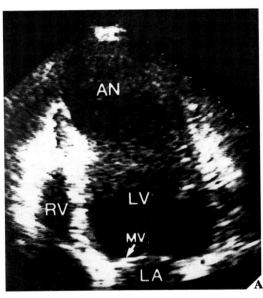
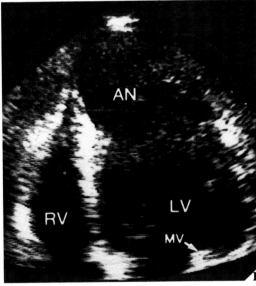
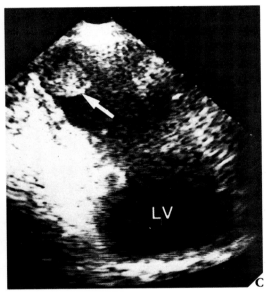

FIG. 6.18 *In these cross-sectional echocardiograms obtained in a patient with a recent anterior myocardial infarction the systolic frame of the apical four-chamber view (**A**) and diastolic frame of the same view (**B**) show a large apical aneurysm (AN). The left ventricle (LV) is moderately dilated at its base, but there is extensive thinning of the apical wall. The aneurysm has* *a wide neck and fundus. (**C**) Apical two-chamber view shows a round mass (arrow) partially filling the aneurysm as it extends from the surface of the akinetic wall, indicative of a mural thrombus (RV, right ventricle; LA, left atrium; MV, mitral valve). (Fig. 120-33, The Heart, 6th ed; see Figure Credits)*

Left Coronary Artery

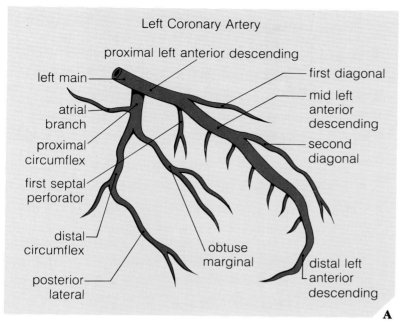

proximal left anterior descending

left main
atrial branch
proximal circumflex
first septal perforator
distal circumflex
posterior lateral

first diagonal
mid left anterior descending
second diagonal
obtuse marginal
distal left anterior descending

A

Right Coronary Artery

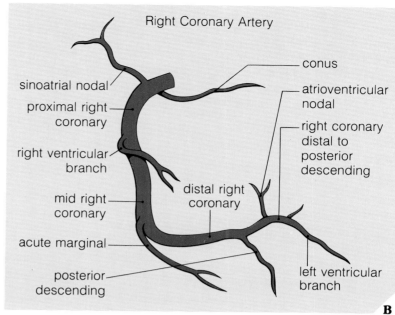

sinoatrial nodal
proximal right coronary
right ventricular branch
mid right coronary
acute marginal
posterior descending

conus
atrioventricular nodal
right coronary distal to posterior descending
distal right coronary
left ventricular branch

B

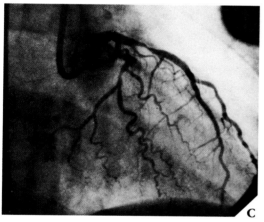

C

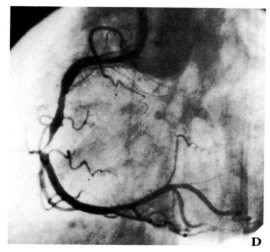

D

FIG. 6.19 (A) *Anatomy of the left coronary artery as seen in the right anterior oblique view.* (B) *Anatomy of the right coronary artery as seen in the left anterior oblique view.* (C) *Right anterior oblique view of the left coronary artery shows high-grade stenosis of the left anterior descending branch proximal to the first septal perforating branch.* (D) *Left anterior oblique view of the right coronary artery shows a high-grade lesion in its midportion.* (A: Fig. 108-37; B: Fig. 108-40; C: Fig. 108-38; D: Fig. 108-41; The Heart, 6th ed; see Figure Credits)

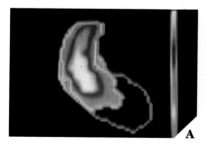

A

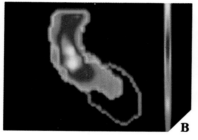

B

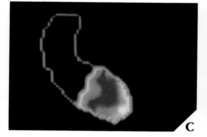

C

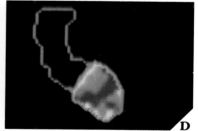

D

FIG. 6.20 *First-pass* ^{99m}Tc *scan of a 45-year-old man shows coronary arteriographic evidence of a 48% diameter narrowing of the left anterior descending artery. The abnormal test result influenced the physicians to conclude that the borderline lesion in the left anterior descending artery was significant.* (A) *In this scan, taken at rest, the blue line represents the end-diastolic contour; the outer limit of the purple area represents the end-systolic contour.* (B) *In this image, taken during exercise, the blue line represents the end-diastolic contour, and the outer limit of the purple area represents the end-systolic contour. Note that the purple area is larger and* the distance between it and the blue line is smaller after exercise. This abnormality represents anterior hypokinesis after exercise. (C,D) *These images reveal that the regional ejection fraction is diminished in the outer myocardial wall during exercise. The left ventricular ejection infraction at rest was 69% and during exercise it declined to 66%; this is abnormal. The left ventricular end-diastolic volume at rest was 122 mL and during exercise it was 151 mL; this is abnormal. The left ventricular end-systolic volume at rest was 38 mL and during exercise it was 51 mL; this is abnormal. (Courtesy of Gordon DePuey, MD, Atlanta, Georgia)*

due to coronary atherosclerosis may have a low resting ejection fraction or one that may not increase with exercise. Patients with cardiomyopathy or elderly subjects who are unaccustomed to exercise may have similar findings.

The exercise ^{201}Tl scan with resting reperfusion studies may demonstrate evidence of infarction or exercise-induced ischemia (Fig. 6.21). Left bundle branch block may give false-positive evidence indicating ischemia.

Nuclear studies do not identify nonobstructive coronary atherosclerosis. Such studies do not become abnormal until the coronary obstruction is sufficiently severe to interfere with coronary blood flow. Even when the coronary disease is sufficiently severe to produce myocardial ischemia, the nuclear tests are only about 85% sensitive and about 90% specific. Nuclear studies have their greatest value as screening tests in patients whose pretest probability of coronary disease is in the intermediate-to-low range. The ^{201}Tl scan may be used following coronary arteriography as a means of judging the significance of borderline lesions.

CARDIAC ENZYMES

The MB band of serum creatine phosphokinase (CK) becomes elevated when a sufficient number of myocardial cells die. Accordingly the test is used when myocardial infarction is suspected.

In general the larger the infarct, the higher the CK and MB band. The prognosis becomes poorer as the levels of CK and MB band increase. It is important to remember, however, that a patient with infarction who has only a little rise in CK and MB band due to a small infarction may have a poor prognosis if there has been a previous infarction. The total amount of myocardial damage determines the prognosis.

It should also be emphasized that there are many serious coronary events that are not associated with permanent myocardial damage. Therefore the failure of the CK and MB band to rise does not imply that an episode of chest pain due to myocardial ischemia is harmless.

OTHER LABORATORY TESTS

Determinations of the fasting blood sugar and lipid profile are often indicated in patients with coronary atherosclerosis.

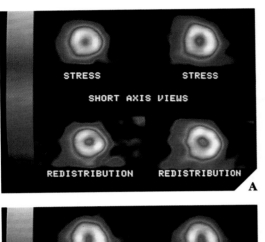

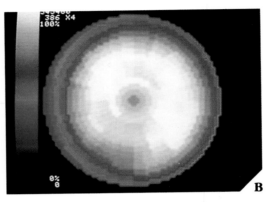

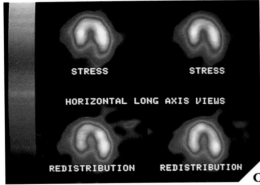

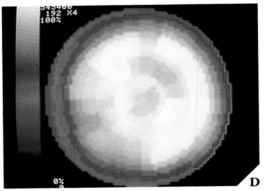

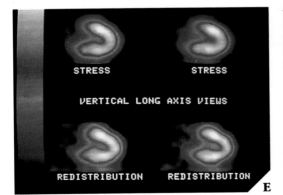

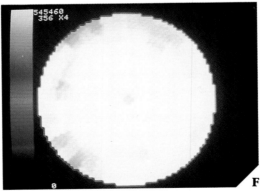

FIG. 6.21 (A–F) *Normal tomographic* ^{201}*Tl study was obtained using a rotating gamma scintillation camera. Selected tomographic slices are shown at stress and redistribution in the short axis* (A), *horizontal long axis* (C), *and vertical long axis* (E). *Note the uniform homogeneous uptake of* ^{201}*Tl in the myocardium.* (B,D,F) *Functional quantitative images ("bull's-eye displays") are also shown. Each short-axis tomographic slice from apex to base is subjected to maximal count circumferential profile analysis. These profiles then are displayed as a series of concentric circles with the apex at the center and the base at the periphery. They are positioned in the same way as are the short-axis tomographic slices shown in part* (A). *The bull's-eye displays in parts* (B) *and* (D) *were obtained from stress and delayed images. Part* (F) *shows the bull's-eye for* ^{201}*Tl washout. Note that there is uniform uptake of* ^{201}*Tl at stress and redistribution and that the washout bull's-eye also is uniform with no abnormal zones depicted* (continued).

NATURAL HISTORY

The prognosis of patients with asymptomatic coronary atherosclerosis who exhibit no other evidence of myocardial ischemia is not known.

The average annual mortality of patients with *stable angina pectoris* who do not have left main coronary artery obstruction is about 3%–4%. When hypertension and abnormal Q waves or ST-segment displacement are present in the ECG, the annual mortality is 8%. The prognosis of patients with stable angina cannot be accurately determined by the severity of the symptoms. Ventricular ectopy probably worsens prognosis, but it is difficult to separate this abnormality from other determinants of survival.

Individuals with an excellent exercise tolerance have a better prognosis than those who do not. If a person can reach a heart rate of 160 beats per minute or attain stage 4 on the Bruce protocol, his or her annual mortality rate will be about 1%–2%. The inability to attain stage 2 because of a cardiac cause is associated with an annual mortality rate of 6%–10%. This predictor is independent of displacement of the ST segment since the absence of ST change does not guarantee a good survival. Also, in patients who have as much as 2 mm of ST-segment displacement in the ECG with exercise, there is a good correlation between the duration of exercise and the five-year survival. The shorter the exercise period required to produce the ECG change, the poorer the prognosis. The development of angina during an exercise test may be an independent marker, while the development of hypotension indicates a poor prognosis.

Kent and co-workers (1982) reported on patients who currently had little or no angina but had a history of previous angina or infarction. They found that the patients who entered the study with triple-vessel disease and a poor exercise performance had 9% annual mortality. In contrast patients with triple-vessel disease who had an excellent exercise performance had an annual mortality of 4%.

Staniloff and colleagues (1982) reported a group of 819 patients who were referred to them for ²⁰¹Tl diagnostic studies. They found that 17% of patients with a severe thallium reperfusion defect had a coronary event during the following years, compared with 1% in patients with no abnormalities. A large reperfusion defect, more than

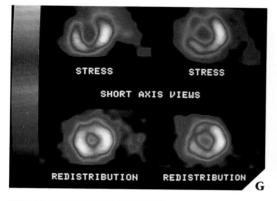
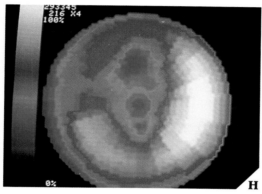

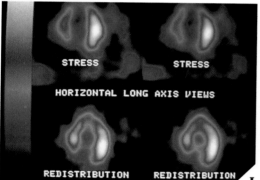
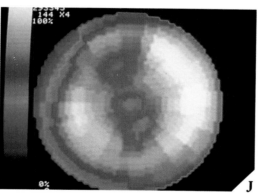

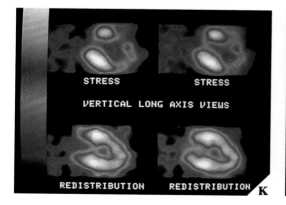
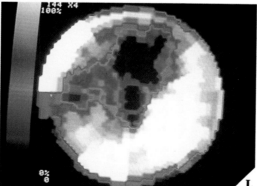

FIG. 6.21 (G–L) *Tomographic* ²⁰¹*Tl images in a patient with critical disease of the left anterior descending coronary artery are shown in the same format as that for parts (A–F). A large perfusion defect is demonstrated in the anterior wall, septum, and apex. Complete redistribution is demonstrated. The bull's eye displays show abnormal* ²⁰¹*Tl uptake at stress with virtually complete normalization at delayed imaging (H,J). In the bull's-eye shown in part (L) there is abnormal* ²⁰¹*Tl washout depicted as dark blue and black, defining the precise zone of myocardial ischemia. (Front and back end papers, The Heart, 6th ed; see also Figure Credits)*

one defect, and hang-up of thallium in the lungs are considered by most workers to be severe defects.

The ejection fraction, determined by ^{99m}Tc ventriculography or the first-pass technique, gives useful information regarding prognosis. Patients with a diminished ejection fraction at rest (or the failure of the ejection to rise with exercise) are in a poor-risk group compared with those with normal ejection fractions at rest that become higher with exercise. There are, of course, other causes of these abnormalities besides coronary disease and this limits the value of the test to some degree. However, ejection fraction as an estimate of ventricular function is a more valuable prognostic marker than the extent of arteriographic narrowing (Fig. 6.22).

Workers at the Cleveland Clinic were the first to present evidence that the anatomic locations of the coronary lesions influenced the survival time of patients with coronary disease (Fig. 6.23).

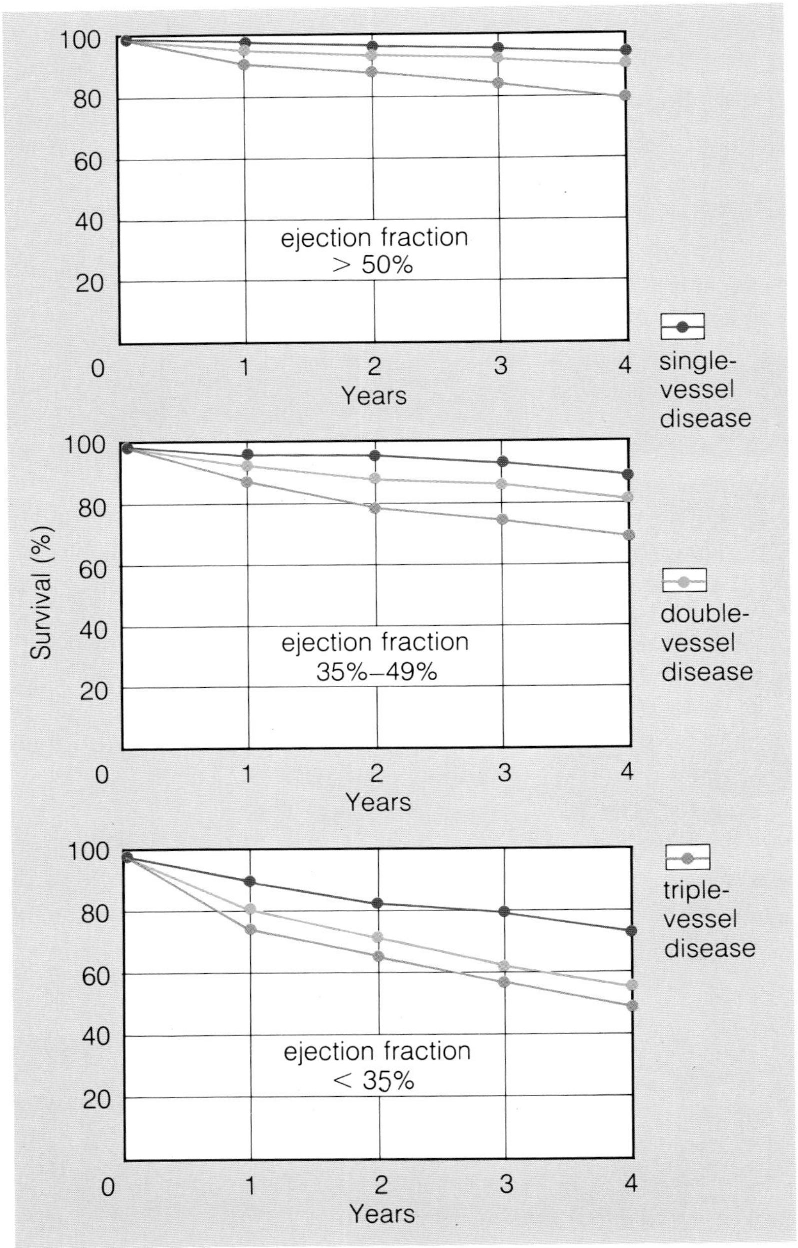

Friesinger has summarized the prognostic implications of angiographic findings in patients with stable angina pectoris as follows:

The data concerning prognostic implications of angiographic findings in stable reversible myocardial ischemia can be summarized. The patient may have stable angina pectoris; no angina but objective evidence of ischemia; or angina equivalents (dyspnea or exhaustion with effort). The prognosis worsens as the extent of arteriographic abnormality increases. The outlook for so-called single-vessel disease and good ventricular function is good, less than 1 to 2 percent mortality rate each year for the 5 years after presentation. Disease localized to the left anterior descending artery carries a poorer prognosis than a similar degree of disease localized to the right coronary artery. Left main coronary artery lesions carry a very poor prognosis. So-called double- and triple-vessel disease are intermediate. The prognosis of patients with

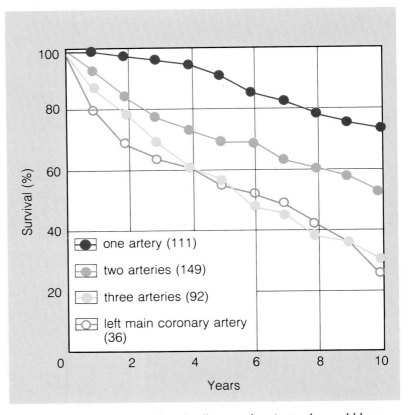

FIG. 6.23 *Survival curves of medically treated patients who could have had coronary bypass surgery but did not. (Redrawn; reproduced with permission of the authors and publisher; see Figure Credits. Also, Fig. 45-30, The Heart, 5th ed, p 1090)*

FIG. 6.22 *Data on the four-year survival in stable patients from the Coronary Artery Surgery Study (CASS) registry involved 6791 patients, 73% with typical angina pectoris. The importance of left ventricular performance, judged on the basis of ejection fraction, is illustrated. Regional wall-motion abnormalities showed a similar trend, i.e., worsening prognosis with increasing wall-motion abnormalities for all grades of coronary arteriosclerosis. (Redrawn; reproduced with permission of the authors and publisher; see Figure Credits. Also, Fig. 45-4, The Heart, 6th ed, p 922)*

PART II: DISEASES OF THE HEART

angina equivalents may be poor because the complaints are sometimes due to severe disease with global myocardial ischemia. There are, however, inadequate reports on such patients. (*The Heart,* 6th ed, p 922)

Patients with *unstable angina pectoris* or prolonged myocardial ischemia without evidence of infarction have a poorer prognosis than patients with stable angina pectoris. The National Cooperative Study (1978) revealed that patients with unstable angina assigned to medical therapy had, at 30 months, a 10% mortality rate, a 19% incidence of infarction, and a 36% cross-over to surgery for unacceptable angina.

Friesinger has summarized the prognostic implication of unstable angina as follows:

The information available regarding the prognosis of patients with the unstable angina syndromes can be summarized. Clinical recognition and *prompt attention to evaluation and therapy are of critical importance in patients with new onset or a change in symptoms since the incidence of sudden cardiac death and myocardial infarction in the 3 to 6 months following onset of an unstable anginal syndrome is higher than in stable patients.* Patients experiencing this presentation of atherosclerotic coronary heart disease represent a broad spectrum. Some will have had stable angina pectoris and/or previous myocardial infarction while others will be experiencing their first manifestation of disease. A higher incidence of left main coronary disease may be present in patients with unstable syndromes. Several studies have reported a 10 to 15 percent incidence of left main coronary artery obstruction which is higher than it is in most reports of stable angina pectoris. Patients who experience ST-segment elevation during episodes or who have episodes persist despite excellent drug therapy or who have had previous symptomatic ischemic heart disease tend to have a worse prognosis than those without such features. Left ventricular function is an important prognostic factor. Finally, the unstable state is a transient phase and judged to persist 3 to 4 months in most patients, following which the patient develops stable angina, and/or becomes asymptomatic. The prognosis then becomes the prognosis of the new clinical subset. A most intriguing area of current research concerns hypotheses which might explain why patients enter the unstable phase of disease. (*The Heart,* 6th ed, pp 923–924)

Patients with *prolonged myocardial pain due to ischemia* without evidence of myocardial infarction may be viewed in another way. Patients with prolonged chest discomfort may not all have coronary disease. If they do, as shown by arteriography, the one to two year prognosis is similar to that of patients who have objective evidence of infarction.

Patients with *Prinzmetal's variant angina* usually have obstructive disease of the epicardial arteries and in addition have coronary artery spasm. A few patients have coronary spasm without coronary atherosclerosis. Waters and colleagues (1982) reported that 18% of patients die during the first three months following the onset of variant angina.

Patients with severe coronary atherosclerosis and left ventricular dysfunction who respond poorly to treatment have the worst prognosis.

Myocardial infarction can be divided into four phases: (1) early myocardial ischemia; (2) evolving infarction; (3) completed infarction; and (4) complicated infarction.

Patients may die with an arrhythmia during the early minutes of an episode of myocardial ischemia; this early phase of infarction is called *very early profound ischemia.* Patients succumbing in this period do not live long enough for infarction to develop. About one fifth of patients with an acute coronary event die within one to two hours.

The period one to six hours after the onset of chest discomfort is designated as the phase of *evolving myocardial infarction.* This distinction is important because early intervention with thrombolytic therapy, coronary angioplasty, or coronary bypass surgery is currently under investigation. The prognostic determinants of an evolving infarct are shown in Table 6.4.

Completed myocardial infarction is defined as the period after the first six hours following the onset of chest pain due to ischemia. In general there is a 6%–10% mortality during the first year after infarction, with more deaths occurring during the first six months than the second six months. The mortality is 3%–4% per year in the second and third year after infarction. In order to identify subsets of patients who are at greater than usual risk, it is necessary to perform either a submaximal exercise ECG, a radionuclide study, or coronary arteriography and ventriculography.

The submaximal exercise ECG stress test performed before the patient with myocardial infarction is discharged from the hospital can be used to determine prognosis. Angina, ST-segment displacement, or poor exercise performance are used as end points in the test. One study of 210 patients revealed that patients who had no ST-segment displacement had a 2.1% mortality the first year after infarction and patients with abnormal ST-segment displacement had a 27% mortality the first year after infarction (Theroux et al, 1979). Patients with a positive response should have a coronary arteriogram because bypass surgery or angioplasty may be needed.

Gibson and collaborators (1983) showed that the results of ^{201}Tl studies in patients after myocardial infarction had higher predictive values for future cardiac events than the results of submaximal exercise ECG testing or arteriography. Leppo and co-workers (1984) used dipyridamole ^{201}Tl scintigraphy in patients prior to discharge after infarction. They noted a much higher mortality in a mean follow-up period of 19 months for patients with transient defects as compared with patients who had no transient defects.

Patients who have complications such as angina or ventricular arrhythmias following infarction should have coronary arteriograms rather than noninvasive tests. Many physicians believe that coronary arteriograms should be performed in most patients following myocardial infarction. Others believe that the procedure should be done only on those patients who are found to be at poor risk by noninvasive means. The ejection fraction is a more powerful predictor of survival than the

---

Table 6.4 Prognostic Determinants: Evolving Myocardial Infarction

Infarct size and ventricular function	Angina pectoris of more than three months' duration
Clinical manifestations (especially left ventricular dysfunction)	Age
ECG changes (especially location of infarct and conduction defects)	Infarct extension
Peak enzyme levels	Heart size (and left ventricular hypertrophy)
Blood pressure	Associated diseases
Previous infarction and scarring	Diabetes
	Hypertension
	Pulmonary disease

(Table 45-4, *The Heart,* 6th ed, p 925)

extent of the coronary disease because most patients with infarction have multivessel disease. The clinician, of course, uses several factors to determine prognosis after infarction (Fig. 6.24).

A *complicated infarction* is defined as one in which certain events occur that alter the prognosis and treatment of the patient. Friesinger's comments highlight the problem of predicting the prognosis of patients with a complicated infarction:

> Several investigators have attempted to utilize the multiplicity and complexity of features involved in estimating prognosis in acute infarction by developing a prognostic index which incorporates those factors that have greatest importance and are additive. In such analyses, objective data are given preference over subjective data (e.g., ECG changes in preference to pain), quantitative information over semiquantitative information (congestion on chest x-ray, or wedge pressure, in preference to rales), and permanent findings over transient figures (e.g., the presence of bundle branch block over rhythm disturbances). (*The Heart*, 6th ed, pp 927–928)

Patients who have angina pectoris, heart failure, shock, or certain arrhythmias after infarct are in a high-risk group. Patients with papillary muscle or septal rupture are at great risk of dying unless surgery is performed without delay. A few patients with external rupture of the heart may be saved by emergency surgery but the number is small. A ventricular aneurysm may develop and be responsible for heart failure, arrhythmias, and systemic emboli.

Sudden death is usually due to an arrhythmia rather than infarction. The one-year mortality of the survivors of sudden death who do not have infarction is 4%, whereas the one-year mortality of the survivors of sudden death associated with infarction is 26%. Ventricular fibrillation occurring in the coronary care unit is not associated with an extremely poor prognosis if it is treated promptly. Such data indicate that ventricular fibrillation that kills early occurs in a pathophysiologic setting that is different from the arrhythmia occurring some hours after infarction.

Patients who have cardiac arrest and are resuscitated outside the hospital should have coronary arteriography. The procedure should also be performed on those patients who had ventricular fibrillation in the coronary care unit.

Heart failure as a result of *ischemic cardiomyopathy* is a serious complication. Half the patients will die within three years. Survival rates of patients with a ventricular aneurysm, mitral regurgitation due to papillary muscle rupture or dysfunction, and even septal rupture may improve with surgery. In contrast patients with diffuse myocardial disease rarely benefit from bypass surgery. Cardiac transplantation may be indicated in some patients with severe ischemic cardiomyopathy.

PREVENTION OF ATHEROSCLEROTIC CORONARY HEART DISEASE

There is evidence to support the view that the elimination or management of risk factors may decelerate the atheromatous process. Many individuals have the disease even when known risk factors are not apparent. This fact suggests that the etiology of the disease may be genetically determined and that the known risk factors are accelerators.

It seems prudent to alter the risk factors, when possible, even though they may only be accelerators. Accordingly tobacco smoking should be curtailed or stopped; hypertension should be controlled; obesity should be avoided; a low-fat, low-cholesterol diet is desirable; a serum cholesterol level of 200 mg/dL or lower should be attained with drugs if dietary control is not successful; diabetes should be controlled; type A personality traits should be altered if possible; and an active exercise program should be pursued. The drug lovastatin has been released for general use. While it reliably lowers the level of serum cholesterol, more research is needed to determine its value and safety.

TREATMENT OF ATHEROSCLEROTIC CORONARY HEART DISEASE

Treatment includes general advice, drug therapy, the use of pacemakers, the use of an intra-aortic balloon, coronary angioplasty, and coronary bypass surgery. These are discussed individually.

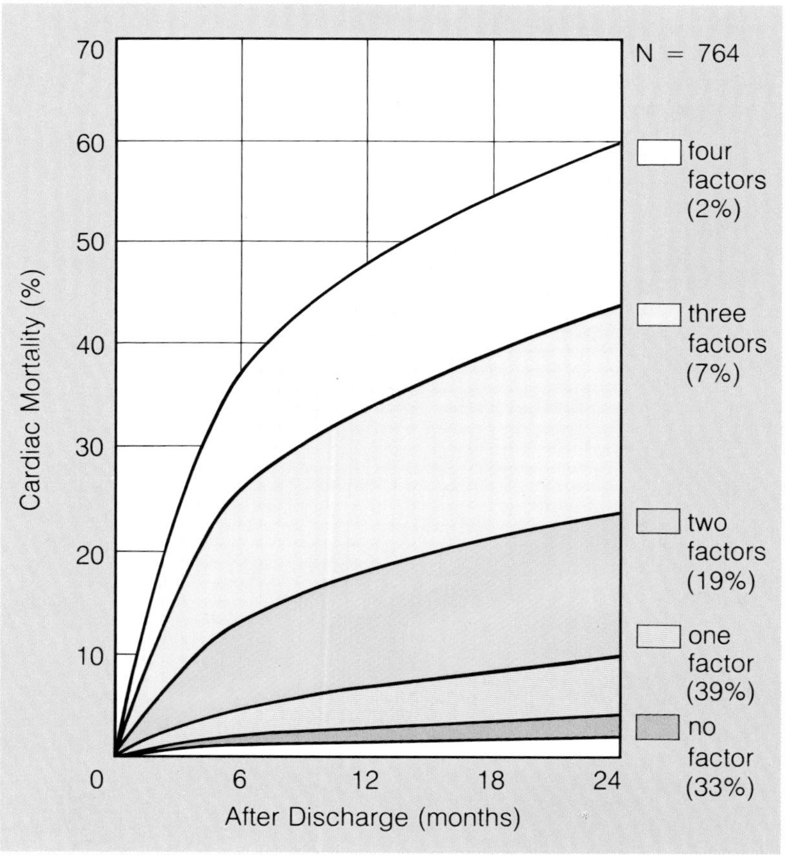

FIG. 6.24 *Risk stratification was graphed for 764 (of 866) patients with completed myocardial infarction. Mortality two years following myocardial infarction varied from 3% for those with none of the factors to 60% if all four factors were present. The four risk factors were (old) New York Heart Association function classes II–IV before admission, pulmonary rales in the upper lung zones during evolving infarction, occurrence of ten or more ventricular ectopic depolarizations per hour, and a radionuclide ejection fraction below 0.40. The data were obtained during the convalescence period and prior to hospital discharge. The numbers in parentheses denote the percentage of the population with the specified number of factors. (Redrawn; reproduced with permission of the authors and publisher; see Figure Credits. Also, Fig. 45-6,* The Heart, *6th ed, p 927)*

GENERAL ADVICE

The reader is referred to the discussion that deals with prevention. The principles discussed there should also be employed in patients who have any evidence of the disease with the hope, but not guarantee, that the disease process may be decelerated.

DRUGS

The reader is referred to Chapter 45, *The Heart* (6th ed) for details on drugs used in treating coronary atherosclerotic heart disease.

NITRATES

Sublingual nitroglycerin for the relief of angina pectoris has been available for decades. Long-acting *transdermal* preparations of nitroglycerin for the prevention of myocardial ischemia have recently become available and, although not totally reliable, they remain popular. A preparation of nitroglycerin for *intravenous* use has also been developed and is used with benefit in patients with frequent episodes of angina. Long-acting *sublingual* and *oral* preparations of nitrates such as isosorbide dinitrate are clearly useful in the prevention of myocardial ischemia and angina.

BETA-BLOCKING DRUGS

Beta-blocking drugs were released for use in the early 1970s. This family of drugs is used to prevent angina pectoris and may prolong the lives of selected categories of poor-risk patients following myocardial infarction. The drugs also are used to treat and prevent atrial and ventricular arrhythmias.

CALCIUM CHANNEL BLOCKING DRUGS

Calcium channel blocking drugs were released for use in the late 1970s for the treatment of patients with angina pectoris due to arteriosclerotic coronary heart disease. These drugs, which include nifedipine, diltiazem, and verapamil, tend to prevent coronary artery spasm.

DIGITALIS

While digitalis has limited application in the treatment of heart failure due to coronary disease, it is still used to control atrial fibrillation.

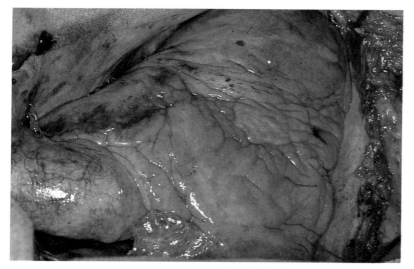

NARCOTICS

Narcotics are used to relieve the pain of infarction; tranquilizers are used to relieve anxiety.

THROMBOLYTIC AGENTS

Thrombolytic agents such as streptokinase and tissue plasmogen activator are used to dissolve the thrombus associated with early infarction.

ANTIARRHYTHMIC DRUGS

Drugs such as beta-blockers, procainamide, lidocaine, quinidine, tocainide, flecainide, maxelitine, amiodarone, and others are used to treat and prevent various arrhythmias that occur in patients with coronary heart disease.

DRUGS USED TO TREAT SHOCK

Drugs such as norepinephrine, dobutamine, and dopamine are used to treat shock due to myocardial infarction.

PACEMAKERS AND INTRA-AORTIC BALLOON PUMPS

Temporary and permanent artificial *pacemakers* are used to treat high-grade atrioventricular block, the sick sinus node syndrome, and certain subsets of bifascicular block. The *intra-aortic balloon* pump is used to treat shock and uncontrolled angina pectoris.

CORONARY BYPASS SURGERY

Coronary bypass surgery relieves angina pectoris and prolongs the lives of carefully selected patients with obstructive coronary disease. The operative risk is about 1% in good-risk patients and up to 4%–5% in certain poor-risk patients. The incidence of perioperative infarction is about 4%. The complications of pericarditis and arrhythmias are easily managed. Major complications, such as stroke and sternal and mediastinal infection, occur in about 1% of patients.

The operative approach to the coronary arteries is almost invariably through a median sternotomy. Though they are surface structures, the coronary arteries are not always easily identifiable, especially in the patient with coronary artery disease (Fig. 6.25). In addition to a covering of epicardial fat, the vessels may lie deep within the atrioventricular groove, and even major branches may take an intramyocardial course.

FIG. 6.25 *The anterior surface of the heart and aorta is viewed through a median sternotomy. The coronary vessels are nearly totally obscured by epicardial fat deposits.*

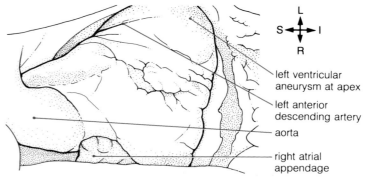

left ventricular aneurysm at apex

left anterior descending artery

aorta

right atrial appendage

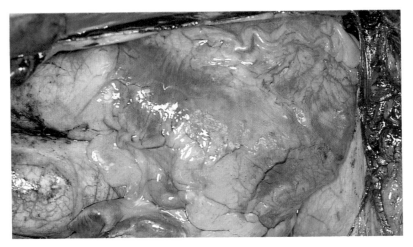

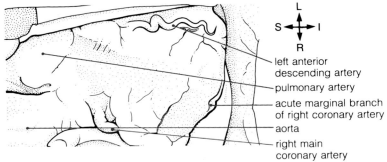

FIG. 6.26 *In this operative view of an adult patient, the coronary arteries are more readily seen. Still, only a portion of the right main coronary artery and the anterior interventricular artery can easily be seen.*

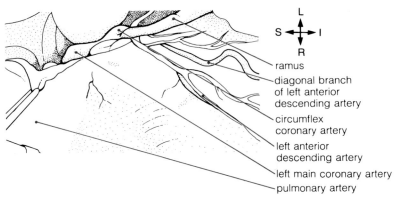

left anterior
descending artery
pulmonary artery
acute marginal branch
of right coronary artery
aorta
right main
coronary artery

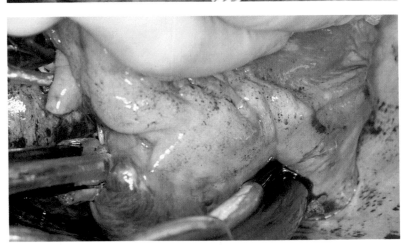

FIG. 6.27 *Tilting the heart slightly out of the pericardium exposes the left main coronary artery and its branches.*

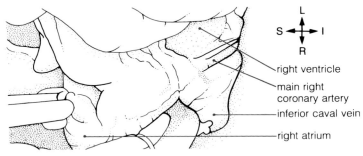

ramus
diagonal branch
of left anterior
descending artery
circumflex
coronary artery
left anterior
descending artery
left main coronary artery
pulmonary artery

FIG. 6.28 *Marked anterior displacement of the apex exposes the distal right main coronary artery in the atrioventricular groove medial to the inferior caval vein.*

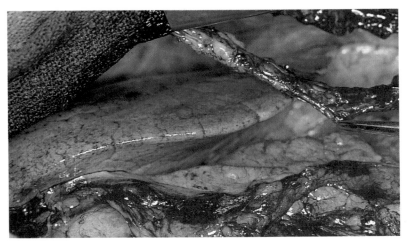

right ventricle
main right
coronary artery
inferior caval vein
right atrium

FIG. 6.29 *Left internal thoracic artery (IMA) is suspended with its pedicle from the anterior chest wall.*

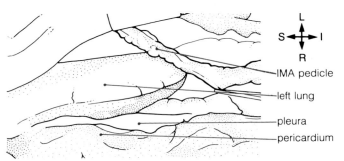

IMA pedicle
left lung
pleura
pericardium

When the heart is viewed through the usual median sternotomy, only a portion of the anterior interventricular branch of the left coronary artery and occasionally a bit of the right coronary may be seen (Fig. 6.26). By lifting the apex of the heart to the right one is afforded a better view of the left-sided branches (Fig. 6.27), and if the apex of the heart is further elevated toward the patient's head, the right coronary artery may be visualized coursing along the right atrioventricular groove (Fig. 6.28). Exposure of these vessels is considerably simplified by induction of car-

dioplegic arrest and emptying the relaxed heart.

Usually multiple grafts are required when performing coronary artery bypass surgery. If possible, one utilizes an internal thoracic artery (i.e., the internal mammary artery, or IMA) (Fig. 6.29) as the bypass of choice because of its superior performance in terms of prolonged patency (Loop et al, 1986). Most often the left IMA is used to bypass lesions in the anterior descending artery (Fig. 6.30). However, with a favorable anatomic arrangement it may be possible to revascularize

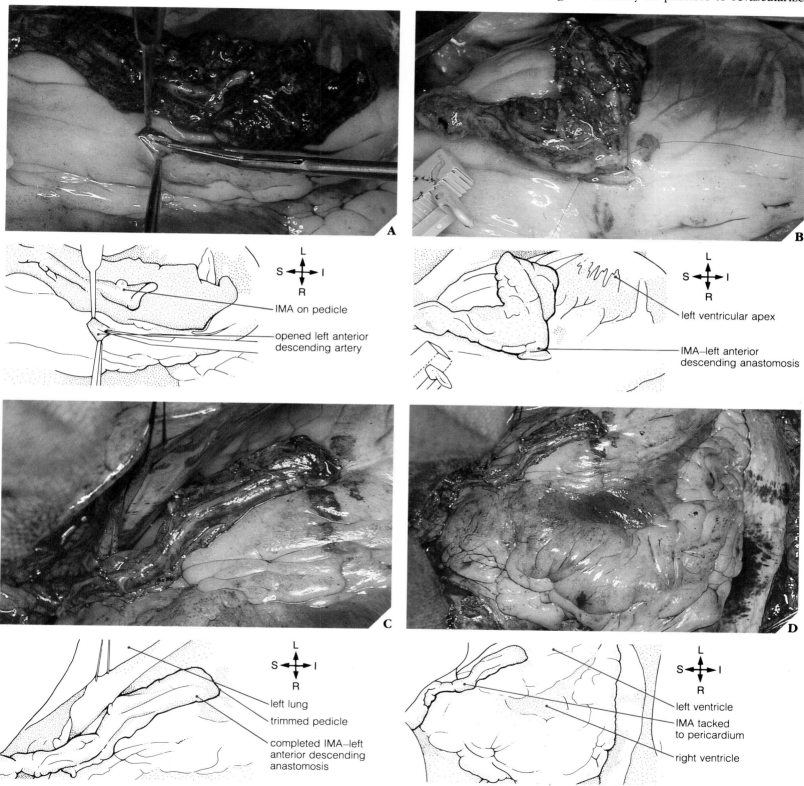

FIG. 6.30 (A–D) *The IMA and its pedicle are transferred to the surface of the heart for anastomosis with the anterior interventricular branch of the left coronary artery.*

almost any aspect of the coronary system utilizing either the right, left, or both internal mammary arteries (IMA) (Fig. 6.31).

The increasing popularity of the IMA graft notwithstanding, the saphenous vein remains as the major conduit available to the surgeon. Indeed absence of a suitable saphenous vein presents a substantial problem, since a satisfactory substitute has not been developed. This could become increasingly worrisome as the number of reoperations for coronary artery disease grows over the ensuing years (Fig. 6.32).

The saphenous vein may be utilized when bypassing a single lesion in one of the coronary subsystems (Fig. 6.33A), or it may be used to revascularize multiple areas of the myocardium. So-called "snake"

grafts, used with the idea that greater flow enhances patency, are less popular than they once were. However, the use of sequential grafting may be the only alternative under certain circumstances (Fig. 6.33B). Occasionally the use of a "Y" vein graft is possible (Fig. 6.33C) if such a vein is available and the runoff in the distal vessels is well matched so that a "steal" does not become a problem.

Coronary artery bypass surgery is not infrequently combined with other cardiac procedures. Usually this does not greatly complicate matters, but it does require careful planning to optimize cardioplegia time and, in the case of aortic valve disease, placement of the proximal anastomoses (Fig. 6.34).

FIG. 6.31 *Operative view shows bilateral IMA implants into the coronary arteries.*

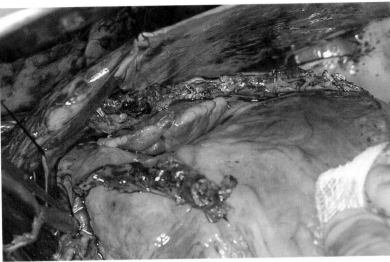

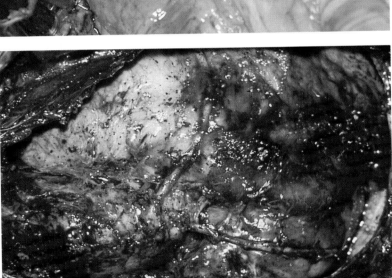

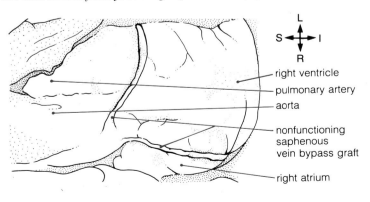

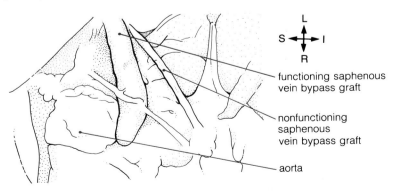

FIG. 6.32 **(A)** *In this operative view, failed saphenous vein bypass grafts are seen several years following implantation.* **(B)** *A similar view contrasts a functioning "snake" graft and a failed saphenous vein bypass graft six years after implantation.*

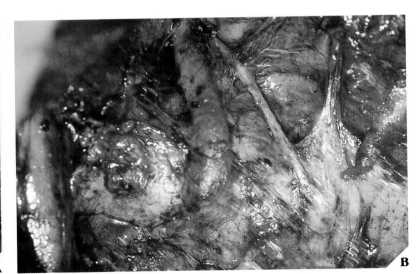

right ventricle
pulmonary artery
aorta
nonfunctioning saphenous vein bypass graft
right atrium

functioning saphenous vein bypass graft
nonfunctioning saphenous vein bypass graft
aorta

PART II: DISEASES OF THE HEART

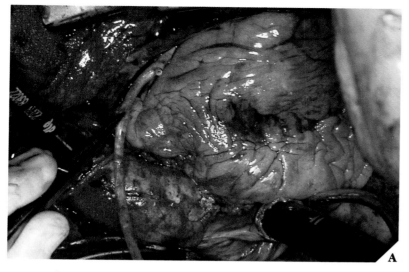

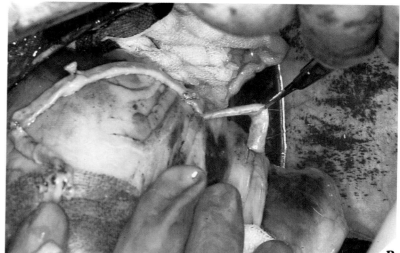

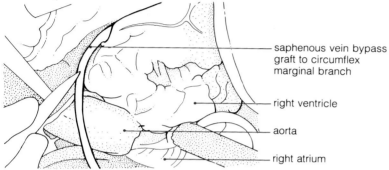

- saphenous vein bypass graft to circumflex marginal branch
- right ventricle
- aorta
- right atrium

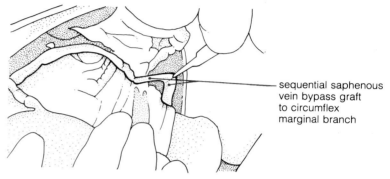

- sequential saphenous vein bypass graft to circumflex marginal branch

FIG. 6.33 **(A)** *In this single-vein bypass to the posterior surface of the heart, the proximal anastomosis has not yet been completed.* **(B)** *A sequential graft is made to distal branches of the circumflex artery. The apparent redundancy is necessary to allow for filling of the heart following discontinuation of cardiopulmonary bypass graft.* **(C)** *A "Y" graft is made to the anterior branches of the left coronary artery.*

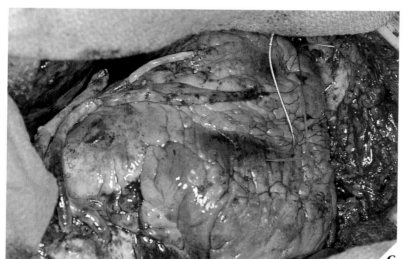

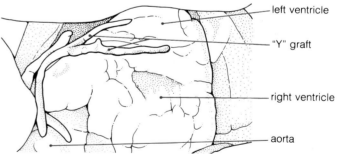

- left ventricle
- "Y" graft
- right ventricle
- aorta

FIG. 6.34 *Operative view of a proximal saphenous vein anastomosis is seen in relationship to the aortotomy in a patient requiring aortic valve replacement and bypass grafting.*

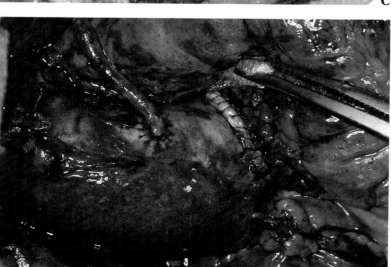

- pulmonary artery
- proximal anastomosis
- aortic suture line
- aorta
- right atrial appendage

The pathology of saphenous vein graft failure relates to several features, including wall laceration at the suture site and ischemia of the vein graft. Thrombosis is often an early complication (Fig. 6.35) and may be enhanced when the graft is placed at the site of preexisting coronary obstruction (Fig. 6.36). Dissections may occur, induced by the procedure, usually at the site of a plaque. Intimal proliferation as a rule is induced by either graft injury or laceration of the grafted artery. It may extend into the venous graft and eventually may lead to total obliteration of the vein graft (Fig. 6.37).

CORONARY ANGIOPLASTY

Gruentzig first performed percutaneous transluminal coronary angioplasty in 1977. He and his colleagues performed about 5000 procedures at Emory University Hospital between 1980 and his death in 1985. Since then Drs. King, Douglas, and Roubin have continued the work. The primary success rate in their hands is about 90%. Infarction occurs in about 3% of cases and a similar number need emergency coronary bypass surgery. The re-stenosis rate, which at six months is about 30%, is the major limitation of the procedure.

The ideal candidate for coronary angioplasty is a patient with angina pectoris or objective evidence of myocardial ischemia who has a short (less than 20 mm) noncalcified lesion in the proximal portion of a single major coronary artery (Fig. 6.38). Although obstructions in two or three arteries have been dilated, more data are needed to formulate indications for the use of angioplasty in such patients. We at Emory have emphasized the need for a randomized trial in which the immediate and long-term results of multivessel coronary angioplasty are compared with the results of coronary bypass surgery. The trial, funded by the National Institutes of Health, began in mid-1987.

Additionally coronary angioplasty is used in patients receiving thrombolytic therapy for evolving infarction (less than three to four hours after onset of pain due to myocardial ischemia). More research is needed before rigid guidelines can be stated for this indication. Angioplasty can also be used to dilate obstructions in saphenous vein grafts.

Because acute closure of a dilated artery can occur and re-stenosis is common, current research efforts are directed toward the prevention of these complications by use of an intracoronary metal coil stent. Early results appear promising.

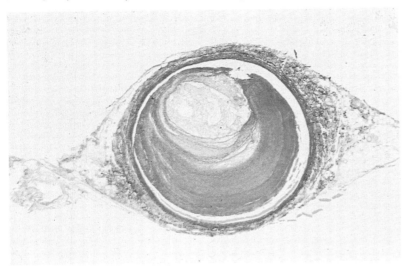

FIG. 6.35 *A venous bypass graft is occluded by a recent thrombus.*

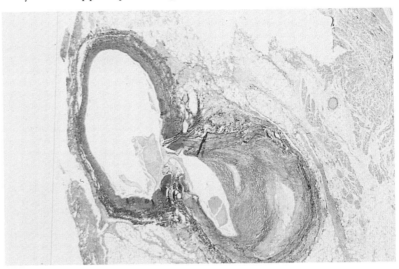

FIG. 6.36 *A venous bypass graft is sutured at the site of a significant preexistent atherosclerotic lesion in the major coronary artery. This often leads to early graft thrombosis.*

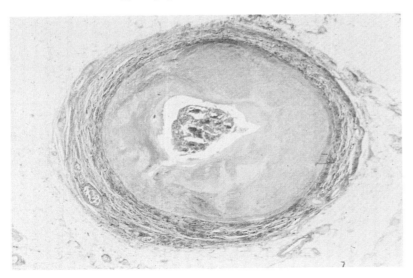

FIG. 6.37 *Fibrocellular intimal proliferation of a venous bypass graft is a complication that eventually may lead to total obliteration of the graft.*

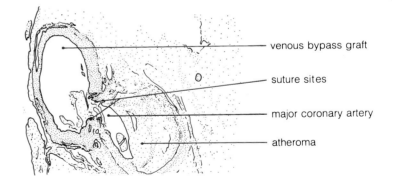

venous bypass graft

suture sites

major coronary artery

atheroma

Definition and Treatment of Various Subsets of Atherosclerotic Coronary Heart Disease

PATIENTS WITHOUT ANGINA OR OBJECTIVE EVIDENCE OF MYOCARDIAL ISCHEMIA
DEFINITION AND RECOGNITION

These patients are identified when a coronary arteriogram, performed because the patient has valve disease, reveals evidence of coronary atherosclerosis.

TREATMENT

Coronary bypass surgery is usually performed in patients who have obstructive lesions in the coronary arteries and are being operated on for valve disease even when there is no evidence of myocardial ischemia. Lesions that obstruct less than 50% of the luminal diameter of a coronary artery are usually not candidates for bypass surgery.

STABLE ANGINA PECTORIS
DEFINITION AND RECOGNITION

The adjective *stable* is used when angina has been present and unchanging for 60 days or more. The frequency of attacks, duration of episodes, and precipitating causes must not have changed during that period. The physician must be certain that the patient has not decreased his or her activity during the period as a means of controlling the angina, because this could signify that the exercise tolerance has decreased and would therefore be an indication that the angina is increasing.

The pathophysiology of stable angina pectoris is usually related to an increase in the demand side of the myocardial perfusion (sup-

ply–demand) system. An increase in work of the myocardium increases the oxygen requirements of the heart cells.

The patient's angina must be categorized as class 1, 2, 3, or 4 using the Canadian Cardiovascular Society recommendations (see Table 6.2).

Most patients under age 70 with stable angina should have a coronary arteriogram and left ventriculogram to be certain of the diagnosis and to determine the need for coronary angioplasty or surgery.

Exceptions are patients whose history has a predictive value of 70%–80% and have negative results in exercise ECGs, ^{201}Tl scans, or exercise ^{99m}Tc tests; who are over the age of 75 and have class 1 or 2 stable angina; or who have another disease that prevents further workup.

TREATMENT

The preventive measures and drug therapy discussed earlier should be used, but the need for angioplasty or bypass surgery must be determined.

Patients with class 1, 2, 3, or 4 stable angina who have obstruction in a single coronary artery should be considered for angioplasty. Patients with single-vessel coronary disease with class 3 or 4 stable angina who are not considered to be candidates for angioplasty should have bypass surgery when the distal vessels permit the procedure.

Patients with left main coronary obstruction should have bypass surgery regardless of the class of angina. Left main coronary artery obstruction is found in less than 2% of patients with stable angina, but in 10% or more of patients with unstable angina. Angioplasty is contraindicated for left main coronary artery obstruction.

Patients with class 1, 2, 3, or 4 stable angina who have triple-vessel coronary disease and an abnormal ejection fraction should have bypass surgery. Moreover bypass surgery should be performed in patients with multivessel coronary disease who also have a poor exercise per-

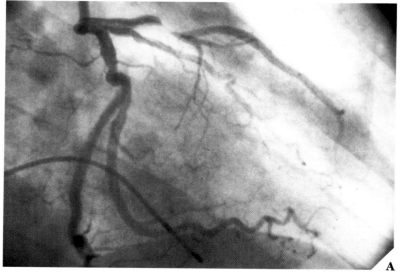

A

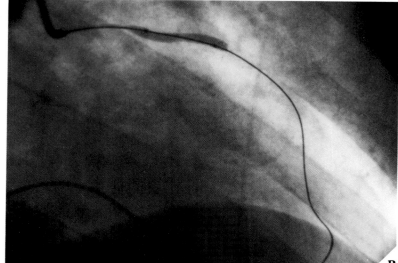

B

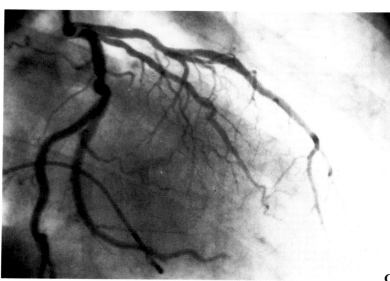

C

FIG. 6.38 *Right anterior oblique projections of the left coronary artery in a 61-year-old man with unstable angina show* (**A**) *a severe concentric stenosis of the proximal left anterior descending coronary artery.* (**B**) *The guidewire is in the distal artery and the inflated balloon is positioned across the stenosis.* (**C**) *Immediate postangioplasty angiogram shows successful dilation.* (Fig. 117-1 A–C, The Heart, 6th ed; see Figure Credits)

formance on the treadmill or have a positive ^{201}Tl scan that reveals a large area or more than one area of reperfusion.

The approach stated above for triple-vessel disease should also be used for most patients with double-vessel disease when one of the vessels involved is the left anterior descending coronary artery.

As stated earlier, many physicians use coronary angioplasty to treat patients with stable angina who have multivessel coronary disease. There are no data at present to support this activity, and Gruentzig believed a randomized trial was needed to compare the results of angioplasty with those of surgery.

Patients with class 1 or 2 stable angina who have obstruction in one, two, or three coronary arteries and who have normal ejection fractions and negative exercise ECGs and ^{201}Tl tests can be treated medically. One must then realize that follow-up must be carefully designed to observe these patients, since about 25% of them will need bypass surgery or angioplasty within five years for unacceptable angina. In fact 7% per year of those with triple-vessel disease will need surgery for unacceptable angina within a five-year follow-up (CASS, 1983).

POSITIVE EXERCISE TEST IN ASYMPTOMATIC PATIENTS
DEFINITION AND RECOGNITION

The asymptomatic patient may develop angina during the treadmill test, because the test demands more effort than the patient expends during his or her daily activities. The patient may, however, develop an abnormal ST-segment displacement, hypotension, or a cardiac arrhythmia during the test but may not develop angina. Most males who exhibit these responses with or without angina should have a coronary arteriogram. Since it is not useful to perform exercise ECGs in middle-aged women because of the high false-positive response, ^{201}Tl scans are indicated when these patients are asymptomatic.

TREATMENT

Treatment depends upon the abnormalities identified in the coronary arteriogram and left ventriculogram. Although data are meager, the approach is similar to that for patients with class 1 or 2 stable angina described in the discussion above. Kent and co-workers (1982) reported that patients who are currently asymptomatic or nearly so but who previously had angina or an infarct, triple-vessel disease, and a poor exercise performance on the treadmill had a 9% annual mortality. There is no surgically treated group with such a high annual mortality.

Admittedly the treatment of asymptomatic patients who exhibit objective signs of myocardial ischemia is controversial. However, when the objective abnormalities noted are similar to those in patients who have class 1 or 2 stable angina, it seems reasonable to improve coronary blood flow with angioplasty or bypass surgery. Drug treatment is used, but its value is not known. The usual rehabilitative and preventive measures should be implemented.

ANGINA EQUIVALENTS
DEFINITION AND RECOGNITION

Angina equivalents are nonanginal signals of myocardial ischemia, including dyspnea on effort, abrupt dyspnea at rest, exhaustion with effort, chronic fatigue, and cardiac arrhythmias. Whereas the predictive value of these symptoms is not as high as it is with angina, such symptoms should not be dismissed without considering myocardial ischemia due to coronary disease.

Patients with angina equivalents should be considered for coronary arteriography. A ^{201}Tl stress test may be diagnostic in some patients, but many times it is unwise to exercise such patients, especially those with dyspnea or arrhythmia.

TREATMENT

Angina equivalents may be stable (unchanged for 60 days or more) or unstable (recent in onset, less than 60 days, or increasing). The choice of treatment depends upon the abnormalities found at coronary arteriography and ventriculography. After review of the film the approach should be that described in the sections dealing with stable (see above) and unstable (see below) angina. The usual rehabilitative and preventive measures should be implemented.

UNSTABLE ANGINA PECTORIS
DEFINITION AND RECOGNITION

The adjective *unstable* signifies that angina pectoris has made its first appearance, has been present for less than 60 days, has increased in frequency or duration, or has occurred with less provocation, or at rest when it did not formerly do so.

The pathophysiology of unstable angina is usually related to further obstruction of the supply end of the myocardial oxygen supply–demand system. Such patients have coronary thrombosis, coronary spasm, or some other cause for the acceleration of the obstructive process. They are more likely to have sudden death or myocardial infarctions within the near future than patients with stable angina.

Unless there is some contraindication, the patient with unstable angina pectoris should have coronary arteriography and left ventriculography. Exercise tests are usually contraindicated.

TREATMENT

When angina occurs several times daily, the patient should be admitted to the coronary care unit. Nitrates, including nitroglycerin ointment and isosorbide dinitrate, should be administered. Intravenous nitroglycerin or calcium blocking agents should be used when the angina occurs frequently. A beta-blocking drug can be added if the preceding approach fails. Heparin is often used in such patients. The intra-aortic balloon pump may be needed when despite medical treatment the episodes of angina occur frequently. Thrombolytic agents are now being used.

Coronary angioplasty should be performed when the conditions are appropriate. The best candidates are those with a short segment of subtotal obstruction in the proximal portion of a single coronary artery. Certain carefully selected patients with multivessel coronary obstruction may have angioplasty, but rigid recommendations cannot be formulated at this time since the research needed for an informed opinion has not yet been completed. Coronary bypass surgery is often used, even in patients with single-vessel disease when angioplasty cannot be performed.

Coronary bypass surgery should be performed in patients with left main coronary artery obstruction. At the present time coronary bypass surgery is usually used in patients with unstable angina who have triple- or double-vessel disease, especially when the proximal portion of the left anterior descending coronary artery is obstructed. Angioplasty may eventually have an application in some of these cases. Rehabilitation and preventive measures should be implemented.

POSTINFARCTION ANGINA PECTORIS
DEFINITION AND RECOGNITION

The term *immediate* postinfarction angina pectoris refers to episodes that occur during the first few days after infarction. The term *delayed* postinfarction angina pectoris refers to episodes that occur days to weeks after infarction. Because dead muscle cannot produce pain, the appearance of postinfarction angina pectoris despite medical treatment is a serious matter, often presaging a more serious coronary event. Most patients with this syndrome should have coronary arteriography.

TREATMENT

Most patients with immediate or delayed postinfarction angina occurring despite medical treatment should have coronary bypass surgery as described in the discussion regarding unstable angina. Some patients may qualify for coronary angioplasty.

PRINZMETAL'S ANGINA (VARIANT ANGINA)
DEFINITION AND RECOGNITION

Prinzmetal's angina is due to coronary artery spasm. Patients usually have coronary spasm superimposed on atherosclerotic lesions, but a small percentage have coronary artery spasm only. The angina usually takes place when the patient is at rest, and it tends to occur at the same time each day. Tobacco, alcohol, and cocaine have been incriminated as precipitating agents. The ECG recorded during an attack of angina may show ST-segment elevation in contrast to the downward ST-segment displacement seen with ordinary angina (Fig. 6.39). Tran-

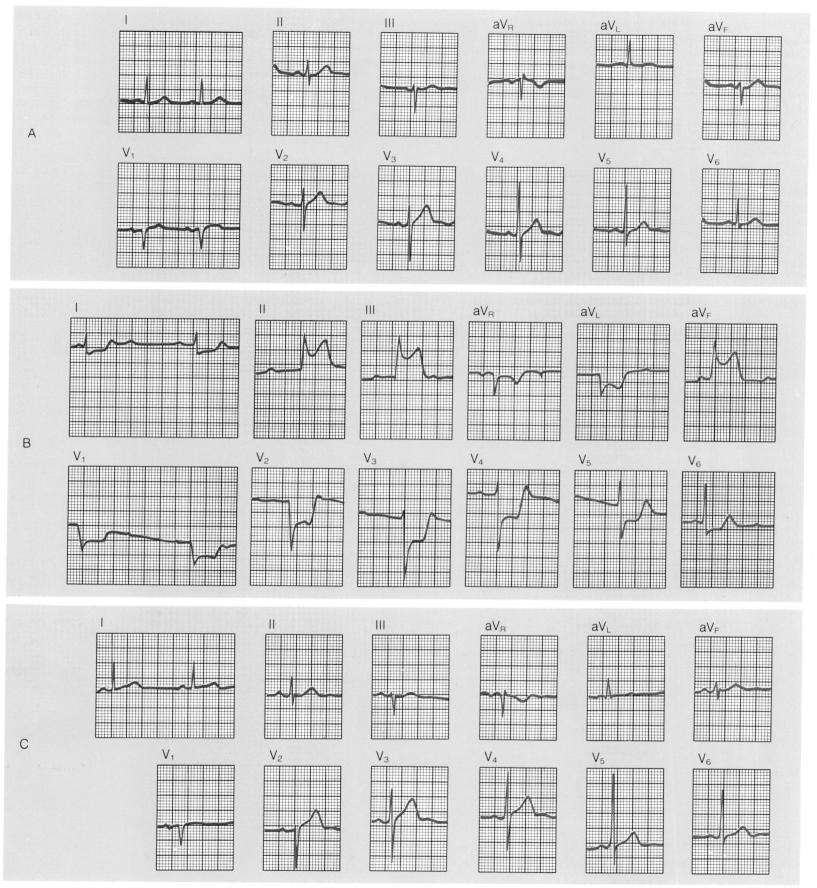

FIG. 6.39 *ECGs recorded from a 59-year-old male with Prinzmetal's angina pectoris who was experiencing repeated bouts of anterior chest discomfort at rest. (A) This ECG was recorded at 10 AM; he was having no chest pain at the time. (B) In an ECG recorded at 5 PM during an episode of chest pain, note the high degree of atrioventricular block and marked ST-segment displacement. The mean ST vector is directed inferoposteriorly.*

(C) The ECG recorded at 6:15 PM the same day is similar to the one recorded at 10 AM. Coronary arteriography revealed a discrete lesion (95% obstruction) in the right coronary artery. Left ventricular function was normal. The patient illustrates destructive coronary disease plus coronary artery spasm. (Redrawn; Fig. 45-17, The Heart, 5th ed; see Figure Credits. Courtesy of Joel M. Felner, MD, Atlanta, Georgia)

sient Q waves, atrioventricular block, and ventricular arrhythmias may occur during an episode.

Stress tests are seldom indicated in such patients. Coronary arteriography is indicated, and intravenous ergonovine may be used to provoke spasm during the procedure. The drug may precipitate persistent coronary spasm, but it does not provoke spasm in all patients with the syndrome.

TREATMENT

Nitrates and calcium channel blocking drugs are used in the treatment of Prinzmetal's angina. Beta-blockers may or may not be helpful.

Coronary angioplasty and coronary bypass surgery cannot be used when coronary spasm alone is the cause of the syndrome. Coronary bypass surgery is usually indicated when obstructing atheroma plus coronary spasm produce the ischemia. Coronary angioplasty may be used in carefully selected patients.

Rehabilitative and preventive measures, as discussed above, should be implemented, when coronary atherosclerosis is present. Smoking *must* be discontinued when spasm is present.

PROLONGED MYOCARDIAL ISCHEMIA WITHOUT OBJECTIVE EVIDENCE OF INFARCTION
DEFINITION AND RECOGNITION

Angina pectoris produced by effort usually lasts one to five minutes after the activity is discontinued. Whenever the chest discomfort is more prolonged, lasting 20–30 minutes, and especially when it occurs at rest, it is highly likely that the pathophysiologic mechanism involved is related to further narrowing of a coronary artery either by spasm, thrombosis, or both. The ECG may show downward displacement of the ST segment and/or T-wave inversion that persists for hours or days. The ST segment may be elevated during the episode of pain; this is referred to as Prinzmetal's phenomenon.

Myocardial necrosis is not evident as measured by serum cardiac enzymes. It is likely, however, that a few myocardial cells die when ischemia persists for 20 minutes.

Stress tests in such patients are usually contraindicated, and coronary arteriography should be performed unless other conditions contraindicate it.

TREATMENT

Management is similar to that for patients who have unstable angina or small infarction. The pain has usually subsided by the time the physician sees the patient, although patients who are already in the hospital may be seen while the pain is present. The pain should be relieved by an opiate. Nitrates, beta-blockers, and calcium antagonists are usually used. When the evidence supports spasm with or without coronary atherosclerosis, it is usually wise to use nitrates and calcium antagonists rather than beta-blockers. Thrombolytic agents are now being used.

Coronary arteriography is indicated in most patients with this syndrome. When coronary arteriography reveals a thrombus in the coronary artery and less than four hours have elapsed since the onset of pain, it is proper to consider the use of a thrombolytic agent if such agents have not been used earlier.

The need for coronary bypass surgery or coronary angioplasty cannot be determined without a coronary arteriogram. When the anatomic conditions in the coronary arteries are appropriate, it is proper to consider bypass surgery or coronary angioplasty. If either bypass surgery or angioplasty is not performed, the patient should be treated as if he or she had a small infarction.

The patient should be rehabilitated after discharge from the hospital, and preventive measures should be implemented.

CORONARY ATHEROSCLEROSIS WITH IRREVERSIBLE MYOCARDIAL ISCHEMIA AND NECROSIS
VERY EARLY PROFOUND ISCHEMIA

DEFINITION AND RECOGNITION. This term is used to designate the first phase of myocardial infarction. The patient may be at home, at work, or participating in other events when the pain occurs. The spouse or bystander decides that emergency help is indicated and calls the rescue squad or physician. Although the ECG and the results of the serum cardiac enzymes test are not available, the patient is treated for myocardial infarction. This stage of infarction is similar to the syndrome of prolonged myocardial ischemia without infarction (see above) and shifts into the stage of early evolving infarction (see below).

In early and profound ischemia the first noticeable changes are

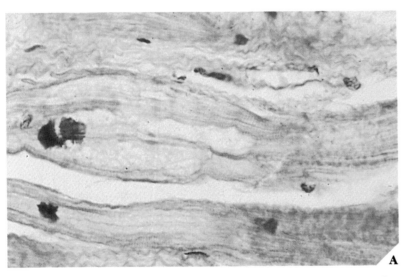
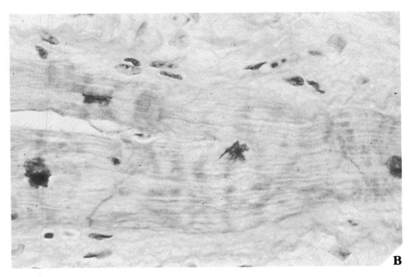

FIG. 6.40 *Early ischemic changes include hydropic cell swelling (A) and additional contraction band changes (B). (Reproduced with permission of the authors and publisher; see Figure Credits)*

depletion of enzymes and disturbances in the functional characteristics of the cells. At a light-microscopic level the Z bands of myofibrils are further apart. Hydropic cell swelling indicates the loss of ability to control osmolality of the cell (Fig. 6.40). This process still may be reversible, but in the early stages it most likely renders the cell vulnerable to reperfusion. The latter may lead to contraction band changes (see Fig. 6.40), most likely due to excessive calcium influx.

TREATMENT. The discomfort should be relieved with an opiate. Paramedics or the physician should begin an intravenous infusion of lidocaine and move the patient to a coronary care unit. The ECG may show signs of definite infarction or only ST-T change. The cardiac enzymes will usually be elevated.

Intravenous thrombolytic therapy may be used as quickly as possible. The patient usually should have a coronary arteriogram and possibly intracoronary thrombolytic therapy (if it had not been instituted earlier), coronary angioplasty, or perhaps coronary bypass surgery (see below).

EARLY EVOLVING MYOCARDIAL INFARCTION

DEFINITION AND RECOGNITION. This term is used to designate the first three to six hours after the onset of chest pain due to myocardial ischemia. It is well established that after a six-hour period most of the myocardial cells that were initially ischemic have either died or returned to normal. Accordingly any intervention designed to save myocardial cells must be instituted during the first three hours—the sooner the intervention the better.

The ECG may show ST-T wave abnormalities and may or may not reveal abnormal Q waves. The result of the determination of serum cardiac enzymes is usually not available when an intervention is implemented.

The earliest changes of myocardial necrosis are eosinophilia of the cell cytoplasm due to an increased acidity within the cells, accompanied by pyknosis of nuclei. Occasionally a wavy appearance of myofibrils can be observed as an indication of overstretched injured cells (Fig. 6.41). An inflammatory response is not yet present. Enzyme staining techniques may reveal the infarct (Fig. 6.42).

TREATMENT. The treatment of these patients has not been standardized. Many physicians believe that intravenous streptokinase or intravenous tissue plasmogen activator (TPA) should be given to all patients. If early thrombolytic treatment is successful in lysing the coronary thrombus, more heart muscle will be saved from necrosis than with intracoronary streptokinase. The latter technique dissolves thrombi more readily but has the disadvantage of delayed administration.

Other interventional approaches may be utilized. Some physicians use coronary angioplasty without thrombolytic therapy in such patients. Others recommend bypass surgery as an emergency measure without thrombolytic therapy. In the future a standardized approach to such patients may be formalized. At present it is not possible to make a specific recommendation regarding treatment except that some type of active intervention seems justified.

During the intervention described above, the pain should be relieved with opiates, nitrates, beta-blockers, or calcium antagonists. After definitive therapy is implemented the rehabilitation process, including preventive measures, should be employed.

UNCOMPLICATED COMPLETED MYOCARDIAL INFARCTION

DEFINITION AND RECOGNITION. Myocardial infarction is characterized by chest pain due to myocardial ischemia that usually lasts longer than 20 minutes, the development of Q waves and/or ST-T wave abnormalities in the ECG, and elevation of the serum cardiac enzymes. All of these features may not be present in all cases and the infarction may be discovered at arteriography and ventriculography or at autopsy.

Completed signifies that most of the ischemic myocardium has become necrotic or has returned to normal. As a rule this occurs within six hours after the onset of pain. *Uncomplicated* signifies that complications such as cardiac arrhythmias, heart failure, or shock have not developed. The designation of uncomplicated should not be made until after the fourth day following the onset of chest pain.

A reactive response to the afflicted injury is seen depending on the time of irreversible ischemic myocardial cell change. Early invasion of polymorphonuclear granulocytes appears at approximately 12 hours following onset of infarction with a maximal concentration seen at

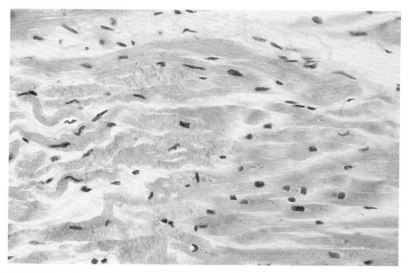

FIG. 6.41 *The earliest indication of myocardial necrosis is eosinophilia of the myocytes. Nuclear pyknosis and so-called wavy appearance of the cells dominate the histology. (Reproduced with permission of the authors and publisher; see Figure Credits)*

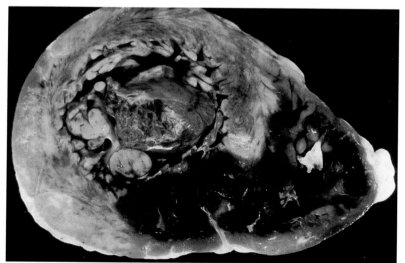

FIG. 6.42 *In the macroenzyme technique on a cross-section of a heart with an acute myocardial infarction, the area containing viable myocardial cells stains dark purple. The infarct is characterized by absent staining.*

about three days (Fig. 6.43). The first signs of macrophage activity appear at approximately three to five days, while the first signs of onset of fibrotic repair occur approximately one week following onset of infarction (Fig. 6.44).

It appears that during the first week following onset of infarction, the myocardium is edematous, and hence prone to mechanically induced complications.

TREATMENT. The chest pain should be relieved by opiates, and the patient should be placed in a coronary care unit. Oxygen should be administered by nasal catheter. Lidocaine is not needed routinely but should be given for ventricular ectopic beats. A Swan-Ganz catheter is not routinely used in patients with uncomplicated completed infarction. Beta-blockers may be used when tachycardia and mild hypertension are present. The patient is usually moved from the coronary care unit to an intermediate unit on about the third day. The cardiac rhythm is monitored while the patient is in the step-down unit, since about one third of the deaths occur after the patient has left the coronary care unit.

The patient can sit in a chair and use the bathroom during the first few days of recovery and can walk in the room and hall after about one week. Many patients with uncomplicated infarction can leave the hospital on the ninth or tenth day for further convalescence at home.

Prior to leaving the hospital, the patient should have either a submaximal exercise ECG test, a ^{201}Tl exercise test, or a coronary arteriogram. If a noninvasive test is performed, a coronary arteriogram is indicated in those patients who do poorly. Many physicians prefer to subject their patients to coronary arteriography rather than screen them first with noninvasive tests. The treatment is then dictated by the results of these tests. Some patients will need coronary angioplasty or coronary bypass surgery. The timing of the procedure must be determined in each patient, rather than applying a general rule. The patient should be rehabilitated following these procedures and can usually return to work in about six weeks.

A cross-sectional echocardiogram should be performed in patients with an anterior myocardial infarction in an effort to identify a left ventricular mural thrombus. When a thrombus is found, the patient should be given the anticoagulant warfarin (Coumadin) for six months.

When bypass surgery or angioplasty is not performed, the patient should be rehabilitated, preventive measures should be instituted, and a beta-blocker and antiplatelet drug may be recommended.

COMPLICATED COMPLETED MYOCARDIAL INFARCTION

The complications of myocardial infarction include cardiac arrhythmias and conduction disturbances, persistent or recurrent chest pain due to myocardial ischemia, heart failure, hypotension, shock, cardiac arrest, pericarditis, pulmonary embolism, systemic embolism, rupture of the ventricular septum, papillary muscle dysfunction and rupture, cardiac rupture, and emotional turmoil. (The brief discussion that follows of each of these complications can be supplemented by the more detailed discussions in *The Heart,* 6th ed, pp 972–987.)

CARDIAC ARRHYTHMIAS AND CONDUCTION DISTURBANCES. Arrhythmias occurring *early* in the course of myocardial infarction include the following:

sinus tachycardia, which may be ominous because it is often associated with, or precedes the development of, left ventricular dysfunction;

sinus bradycardia, which, when treated properly, does not alter hospital mortality to a significant degree;

sinus node dysfunction, which occurs in a small percentage of patients and may require treatment;

atrial premature depolarizations, which occur in about half of patients with myocardial infarction;

atrial tachycardia, which is defined as three or more ectopic P waves occurring at a rate greater than 100 beats per minute, and is seen in about 20% of patients;

atrial flutter, which occurs in about 5% of the patients

atrial fibrillation, which is a common complication of myocardial infarction;

accelerated atrioventricular junctional rhythm and atrioventricular tachycardia;

premature ventricular depolarizations, which occur in 80% of patients;

ventricular tachycardia and ventricular fibrillation;

first- and second-degree atrioventricular block, varying atrioventricular block, and complete heart block;

right and left bundle branch block and bifascicular block.

Arrhythmias may also occur *late* in the course of myocardial infarction. Premature ventricular depolarizations, ventricular tachycardia, ventricular fibrillation, and cardiac arrest may develop days, weeks, or months after the patient has been discharged from the hospital. (For a discussion of the treatment of arrhythmias and conduction disturbances that occur early and late in the course of myocardial infarction the reader is referred to *The Heart,* 6th ed, Chapters 25–28.)

POSTINFARCTION ANGINA PECTORIS. When angina pectoris occurs *early* after myocardial infarction, it signifies that myocardial ischemia is continuing, since dead tissue does not produce pain. When drug therapy fails to relieve recurrent angina, it is a signal for the

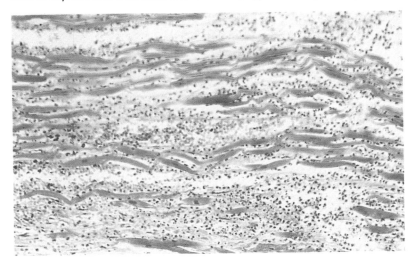

FIG. 6.43 *Necrosis of myocardial cells is evident with edema and a heavy infiltration of polymorphonuclear leukocytes in this myocardial infarct of three to five days' duration. (Reproduced with permission of the authors and publisher; see Figure Credits)*

physician to obtain a coronary arteriogram and left ventriculogram. If suitable coronary anatomy is found, it may be necessary to have coronary bypass surgery or coronary angioplasty.

When angina pectoris occurs *late* in the course of infarction, weeks or months after discharge from the hospital, the patient should have coronary arteriography and left ventriculography. In addition, when suitable anatomy is identified, the patient should have coronary bypass surgery or coronary angioplasty.

VENTRICULAR DYSFUNCTION. About two thirds of patients with acute myocardial infarction have elevations of left ventricular filling pressure but may exhibit no clinical signs of heart failure. About one half of patients with acute infarction have a decrease in resting cardiac output. The stroke volume and ejection fraction decrease and the end-systolic volume increases when there is considerable myocardial destruction.

The patient with left ventricular infarction may have mild to severe dyspnea. A left ventricular gallop (S_3) is associated with a pulmonary wedge pressure of more than 12 mmHg. Abnormal neck vein distention or pulsation may be present when the pulmonary arterial wedge pressure is normal in patients with right ventricular infarction or severe lung disease. In contrast these signs may not be seen when there is early left ventricular dysfunction. Rales may not be heard in patients with interstitial pulmonary edema. Because of this, physical examination of the lungs is not as useful as the chest x-ray film in identifying heart failure with pulmonary congestion.

Radionuclide ventriculography can be used to study ventricular function in patients with acute infarction. Furthermore it can be used to determine serial changes. The procedure is not used routinely but may be indicated when right ventricular infarction is suspected.

It is not necessary to insert a Swan-Ganz catheter into the pulmonary artery of patients with uncomplicated myocardial infarction, but patients with heart failure, right ventricular infarction, persistent pain, hypotension, and shock should have continuous hemodynamic monitoring. (See Figure 45-10 in *The Heart*, 6th ed, for an algorithmic approach to the management of such patients based on hemodynamic measurements and clinical features.)

Right ventricular infarction may occur in patients with inferior wall infarction of the left ventricle that extends beyond the crux into the right ventricular wall (Fig. 6.45). Isolated right ventricular infarction is rare, but when it occurs, it usually presents in the setting of chronic lung disease with resultant right ventricular hypertrophy and dilation.

The clinical picture is that of "right heart failure" with abnormal neck veins and is characterized by distention of the external jugular veins and abnormal pulsations of the internal jugular veins because of a large V wave and rapid y descent; right ventricular S_3 and S_4 gallop sounds; arterial hypotension; clear lung fields on the chest film; and evidence of an inferior infarction with elevation of the ST segments in lead V_{4R}. The right-sided filling pressure is greater than the left-sided filling pressure, and the systolic pressure in the right ventricle and pulmonary arteries is about normal. The clinical picture resembles constrictive pericarditis, including the equalization of diastolic pressures and a diastolic dip and plateau in the right ventricular pressure curve. Cor pulmonale may be clinically similar, but the systolic and diastolic pulmonary artery pressures are elevated with a normal wedge pressure.

The treatment for right ventricular infarction is blood volume expansion and inotropic agents; diuretics are not indicated. Such patients may also have atrioventricular block, which may require temporary pacing. The patient with right ventricular infarction may have a benign course or may have a poor outlook when atrioventricular block and shock develop. If left ventricular function is adequate, right ventricular function may gradually improve.

Late or *chronic* heart failure due to atherosclerotic coronary heart disease is treated with diuretics, drugs to alter the preload and afterload, and digitalis. There is little evidence to support the use of digitalis in patients without atrial fibrillation since toxicity from the drug is increased in this setting.

Physicians now realize that evidence of myocardial dysfunction may be identified by hemodynamic measurements and radionuclide ventriculography in patients without clinical symptoms. The clinician must also exclude ventricular aneurysm whenever heart failure is detected by using echocardiography or radionuclear ventriculography.

The surgical removal of complicating ventricular aneurysm along with coronary bypass grafting may relieve heart failure and prolong life. Some patients with chronic, progressive heart failure may be candidates for cardiac transplantation.

REVERSIBLE HYPOTENSIVE STATES. The *bradycardia–hypotensive syndrome* is usually seen in patients with an inferoposterior infarction. The ischemic area stimulates the vagal afferent fibers and produces bradycardia and hypotension. The skin is warm, and at least early in the course the signs of systemic hypoperfusion are not present. The treatment is intravenous atropine, elevation of the legs, and intravenous infusion of glucose in water. Occasionally volume expansion may not correct the low cardiac output and inotropic agents may be needed. Occasionally a pacemaker may be required when heart block complicates the clinical picture.

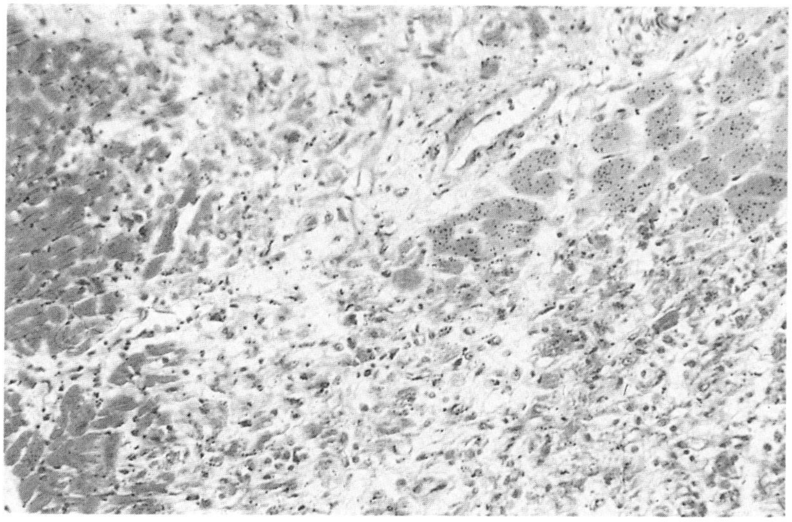

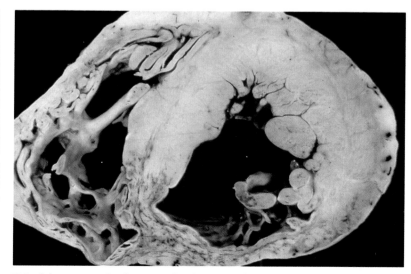

FIG. 6.44 *In the early stages of repair following myocardial infarction there is an abundance of macrophages and early fibroblastic proliferation. The changes are in accord with an infarction of approximately seven to ten days' duration. (Reproduced with permission of the authors and publisher; see Figure Credits)*

FIG. 6.45 *Scarred inferior wall infarction of the left ventricle extends onto the posterior ventricular septum and inferior wall of the right ventricle. (Reproduced with permission of the authors and publisher; see Figure Credits)*

CARDIOGENIC SHOCK. Many patients have all the signs of shock when they reach the hospital. Systolic blood pressure is usually below 100 mmHg and sinus tachycardia is present. Pulmonary edema is usually evident. The skin is pale and moist, and urine output is diminished. There is evidence of massive infarction, the cardiac output is low, and the pulmonary wedge pressure is high. Most patients do not survive.

Some patients develop the shock state more gradually as a result of a slow and steady increase in myocardial destruction. Hemodynamic monitoring is instituted and treatment consists of intravenous nitroglycerin, inotropic agents, and intra-aortic balloon counterpulsation. Surgical intervention may be needed when papillary muscle or interventricular septal rupture is present. Unfortunately the prognosis is poor. (The reader is referred to *The Heart,* 6th ed, Chapters 22 and 23 for discussions, respectively, of the pathophysiology and recognition and management of hypotension and shock.)

NONARRHYTHMIC CARDIAC ARREST. Sudden death in patients with acute myocardial infarction is usually the result of ventricular fibrillation, although asystole may occur. Sudden death may also occur as a result of electromechanical dissociation. These patients have such feeble contractions of the heart due to global myocardial ischemia that no heart sounds are produced and no blood pressure is generated. The ECG, however, shows QRS complexes. Treatment is unsatisfactory because resuscitative measures usually fail.

PERICARDITIS. Acute pericarditis may occur during the first few days after the onset of myocardial infarction (Fig. 6.46). The pain of pericarditis is aggravated by inspiration, and a pericardial rub may or may not be heard. Alternately a pericardial rub may be heard without associated pain. The ECG may not reveal the usual signs of pericarditis. The treatment consists of a short course of corticosteroids. Anticoagulants should not be used.

Dressler's syndrome may develop several weeks or months after myocardial infarction. The condition is characterized by fever, chest pain aggravated by inspiration, pericardial rub, left pleural effusion, and pleural rub. Cardiac tamponade is rare. The syndrome is considered to be the result of an immunologic response to the damaged myocardium. Corticosteroids and nonsteroidal anti-inflammatory drugs such as indomethacin are used in treatment.

PULMONARY EMBOLISM. About 30% of patients with acute myocardial infarction have thrombi in the veins of the calves as determined by ^{125}I-labeled fibrinogen scanning. Pulmonary embolism is unlikely unless the thrombi are located in veins that are proximal to the calf (Fig. 6.47). Leg exercise and early ambulation decrease the thrombi in the leg veins and also decrease pulmonary emboli. Pulmonary emboli are responsible for about 1% of deaths.

Pulmonary emboli may produce episodes of dyspnea, tachycardia, cyanosis, and, as pulmonary infarction develops, a pleural friction rub. The Pao_2 may diminish and the $Paco_2$ may remain normal. A definite diagnosis may not be established without a pulmonary scan, but it may not be wise to move the patient from the coronary care unit to the radiology department in order to perform the examination. An echocardiogram should be performed on patients with pulmonary emboli to determine if the thrombus from the legs has been retained in the right ventricle.

Anticoagulation with heparin or coumadin is not used routinely in every patient with myocardial infarction. Heparin and oral anticoagulants should be given to patients who are at high risk for pulmonary embolism. Such patients include those with chronic heart failure, inactive patients, obese patients, and those with previous evidence of venous disease of the legs.

Patients with pulmonary emboli should be treated with heparin followed by coumadin for three to six months. When anticoagulation

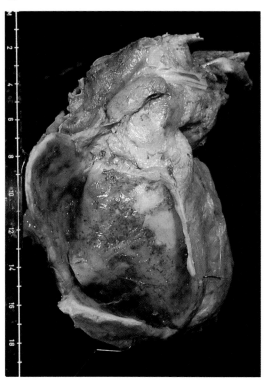

FIG. 6.46 *Fibrinous pericarditis is seen in this case of acute myocardial infarction.*

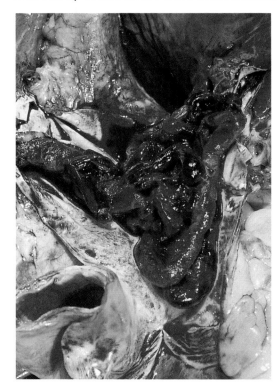

FIG. 6.47 *Saddle thromboembolus in the bifurcation of the pulmonary trunk is a complication of deep vein thrombosis of the legs.*

fails to prevent pulmonary emboli, it may be necessary for a surgeon to place a filter in the inferior caval vein (Fig. 6.48).

SYSTEMIC ARTERIAL EMBOLISM. Although the incidence of systemic emboli has decreased in recent years, new data obtained using cross-sectional echocardiography have stimulated a new approach to this problem.

Systemic emboli following myocardial infarction are the result of thrombi located in the left ventricle (Fig. 6.49). The thrombi are more likely to form in akinetic or dyskinetic areas of the left ventricle of patients who have had a large anterior myocardial infarction. Accordingly it seems wise to obtain a cross-sectional echocardiogram on such patients.

The treatment for a mural thrombus found by echocardiography is anticoagulation with coumadin for about six months. The treatment of systemic emboli to the brain, extremities, bowel, kidney, or other organs is determined by the extent and location of the end-organ damage.

VENTRICULAR SEPTAL RUPTURE. This complication occurs in about 1%–3% of patients with myocardial infarction (Fig. 6.50). It usually occurs during the first week in patients who have experienced their first transmural infarction.

Septal rupture is usually recognized by the appearance of a systolic murmur located in the third and fourth intercostal space near the sternum, although the murmur may occasionally be louder at the apex. The event usually is associated with pulmonary edema and shock. The bedside use of the Swan-Ganz catheter has made it possible to identify the presence and magnitude of a left-to-right shunt and to separate it from mitral regurgitation due to rupture of a papillary muscle.

The treatment of septal rupture is surgical repair, and the current

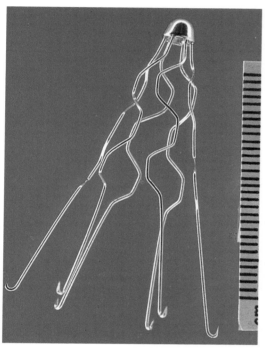

FIG. 6.48 An "umbrella" or Greenfield filter, placed in the inferior caval vein, may be necessary in cases of pulmonary emboli. (Courtesy of Robert B. Smith III, MD, Atlanta, Georgia)

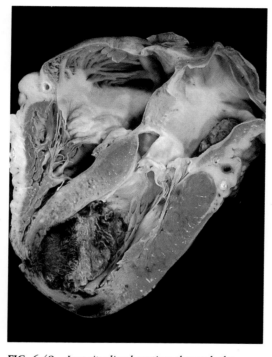

FIG. 6.49 Longitudinal section through the heart shows an intracavitary left ventricular thrombosis complicating myocardial infarction.

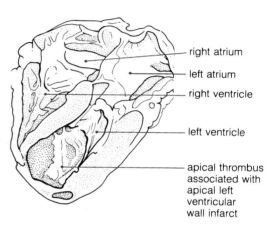

right atrium
left atrium
right ventricle
left ventricle
apical thrombus associated with apical left ventricular wall infarct

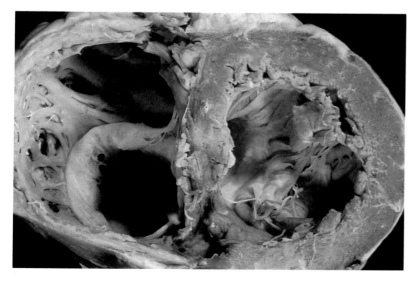

FIG. 6.50 Ventricular septal rupture may complicate acute myocardial infarction.

trend is toward early operation for such patients. Formerly the approach to this serious problem was to wait as long as possible to allow damaged myocardium to heal to some degree so that repair was more easily accomplished. Today the surgical technique has improved so that early intervention seems to be desirable.

PAPILLARY MUSCLE DYSFUNCTION. This condition is due to infarction or ischemia of a papillary muscle of the mitral valve (Fig. 6.51). The associated segment of the ventricular wall is usually infarcted. The condition is recognized by the development of a new systolic murmur at the apex, either holosystolic or mid- to late systolic in duration. A V wave may be noted in the pressure curve recorded when the Swan-Ganz catheter is in the pulmonary artery wedge position. Cross-sectional echocardiography may differentiate between papillary muscle dysfunction and rupture.

The treatment depends on the state of the myocardium and the degree of mitral regurgitation. With severe mitral regurgitation and heart failure, the mitral valve may be replaced unless myocardial contractility is too poor to permit it.

PAPILLARY MUSCLE RUPTURE. Complete rupture of the belly of a papillary muscle produces severe mitral regurgitation, pulmonary edema,

shock, and death. If the infarction does not produce complete severance of the muscle or when there is rupture of one or two of the heads of the muscle, the situation may be less serious, allowing time for surgical correction. The posteromedial papillary muscle is more commonly involved than the anterolateral one (Fig. 6.52). About one third or more patients with papillary muscle rupture have single-vessel coronary disease.

The condition is recognized by the identification of a new systolic murmur at the apex, pulmonary congestion, and hypotension. A systolic murmur may not be heard if the patient is in shock, myocardial contractility is markedly diminished, or there is complete separation of the muscle from the ventricular wall. An abnormal V wave may be seen in the pressure curve recorded with the Swan-Ganz catheter in the pulmonary wedge position. The cross-sectional echocardiogram may detect a flail leaflet of the mitral valve leaflets.

Treatment with vasodilator drugs and intra-aortic balloon pump may be temporarily helpful but most patients will require mitral valve replacement soon after the diagnosis is made.

EXTERNAL CARDIAC RUPTURE. Rupture of the myocardial wall is responsible for about 10% of deaths due to myocardial infarction (Fig. 6.53). Patients with cardiac rupture are usually in their 60s and have

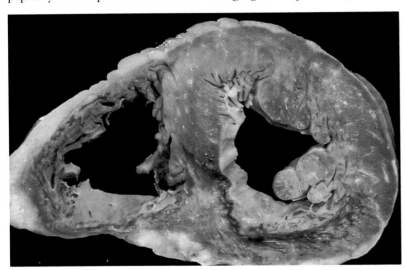

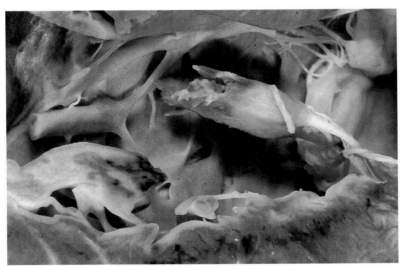

FIG. 6.51 *Papillary muscle dysfunction in this cross-section of the heart is due to extensive myocardial infarction involving the area at the base of the posteromedial papillary muscle group of the left ventricle.*

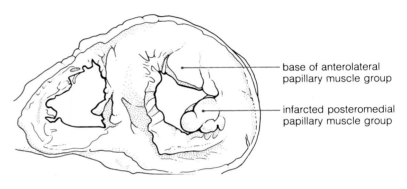

base of anterolateral papillary muscle group

infarcted posteromedial papillary muscle group

FIG. 6.52 *Rupture of the posteromedial papillary muscle may be a complication in the acute phase of inferior-wall myocardial infarction.*

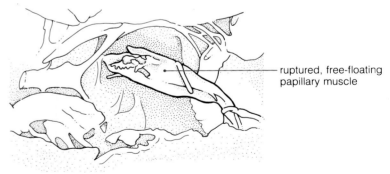

ruptured, free-floating papillary muscle

a transmural infarction with poor collateral circulation, as well as hypertension.

External rupture of the heart produces sudden death, signs of cardiac tamponade due to hemorrhage into the pericardial space, and abrupt severe pericardial pain and rub. The ECG may show no new changes from those of myocardial infarction.

Treatment fails because death usually occurs quickly. On rare occasion pericardial aspiration during the time the patient is being moved to the operating room for emergency cardiac surgery may be successful.

EMOTIONAL RESPONSES.   Patients with coronary disease, especially those with an acute event such as myocardial infarction, may pass through several identifiable phases of emotional reaction: denial, acceptance, fear and anxiety, depression, and realistic adaptation. The physician must be able to recognize each of these stages, even when minor diagnostic clues are present.

The treatment of emotional reactions ordinarily is not difficult. The perceptive physician can usually reassure the patient since many new approaches to therapy are available. Treatments such as proper drugs, angioplasty, and coronary bypass surgery should be implemented without delay, since procrastination leads to disability. A rehabilitation and

health-enhancement program should be implemented as soon as possible. The exact program employed for the patient must be determined on an individual basis.

VENTRICULAR ANEURYSM.   Ventricular aneurysms are usually associated with transmural infarction of the anterior and apical region of the heart (Fig. 6.54). Common complications include ventricular arrhythmias, congestive heart failure, or peripheral emboli. A ventricular aneurysm rarely ruptures.

The aneurysm may produce an abnormal ectopic pulsation on the surface of the chest or a large apical impulse. A systolic murmur and ventricular gallop may be heard at the apex. The ECG usually shows the Q waves of anterior infarction and persistent shift of the ST segments. An abnormal bulge of the myocardium may be seen on the chest radiograph, and calcium may be noted in the wall of the aneurysm. It is surprising, however, how often the chest film reveals no abnormality. A ventricular aneurysm and thrombus may be detected by cross-sectional echocardiography.

A nuclear ventriculogram can be used to identify the presence and extent of a ventricular aneurysm, as well as determine the ejection fraction. This method of examination can be used to screen patients who are suspected of having an aneurysm.

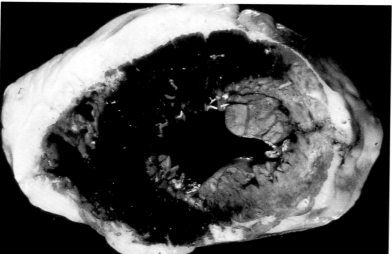
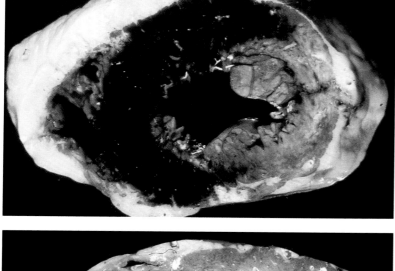

FIG. 6.53   *Cardiac rupture of the left ventricular lateral free wall in the setting of an acute myocardial infarction causes sudden death. The macroenzyme stain of the cross-section of the heart shows the infarcted area as a pale-brown zone; the dark-purple area represents viable myocardium. (Reproduced with permission of the authors and publisher; see Figure Credits)*

FIG. 6.54   *Ventricular aneurysm of the left ventricular lateral free wall in this cross-section of the heart is located between both papillary muscle groups.*

A ventricular aneurysm is best studied by left ventriculography (Fig. 6.55). The size, location, and presence of a thrombus can be detected with this technique. A coronary arteriogram can be performed at the same time, and a decision can be made regarding cardiac surgery. A ventricular aneurysm should be treated surgically when there is persistent heart failure due to the aneurysm, ventricular arrhythmias not controlled with medical treatment, uncontrolled angina pectoris, or peripheral emboli despite adequate anticoagulation. Coronary bypass surgery may be carried out at the same time when the conditions are proper. Electrophysiologic mapping is now being used to guide the surgeon during removal of a ventricular aneurysm in a patient with uncontrolled ventricular arrhythmias.

A *false aneurysm* of the left ventricle may result from myocardial infarction when there is a small rupture and slow leakage of blood into the pericardial space (Fig. 6.56). The pericardium becomes adherent to the infarct and contains the hematoma. False aneurysms, which may be detected by cross-sectional echocardiography, should be repaired surgically.

SHOULDER–HAND SYNDROME. The shoulder–hand syndrome has almost disappeared since patients with myocardial infarction are permitted to perform more physical acts including the use of their arms early after the event. Formerly patients developed pain, stiffness, and decreased motion of the shoulders and arms because of inactivity. In this syndrome the skin of the fingers becomes shiny and swollen. The treatment is physiotherapy and corticosteroids.

SUDDEN DEATH

Atherosclerotic coronary|heart disease is the most common cause of sudden death, usually due to ventricular fibrillation. Cardiac asystole and electrical-mechanical dissociation may also be causes. Less than 50% of patients who experience cardiac arrest and are resuscitated give a history of angina pectoris; the death or the episode resulting in resuscitation is the first evidence of disease.

Treatment consists of resuscitation. When resuscitation is successful, coronary arteriography should be performed. Following coronary arteriography a decision must be made regarding medical therapy, coronary angioplasty, or bypass surgery.

SYNCOPE

Some of the mechanisms responsible for sudden death may produce syncope or near-syncope. Patients with atherosclerotic coronary heart disease may have syncope due to ventricular arrhythmias. Ischemia is the usual cause of arrhythmias, but nonischemic reasons do exist. Some patients with Prinzmetal's syndrome may have a combination of atherosclerotic obstruction plus spasm of the right coronary artery, which may produce high-grade atrioventricular block and syncope.

The treatment for syncope due to ventricular arrhythmia is usually medical. A small percentage of patients who do not respond to medical therapy may require surgical intervention including coronary bypass surgery and electrical mapping of the heart with surgical removal of the arrhythmogenic focus. A permanent internal defibrillator may occasionally be needed. The treatment of syncope related to Prinzmetal's syndrome due to obstructive disease plus coronary spasm is usually coronary bypass surgery and a cardiac pacemaker.

CARDIAC ARRHYTHMIAS

Cardiac arrhythmia may occur with all types of heart disease and may be seen in patients with no other evidence of heart disease. All arrhythmias and conduction disturbances may be seen in patients with atherosclerotic coronary heart disease. It is not always possible to determine whether the arrhythmia is actually due to the ischemia and

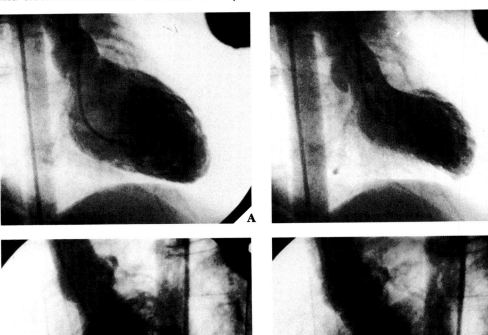

FIG. 6.55 *Left ventriculography was performed with a biplane technique in this case of ventricular aneurysm. Right anterior oblique views show the left ventricle at end diastole (**A**) and at end systole (**B**). Note the contraction abnormality of the anterior wall. Left anterior oblique views show the left ventricle at end diastole (**C**) and at end systole (**D**). (Fig. 108-46,* The Heart, *6th ed; see Figure Credits)*

scarring of atherosclerotic coronary disease or due to an unrelated disease such as Lenegre's or Lev's disease. In addition an abnormal rhythm such as atrial fibrillation may be due to hemodynamic alterations produced by complications of atherosclerotic coronary heart disease rather than by ischemia itself. It should be obvious that the difference among syncope, sudden death, and cardiac arrhythmias without symptoms is determined by the type of arrhythmia and its duration.

The arrhythmia may be discovered on routine ECG, but Holter monitoring is often necessary. Most arrhythmias are managed with simple drug therapy, but some patients with refractory arrhythmias need special electrophysiologic testing and coronary arteriography in order to determine the best approach to treatment. This may be drug therapy, coronary angioplasty, coronary bypass surgery, surgery for arrhythmias, a pacemaker, or a permanent internal defibrillator. The exact treatment is determined by the type and mechanism of the rhythm disturbance.

ISCHEMIC CARDIOMYOPATHY

Atherosclerotic coronary heart disease is a major cause of cardiomyopathy (Fig. 6.57); heart failure is the usual consequence. It is often difficult to separate other causes of cardiomyopathy from ischemic cardiomyopathy. Ischemic and nonischemic cardiomyopathies may produce heart failure, arrhythmias, peripheral emboli, angina pectoris, or diagnostic ECG signs of infarction. Ischemic cardiomyopathy due to coronary disease and idiopathic cardiomyopathy may occur in the same patient.

The presence of ischemic cardiomyopathy is determined with certainty by coronary arteriography and left ventriculography. Medical treatment is usually employed, but an increasing number of patients now are treated by cardiac transplantation.

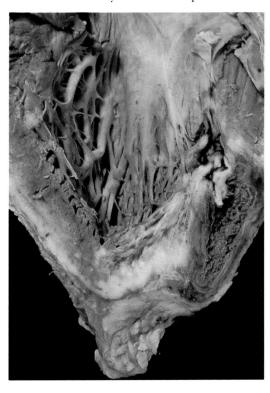

FIG. 6.56 *False aneurysm of the left ventricle is due to incomplete rupture in the setting of an acute myocardial infarction.*

ATHEROSCLEROTIC CORONARY HEART DISEASE IN PATIENTS WITH OTHER DISEASES
CHEST PAIN FOLLOWING CORONARY BYPASS SURGERY

Nonischemic chest pain often appears after bypass surgery. The pain may be due to pericarditis, chest wall problems, sternal infection, or anxiety. The discomfort is usually easy to separate from angina pectoris or prolonged pain due to myocardial ischemia. At times, however, the pain is clearly due to myocardial ischemia or cannot be differentiated from it. Then it is necessary to consider the possibilities of graft closure or progression of atherosclerosis in the native coronary arteries.

An exercise ECG or a ^{201}Tl stress test may solve the diagnostic problem when the pretest probability for cardiac ischemia is low. A coronary arteriogram is usually indicated when the pretest probability for cardiac ischemia is high.

The treatment varies according to the cause. Pericarditis is treated with indomethacin or prednisone; sternal infection is treated by antibiotics, debridement, and plastic surgery. Patients with chest wall pain can be assured it will diminish as time passes. Patients with myocardial ischemia may be treated with angioplasty of an obstructed native vessel or graft, by coronary bypass surgery, or by medical means if the results of the coronary arteriogram do not demand more active intervention.

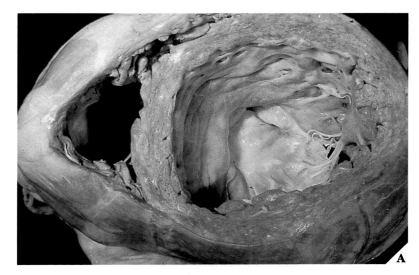

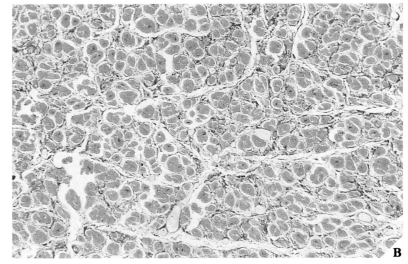

FIG. 6.57 *In ischemic cardiomyopathy the left ventricular cavity may be widely dilated with a hypertrophic wall (A). (B) Histologically there is extensive lacelike myocardial fibrosis.*

CAROTID ARTERY DISEASE IN COMBINATION WITH CORONARY DISEASE

A male patient with a carotid bruit due to carotid artery disease (Fig. 6.58) is more likely to have overt coronary atherosclerosis in the future. It is important to question a patient with coronary disease for symptoms of transient ischemic attacks and to listen for carotid bruits that may be related to occlusive carotid disease. It is equally important to question patients who are to undergo carotid artery surgery for symptoms of coronary disease such as angina pectoris.

Rigid guidelines for the treatment of patients with carotid artery disease who also have evidence of coronary atherosclerotic heart disease have not been developed. Asymptomatic carotid bruits in patients who are to undergo coronary bypass surgery are usually investigated with noninvasive tests of the carotid arteries. If these studies show that the carotid arteries are not occluded to a significant degree, coronary bypass surgery is performed without carotid artery surgery. The patient with transient ischemic attacks should usually have additional studies of the carotid arteries including a carotid arteriogram prior to coronary bypass surgery. When surgery is indicated for carotid disease and coronary disease, it is customary to do both operations at one time, carotid surgery immediately before coronary bypass surgery.

ABDOMINAL AORTIC ANEURYSM OR PERIPHERAL VASCULAR DISEASE IN COMBINATION WITH ATHEROSCLEROTIC HEART DISEASE

Workers at the Cleveland Clinic have performed the best clinical study of patients who have coronary artery disease and peripheral vascular disease (Hertzer et al, 1984). Patients who have an atherosclerotic abdominal aortic aneurysm or have intermittent claudication due to atherosclerotic lesions of the peripheral arteries usually have atherosclerotic coronary heart disease even if they are asymptomatic (Fig. 6.59).

It is wise to perform a stress ECG or a ^{201}Tl scan in patients who have no angina before surgery for an abdominal aortic aneurysm or obstructive arterial disease of the lower extremities is performed. Patients who have angina or positive stress tests should have a coronary arteriogram prior to surgery for an abdominal aortic aneurysm or atherosclerotic disease of the arteries to the legs. Patients who cannot exercise may require the dipyridamole ^{201}Tl test (Boucher et al, 1985).

Patients who need surgical treatment of an abdominal aortic aneurysm and/or obstructive arterial disease of the lower extremities and who have symptomatic coronary disease or positive stress tests with coronary arteriographic evidence of compelling obstructive coronary artery disease should have coronary bypass surgery or angioplasty

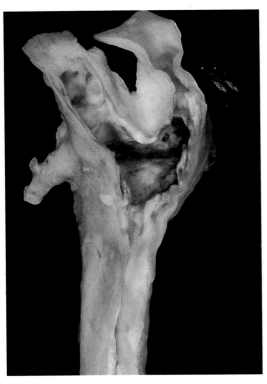

FIG. 6.58 *Obstructive atherosclerosis of the carotid artery is found at the site of the bifurcation of internal and external arteries.*

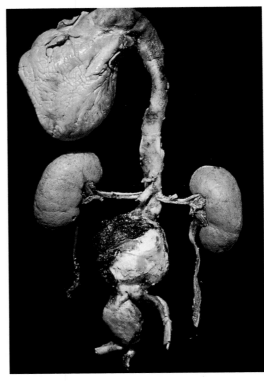

FIG. 6.59 *An atherosclerotic aneurysm of the abdominal aorta is located distal to the renal arteries, with an additional aneurysm in the right common iliac artery. The atherosclerosis of the aorta is associated with obstructive atherosclerotic coronary artery disease.*

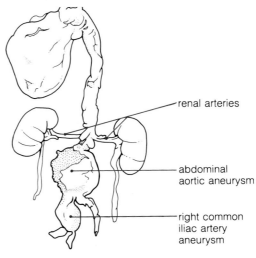

renal arteries

abdominal aortic aneurysm

right common iliac artery aneurysm

performed several weeks prior to surgery for the abdominal aortic aneurysm or obstructive disease of the arteries to the legs. Failure to heed this advice invites the occurrence of myocardial infarction during the perioperative period associated with surgery for the aneurysm or obstructive disease of the arteries to the legs.

CARDIAC VALVE DISEASE IN COMBINATION WITH ATHEROSCLEROTIC CORONARY DISEASE

Many patients with cardiac valve disease also have coronary atherosclerosis, and some have angina pectoris without coronary atherosclerosis. This is common in patients with aortic valve disease (Fig. 6.60). Some patients with valve disease also have significant asymptomatic coronary disease. It is not possible without a coronary arteriogram to determine the contribution that valve or coronary disease makes to produce myocardial ischemia. Accordingly all adult candidates for valve surgery should have a coronary arteriogram.

The indications for cardiac valve surgery are discussed in Chapter 4. Patients with angina pectoris or abnormal stress tests who have coronary disease with obstructions greater than 50% diameter narrowing should have coronary bypass surgery at the time of valve surgery. Patients who undergo valve surgery, having no angina and less than 40%–50% diameter narrowing on coronary arteriogram, are not candidates for coronary bypass surgery.

Patients who undergo coronary bypass surgery may have aortic stenosis with an aortic-ventricular gradient of 50 mmHg. Aortic stenosis of this severity is not usually treated with aortic valve replacement. If,

however, the patient is to have coronary bypass surgery, it may be wise to replace the aortic valve since a significant number will require aortic valve replacement within a few years.

The operative risk for patients who are operated on for aortic stenosis or insufficiency and coronary disease is higher than that of aortic valve surgery performed in the absence of coronary disease. The risk of valve surgery in a patient without obstructive coronary disease is 2%–3%, whereas the risk is in the range of 5% when coronary bypass surgery is also performed.

The operative risk for patients undergoing mitral valve surgery without coronary disease is about 5%. When coronary bypass surgery is also performed, the operative risk increases to perhaps 8%. When mitral regurgitation is due to coronary disease such as papillary muscle rupture or dysfunction, the operative risk is as high as 50%. Obviously the operative risks depend on the stage of the disease, the cause of the valve lesions, and the skill of the operating and nursing teams.

ATHEROSCLEROTIC CORONARY DISEASE AND NONCARDIOVASCULAR PROBLEMS REQUIRING SURGERY

It is not uncommon for patients with coronary atherosclerotic heart disease to require surgery for noncardiovascular problems. Common examples are patients with angina or objective evidence of myocardial ischemia who need cholecystectomy or prostate surgery. Coronary arteriography may be indicated in such patients; when the coronary arterial anatomy is favorable, it is usually wise for coronary bypass surgery to precede nonurgent surgery on the gallbladder or prostate.

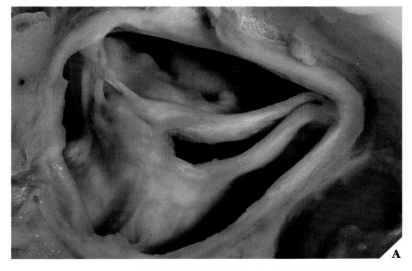

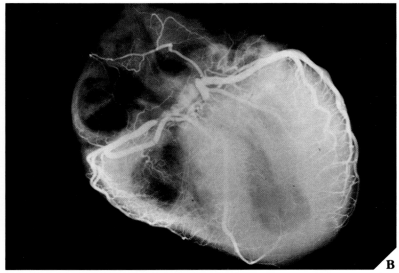

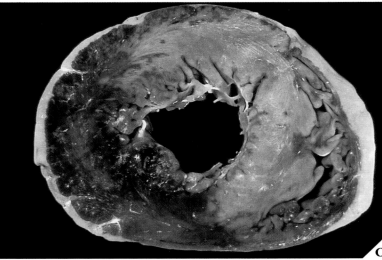

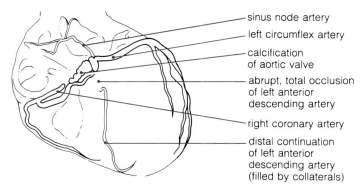

sinus node artery
left circumflex artery
calcification of aortic valve
abrupt, total occlusion of left anterior descending artery
right coronary artery
distal continuation of left anterior descending artery (filled by collaterals)

FIG. 6.60 *Valve disease, such as this example of isolated calcific aortic stenosis (A), may be associated with coronary atherosclerotic heart disease. (B) Postmortem coronary arteriogram shows calcifications at the aortic valve level and abrupt total occlusion of the left anterior descending coronary artery. (C) Macroenzyme technique in a cross-section of the heart shows recent transmural myocardial infarction of the anterior wall of the left ventricle and the ventricular septum, which corresponds with the occluded anterior descending artery seen on the arteriogram.*

REFERENCES

Boucher CA, Brewster DC, Darling RC, Okada RD, Strauss HW, Pohost GM (1985) Determination of cardiac risks by dipyridamole-thallium imaging before peripheral vascular surgery. *N Engl J Med* 312:389

CASS Principal Investigators and their Associates (1983) Coronary artery surgery study (CASS): A randomized trial of coronary artery bypass surgery. survival data. *Circulation* 68(5):939

Gibson RS, Watson DD, Crampton RS, Craddock GB, Beller GA (1983) Predischarge [201]thallium scintigraphy to identify post-infarction patients at high risk for future cardiac events. *Circulation* 68(2):321

Hertzer NR, Beven EG, Young JR, et al (1984) Coronary artery disease in peripheral vascular patients: A classification of 1000 coronary angiograms and results of surgical management. *Ann Surg* 199(2):223

Kent KM, Rosing DR, Ewels CJ, Lipson L, Bonow R, Epstein SE (1982) Prognosis of asymptomatic or mildly symptomatic patients with coronary artery disease. *Am J Cardiol* 49(8):1823

Leppo JA, O'Brien J, Rothendler JA, Getchell JD, Lee VW (1984) Dipyridamole-thallium-201 scintigraphy in the prediction of future cardiac events after acute myocardial infarction. *N Engl J Med* 310:1014

National Cooperative Study Group to Compare Medical and Surgical Therapy (1978) Unstable Angina Pectoris. I. Report of protocol—patient population. *Am J Cardiol* 42:839

Staniloff H, Diamond G, Forrester J, Berman D, Swan HJC (1982) Prediction of death, infarction, and worsening chest pain with exercise electrocardiography and thallium scintigraphy. *Am J Cardiol* 49:967

Theroux P, Waters DD, Halphen C, Debaisieux JC, Mizgala HF (1979) Prognostic value of exercise testing soon after myocardial infarction. *N Engl J Med* 30(7):341

Waters DD, Szlachcic J, Miller D, Theroux P (1982) Clinical characteristics of patients with variant angina complicated by myocardial infarction or death within 1 month. *Am J Cardiol* 49:658

FIGURE CREDITS

FIG. 6.5 From Becker AE, Anderson RH: *Cardiac Pathology.* New York, Raven Press, 1983, p 3.4.

FIG. 6.8 From Becker AE, Anderson RH: *Cardiac Pathology.* New York, Raven Press, 1983.

FIG. 6.9 Adapted from Becker AE, Hoedemaeker PJ: *Pathologie.* Utrecht, Wetenschappelijke Uitgeverij Bunge, 1984.

Table 6.2 From Campeau L: Letter to the editor. *Circulation* 54:522, 1976; with permission of the American Heart Association, Inc.

FIG. 6.10 (A,B) Redrawn from Hurst JW, Woodson GC: *Atlas of Spatial Vector Electrocardiography.* New York, The Blakiston Company, 1952, pp 124, 125, 138, 139.

FIG. 6.11 (A–I) Redrawn from Silverman ME, Myerburg RJ, Hurst JW: *Electrocardiography: Basic Concepts and Clinical Application.* New York, McGraw-Hill, 1983, pp 140–148.

FIG. 6.12 Redrawn from Castellanos A, Myerburg RJ: The resting electrocardiogram, Chapter 14 in Hurst JW (ed): *The Heart,* 6th ed. New York, McGraw-Hill, 1986, p 221.

FIG. 6.13 Redrawn from Hurst JW, Wenger NK (eds): *Electrocardiographic Interpretation.* New York, McGraw-Hill, 1963, p 153.

FIG. 6.14 Redrawn from Hurst JW, Woodson GC: *Atlas of Spatial Vector Electrocardiography.* New York, The Blakiston Company, 1952, pp 202, 203.

FIG. 6.15 Redrawn from Hurst JW, Wenger NK (eds): *Electrocardiographic Interpretation.* New York, McGraw-Hill, 1963, p 217.

FIG. 6.16 Redrawn from Hurst JW, Wenger NK (eds): *Electrocardiographic Interpretation.* New York, McGraw-Hill, 1963, p 289.

FIG. 6.17 Redrawn from DeBusk RF: Techniques of exercise testing, Chapter 98 in Hurst JW (ed): *The Heart,* 6th ed. New York, McGraw-Hill, 1986, p 1707.

FIG. 6.18 From Felner JM: Echocardiography, Chapter 120 in Hurst JW (ed): *The Heart,* 6th ed. New York, McGraw-Hill, 1986, p 1962.

FIG. 6.19 (A–D) From Franch RH, King III SB, Douglas JS Jr: Techniques of cardiac catheterization, Chapter 108 in Hurst JW (ed): *The Heart,* 6th ed. New York, Mc-Graw Hill, 1986, pp 1798–1800.

FIG. 6.21 (A–L) From Zaret BL, Berger HJ: Techniques of nuclear cardiology, Chapter 109 in Hurst JW (ed): *The Heart,* 6th ed. New York, McGraw-Hill, 1986, pp 1809–1858.

FIG. 6.22 Redrawn from Mock MB, Ringqvist I, Fisher LD, et al: Survival of medically treated patients in the coronary artery surgery study (CASS) Registry. *Circulation* 66:562, 1982; with permission of the American Heart Association, Inc.

FIG. 6.23 Redrawn from Proudfit WL, Bruschke AVG, Sones FM Jr.: Natural history of obstructive coronary artery disease: Ten-year study of 601 non-surgical cases. *Prog Cardiovasc Dis* XXI (1):61, 1978.

FIG. 6.24 Redrawn from Multicenter Postinfarction Research Group: Risk stratification and survival after myocardial infarction (Arthur J. Moss, MD, Principal Investigator). *N Engl J Med* 308:331, 1983.

FIG. 6.38 (A–C) From Hall DP, Gruentzig AR: Technique of percutaneous transluminal angioplasty of the coronary, renal, mesenteric, and peripheral arteries, Chapter 117 in Hurst JW (ed): *The Heart,* 6th ed. New York, McGraw-Hill, 1986, p 1902.

FIG. 6.39 From Hurst JW, King III SB, Walter PF, Friesinger GC, Edwards JE: Atherosclerotic coronary heart disease: Angina pectoris, myocardial infarction, and other manifestations of myocardial ischemia, Chapter 45, in Hurst JW (ed): *The Heart,* 5th ed. New York, McGraw-Hill, 1982, p 1090.

FIG. 6.40 From Becker AE, Anderson RH: *Cardiac Pathology.* New York, Raven Press, 1983, p 3.13.

FIG. 6.41 From Becker AE, Anderson RH: *Cardiac Pathology.* New York, Raven Press, 1983, p 3.17.

FIG. 6.43 From Becker AE, Anderson RH: *Cardiac Pathology.* New York, Raven Press, 1983, p 3.18.

FIG. 6.44 From Becker AE, Anderson RH: *Cardiac Pathology.* New York, Raven Press, 1983, p. 3.18.

FIG. 6.45 From Becker AE, Anderson RH: *Cardiac Pathology.* New York, Raven Press, 1983.

FIG. 6.53 From Becker AE, Anderson RH: *Cardiac Pathology.* New York, Raven Press, 1983, p 3.22.

FIG. 6.55 From Franch RH, King III SB, Douglas JS Jr. Techniques of cardiac catheterization, Chapter 108 in Hurst JW (ed): *The Heart,* 6th ed. New York, McGraw-Hill, 1986, p 1804.

7
PERICARDIAL DISEASE

J. Willis Hurst, MD
Ralph Shabetai, MD
Anton E. Becker, MD
Benson R. Wilcox, MD

Abstracted with permission of the author and publisher from Shabetai R: Diseases of the pericardium, Chapter 59, pp 1249–1275, in Hurst JW (ed): *The Heart,* 6th ed. New York, McGraw-Hill, 1986. Figures and the tables reproduced in this chapter from the above chapter, other chapters in *The Heart*, or other sources are also reprinted with permission of the authors and publishers. For the full bibliographic citations of the sources of figures other than the above chapter, see Figure Credits at the end of this chapter.

While the principal causes of pericardial disease are numerous (Table 7.1), four clinical syndromes may be defined: acute pericarditis, recurrent pericarditis, pericardial effusion with or without cardiac tamponade, and constrictive pericarditis.

ACUTE PERICARDITIS
ETIOLOGY AND PATHOLOGY

Acute pericarditis is usually due to a viral infection, commonly by echovirus or coxsackievirus. The term idiopathic pericarditis is used when clinical features are similar to those of a viral infection, but a viral etiology is not demonstrated (see Table 7.1).

The pathology of acute pericarditis is determined by the exudative response as it relates to the underlying cause. The pericardial layers are often coated with fibrinous depositions (Fig. 7.1). Cultures of the fibrin deposits and fluid may reveal the etiology. Purulent pericarditis indicates a bacterial cause, often due to direct spread of the infection from other sites in the heart (Figs. 7.2, 7.3) or surrounding structures, such as the lung. A hemorrhagic exudate often indicates a neoplasm as the underlying cause; it may also occur in patients with tuberculosis or in those receiving anticoagulant therapy for chronic renal disease. Pericarditis may occur after myocardial infarction or following cardiac surgery. Lupus erythematosus may be the cause, especially in young women. Occasionally cytology of the exudate may indicate the proper

---

Table 7.1 Etiology of Pericarditis*

I. Trauma
  A. Pericardiotomy
  B. Indirect trauma to chest
  C. Transeptal catheterization
  D. Pressure injection of contrast medium
  E. Perforation of right ventricle by indwelling catheter
  F. Implantation of epicardial pacemaker
  G. Blow to chest
  H. Perforation of right ventricle with catheter for parenteral nutrition

II. Viral infections
  A. Coxsackieviruses B5, B6
  B. Echovirus
  C. Adenovirus
  D. Infectious mononucleosis
  E. Influenza
  F. Lymphogranuloma venereum
  G. Chickenpox
  H. Mycoplasma pneumoniae

III. Bacterial infections
  A. Staphylococcus
  B. Pneumococcus
  C. Meningococcus
  D. Streptococcus
  E. Haemophilus influenzae
  F. Psittacosis
  G. Salmonella
  H. Tuberculosis

IV. Amebiasis
V. Echinococcus cysts
VI. Fungus infections—histoplasmosis, aspergillosis, blastomycosis, coccidioidomycosis
VII. Rickettsia
VIII. Radiation
IX. Amyloidosis

X. Tumors
  A. Primary
    1. Mesothelioma
    2. Rhabdomyosarcoma
    3. Teratoma
    4. Fibroma
    5. Leiomyofibroma
    6. Lipoma
    7. Angioma
  B. Metastatic
    1. Bronchogenic carcinoma
    2. Carcinoma of breast
    3. Lymphoma
    4. Leukemia
    5. Melanoma

XI. Sarcoid
XII. Collagen disease
  A. Rheumatic fever
  B. Lupus erythematosus
  C. Rheumatoid arthritis
  D. Vasculitis
  E. Polyarteritis nodosa
  F. Scleroderma
  G. Dermatomyositis

XIII. Anticoagulants
  A. Heparin
  B. Warfarin

XIV. Myocardial infarction
  A. Acute myocardial infarction
  B. Postmyocardial infarction (Dressler's syndrome)

XV. Idiopathic thrombocytopenic purpura
XVI. Drugs
  A. Procainamide
  B. Cromolyn sodium
  C. Hydralazine
  D. Dantrolene
  E. Methysergide

XVII. Dissecting aneurysm
XVIII. Infective endocarditis with valve ring abscess
XIX. Thymic cyst

(Modified from Table 59-1, *The Heart,* 6th ed, p. 1252)
*Principal causes of pericardial disease and pericardial heart disease. Many of these conditions can cause pericardial effusion, cardiac tamponade, and/or constrictive pericarditis. The more common causes of these syndromes are mentioned under the syndromes and under specific disorders.

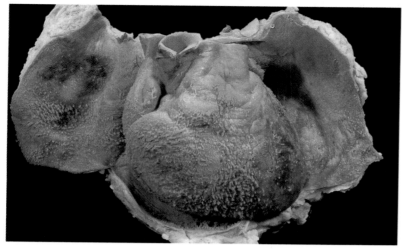

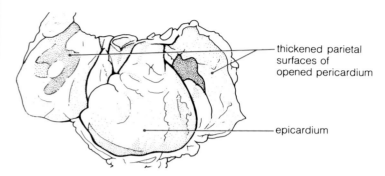

FIG. 7.1 *This heart with the pericardium opened shows fibrinous pericarditis, which is most likely of viral origin.*

thickened parietal
surfaces of
opened pericardium

epicardium

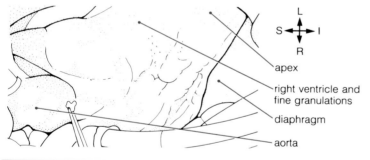

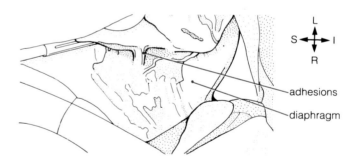

FIG. 7.2 (A) *The epicardial surface in this operative view of the heart has a fine granular appearance. Bacterial endocarditis extends into the pericar-*

dium. (B) *Adhesions extend to the diaphragmatic surface of the heart.*

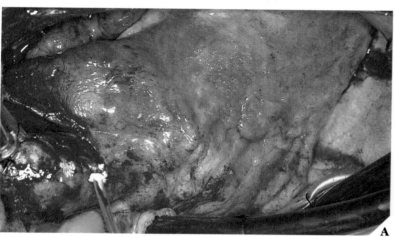

apex

right ventricle and
fine granulations

diaphragm

aorta

adhesions

diaphragm

FIG. 7.3 *Chronic purulent pericarditis in this heart was caused by bacterial infection.*

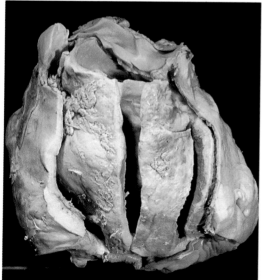

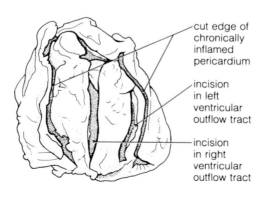

cut edge of
chronically
inflamed
pericardium

incision
in left
ventricular
outflow tract

incision
in right
ventricular
outflow tract

diagnosis, such as lymphoma or Pfeiffer's disease (infectious mononucleosis). In rare cases the histology identifies the underlying cause as fungi or caseous granulomata suggesting tuberculosis (Fig. 7.4).

ABNORMAL PHYSIOLOGY

The amount of pericardial fluid may slightly increase with acute pericarditis, but patients who have considerable fluid are excluded from this discussion. By definition, therefore, hemodynamic alterations do not occur in patients with uncomplicated acute pericarditis. The chest pain produced by pericarditis is due to stimulation of the phrenic and intercostal nerves.

CLINICAL MANIFESTATIONS
SYMPTOMS

Patients may develop myalgia and fever a few days before the onset of chest pain. Usually located in the anterior portion of the chest or precordium, the pain may radiate to the top of the shoulders. It may be either sharp or crushing, and may be aggravated by inspiration, turning, or swallowing. Patients may also have pericarditis without chest pain.

PHYSICAL EXAMINATION

While the physical examination may be normal, it is possible to detect that the patient is trying to avoid deep inspirations that produce pain. A pericardial friction rub is sometimes detected. It is best heard with the patient in a sitting position; the stethoscope is placed on the precordium between the left sternal border and the apex. The rub may be louder during inspiration. It is often triphasic; the components occur with atrial systole, ventricular systole, and ventricular diastole (Spodick, 1971). However, the rub may consist of only one or two of these components. Atrial arrhythmias may occur, possibly due to inflammation of the sinus node (Spodick, 1984).

LABORATORY STUDIES

CHEST RADIOGRAPHY. The chest film is usually normal in patients with acute pericarditis with little pericardial fluid and no myocarditis.

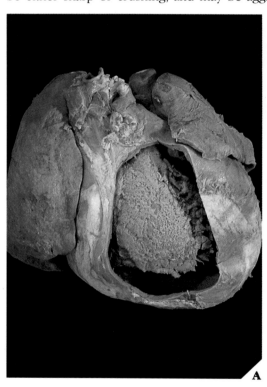
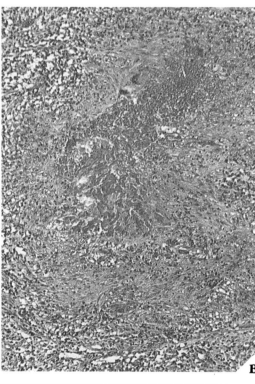

FIG. 7.4 (**A**) *A window cut into the pericardium of this grossly enlarged heart exposes fibrinous pericarditis due to tuberculosis.* (**B**) *Histologic section of the pericardium shows caseous necrosis indicative of tuberculosis. (Reproduced with permission of the authors and publisher; see Figure Credits)*

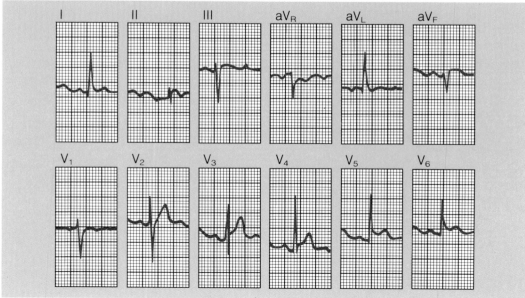

FIG. 7.5 *ECG from a patient with acute pericarditis shows PR-segment depression and ST-segment elevation. (Redrawn; reproduced with permission of the author and publisher; see Figure Credits. Also, Fig. 59-2, The Heart, 6th ed, p 1253)*

The film may show the disease process etiologically related to the pericarditis, such as pneumonia or neoplastic disease.

ELECTROCARDIOGRAPHY.   The electrocardiogram (ECG) of acute pericarditis is characterized by PR-segment depression, normal QRS complexes, and a mean ST-segment vector that is directed toward the cardiac apex (Fig. 7.5). Later in the disease course the ST-segment vector becomes smaller, and as it does, the T wave vector is abnormally directed away from the cardiac apex (Spodick, 1973). These changes are due to inflammation of the epicardium of the heart. Myocarditis should be considered when atrioventricular block or bundle branch block occurs. Electrocardiographic changes may not appear in uremic pericarditis.

ECHOCARDIOGRAPHY.   The echocardiogram is normal unless pericardial fluid or myocarditis is present.

OTHER LABORATORY ABNORMALITIES.   The erythrocyte sedimentation rate is usually elevated. Leukocytosis or lymphocytosis may be present. Cardiac enzyme levels are usually normal. Skin tests for tuberculosis and fungi may be performed.

NATURAL HISTORY
The natural history of acute pericarditis often depends on the etiology. The prognosis of pericarditis follows that of the causative disease itself in the following: uremia, collagen disease, acute myocardial infarction, and dissection of the aorta.

The natural history of bacterial pericarditis is very different from that of viral pericarditis. Bacterial causes may be fatal unless recognized with subsequent drainage of the pericardium. The natural history of viral or idiopathic pericarditis is usually predictable due to the self-limiting nature of viral infections. Fever and pericardial rub usually subside within two weeks; however, the disease may recur. When the illness lasts longer than two weeks, it is wise to consider a more serious etiology.

TREATMENT
There are two approaches to the relief of pain due to pericarditis. Some physicians use aspirin, ibuprofen, or indomethacin to relieve the pain, resorting to corticosteroids only if nonsteroidal therapy fails. Other physicians use corticosteroids initially. However, it is important to consider the etiology of the condition before utilizing either therapeutic modality. Corticosteroids are contraindicated in patients who have bacterial pericarditis. Whenever corticosteroids are used it is wise to use the smallest dose of corticosteroids allowing pain relief, and the drugs are discontinued as soon as possible (Connoly and Burchell, 1961).

RECURRENT PERICARDITIS
Regardless of the etiology acute pericarditis may recur after varying intervals (Burchell, 1954), possibly due to immunologic causes. Therapy consists of nonsteroidal drugs and corticosteroids, although long-term use of corticosteroids should be avoided. Immunosuppressive therapy has been used. A few patients will require pericardiectomy for relief of recurrent pericardial pain.

PERICARDIAL EFFUSION
ETIOLOGY AND PATHOLOGY
Pericardial effusion may be clinically associated with acute or recurrent pericarditis. It may be discovered on routine examination or during the workup of an ill patient. The effusion may be asymptomatic, or it may produce cardiac tamponade.

The common causes of pericarditis with effusion are acute viral or idiopathic pericarditis, collagen disease (especially lupus and rheumatoid arthritis), neoplastic disease (especially breast cancer, bronchogenic carcinoma, and lymphoma), and postpericardiotomy or Dressler's (postmyocardial infarction) syndrome (see Table 7.1). Most commonly transmural myocardial infarction results in effusion (Fig. 7.6), but in this situation the pathology of the epicardium and pericardium is not specific. Hemorrhagic pericardial effusion may be caused by rupture of the heart due to myocardial infarction or dissecting aortic aneurysm. Pyogenic effusion must not be overlooked, since specific therapy is necessary for cure.

ABNORMAL PHYSIOLOGY
The normal amount of pericardial fluid is approximately 50 mL. The characteristics of the pericardial pressure–volume curve shown in Figure 7.7 (Holt, 1970) are determined by the elastic properties of the pericardium and the speed at which pericardial fluid accumulates. The initial flat portion of the curve indicates fluid accumulation; during

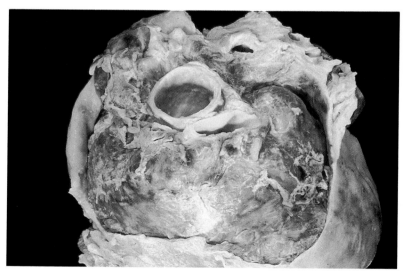

FIG. 7.6   *This example of fibrinous pericarditis occurred as a consequence of acute myocardial infarction. (Reproduced with permission of the authors and publisher; see Figure Credits)*

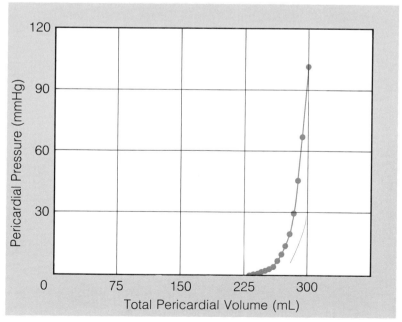

FIG. 7.7   *Pericardial pressure–volume curve (canine). (Redrawn; reproduced with permission of the author and publisher; see Figure Credits. Also, Fig. 59-1, The Heart, 6th ed, p 1250)*

this phase the pericardium stretches and adapts to the increasing volume. The intrapericardial pressure is lower than the atrial or ventricular diastolic pressure.

As more fluid accumulates, stretching of the pericardium reaches a limit; at that point the intrapericardial pressure may rise to dangerous levels. The normal filling pressures of the heart are then exceeded and must increase to allow continued circulation. When fluid accumulates slowly, the cardiac silhouette may become quite large with no signs of tamponade. When fluid accumulates abruptly, the cardiac silhouette may increase only slightly in size, yet serious tamponade may be present.

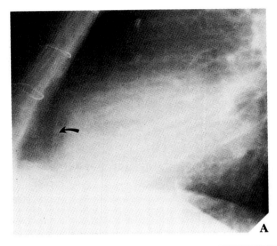
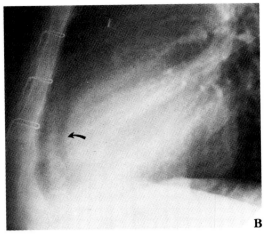

A

B

FIG. 7.8 **(A)** *Lateral radiograph of a patient three weeks after a coronary bypass procedure shows normal pericardium as a hairline density* (arrow) *sandwiched between the subepicardial fat stripe interiorly and the mediastinal fat exteriorly. Metallic sutures are evident in the sternum, and a surgical clip marks the origin of a venous graft in the ascending aorta.* **(B)** *The same patient developed postpericardiotomy syndrome five weeks postoperation. In this lateral radiograph the subepicardial fat stripe* (arrow) *is more distinct because of pericardial effusion, and is displaced interiorly by the widened pericardium.* (Fig. 107-4, The Heart, 6th ed; see Figure Credits)

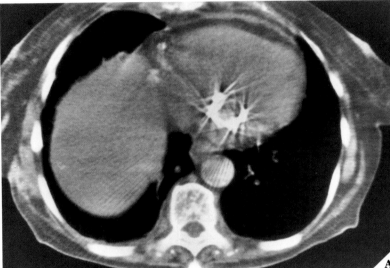

A

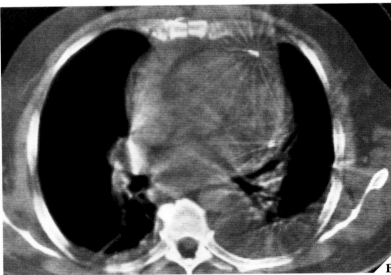

B

FIG. 7.9 **(A)** *CT scan at the level of a mitral heterograft in a 77-year-old female following mitral valve replacement shows anterior pericardial thickening between the more lucent epicardial fat and retrosternal fat.* **(B)** *A scan of a 53-year-old male examined because of suspected mediastinitis two weeks following coronary bypass surgery reveals loculated pericardial effusion in the right side of the pericardial space, outlined by the air-containing lung laterally and the epicardial fat medially. Bilateral pleural effusions are also present. The two densities with streak artifacts are surgical clips.* (Figs. 111-3, 111-4, The Heart, 6th ed; see Figure Credits)

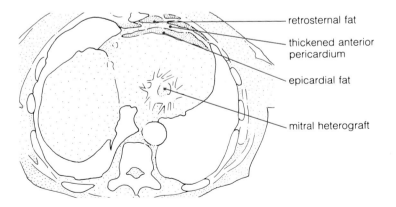

retrosternal fat

thickened anterior pericardium

epicardial fat

mitral heterograft

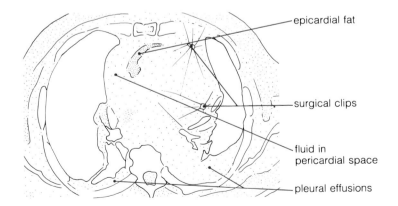

epicardial fat

surgical clips

fluid in pericardial space

pleural effusions

CLINICAL MANIFESTATIONS
Pericardial Effusion Without Cardiac Tamponade

Pericardial effusion should be considered when a patient has a disease that may involve the pericardium. Effusion should be suspected especially when there is any evidence of pericarditis.

SYMPTOMS

There may be no symptoms resulting from pericardial effusion unless tamponade is present.

PHYSICAL EXAMINATION

The physical examination does not usually reveal any evidence of fluid. The neck veins do not show abnormal distention or pulsation. Heart sounds are not usually diminished in intensity by the presence of pericardial fluid; a friction rub may be heard even when there is considerable effusion.

LABORATORY STUDIES

CHEST RADIOGRAPHY.   Pericardial fluid may be suspected when the chest film is reviewed. An epicardial fat stripe may occasionally be seen in patients with pericardial effusion (Fig. 7.8). However, the typical appearance is an enlarged cardiac shadow with smooth borders and no evidence of pulmonary congestion. The problem, however, is to differentiate among pericardial fluid alone, cardiac enlargement alone, and the presence of both pericardial effusion and cardiac enlargement. Computed tomography (CT) may be used to identify pericardial disease and pericardial effusion (Fig. 7.9).

ELECTROCARDIOGRAPHY.   The ECG may reveal low voltage. Electrical alternans is occasionally present when the effusion is large (Fig. 7.10).

ECHOCARDIOGRAPHY.   The cross-sectional echocardiogram is both sensitive and specific in identifying pericardial effusion (Fig. 7.11)

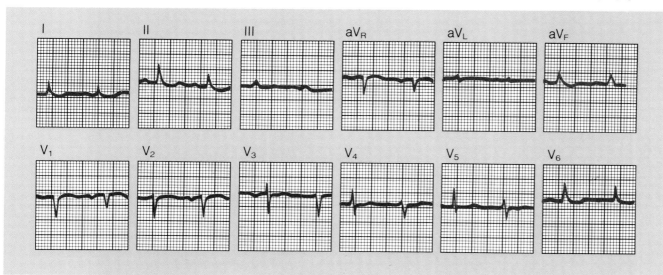

FIG. 7.10 *Electrical alternans of the QRS complex may occur with pericardial effusion. This particular patient also had cardiac tamponade. (Redrawn; reproduced with permission of the authors and publisher; see Figure Credits. Also, Fig. 59-6, The Heart, 6th ed, p 1261)*

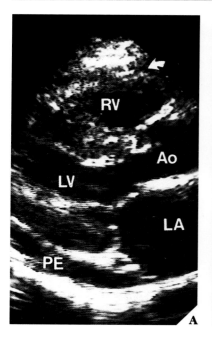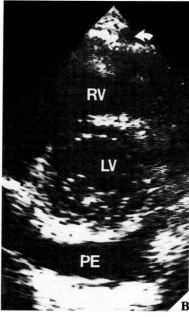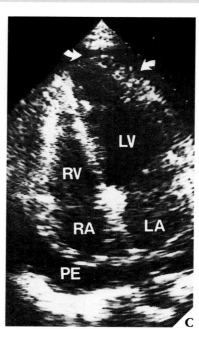

FIG. 7.11 *Parasternal long axis (A) and short axis (B) cross-sectional echocardiograms show moderate-sized posterior (PE) and small anterior pericardial effusions (arrows). Apical four-chamber view (C) shows fluid completely surrounding the heart (RV, right ventricle; LV, left ventricle; Ao, aorta; LA, left atrium; RA, right atrium) (Courtesy of Joel Felner, MD, Atlanta, Georgia)*

(Teicholz, 1978; Haaz et al, 1980); in addition it may be used to identify chamber enlargement when present.

CARDIAC CATHETERIZATION. Pericardial effusion without tamponade is occasionally detected when cardiac catheterization and angiography are performed (Fig. 7.12).

PERICARDIAL ASPIRATION. Pericardial aspiration (Fig. 7.13) is not usually indicated in patients who have either viral or self-limited pericarditis with effusion. This technique should be performed when the clinical course runs longer than two weeks despite medical therapy, and bacterial or nonviral infection is considered a possible cause. It is, for example, used to distinguish between neoplastic effusion and

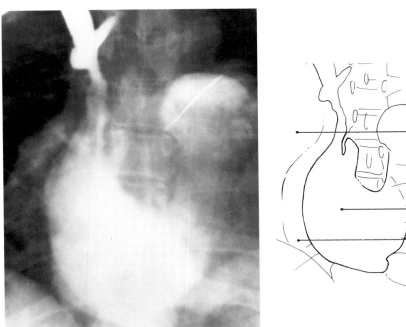
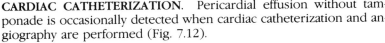

FIG. 7.12 *Pericardial effusion is demonstrated by contrast medium injected into the right side of the heart. Note the distance between contrast medium located in the right atrium and the right border of the pericardium. (Courtesy of Murray Baron, MD, Atlanta, Georgia)*

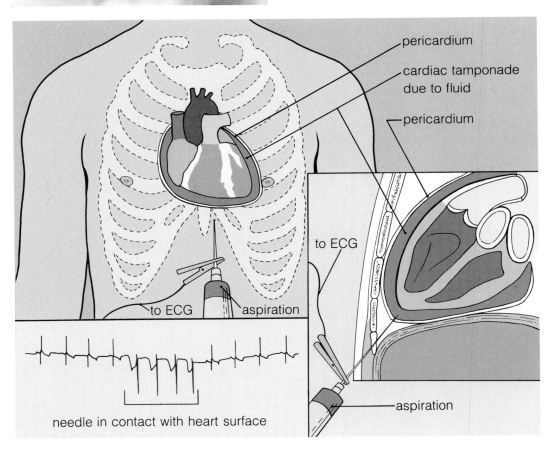

FIG. 7.13 *In the subxiphoid pericardiocentesis technique, the needle is inserted to the left of the xiphoid and directed toward the midscapular area. The ECG lead is attached to the needle. Negative deflection of the QRS complex represents contact with the heart surface. As the needle is slowly withdrawn, the ECG reverts to normal when the needle loses contact with the myocardium. (Redrawn; reproduced with permission of the authors and publisher; see Figure Credits. Also, Fig. 126-1, The Heart, 6th ed, p 2009)*

radiation pericarditis in patients with cancer of the breast or lung. Aspiration is also indicated when tamponade from any cause is suspected.

Pericardial Effusion With Cardiac Tamponade

Any disease affecting the pericardium may cause pericardial effusion, which in turn may potentially produce cardiac tamponade. The common causes of tamponade are trauma (including surgical procedures on the heart), cardiac rupture from infarction, dissecting aneurysm, viral or idiopathic pericarditis, neoplastic pericarditis, collagen disease, dialysis-related pericardial disease, and, rarely, Dressler's syndrome.

SYMPTOMS

Severe symptoms or death may result from acute cardiac tamponade that occurs rapidly, as in cardiac rupture. In less dramatic examples the patient may complain of dyspnea, chest tightness, or pericardial pain.

PHYSICAL EXAMINATION

The external jugular veins are distended, and the systemic arterial pressure may be abnormally low. When the tamponade does not occur rapidly, abnormal pulsations of the internal jugular veins may be identified. The x descent becomes prominent and coincides with the carotid pulse. A paradoxical pulse may be detected with the blood pressure cuff unless hypotension is severe (Cohn et al, 1967). The apex impulse of the heart is decreased in size, but heart sounds may not be diminished in intensity (Beck, 1935).

LABORATORY STUDIES

ELECTROCARDIOGRAPHY.   No signs of cardiac tamponade are detected in the ECG. Electrical alternans may occur with pericardial effusion, but it does not necessarily imply that tamponade is present.

ECHOCARDIOGRAPHY.   Cross-sectional echocardiography is extremely useful in identifying pericardial effusion with cardiac tamponade (Fig. 7.14). It reveals evidence of compression of the right atrium and diastolic collapse of the right ventricle (Gillam et al, 1983; Leimgruber et al, 1983).

CARDIAC CATHETERIZATION.   Cardiac catheterization reveals equal diastolic pressure in the two sides of the heart and decreased ventricular volumes. This procedure is usually not necessary, but it is occasionally useful to measure the right atrial and pulmonary wedge pressures. However, echocardiographic studies may be adequate to supply this information.

PERICARDIAL ASPIRATION.   See the sections "Pericardial Effusion Without Cardiac Tamponade" (above) and "Treatment" (below).

SKIN TESTS AND OTHER LABORATORY TESTS.   Skin tests for tuberculosis and fungi aid in defining the etiology of pericarditis with effusion. Blood may also be tested for evidence of collagen disease or prior viral infections.

NATURAL HISTORY

The natural history of pericardial effusion with or without tamponade is determined by the promptness of the diagnosis, the etiology of the disease, and the therapy employed. Viral or idiopathic pericarditis with effusion is usually self-limiting and benign; however, it may recur or lead to constriction. Pericarditis due to bacteria, including the tubercle bacillus, is always serious, but it may be successfully treated when recognized. Effusion due to neoplasm is obviously serious and may contribute to the death of the patient. Effusion due to collagen disease can usually be managed on a long-term basis, although cardiac tamponade may ensue. In general, however, the patient's clinical course is related to the collagen disease. Acute hemorrhagic effusion with tamponade is often lethal when caused by rupture of the heart or aorta.

TREATMENT

The treatment of pericardial effusion depends on the etiology of the effusion and the presence or absence of tamponade. When no tamponade is present, the patient with viral or idiopathic pericarditis may be treated with nonsteroidal drugs or corticosteroids. Effusions caused by bacteria are treated with appropriate antibiotics and pericardial drainage. Tuberculous pericarditis with effusion should be treated with long-term antituberculous therapy.

Patients with pericardial effusion and tamponade must be treated promptly. Intravenous fluid is often needed to maintain an adequate

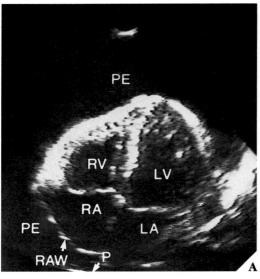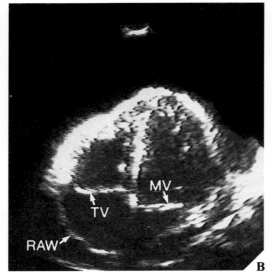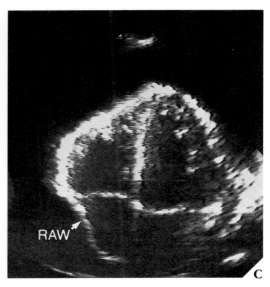

FIG. 7.14   (A–C) *Apical four-chamber views from cross-sectional echocardiography of a patient with cardiac tamponade reveal a large pericardial effusion* (PE) *surrounding the entire heart. The right atrial wall* (RAW) *is seen to collapse inwardly on each view* (RV, *right ventricle;* RA, *right atrium;* LV, *left ventricle;* LA, *left atrium;* TV, *tricuspid valve;* MV, *mitral value*). *(Courtesy of Joel Felner, MD, Atlanta, Georgia)*

filling pressure. Isoproterenol may be used to increase contractility, while nitroprusside is used to decrease peripheral arterial resistance. Medical management is not, however, a permanent solution to the problem of tamponade. More definitive treatment with aspiration or surgery is usually needed. Pericardial aspiration of even a small amount of fluid may reverse the hemodynamic abnormalities (Krikorian and Hancock, 1978). If repeated aspirations are needed, surgical drainage is indicated. If the etiology is not clear after drainage, a pericardial biopsy may be helpful.

CONSTRICTIVE PERICARDITIS
ETIOLOGY AND PATHOLOGY
Constrictive pericarditis may develop following pericarditis due to any cause. The majority of cases are idiopathic or postviral, posttraumatic (including surgery on the heart), neoplastic, postradiation treatment to the mediastinum, due to collagen disease (i.e., rheumatoid arthritis), or due to bacterial infections including tuberculosis. Constrictive pericarditis due to bacterial causes is becoming less common (Andrews et al, 1948).

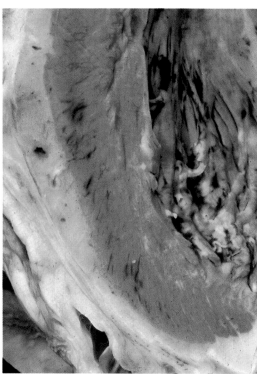

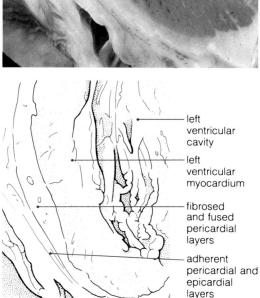

left ventricular cavity

left ventricular myocardium

fibrosed and fused pericardial layers

adherent pericardial and epicardial layers producing constriction

Constrictive pericarditis is characterized by fibrous tissue encapsulating the heart either locally or diffusely (Fig. 7.15) The cause of injury cannot usually be determined from the current pathological state; an exception is constriction due to massive growth of a tumor. The creamy pericardial fluid found in some examples of constrictive pericarditis may contain calcium (Fig. 7.16); in these cases one may overestimate the amount of calcification of the epicardium, when viewing the chest film.

ABNORMAL PHYSIOLOGY
The inflammation of pericarditis produces a fibrous tissue response in the pericardium and epicardium, eventually leading to a tight pericardium and poor compliance. The fibrous tissue gradually limits diastolic filling of the heart; when a critical point is reached, the hemodynamics of the heart are altered.

The altered physiology of cardiac tamponade and constrictive pericarditis is similar, but there are some distinct differences, as illustrated in Figure 7.17. Cardiac catheterization shows abnormalities associated with cardiac tamponade (Fig. 7.18) and with constrictive pericarditis (Fig. 7.19).

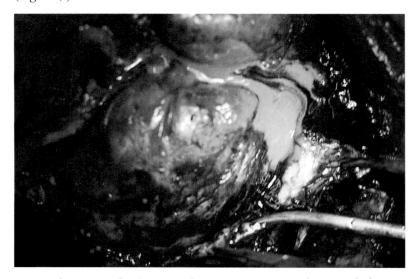

FIG. 7.15 *Fibrosed pericardial layers encapsulating the heart characterize constrictive pericarditis. (Reproduced with permission of the authors and publisher; see Figure Credits)*

FIG. 7.16 *Creamy fluid, seen in this operative view, in chronic calcific constrictive pericarditis contains calcium crystals. The radiographic appearance of this heart suggested more extensive calcification than was actually found.*

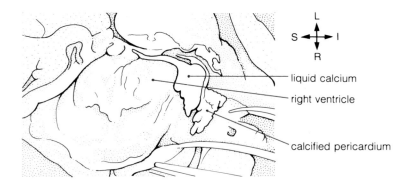

liquid calcium

right ventricle

calcified pericardium

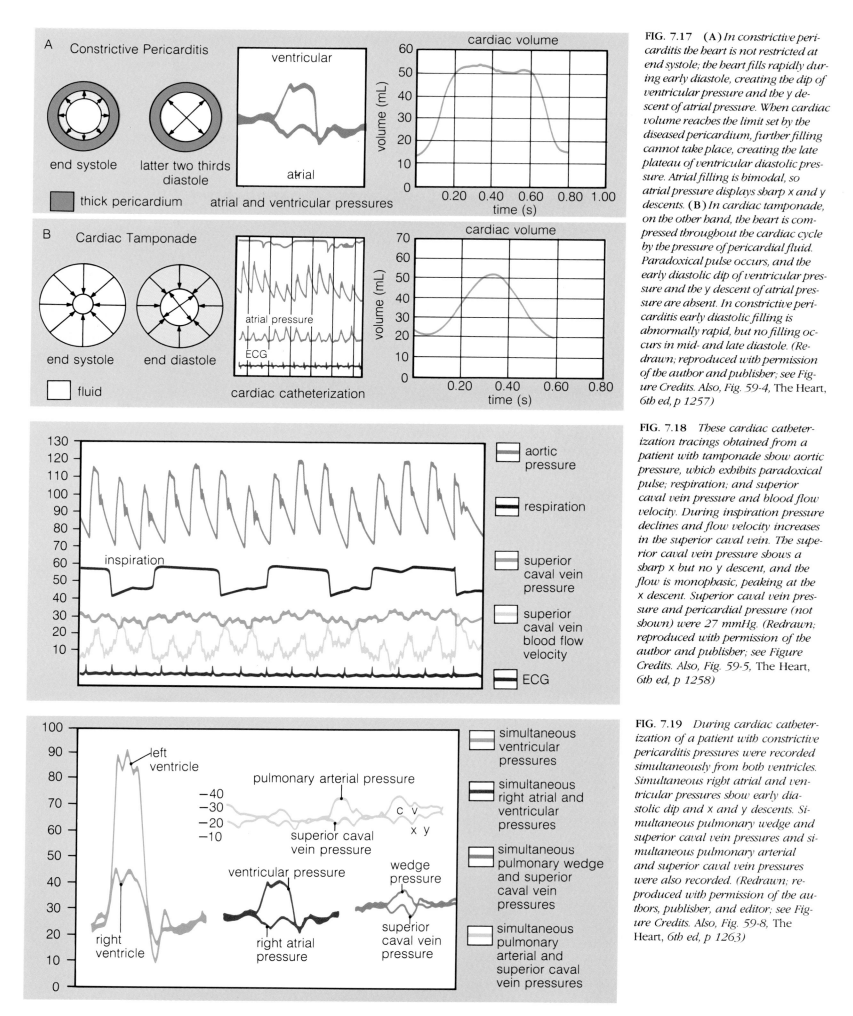

A Constrictive Pericarditis

end systole   latter two thirds diastole

■ thick pericardium

ventricular

atrial

atrial and ventricular pressures

cardiac volume

volume (mL)
60
50
40
30
20
10
0

0.20   0.40   0.60   0.80   1.00
time (s)

B Cardiac Tamponade

end systole   end diastole

□ fluid

atrial pressure

ECG

cardiac catheterization

cardiac volume

volume (mL)
70
60
50
40
30
20
10
0

0.20   0.40   0.60   0.80
time (s)

FIG. 7.17 (**A**) *In constrictive pericarditis the heart is not restricted at end systole; the heart fills rapidly during early diastole, creating the dip of ventricular pressure and the y descent of atrial pressure. When cardiac volume reaches the limit set by the diseased pericardium, further filling cannot take place, creating the late plateau of ventricular diastolic pressure. Atrial filling is bimodal, so atrial pressure displays sharp x and y descents. (**B**) In cardiac tamponade, on the other hand, the heart is compressed throughout the cardiac cycle by the pressure of pericardial fluid. Paradoxical pulse occurs, and the early diastolic dip of ventricular pressure and the y descent of atrial pressure are absent. In constrictive pericarditis early diastolic filling is abnormally rapid, but no filling occurs in mid- and late diastole. (Redrawn; reproduced with permission of the author and publisher; see Figure Credits. Also, Fig. 59-4, The Heart, 6th ed, p 1257)*

130
120
110
100
90
80
70
60
50
40
30
20
10

inspiration

— aortic pressure

— respiration

— superior caval vein pressure

— superior caval vein blood flow velocity

— ECG

FIG. 7.18 *These cardiac catheterization tracings obtained from a patient with tamponade show aortic pressure, which exhibits paradoxical pulse; respiration; and superior caval vein pressure and blood flow velocity. During inspiration pressure declines and flow velocity increases in the superior caval vein. The superior caval vein pressure shows a sharp x but no y descent, and the flow is monophasic, peaking at the x descent. Superior caval vein pressure and pericardial pressure (not shown) were 27 mmHg. (Redrawn; reproduced with permission of the author and publisher; see Figure Credits. Also, Fig. 59-5, The Heart, 6th ed, p 1258)*

100
90
80
70
60
50
40
30
20
10
0

left ventricle

pulmonary arterial pressure

—40
—30
—20
—10

superior caval vein pressure

c v
x y

ventricular pressure

wedge pressure

right ventricle

right atrial pressure

superior caval vein pressure

— simultaneous ventricular pressures

— simultaneous right atrial and ventricular pressures

— simultaneous pulmonary wedge and superior caval vein pressures

— simultaneous pulmonary arterial and superior caval vein pressures

FIG. 7.19 *During cardiac catheterization of a patient with constrictive pericarditis pressures were recorded simultaneously from both ventricles. Simultaneous right atrial and ventricular pressures show early diastolic dip and x and y descents. Simultaneous pulmonary wedge and superior caval vein pressures and simultaneous pulmonary arterial and superior caval vein pressures were also recorded. (Redrawn; reproduced with permission of the authors, publisher, and editor; see Figure Credits. Also, Fig. 59-8, The Heart, 6th ed, p 1263)*

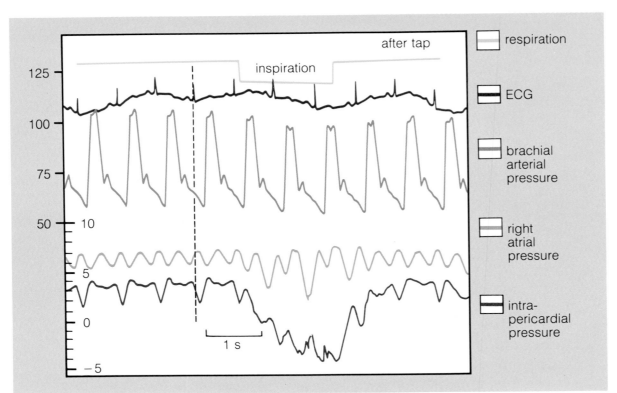

FIG. 7.20 *These recordings were made during cardiac catheterization of a patient with effusive constrictive pericarditis due to bronchogenic carcinoma. The tracings were obtained during pericardiocentesis, which lowered pericardial pressure. However, right atrial pressure elevation persists, and the tracing shows prominent x and y descents and absent respiratory variation. (Redrawn; reproduced with permission of the author and publisher; see Figure Credits. Also, Fig. 59-9, The Heart, 6th ed, p 1265)*

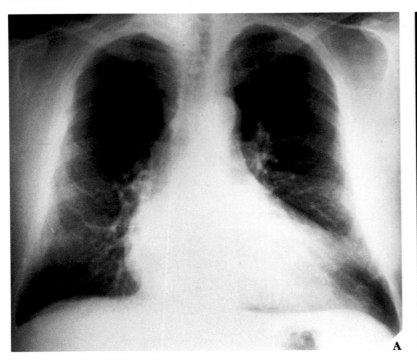 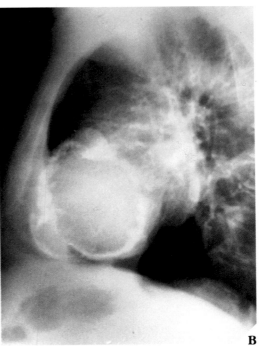

FIG. 7.21 **(A)** *Posteroanterior chest radiograph of a patient with calcific pericarditis does not clearly show the calcified pericardium.* **(B)** *Lateral view demonstrates the calcified pericardium surrounding the heart. The etiology was never established; however, tuberculous pericarditis was suspected. (Courtesy of Stephen D. Clements, Jr., MD, and William J. Casarella, MD, Atlanta, Georgia)*

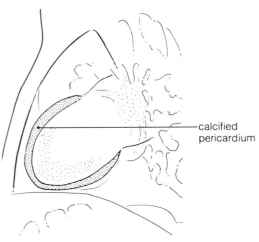

PART II: DISEASES OF THE HEART

Effusive constrictive pericarditis occurs when pericardial fluid is present while the pericardium constricts (Fig. 7.20) (Hancock, 1971).

CLINICAL MANIFESTATIONS
SYMPTOMS

Early in the disease process the patient may not have symptoms. There may be a history of prior pericarditis. As constriction progresses, the patient complains of dyspnea, edema of the extremities, and a large abdomen due to ascites; the edema and ascites are often out of proportion to the dyspnea.

PHYSICAL EXAMINATION

A paradoxical pulse is occasionally found in patients with constrictive pericarditis. The neck veins are distended, and the x and y descents may be prominent in the internal jugular venous pulse. The apex impulse is not prominent, and a pericardial knock may be heard. An enlarged liver, ascites, and severe peripheral edema may be encountered.

LABORATORY STUDIES

CHEST RADIOGRAPHY. The size of the heart may be normal, or it may be slightly enlarged when the pericardium is thick. Pericardial calcification may be seen on the lateral view (Fig. 7.21).

ELECTROCARDIOGRAPHY. Atrial fibrillation may be detected on ECG. The voltage is often diminished, and nonspecific ST-T waves may be present. Less commonly scars and calcium may involve the myocardium, producing bundle branch block and atrioventricular conduction defects.

ECHOCARDIOGRAPHY. The echocardiogram may reveal evidence of pericardial calcification and clues to the presence of constrictive pericarditis (Fig. 7.22).

CARDIAC CATHETERIZATION. Cardiac catheterization reveals equalization of the pulmonary arterial wedge pressure, diastolic pulmonary arterial pressure, diastolic right ventricular pressure, and right atrial

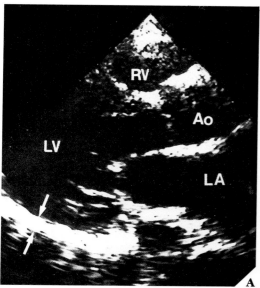 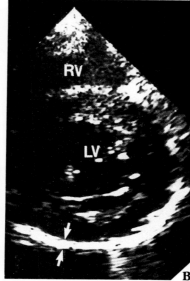 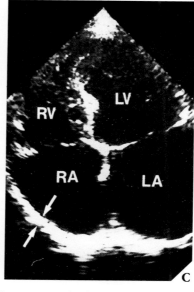

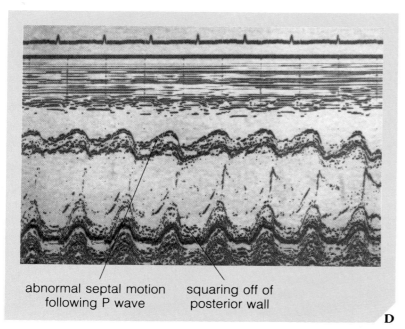

abnormal septal motion following P wave

squaring off of posterior wall

FIG. 7.22 *Cross-sectional echocardiograms in a patient with pericardial calcification show an increase in the intensity and width of the pericardial echo* (opposing arrows) *in each of the standard views:* (**A**) *parasternal long-axis view;* (**B**) *parasternal short-axis view;* (**C**) *apical four-chamber view* (LV, *left ventricle;* RV, *right ventricle;* Ao, *aorta;* LA, *left atrium;* RA, *right atrium*). (**D**) *In this M-mode echocardiogram from a patient with constrictive pericarditis following radiation to the mediastinum for malignancy, septal motion is abnormal beginning after the P wave. The posterior wall abruptly squares off in diastole as filling of the ventricle is limited by the scarred pericardium.* (**A–C**: *Courtesy of Joel M. Felner, MD, Atlanta, Georgia;* **D**: *Courtesy of Stephen D. Clements, Jr, MD, Atlanta, Georgia*)

mean pressure. The right ventricular pressure curve shows an early diastolic dip and late diastolic plateau (see Fig. 7.19).

DIFFERENTIAL DIAGNOSIS

Constrictive pericarditis must be differentiated from cirrhosis of the liver, chronic cor pulmonale, and restrictive cardiomyopathy by the techniques described above. It may not be possible, however, to differentiate restrictive cardiomyopathy from constrictive pericarditis (Meany et al, 1976; Goodwin and Oakley, 1972); an exploratory thoracotomy may be necessary. Endocardial biopsy may identify myocardial disease (Swanton et al, 1977).

NATURAL HISTORY

Without surgical intervention the patient with constrictive pericarditis shows slowly progressive deterioration with the development of atrial fibrillation, cardiac cirrhosis, nephrosis, and all of the consequences of low cardiac output.

TREATMENT

Digitalis may be needed to control atrial fibrillation. Diuretics may not be helpful in treatment of constrictive pericarditis, since a high filling pressure is required to maintain an adequate cardiac output.

Surgical removal of the pericardium is the treatment of choice (Carson et al, 1974). This is accomplished most effectively through a full median sternotomy (Fig. 7.23), which offers excellent exposure, allowing the pericardium to be removed from all surfaces of the ventricular mass. In addition this approach offers the added safety of access to institute cardiopulmonary bypass if necessary. Access to the heart can be gained through a left anterolateral thoracotomy (Fig. 7.24).

Although this affords excellent exposure of the left ventricle, the right heart is difficult to see.

The hospital mortality associated with surgical intervention for chronic constrictive pericarditis is in the range of 5%–15%. Operative risk relates to the degree of physiologic impairment of the individual patient, the presence of ascites and edema, or a depressed cardiac index (McCaughan et al, 1985).

REFERENCES

Andrews GWS, Pickering GW, Sellors TH (1948) The aetiology of constrictive pericarditis with special reference to tuberculosis pericarditis, together with a note on polyserositis. *Q J Med* 17:291.

Beck CS (1935) Two cardiac compression triads. *JAMA* 104:714.

Burchell HB (1954) Problems in the recognition and treatment of pericarditis. *Lancet* 74:465.

Carson TJ, Wilcox BR, Murray GF, Starek PJK (1974) The role of surgery in tuberculous pericarditis. *Ann Thorac Surg* 17:163.

Cohn JN, Pinkerson AL, Tristani FE (1967) Mechanism of pulsus paradoxus in clinical shock. *J Clin Invest* 46:1744.

Connoly DC, Burchell HB (1961) Pericarditis: a ten-year survey. *Am J Cardiol* 7:7.

Gillam LD, Guyer DE, Gibson TC, et al (1983) Hemodynamic compression of the right atrium, a new echocardiographic sign of cardiac tamponade. *Circulation* 68:294.

Goodwin JF, Oakley CM (1972) The cardiomyopathies. *Br Heart J* 34:345.

Haaz WS, Mintz GS, Kotler MN, Parry W, Segal BL (1980) Two-dimensional echocardiographic recognition of the descending thoracic aorta: value in differentiating pericardial from pleural effusion. *Am J Cardiol* 46:739.

Hancock EW (1971) Subacute effusive–constrictive pericarditis. *Circulation* 43:183.

Holt JP (1970) The normal pericardium. *Am J Cardiol* 26:455.

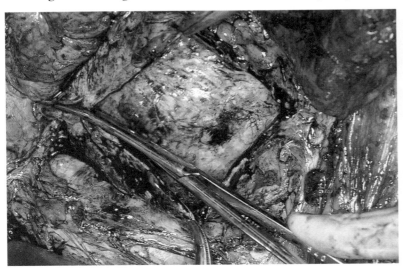

FIG. 7.23 *The bulging surface of the right ventricle is seen in the center of this operative view. A chronically constricting pericardium was excised through a median sternotomy.*

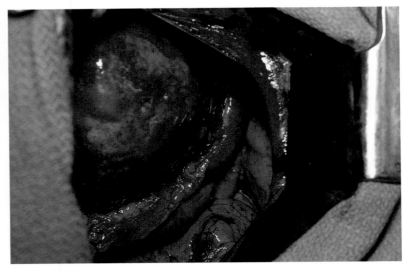

FIG. 7.24 *The apex of the heart after resection of grossly thickened pericardium can be seen through a left anterolateral thoracotomy.*

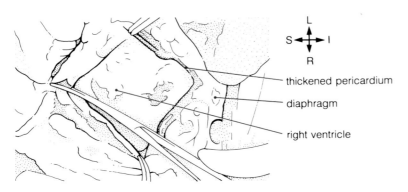

thickened pericardium

diaphragm

right ventricle

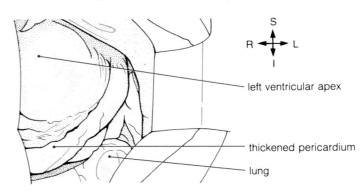

left ventricular apex

thickened pericardium

lung

Krikorian JG, Hancock EW (1978) Pericardiocentesis. *Am J Med* 65:808.

Leimgruber PP, Klopfenstein HS, Wann LS, Brooks HL (1983) The hemodynamic derangement associated with right ventricular diastolic collapse in cardiac tamponade: an experimental echocardiographic study. *Circulation* 68:612.

McCaughan BC, Schaff HV, Piehler JM, et al (1985) Early and late results of pericardiectomy for constrictive pericarditis. *J Thorac Cardiovasc Surg* 89:340.

Meany E, Shabetai R, Bhargava V, et al (1976) Cardiac amyloidosis, constrictive pericarditis and restrictive cardiomyopathy. *Am J Cardiol* 38:547.

Spodick DH (1984) Frequency of arrhythmias in acute pericarditis determined by Holter monitoring. *Am J Cardiol* 53:842.

Spodick DH (1973) Diagnostic electrocardiographic sequences in acute pericarditis: significance of PR segment and PR vector changes. *Circulation* 48:575.

Spodick DH (1971) Acoustic phenomena in pericardial disease. *Am Heart J* 81:114.

Swanton RH, Brooksby IAB, Davies MJ, et al (1977) Systolic and diastolic ventricular function in cardiac amyloidosis. *Am J Cardiol* 39:658.

Teicholz LE (1978) Echocardiographic evaluation of pericardial diseases. *Prog Cardiovasc Dis* 21:133.

FIGURE CREDITS

FIG. 7.4 (A,B) From Becker AE, Anderson RH: *Cardiac Pathology*. New York, Raven Press, 1983, p 5.4.

FIG. 7.5 Redrawn from R. Shabetai: *The Pericardium*. New York, Grune & Stratton, 1981, p 359.

FIG. 7.6 From Becker AE, Anderson RH: *Cardiac Pathology*. New York, Raven Press, 1983, p 3.17.

FIG. 7.7 Redrawn from Holt JP: The normal pericardium. *Am J Cardiol* 26:455, 1970.

FIG. 7.8 (A,B) From Chen JTT: Technique of cardiac fluoroscopy, Chapter 107 in Hurst JW (ed): *The Heart,* 6th ed. New York, McGraw-Hill, 1986, p 1766.

FIG. 7.9 (A,B) From Baron MG: Computed tomography of the heart, Chapter 111 in Hurst JW (ed): *The Heart,* 6th ed. New York, McGraw-Hill, 1986, pp 1869, 1870.

FIG. 7.10 Redrawn from Surawicz B, Lasseter KC: Electrocardiogram in pericarditis. *Am J Cardiol* 26:472, 1970.

FIG. 7.13 Redrawn from Ebert PA: The pericardium, in Sabiston DC (ed): *Gibbon's Surgery of the Chest,* 4th ed. Philadelphia, WB Saunders, 1983, p 996.

FIG. 7.15 From Becker AE, Anderson RH: *Cardiac Pathology*. New York, Raven Press, p 5.5.

FIG. 7.17 Redrawn from Shabetai R: *The Pericardium*. New York, Grune & Stratton, 1981, p 1257.

FIG. 7.18 Redrawn from Shabetai R: *The Pericardium*. New York, Grune & Stratton, 1981, p 1258.

FIG. 7.19 Redrawn from Shabetai R, Grossman W: Profiles in constrictive pericarditis, restrictive cardiomyopathy and cardiac tamponade, in Grossman W (ed): *Cardiac Catheterization and Angiography,* 2d ed. Philadelphia, Lea & Febiger, 1980, p 360.

FIG. 7.20 Redrawn from Shabetai R: *The Pericardium*. New York, Grune & Stratton, 1981, p 273.

8
HEART DISEASE DUE TO LUNG DISEASE AND PULMONARY HYPERTENSION

CHRONIC COR PULMONALE

J. Willis Hurst, MD
Joseph C. Ross, MD
John H. Newman, MD
Anton E. Becker, MD

PULMONARY EMBOLISM

J. Willis Hurst, MD
James E. Dalen, MD
Joseph S. Alpert, MD
Anton E. Becker, MD

SPECIAL TYPES OF PULMONARY EMBOLI

J. Willis Hurst, MD
Robert C. Schlant, MD

PRIMARY PULMONARY HYPERTENSION

J. Willis Hurst, MD
Hiroshi Kuida, MD
Anton E. Becker, MD

This chapter deals with three pulmonary problems that may produce heart disease: chronic lung disease of various types, special types of pulmonary embolism, and primary pulmonary hypertension.

CHRONIC COR PULMONALE*

The term chronic cor pulmonale is used to designate the effect of chronic lung disease on the right side of the heart. Many different types of chronic lung disease cause chronic cor pulmonale; the common denominator is pulmonary hypertension and its effect on the right ventricle. The term cor pulmonale should not be applied to right-sided heart disease due to congenital heart disease, to diseases causing elevation of the left atrial pressure, or to primary pulmonary hypertension.

ETIOLOGY AND PATHOLOGY

Emphysema and chronic bronchitis cause at least half of the cases of chronic cor pulmonale in the United States. In turn cor pulmonale is responsible for about 20%–30% of hospital admissions for heart failure. The condition occurs more frequently in males who smoke tobacco and who are between the ages of 50 and 60 years. The major causes of chronic cor pulmonale are shown in Table 8.1.

---

*Abstracted with permission of the authors and publisher from Ross JC, Newman JH: Chronic cor pulmonale, Chapter 55, pp 1120–1129, in Hurst JW (ed): *The Heart,* 6th ed. New York, McGraw-Hill, 1986. Figures and tables reproduced in this section from the above chapter, other chapters in *The Heart,* or other sources are also reproduced with permission of the authors and publishers. For the full bibliographic citations of the sources of figures and tables other than the above chapter, see Figure Credits at the end of this chapter.

In pulmonary emphysema the main pathologic features are loss of elasticity, accompanied by destruction of the wall of the terminal bronchioli in the case of centrilobular emphysema (Fig. 8.1) or of the distal terminal airways in the case of panacinar emphysema. As a result air spaces are dilated and the total alveolar surface area is decreased. Alveolar hypoxia underlies constriction of the arterioles, which is often accompanied by a longitudinally oriented smooth-muscle cell proliferation within the intima (Fig. 8.2). Under these circumstances pulmonary hypertension may result. In long-standing disease the major pulmonary arteries often display atherosclerosis (Fig. 8.3), a hugely dilated pulmonary trunk, and a markedly enlarged right heart (Fig. 8.4). Right ventricular wall hypertrophy is often accompanied by dilation of the chamber, leading to a marked distortion of ventricular geometry (Fig. 8.5). The ventricular septum is "pushed" toward the left side, thereby distorting the left ventricular contour (Fig. 8.6). Under such circumstances myocardial ischemia and infarction may occur despite minimal obstructive coronary atherosclerotic disease.

PATHOPHYSIOLOGY
NORMAL PULMONARY CIRCULATION

The pulmonary vascular system in a healthy person receives the entire cardiac output in order to permit the exchange of O_2 and CO_2 between the capillaries and the alveolar spaces. The normal mean pulmonary arterial pressure is about 12–17 mmHg. The pulmonary vascular resistance is 10- to 20-fold less than the vascular resistance in the systemic circuit. This is possible because the pulmonary arteries are thin-walled with little resting muscle tone, because there is little vasomotor control by the autonomic nervous system in adults, and because many arterioles and capillaries are nonperfused at rest but are recruited when needed.

Table 8.1 Etiologies of Chronic Cor Pulmonale by Mechanism of Pulmonary Hypertension

Hypoxic vasoconstriction
   Chronic bronchitis and emphysema, cystic fibrosis
   Chronic hypoventilation
      Obesity
      Sleep apnea
      Neuromuscular disease
      Chest wall dysfunction
      High-altitude dwelling and chronic mountain sickness
Occlusion of the pulmonary vascular bed
   Pulmonary thromboembolism, parasitic ova, tumor emboli
   Veno-occlusive disease
   Pulmonary angiitis from systemic disease
      Collagen vascular diseases
      Drug-induced lung disease
Parenchymal disease with destruction of vascular surface area
   Chronic bronchitis and emphysema
   Bronchiectasis, cystic fibrosis
   Diffuse interstitial disease
      Pneumoconioses
      Sarcoid, idiopathic pulmonary fibrosis, histiocytosis X
      Tuberculosis, chronic fungal infection
      Acute respiratory distress syndrome
      Collagen vascular diseases

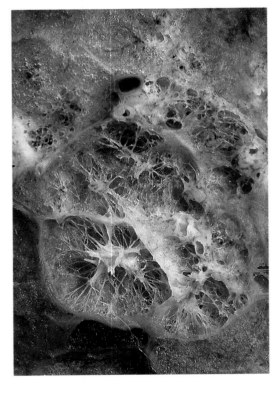

FIG. 8.1 *Gross aspect of a lung with pulmonary emphysema shows centrally dilated air spaces surrounded by a rim of less affected parenchyma; this is a classic example of centrilobular emphysema.*

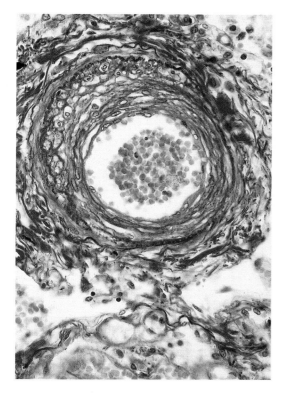

FIG. 8.2 *Histologic section of a pulmonary arteriole depicts eccentric intimal thickening due to a proliferation of longitudinally oriented smooth muscle cells, as often seen in hypoxic pulmonary hypertension (elastic tissue stain).*

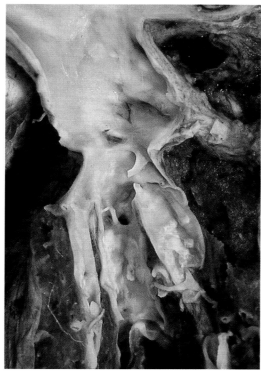

FIG. 8.3 *The central pulmonary artery with its main branches displays extensive atherosclerosis as an effect of long-standing pulmonary hypertension. (Reproduced with permission of the authors and publisher; see Figure Credits)*

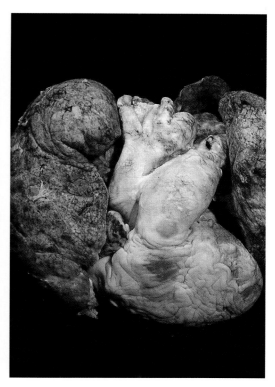

FIG. 8.4 *A heart-lung specimen from a patient with chronic cor pulmonale shows a dilated pulmonary trunk. In addition the right heart size is markedly increased.*

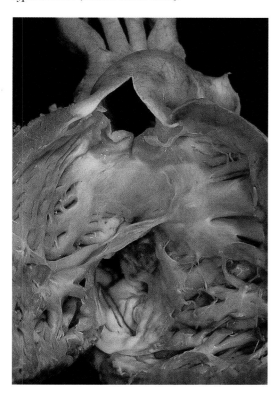

FIG. 8.5 *The right side of the heart is opened to show marked right ventricular hypertrophy and a dilated right ventricular chamber in a case of chronic cor pulmonale.*

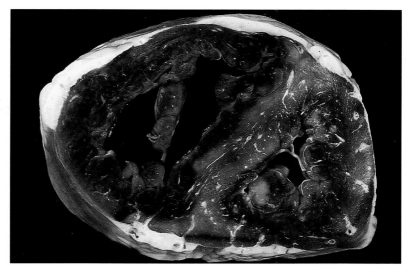

FIG. 8.6 *A cross-section of a heart in a case of long-standing pulmonary hypertension shows massive right ventricular wall hypertrophy with a displaced ventricular septum, which distorts left ventricular geometry. Diffuse, patchy myocardial infarction (pale-staining areas) contrasts with the dark-blue zones of viable myocardium (macroenzyme staining technique).*

Different factors may cause dilation and constriction of the pulmonary arterioles (Table 8.2). Hypoxia is the most important clinical cause of vasoconstriction (Fig. 8.7).

Other factors may elevate the pulmonary arterial blood pressure. When a large area of the lungs is reduced because of pulmonary disease, there is an increase in cardiac output, heart rate, and blood volume, which increases the pulmonary arterial pressure. Acidosis, increased blood viscosity, and left ventricular failure also increase the likelihood of pulmonary hypertension. Pulmonary hypertension due to hypoxia leads to irreversible pulmonary hypertension due to the gradual increase in the muscular component of the arterioles; this elevates the resting pulmonary arterial pressure and also the vasoconstrictive response to stimuli.

RESPONSE OF THE HEART TO PULMONARY HYPERTENSION
The right ventricle, because of its thin wall and relatively large radius of curvature, tolerates a volume load better than it tolerates a pressure load. The hypoxia of chronic lung disease leads to chronic pulmonary hypertension, which in turn leads to right ventricular dilation, hypertrophy, and eventually heart failure. Modifying factors include alteration in ventilatory function, alteration in the degree of hypoxia, hypercapnia, acidosis, and alteration in volume load on the right ventricle.

Left ventricular dysfunction may also occur as a result of chronic lung disease. The cause is unclear and has been the stimulus for much investigation. In most instances dysfunction is due to some other cause of left ventricular disease, such as unrecognized coronary artery disease. Regardless of the cause chronic left ventricular failure aggravates pulmonary arterial hypertension and right ventricular dysfunction. In the minority of patients with chronic cor pulmonale there is evidence of left ventricular dysfunction, with no evidence of primary left ventricular disease. There is some evidence that right ventricular hypertrophy and elevation of the end-diastolic pressure of the right ventricle may reduce left ventricular compliance. In addition the wide swing in transpulmonary pressure in patients with obstructive lung disease may result in a decrease in left ventricular filling and an increase in left ventricular afterload.

Peripheral edema occurs in some, but not all, patients with chronic cor pulmonale. The mechanism of production of edema is not clear, but it is related to increased venous pressure, an increase in Pco_2, and a decrease in Po_2. Once the liver is congested, there is a decrease in the clearance of aldosterone. Pleural effusion and pulmonary edema are not a consequence of cor pulmonale.

CLINICAL MANIFESTATIONS
The initial diagnostic problem is to identify the presence and the type of chronic lung disease. The next step is to search for clues to the diagnosis of the heart disease that results from the lung disease.

SYMPTOMS
The physician must remember that heart failure or chronic hypoxia may occur in any patient with pulmonary hypertension. Heart failure is often overlooked because it occurs gradually and imperceptibly. There is no history that is specific for heart failure in patients with cor pulmonale, but the development of heart failure should be considered whenever there is an increase in dyspnea in a patient with chronic lung disease.

PHYSICAL EXAMINATION
The pulmonary component of the second sound may be accentuated. An anterior lift of the sternum may be detected during systole, except when severe pulmonary emphysema prevents it from being observed. Abnormal right ventricular movement may be felt in the epigastrium when severe emphysema is present. The neck veins may be abnormally distended, and they may reveal the systolic wave form of tricuspid

Table 8.2 Pulmonary Vasomotor Tone

DILATOR	CONSTRICTOR
Beta-adrenergic agonists	Alpha-adrenergic agonists
Histamine H_2	Histamine H_1
Prostacyclin (PGI_2)	PGE_2, $PGF_{2\alpha}$, thromboxane A_2
Acetylcholine	Serotonin
O_2	Hypoxia
Bradykinin	Angiotensin II

(Table 55-2, *The Heart*, 6th ed, p 1122)

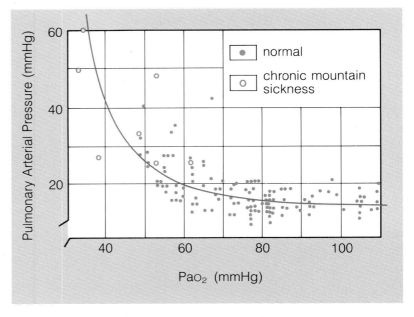

FIG. 8.7 *This graph displays pulmonary arterial pressure as a function of* Pao_2 *in healthy residents of cities of different altitudes and in patients with chronic mountain sickness. Pulmonary arterial pressure rises steeply as* Pao_2 *decreases below 55 torr. (Redrawn; reproduced with permission of the authors and publisher; see Figure Credits. Also, Fig. 55-2,* The Heart, *6th ed, p 1121)*

regurgitation. Peripheral edema may also be present. While cyanosis may be evident, the extremities may be warm because of peripheral arteriolar dilation due to hypercapnia. Many of the signs of heart failure may occur without evidence of a failing right ventricle. In most patients such signs indicate that the right ventricle cannot respond to the load even if the cardiac output is normal.

LABORATORY STUDIES

CHEST RADIOGRAPHY. Evidence of pulmonary disease and pulmonary hypertension is seen on chest films (Fig. 8.8). Pulmonary hypertension should be suspected when there is enlargement of the pulmonary trunk and its right and left branches, or when the right descending pulmonary artery is greater than 16 mm in diameter. The heart may not be increased in size when viewed in the anteroposterior projection, while the right ventricle may or may not appear to be enlarged when viewed in the left lateral projection.

ELECTROCARDIOGRAPHY. The classic signs of right ventricular hypertrophy are usually not evident in the electrocardiogram (ECG) in patients with cor pulmonale due to parenchymal pulmonary lung disease, such as emphysema and chronic bronchitis. The classic signs of right ventricular hypertrophy are generally limited to conditions associated with an anatomic restriction of the pulmonary arteriolar vascular bed. ECGs of patients with chronic cor pulmonale due to emphysema and chronic bronchitis may reveal low QRS voltage, right atrial abnormalities of the P waves, and right axis deviation of the mean QRS vector. Right bundle branch block may be present, and atrial and ventricular arrhythmias may occur. When the electrical field is distorted by emphysema, the mean QRS vector may be superiorly directed.

OTHER LABORATORY ABNORMALITIES. The *echocardiogram* is not useful in assessing the function of the right ventricle in patients with cor pulmonale.

The *first-pass radionuclear angiogram* using ^{99m}technetium (^{99m}Tc) reveals a decrease in right ventricular ejection fraction.

Cardiac catheterization reveals an increase in diastolic pulmonary arterial pressure. The wedge pressure in such patients is significantly lower than the diastolic pulmonary arterial pressure; this excludes left ventricular failure as a cause of the pulmonary hypertension. The pulmonary arterial pressure may be severely elevated when patients have obliterative arteriolar disease, but it is only moderately increased when the pulmonary hypertension is due to disease of the lung parenchyma. The pressure may rise abruptly, however, when there is superimposed hypoxemia or when the patient exercises.

TREATMENT

The treatment of cor pulmonale due to chronic lung disease is directed for the most part toward improving the lung disease. This is not always successful; when it is not, treatment of heart failure is limited.

The elevated pulmonary arterial pressure can be lowered by the judicious use of oxygen to attain an arterial P_{O_2} of 60 torr. Bronchospasm should be treated. Mechanical ventilation may be needed in extreme cases in an effort to relieve hypoxia and hypercarbia.

Digitalis is not helpful, and toxicity is more likely to occur in this setting. Vasodilator therapy may help, but it obviously will not be continuously helpful. Diuretics usually are helpful. Phlebotomy of 200–300 mL of blood may also be helpful when the hematocrit is above 55%–60%.

Heart–lung transplant is currently being used in carefully selected patients.

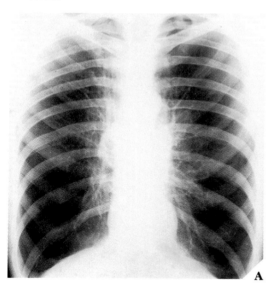 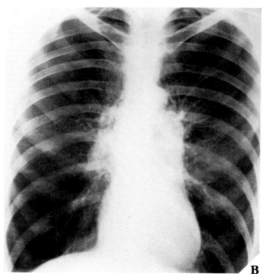

A   B

FIG. 8.8 (**A**) *Chest film of a patient with severe obstructive emphysema shows overaeration of the lungs, a centralized flow pattern, and a small heart size.* (**B**) *Three years later the same patient was in frank right-sided heart failure. The heart enlarged as the emphysema worsened, and the centralized flow pattern became more severe.* (*Figure 15-7A,B,* The Heart, *6th ed; see Figure Credits*)

PULMONARY EMBOLISM*

Pulmonary embolism is a common problem and a feared cause of death. This condition is often undiagnosed.

ETIOLOGY AND PATHOLOGY

Most pulmonary emboli originate as thrombi in the proximal deep venous system of the legs. The risk factors favoring deep venous thrombosis are listed in Table 8.3. Accordingly the prevention of pulmonary emboli is achieved by preventing deep venous thrombosis (Table 8.4). Certain operative procedures are more likely to be complicated by deep venous thrombosis, including hip replacement, hip fractures, and urological procedures. The thrombi begin to develop in the venous system while the patient is anesthetized in the operating room. Accordingly prophylactic treatment should begin prior to the use of anesthesia.

DIAGNOSIS OF DEEP VENOUS THROMBOSIS

The minority of patients with deep venous thrombosis have swelling of the leg and physical signs of the condition are not commonly present. Venography or noninvasive tests must be used to identify the condition. Since such tests are not performed without indications, deep vein thrombosis is underdiagnosed.

---

*Abstracted with permission of the authors and publisher from Dalen JE, Alpert JS: Pulmonary embolism, Chapter 54, pp 1105–1119, in Hurst JW (ed): *The Heart,* 6th ed. New York, McGraw-Hill, 1986. Additional contributions on special types of pulmonary emboli were written by Robert C. Schlant, MD. Figures and tables reproduced in this section from the above chapter, other chapters in *The Heart,* or other sources are also reproduced with permission of the authors and publishers. For the full bibliographic citations of the sources of figures and tables other than the above chapter, see Figure Credits at the end of this chapter.

Venography is the most sensitive and specific test. Scanning of the legs injected with [125]iodine-labeled fibrinogen, the Doppler technique, and impedance plethysmography (IPG) are also useful when properly performed.

When identified, the patient with deep venous thrombosis should be treated with heparin for 7–10 days in an effort to prevent pulmonary emboli. Streptokinase and urokinase have also been used in the hope that the postphlebitic syndrome will be lessened by such treatment.

DIAGNOSIS OF ACUTE PULMONARY EMBOLISM

Acute pulmonary embolism may produce three clinical syndromes: acute unexplained dyspnea, acute cor pulmonale, and pulmonary infarction.

ACUTE UNEXPLAINED DYSPNEA

Pulmonary embolism does not produce acute cor pulmonale unless approximately 60% of the pulmonary circulation is obstructed. Accordingly pulmonary embolism may not produce abnormalities detectable on the ECG or on physical examination of the lungs. When pulmonary infarction does not occur, pleuritic chest pain and abnormalities on the chest radiograph are absent. Pulmonary embolism may be difficult to diagnose, since the only clue to its occurrence may be an acute episode of dyspnea. The physician may consider acute left ventricular failure, pneumonia, or anxiety in the differential diagnosis of patients with acute dyspnea. The existence of a clinical setting where deep venous thrombosis is likely to occur should always stimulate the physician to consider the possibility of pulmonary embolism. Left ventricular failure and pneumonia can usually be identified by abnormalities elicited from further history, physical examination, and chest radiography. Hyperventilation related to anxiety is associated with a decrease in arterial P_{CO_2} and normal P_{O_2}. The diagnosis of

---

Table 8.3 Risk Factors for Deep Venous Thrombosis

Prior history of venous thrombosis
Surgical procedures
Trauma to lower extremities
Bed rest, immobility
Congestive heart failure
Malignancy (including occult malignancy)
Pregnancy
Oral contraceptive agents
Obesity
Advanced age

(Table 54-1, *The Heart,* 6th ed, p 1105)

Table 8.4 Prevention of Deep Venous Thrombosis

Anticoagulation
    Low-dose subcutaneous heparin
    Warfarin
Platelet-active agents
    Aspirin
    Dextran
Other agents
    Dihydroergotamine
Prevention of venous stasis
    Graded compression stockings
    Intermittent pneumatic compression

(Table 54-2, *The Heart,* 6th ed, p 1105)

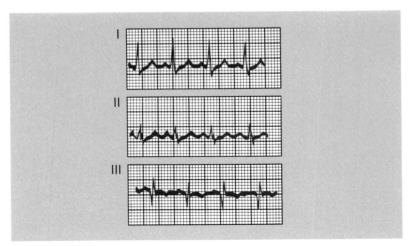

FIG. 8.9 *This ECG was recorded two hours after an attack of pulmonary embolism. Note the Q wave and inverted T waves in lead III. At times this abnormality simulates inferior myocardial infarction. (Redrawn; reproduced with permission of the publisher; see Figure Credits)*

pulmonary embolism can be confirmed with a ventilation/perfusion lung scan.

ACUTE COR PULMONALE

Acute cor pulmonale occurs when more than 60%–75% of the pulmonary circulation is obstructed by pulmonary embolism. Such a catastrophe leads to an increase in the systolic pressure of the right ventricle, which dilates when the systolic pressure is increased beyond 50–60 mmHg. When this occurs, the right ventricle fails, the stroke output diminishes, and the cardiac output and the systolic blood pressure fall.

The patient may experience acute dyspnea, syncope, or sudden death. Tachycardia, tachypnea, and hypotension usually occur. The neck veins are distended, and a right ventricular S_3 gallop may be heard. An abnormal anterior movement of the sternal area due to dilation of the right ventricle is often present. Signs of deep venous thrombosis may or may not be apparent.

The ECG may show the $S_1Q_3T_3$ pattern described by McGinn and White (1935) (Fig. 8.9). These electrocardiographic abnormalities may simulate inferior myocardial infarction. Anterior ischemia may be noted and may be confused with an acute coronary event. Incomplete right bundle branch block or atrial arrhythmias may occur.

When hypotension is present, the central venous pressure and the right atrial pressure are usually elevated. Myocardial infarction or hypovolemia are more likely to be present when hypotension is associated with normal right atrial and central venous pressures.

The arterial Po_2 and Pco_2 are abnormally diminished in patients with acute cor pulmonale. A ventilation/perfusion scan reveals the pulmonary embolism in almost all instances (Fig. 8.10). Pulmonary angiography may be needed when the diagnosis remains uncertain.

PULMONARY INFARCTION

The diagnosis of pulmonary embolism is most frequently made when the complication of pulmonary infarction is recognized.

Patients with pulmonary venous congestion, such as those with mitral stenosis or following myocardial infarction, are particularly susceptible to pulmonary infarction (Fig. 8.11). Pulmonary emboli in middle-sized pulmonary arteries do not necessarily lead to infarcts because of collateral blood supply. The same mechanism underlies the hemorrhagic nature of the infarct, once it occurs. Fibrinous pleuritis is a reactive phenomenon to the infarcted lung.

Pulmonary infarction should be suspected when the patient experiences pleuritic chest pain. Dyspnea and hemoptysis may or may not be present. The physical examination may reveal tachypnea, rales, pulmonary wheezes, pleural friction rub, pleural effusion, and evidence of deep venous thrombosis. The chest radiograph may show an elevation of the diaphragm on one side, a small pleural effusion, or a pulmonary infiltrate.

This condition must be separated from pulmonary infection. The sputum examination, white blood cell count, and differential all aid in the identification of bacterial infection of the lung. The arterial Pco_2 may be diminished, while the arterial Po_2 may be normal. Pulmonary angiography may be needed when the diagnosis remains uncertain.

LABORATORY STUDIES

The chest film, the ECG, arterial blood gases, ventilation/perfusion lung scans, and pulmonary angiography are useful in the diagnosis of pulmonary embolism and infarction. An echocardiogram should be performed on patients with pulmonary embolism; a thrombus may be lodged in the right side of the heart, and emboli may be fed to the lung from that site.

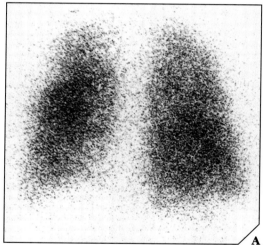

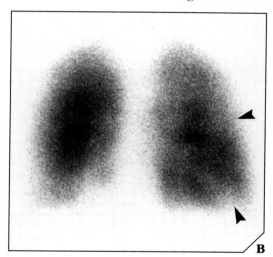

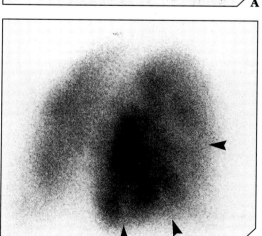

FIG. 8.10 *Ventilation/perfusion scan was performed in a patient with chest pain.* (**A**) *Posterior view of a ventilation scan is normal.* (**B**) *Posterior view of a perfusion scan demonstrates subsegmental defects* (arrows). (**C**) *Right posterior view of a perfusion scan shows multiple subsegmental defects* (arrows). *(Fig. 113-1A–C, The Heart, 6th ed; see Figure Credits)*

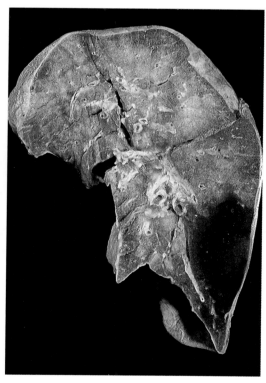

FIG. 8.11 *Grossly an infarct of the lung shows the hemorrhagic aspect due to the collateral supply. The infarct is wedge-shaped with a broad base at the pleural surface.*

PULMONARY EMBOLISM AND CANCER

The patient with pulmonary embolism, with or without infarction, should be screened for cancer of the gastrointestinal tract, pancreas, lung, breast, uterus, and prostate, since pulmonary emboli may occur as a consequence of all these diseases. Such patients may also have thrombophlebitis migrans of the arms, although deep venous thrombosis is more common.

TREATMENT

One must assume that a patient with deep vein thrombosis is likely to have a pulmonary embolus, and that if one pulmonary embolus has occurred, another is likely. Accordingly prophylactic therapy is indicated in these circumstances (Table 8.5).

Surgical treatment to prevent further emboli consists of interruption of the inferior caval vein by the placement of a Mobin–Uddin or Greenfield filter (see Fig. 6.48). An echocardiogram should be made before a surgical procedure is performed on the caval vein because the thrombus, originally located in the deep venous system of the lower extremities, may be coiled up in the right side of the heart. Emboli may pass from this site to the lungs.

DIRECT THERAPY

The surgical removal of a pulmonary embolus may be necessary in some patients. The surgical mortality is high, because patients who need this procedure are usually in shock prior to surgery. A long thrombus that has lodged in the right atrium and the right ventricle usually requires surgical removal.

Fibrinolytic therapy with urokinase or streptokinase has been used in the treatment of pulmonary embolism. The Urokinase Pulmonary Embolism Study Group (1973) compared the results of urokinase with those of heparin. This study showed that urokinase produced a modest degree of resolution of the embolus, but the treatment was associated with major bleeding complications. The second National Institutes of Health (NIH)-sponsored trial compared the results produced by urokinase with those of streptokinase. The resolution of the embolus was equal in the two groups at 12 hours, but significant bleeding occurred in one third of patients in each group. Although the NIH Consensus Development Conference (1980) recommended the use of thrombolytic therapy in patients with pulmonary embolism and hemodynamic abnormalities, the mortality secondary to pulmonary embolism remained the same. Furthermore patients treated with heparin did as well as those treated with thrombolytic therapy. Other investigators recommend thrombolytic therapy for pulmonary embolism when there is proof of embolism and severe hemodynamic complications (Dalen and Alpert, 1986; Genton, 1979).

SPECIAL TYPES OF PULMONARY EMBOLISM

FAT EMBOLISM

The occurrence of dyspnea, mental confusion, and petechiae should stimulate the physician to consider fat emboli. These may occur in patients who have fractures of their long bones, who have injured the subcutaneous fat tissue by contusion, burns, or childbirth, or who have undergone the use of the pump oxygenator. The clinical syndrome may simulate the acute respiratory distress syndrome. Many therapies have been tried without definite benefit; however, corticosteroid therapy may prevent alveolar damage. The goal of therapy is to maintain pulmonary function and to avoid hypoxia with assisted respiration.

AIR EMBOLISM

This dreaded event occurs when air gains access to the circulation; this may occur during intravenous infusions, uterine douches, knee–chest position in puerperium, surgical procedures on the head and neck, retroperitoneal air injection, irrigation of nasal sinuses, tubal or vaginal insufflation, pneumoperitoneum, heart–lung bypass, or orogenital sex. The amount of air required to cause death varies with the amount, the speed of entry into the circulation, age, the position of the patient, and any associated illness. Five-to-fifteen mL/kg of air produces an "air-lock" in the right ventricle or obstructs the pulmonary vascular bed.

Air embolism results in the sudden onset of shock, dyspnea, and cyanosis. The mixture of air and blood in the right ventricle produces a characteristic churning sound. A condition simulating the adult respiratory syndrome may be produced as a result of pulmonary injury. Severe ventilation–perfusion abnormalities may develop as a result of air in the pulmonary vascular bed. Air bubbles may be detected on the echocardiogram.

Treatment consists of turning the patient on the left side with the head in a dependent position. This maneuver tends to dislodge the air from the outflow tract of the right ventricle. Entrapped air can be aspirated with a needle or by a catheter inserted into the right ventricle. Oxygen should be administered, and closed-chest cardiac massage may be needed.

AMNIOTIC FLUID EMBOLISM

This rare complication of delivery is more likely to occur in patients who have predisposing factors, such as increased age, parity, premature separation of the placenta, intrauterine fetal death, a large baby, vigorous and prolonged labor, rupture of the uterus, large doses of oxytocin, meconium leakage into amniotic fluid, or abortion attempted by intra-amniotic injection of saline or glucose. The amniotic fluid enters the maternal circulation through the venous sinuses of the uteroplacental site or through the endocervical veins. The pulmonary embolic manifestations are caused by the solid contents of the fluid.

Later, if the patient survives the pulmonary embolic syndrome, she may develop disseminated intravascular coagulation due to activity of the thromboplastic-like substances from the amniotic fluid. The clinical features include an abrupt onset of dyspnea near the end of the first stage of labor, hypotension, shock, cyanosis, acute cor pulmonale, pulmonary edema, semicoma, coma, convulsions, and cardiac arrest. About 80% of patients die. Those who live may have severe bleeding from all body orifices or into the skin and mucosa due to disseminated intravascular coagulation.

Laboratory test results show abnormalities of most coagulation factors, including factors V and VIII, prothrombin, and fibrinogen. The platelet count is usually decreased.

Treatment consists of supportive measures, evacuation of the uterus, and the administration of fresh-frozen plasma and platelets, packed red cells, and cyroprecipitate.

TUMOR EMBOLISM

Acute and subacute cor pulmonale may be the result of embolization of malignant cells, which may originate from a primary or a metastatic site. This condition is more common in patients with carcinoma of the liver, stomach, or kidney, or with the chorioepithelioma.

The presence of trophoblastic tumors with embolization to the lungs should be considered in any postpartum female who has evidence of pulmonary emboli. The abnormalities on chest radiography may include discrete and rounded opacities, multiple, small, poorly defined opacities, and the changes of obstructed pulmonary arteries.

Outcome of the treatment of cor pulmonale due to tumor emboli is poor, because the prognosis of the underlying cancer is correspondingly grave. The exception is chorioepithelioma, which may respond well to chemotherapy, even with extensive spread to the lungs.

PRIMARY PULMONARY HYPERTENSION*

Pulmonary hypertension is a secondary event in most patients. The conditions that are responsible for it include lesions that produce elevated left atrial pressure, such as mitral stenosis; heart failure with elevated left ventricular diastolic pressure; congenital heart disease with a left-to-right shunt and pulmonary arteriolar disease; and pul-

---

*Abstracted with permission of the author and published from Kuida H: Pulmonary hypertension: Mechanism and recognition, Chapter 52, pp 1091–1099; and Kuida H: Primary pulmonary hypertension, Chapter 53, pp 1099–1104; both in Hurst JW (ed): *The Heart,* 6th ed. New York, McGraw-Hill, 1986.

PART II: DISEASES OF THE HEART

monary disease of various types. Primary pulmonary hypertension, which affects a small percentage of patients with pulmonary hypertension, usually has no identifiable cause.

ETIOLOGY AND PATHOLOGY

The etiology of primary pulmonary hypertension is unknown. Predisposing factors are the female gender, pregnancy (suggesting a relationship to amniotic fluid or thromboplastin-induced fibrin emboli), Raynaud's phenomenon (suggesting a relationship to collagen disease), family history (suggesting a genetic predetermination), and ingestion of drugs, such as aminorex and colsa oil (implicating environmental factors). An unknown number of patients with primary pulmonary hypertension have silent pulmonary emboli. (The reader is referred to Miller, 1985, in *Clinical Essays on The Heart* for a complete discussion of the etiology of primary pulmonary hypertension.)

In the vast majority of patients with secondary pulmonary hypertension a firm diagnosis can be made. In a minority of patients the clinician may have great difficulties in establishing the precise cause of the pulmonary hypertension. Three conditions should be taken into consideration. First, chronic silent pulmonary emboli may eventually lead to increased pulmonary vascular resistance and pulmonary hypertension. Since most patients with this abnormality show no signs of venous thrombosis or other signs indicative of a chronic thrombotic process, the definitive diagnosis is often clinically difficult to ascertain. A second category to be taken into account is the rare anomaly of pulmonary veno-occlusive disease. Diffuse obliteration of small venules throughout the lungs, usually with a normal arterial wedge pressure, leads to pulmonary hypertension most likely through a process of arteriolar vasoconstriction. In the third category there is no detectable cause for the pulmonary vascular disease, even at pathologic study. In such instances there is a diffuse and abrupt narrowing of the caliber of the smaller-sized pulmonary arteries, underlying the changes seen on the chest radiograph and the "winter-tree" aspect on a postmortem pulmonary angiogram (Fig. 8.12). The muscular pulmonary arteries show an edematous concentric intimal layering, often referred to as onion skinning (Fig. 8.13); this is the morphologic counterpart of the increased vascular resistance. In its most extreme form advanced lesions occur; these are characterized by fibrinoid necrosis of the

Table 8.5 Prophylactic Therapy for Treatment of Thrombophlebitis and Pulmonary Embolism	
DIAGNOSIS	HEPARIN DOSAGE
Deep venous thrombosis without pulmonary embolism or with minor pulmonary embolism	5000 U IV loading dose followed by 1000–1500 U IV per hour (24,000 U/24 h); check partial thromboplastin time (PTT) 4 h after initiating infusion and adjust heparin dose to prolong PTT to 1.5–2 times control. Warfarin is started on approximately day 2–3 with changeover from heparin occurring approximately on day 7–10.
Major pulmonary embolism with or without right ventricular failure and hypotension	10,000–15,000 U IV loading dose followed by 1500–2000 U IV per hour (36,000 U/24 h); check PTT 4 h after initiating infusion and adjust heparin dose to prolong PTT to 1.5–2 times control (employ smaller loading and infusion dosage for smaller individuals or patients with hepatic and/or renal insufficiency). Warfarin is started on approximately day 5–6 (if patient is stable) with changeover from heparin occurring approximately on day 8–12.

(Table 54-4, *The Heart*, 6th ed, p 1110)

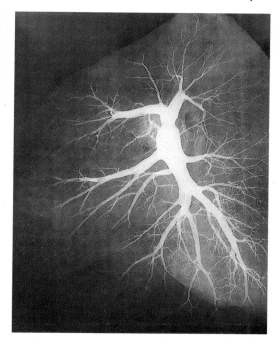

FIG. 8.12 *Postmortem pulmonary angiogram shows the "winter-tree" aspect due to structural changes at the level of the smaller-sized muscular pulmonary arteries in pulmonary vascular disease.*

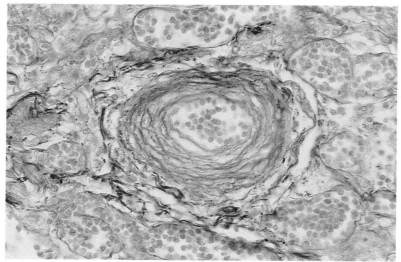

FIG. 8.13 *Histologic section of a muscular pulmonary artery from a patient with pulmonary vascular disease displays lamellar intimal fibrosis, also known as onion skinning (elastic tissue stain).*

arterial walls with plexiform lesions (Fig. 8.14). The latter form of pulmonary hypertension with unknown etiology is usually referred to as primary pulmonary hypertension.

CLINICAL MANIFESTATIONS

The patient with primary pulmonary hypertension may complain of dyspnea on effort, syncope, or chest pain; sudden death may occur. The physical abnormalities include a large a wave in the neck veins, an anterior lift of the sternum due to right ventricular hypertrophy, a palpable pulmonary trunk pulse, a loud pulmonary valve closure sound, and a murmur of pulmonary valve regurgitation.

The chest radiograph reveals right ventricular hypertrophy and large pulmonary arteries that taper quickly. The ECG demonstrates evidence of right ventricular hypertrophy with prominent P waves consistent with right atrial abnormality (Fig. 8.15). Right ventricular hypertrophy

and pulmonary valve regurgitation are also evident from the echocardiogram, while evidence of pulmonary hypertension and normal pulmonary wedge pressure without other evidence of disease is demonstrated at cardiac catheterization. The P_{O_2} may be diminished when there is a right-to-left shunt through the oval foramen.

TREATMENT

The prognosis is poor. Vasodilator drugs, such as hydralazine, do not solve the problem because of their effect on the peripheral circulation. Nifedipine may be more useful, but insufficient data are available to make a strong recommendation. Oxygen therapy helps, and the avoidance of high altitude is recommended. Anticoagulation therapy may be useful in patients with microemboli, but hemoptysis is more likely to occur. The benefit of anticoagulation therapy is unknown at this time.

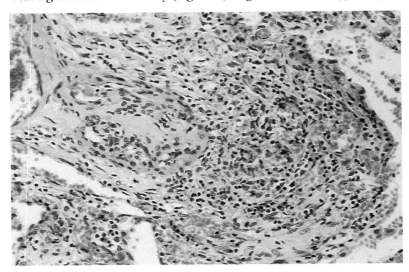

FIG. 8.14 *Histologic section of a plexiform lesion from a patient with advanced pulmonary vascular disease is characterized by multiple, often slit-like, endothelial-lined vascular spaces, most likely due to fibrinoid necrosis of the wall of preexistent arterioles (H&E stain).*

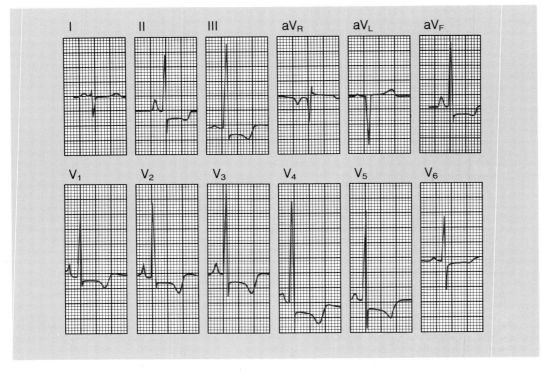

FIG. 8.15 *In this ECG of a patient with primary pulmonary hypertension the mean QRS vector is directed to the right and anteriorly and there is a right atrial abnormality. The QRS voltage is larger than it usually is when the right ventricular hypertrophy is due to pulmonary emphysema. (Redrawn; reproduced with permission of the authors and publisher; see Figure Credits. Also, Fig. 55-4, The Heart, 6th ed, p 1125)*

REFERENCES

Bagshawe KD, Noble MIM (1966) Cardiorespiratory aspects of trophoblastic tumors. *Q J Med* 35:39.

Buda AJ, Pinsky MR, Ingels NG, Daughters GT, Stinson EB, Alderman EL (1979) Effect of intrathoracic pressure on left ventricular performance. *N Engl J Med* 301:453.

Burwell CS, Robin ED, Whaley RD, Bickleman AG (1956) Extreme obesity associated with alveolar hypoventilation—A pickwickian syndrome. *Am J Med* 21:811.

Chang CH (1962) The normal roentgenographic measurement of the right descending pulmonary artery in 1085 cases. *Am J Roentgenol* 87:929.

Consensus Development Conference Report (1980) Thrombolytic therapy in thrombosis: A National Institutes of Health consensus development conference. *Ann Intern Med* 93:141.

Dalen JE, Alpert JR (1986) Pulmonary embolism, in Hurst JW (ed): *The Heart*, 6th ed. New York, McGraw-Hill, pp 1105–1119.

Ence TJ, Gong H Jr (1979) Adult respiratory distress syndrome after venous air embolism. *Am Rev Resp Dis* 119:1033.

Felner JM, Churchwell A, Murphy D (1984) Right atrial thromboemboli: Clinical, echocardiographic and pathophysiological manifestations. *J Am Coll Cardiol* 4:1041.

Gazes PC (1975) *Clinical Cardiology: A Bedside Approach,* Chicago, Year Book Medical Publishers, p 171.

Genton E (1979) Thrombolytic therapy of thromboembolism. *Progr Cardiovasc Dis* 21:333.

Harvey RM, Ferrer MI, Richards DW, Cournand A (1951) Influence of chronic pulmonary disease on the heart and circulation. *Am J Med* 10:719.

Hlastala MP, Robertson HT, Ross BK (1979) Gas exchange abnormalities produced by venous gas emboli. *Resp Physiol* 36:1.

Li MC (1971) Trophoblastic disease: Natural history, diagnosis and treatment. *Ann Intern Med* 74:102.

McGinn S, White PD (1935) Acute cor pulmonale resulting from pulmonary embolism. *JAMA* 104:1473.

Miller DD (1985) The environmental causes of pulmonary hypertension, in Hurst JW (ed): *Clinical Essays on The Heart,* vol 5. New York, McGraw-Hill, p 61.

Morgan M (1979) Amniotic fluid embolism. *Anaestia* 34:20.

Szucs MM Jr, Brooks HL, Grossman W, et al (1971) Diagnostic sensitivity of laboratory findings in acute pulmonary embolism. *Ann Intern Med* 74:161.

Urokinase Pulmonary Embolism Study Group (1973) The urokinase pulmonary embolism trial. *Circulation* 47(Suppl II):1.

FIGURE CREDITS

FIG. 8.3 From Becker AE, Anderson RH: *Cardiac Pathology.* New York, Raven Press, 1983, p2.10.

FIG. 8.7 Redrawn from Reeves JT, Grover RE: High-altitude pulmonary edema. *Prog Cardiol* 4:105, 1975.

FIG. 8.8. From Chen JTT: The chest roentgenogram, in Hurst JW (ed): *The Heart,* 6th ed. New York, McGraw-Hill, 1986, p 237.

FIG. 8.9 Redrawn from Figure 1 in McGinn S, White PD: Acute cor pulmonale resulting from pulmonary embolism. *JAMA* 104(17):1475, 1935.

FIG. 8.10 From Sones PJ, Fajaman WA: Radionuclide lung imaging and pulmonary angiography, in Hurst JW (ed): *The Heart,* 6th ed. New York, McGraw-Hill, 1986, p 1883.

FIG. 8.15 Redrawn from Voelkel NF, Reeves JT: Primary pulmonary hypertension, in *Pulmonary Vascular Diseases.* New York, Marcel Dekker, p 612; courtesy of J. Ray Pryor and Marcel Dekker, Inc.

9
ENDOCARDITIS

J. Willis Hurst, MD
David T. Durack, MD
Anton E. Becker, MD
Benson R. Wilcox, MD

Abstracted with permission of the author and publisher from Durack DT: Infective and non-infective endocarditis, Chapter 56, pp 1130–1157, in Hurst JW (ed): *The Heart,* 6th ed. New York, McGraw-Hill, 1986. Figures, tables, and extracts of text reproduced in this chapter from *The Heart* or other sources are also reproduced with permission of the authors and publishers. For the full bibliographic citations of the sources of figures and tables other than the above chapter, see Figure Credits at the end of this chapter.

When the endothelial surface of the heart or the arteries is infected by bacteria or fungi, the patient is said to have infective endocarditis. Noninfective endocarditis is not produced by microbes; it presents as thrombotic lesions rather than as inflammation. However, these lesions are sometimes colonized by circulating organisms, which convert this condition to infective endocarditis.

Subacute bacterial endocarditis (SBE) is chronic, evolving over weeks to months, and it is caused by organisms of relatively low virulence. Acute bacterial endocarditis (ABE), evolving over a period of days to weeks, is due to organisms of high virulence.

Endocarditis remains a serious and often lethal disease.

ETIOLOGY AND PATHOLOGY

Most patients with infective endocarditis have preexisting heart disease (Tables 9.1, 9.2). The frequency of various organisms causing endocarditis is shown in Table 9.3.

The pathology of infective endocarditis is characterized by the adherence of bacteria to the surface of cardiac valves with an altered endothelial coating.

The approximate frequency of anatomic location of infective endocarditis is shown in Table 9.4. This process is accompanied by fibrin–platelet depositions, which together with the affected valve tissue produce vegetations.

Table 9.1 Approximate Frequency of the Major Preexisting Cardiac Lesions in Patients with Infective Endocarditis

	CHILDREN		ADULTS		
	<2 YEARS OLD (%)	2–15 YEARS OLD (%)	15–50 YEARS OLD (%)	>50 YEARS OLD (%)	IV DRUG ABUSERS (%)
No known heart disease	50–70	10–15	10–20	10	50–60
Congenital heart disease	30–50	70–80	20–30	10–20	10
Rheumatic heart disease	Rare	10–20	30–40	20–30	10
Degenerative heart disease	0	0	Rare	10–20	Rare
Previous cardiac surgery	5	10–15	10–20	10–20	10–20
Previous endocarditis	Rare	5	5	5–10	10–20

(Table 56-1, *The Heart,* 6th ed, p 1132. Information compiled from references 33–51 in *The Heart,* 6th ed, p 1154)

Table 9.2 Estimates of the Relative Risk for Infective Endocarditis Posed by Various Cardiac Lesions

RELATIVELY HIGH RISK	INTERMEDIATE RISK	VERY LOW OR NEGLIGIBLE RISK
Prosthetic heart valves	Mitral valve prolapse	Atrial septal defects
Aortic valve disease	Pure mitral stenosis	Arteriosclerotic plaques
Mitral insufficiency	Tricuspid valve disease	Coronary artery disease
Patent arterial duct	Pulmonary valve disease	Syphilitic aortitis
Ventricular septal defect	Previous infective endocarditis	Cardiac pacemakers
Coarctation of the aorta	Asymmetric septal hypertrophy	Surgically corrected cardiac lesions
Marfan's syndrome	Calcific aortic sclerosis	(without prosthetic implants, more
	Hyperalimentation or pressure-	than six months after operation)
	monitoring lines that reach the right	
	atrium	
	Nonvalvar intracardiac prosthetic	
	implants	

(Table 56-2, *The Heart,* 6th ed, p 1132. Information compiled from references 33, 41, 50–57 in *The Heart,* 6th ed, p 1154)

PART II: DISEASES OF THE HEART

Table 9.3 Frequency of Various Organisms Causing Infective Endocarditis*

	NATIVE VALVE ENDOCARDITIS (%)	IV DRUG ABUSERS (%)	EARLY PROSTHETIC VALVE ENDOCARDITIS (%)	LATE PROSTHETIC VALVE ENDOCARDITIS (%)
Streptococci	65	15	10	35
Viridans, alpha-hemolytic	35	5	<5	25
Strep. bovis (group D)	15	<5	<5	<5
Strep. faecalis (group D)	10	8	<5	<5
Other streptococci	<5	<5	<5	<5
Staphylococci	25	50	50	30
Coagulase-positive	23	50	20	10
Coagulase-negative	<5	<5	30	20
Gram-negative aerobic bacilli	<5	5	20	15
Fungi	<5	5	10	5
Miscellaneous bacteria	<5	5	5	5
Diphtheroids, propionibacteria	<1	<5	5	<5
Other anaerobes	<1	<1	<1	<1
Rickettsia	<1	<1	<1	<1
Chlamydia	<1	<1	<1	<1
Polymicrobial infection	<1	5	5	5
Culture-negative endocarditis	5–10	5	<5	<5

(Table 56-3, *The Heart,* 6th ed, p 1133. Information compiled from references 33, 35, 41, 46–51, 61–64 in *The Heart,* 6th ed, p 1154)
*These are representative figures collated from the literature; wide local variations in frequency are to be expected.

Table 9.4 Approximate Frequency of Anatomic Location of Vegetations in Subacute and Acute Bacterial Endocarditis, and Endocarditis Associated with IV Drug Abuse

	SUBACUTE BACTERIAL ENDOCARDITIS (%)	ACUTE BACTERIAL ENDOCARDITIS (%)	ENDOCARDITIS IN IV DRUG ABUSERS (%)
Left-sided valves	85	65	40
Aortic	15–26	18–25	25–30
Mitral	38–45	30–35	15–20
Aortic and mitral	23–30	15–20	13–20
Right-sided valves	5	20	50
Tricuspid	1–5	15	45–55
Pulmonary	1	Rare	2
Tricuspid and pulmonary	Rare	Rare	3
Left- and right-sided sites	Rare	5–10	5–10
Other sites (patent duct, VSD, coarctation, jet lesions)	10	5	5

(Table 56-4, *The Heart,* 6th ed, p 1138. Information compiled from references 41, 46–51, 95, 122 in *The Heart,* 6th ed, pp 1154–1156)

Endocarditis is a destructive disease. In semilunar valves, such as the aortic valve, the infective process is particularly prominent along the line of closure (Fig. 9.1). The mitral valve shows a distinct tendency for cordal rupture (Fig. 9.2). From a clinical point of view, therefore, valve regurgitation is the leading complication of infective endocar- ditis. Complications are largely determined by the site of the primary infection. Endocarditis of the aortic root may spread onto neighboring structures, such as the epicardial surface, the right ventricular outflow tract, both atria, and the mitral valve (Fig. 9.3). Aortic valve regurgitation may cause secondary and remote infection of the mitral valve

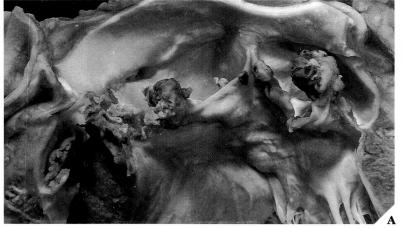

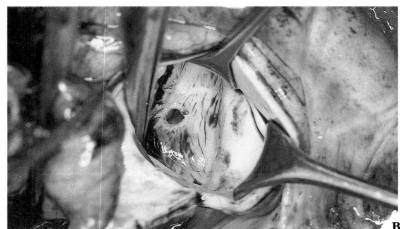

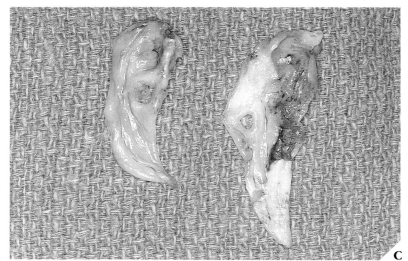

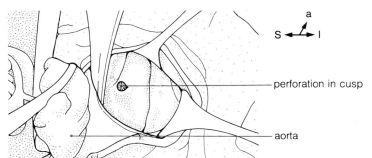

perforation in cusp

aorta

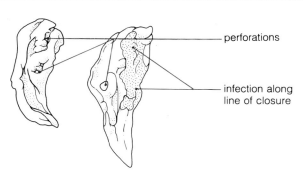

perforations

infection along line of closure

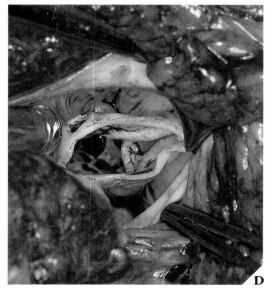

FIG. 9.1 (A) *Infective endocarditis of the aortic valve exhibits massive destruction of the leaflets with vegetations.* (B,C) *A "healing" perforation is seen in a bicuspid aortic valve with small vegetations.* (D) *A healed perforation is exposed in this patient with a bicuspid aortic valve and congenital subaortic stenosis. The perforation was repaired and the subaortic ring was excised, obviating the necessity for valve replacement.*

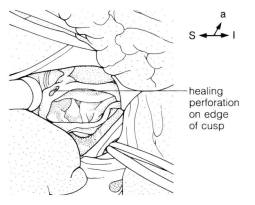

healing perforation on edge of cusp

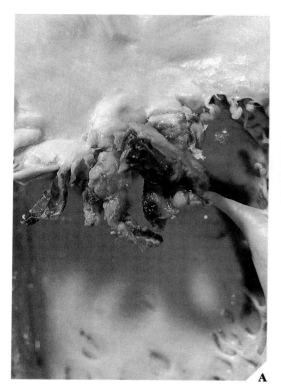

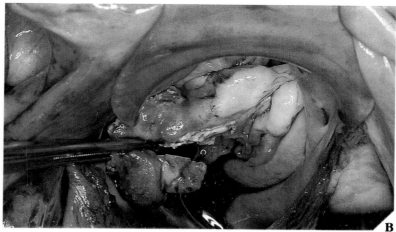

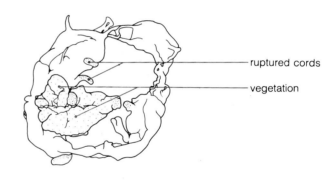

FIG. 9.2 (A) This mitral valve with multiple ruptured cords is coated by thrombotic vegetations due to infective endocarditis. (B,C) A detached mitral valve from an intravenous drug abuser shows a large vegetation.

A
S ← → I
P

mitral valve
with vegetations

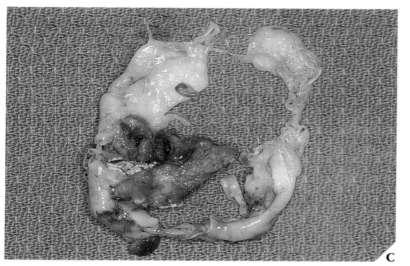

ruptured cords

vegetation

FIG. 9.3 The spread of infection from the aortic root onto the mitral valve can be seen in the area of aortic–mitral valve continuity, as viewed from the atrial aspect.

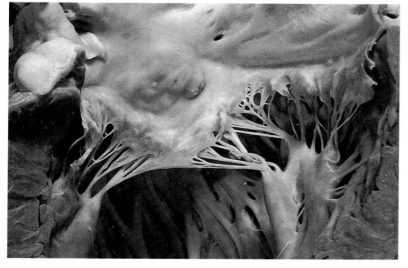

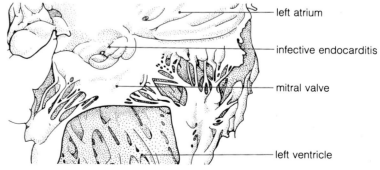

left atrium

infective endocarditis

mitral valve

left ventricle

as part of the regurgitant flow (Fig. 9.4). It may also cause massive left ventricular dilation with secondary myocardial ischemia (Fig. 9.5). The vegetations may cause thromboemboli, which are often infected (Fig. 9.6). Septic myocarditis is a common complication in patients with aortic valve endocarditis (Fig. 9.7).

CLINICAL MANIFESTATIONS
SYMPTOMS

The patient may give a history of dental work or a recent infection, and reports fever, chills, anorexia, weakness, headache, myalgia, and arthralgia. The patient may complain of flu-like symptoms. Symptoms may relate to systemic emboli to the brain, kidney, intestinal tract, extremities, spleen, eye, coronary artery, or other areas. Symptoms of heart failure may appear; if failure was present before the infection, it may worsen due to damage to the aortic or the mitral valve, rupture of tendinous cords, or myocarditis. Table 9.5 summarizes the major clinical manifestations of endocarditis and the investigative tests that aid in diagnosis.

PHYSICAL EXAMINATION

The patient may appear chronically or acutely ill; temperature is usually elevated. Petechial hemorrhages of the skin and the mucous membranes may be evident. Splinter hemorrhages, Osler's nodes, Janeway

lesions, retinal hemorrhages, Roth's spots, endophthalmitis, clubbing of the fingers, signs of peripheral emboli, and splenomegaly may all be identified.

Most patients have a heart murmur due either to stenosis, and/or regurgitation of the aortic, mitral, pulmonary, or tricuspid valves, an interventricular septal defect, patent arterial duct, coarctation, ostium primum atrioventricular septal defect, or prosthetic valves in any valve area.

The physical findings associated with heart failure, embolization to any area, or mycotic aneurysm may be detected.

LABORATORY ABNORMALITIES

Anemia develops in most patients with subacute endocarditis; in many patients with acute infection it develops after the first week. The anemia is usually normochromic and normocytic, but it may be hemolytic when acute infection occurs. Leukocytosis may develop; an extremely high white blood count suggests an abscess. The erythrocyte sedimentation rate is usually elevated. Hematuria may be present. Red cell casts and proteinuria may be found in patients with glomerulonephritis due to endocarditis.

Blood cultures should be obtained from all patients with a heart murmur and fever. Although there are reports that arterial blood is more likely to yield positive cultures than venous blood, most physicians continue to use venous blood. Durack suggested the following approach:

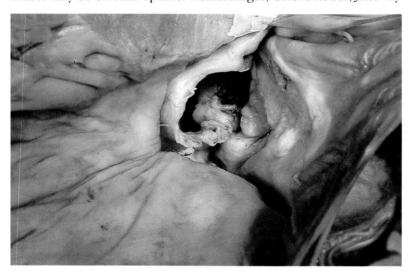

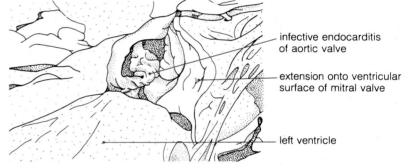

FIG. 9.4 *In this heart infective endocarditis of the aortic valve led to valve destruction and regurgitation. The regurgitant flow caused secondary infection of the ventricular aspect of the adjoining mitral valve leaflet.*

infective endocarditis of aortic valve

extension onto ventricular surface of mitral valve

left ventricle

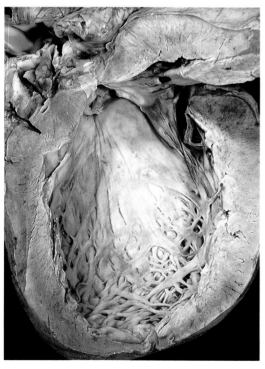

FIG. 9.5 *In the same heart shown in Figure 9.4 aortic valve regurgitation led to massive left ventricular chamber dilation as an adaptive phenomenon. Subendocardial ischemia and infarction are also present.*

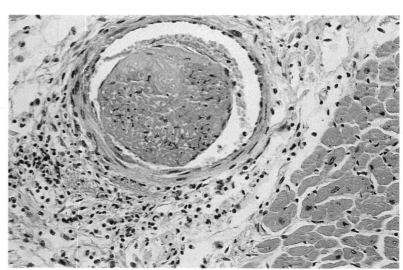

FIG. 9.6 *Histologic section of an intramyocardial coronary artery branch displays an infected thromboembolus. Some inflammatory infiltrate is detectable in the immediate vicinity (H&E stain).*

Katsu [1978] found that arterial cultures were positive slightly more often than venous cultures (72 percent versus 64 percent of 313 cases), and reported 40 cases in which arterial but not venous cultures were positive. Although this difference was significant, it seems too small to justify obtaining arterial cultures in every case. The following practical approach is suggested: for SBE, draw three separate venous blood cultures on the first day. If these cultures show no growth by the second day, draw two more venous cultures. If all are negative on the third day *but the diagnosis of endocarditis still seems likely,* draw two more venous cultures and one arterial blood culture. If the patient had received prior antibiotic therapy, three more venous samples may be taken over the following week, looking for a late recrudescence of bacteremia after partial treatment. For ABE, draw three venous blood cultures and begin empirical antibiotic therapy, because treatment should not be delayed until culture results are available in acute endocarditis.

Because *Staph. epidermidis* [Keys and Hewitt, 1973] and diphtheroids [Gerry and Greenough, 1976] can cause endocarditis, special care must be taken during venipuncture to avoid contamination of the specimen with these common skin organisms, which would result in diagnostic confusion. For each culture, 10 to 20 ml of blood should be drawn and divided equally between one unvented anaerobic bottle of medium and one vented bottle. Media should be adequately supplemented to allow growth of fastidious, nutritionally variant bacteria [Carey et al, 1975; Ellner et al, 1979; Washington, 1982]. Cultures should be incubated for at least 3 weeks, and Gram stains made at intervals even if no growth is apparent on inspection. Pour plates can help to distinguish contaminants from true positive cultures. (*The Heart,* 6th ed, pp 1144–1145)

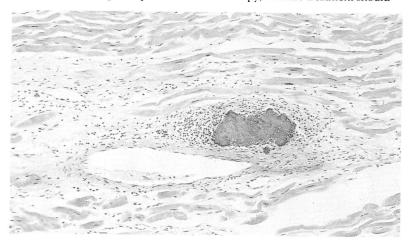

FIG. 9.7 *Septic myocarditis is exemplified by a colony of bacteria surrounded by an inflammatory infiltrate (H&E stain).*

Table 9.5 Summary of the Major Clinical Manifestations of Infective Endocarditis

MANIFESTATIONS OF	HISTORY	EXAMINATION	INVESTIGATIONS
Systemic infection	Fever, chills, rigors, sweats, malaise, weakness, lethargy, delirium, headache, anorexia, weight loss, backache, arthralgia, myalgia Portal of entry: Oropharynx, skin Urinary tract Drug addiction Nosocomial bacteremia	Fever Pallor Weight loss Asthenia Splenomegaly	Anemia Leukocytosis (variable) Raised erythrocyte sedimentation rate Blood cultures positive Abnormal cerebrospinal fluid
Intravascular lesion	Dyspnea, chest pain, focal weakness, stroke, abdominal pain, cold and painful extremities	Murmurs Signs of cardiac failure Petechiae—skin, eye, mucosae Roth's spots, Osler's nodes Janeway lesions Splinter hemorrhages Stroke Mycotic aneurysm Ischemia or infarction of viscera or extremities	Blood in urine Chest radiograph Echocardiography Arteriography Liver–spleen scan Lung scan, brain scan, CT scan Histology, culture of emboli
Immunologic reactions	Arthralgia, myalgia, tenosynovitis	Arthritis Signs of uremia Vascular phenomena Finger clubbing	Proteinuria, hematuria, casts, uremia, acidosis Polyclonal increases in gamma globulins Rheumatoid factor, decreased complement, and immune complexes in serum Antistaphylococcal teichoic acid antibodies

(Table 56-5, *The Heart,* 6th ed, p 1141. Information compiled from references 33, 41, 50, and 148 in *The Heart,* 6th ed, pp 1154, 1156)

The electrocardiogram (ECG) may be normal. However, it may reveal the anatomic features of the underlying heart disease, infarction due to a coronary embolism, or a new conduction defect caused by a small abscess involving the conduction system.

The chest film may reveal the anatomic consequences of the underlying heart disease and, with tricuspid valve endocarditis, evidence of septic pulmonary emboli.

Echocardiography may be used to identify vegetations (Fig. 9.8). The sensitivity of M-mode echocardiography for identification of vegetations is about 50%. Cross-sectional echocardiography is more sensitive, but a negative echocardiogram does not exclude the disease. Vegetations less than 3–4 mm in size cannot be detected, and all valves cannot always be visualized. The tricuspid valve, for example, is difficult to study. False-positive echocardiograms for vegetations do occur, commonly in patients with myxomatous degeneration of the mitral valve. The echocardiogram usually reveals evidence of the underlying heart disease.

Cardiac catheterization is reserved for those patients in whom surgical intervention is planned.

Radionuclide imaging of the liver and spleen may reveal emboli. Computed tomographic scanning of the brain may demonstrate emboli to the brain.

MINIMUM DIAGNOSTIC CRITERIA

The disease should be considered whenever fever of unknown cause develops in a patient with a heart murmur. Blood cultures should be drawn; they are usually positive in the patient who has not received antibiotics. The echocardiogram may be helpful, but a negative study does not exclude the disease.

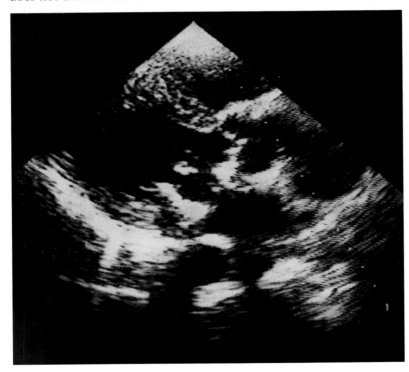

NATURAL HISTORY AND PROGNOSIS

The disease is usually fatal if unrecognized and untreated. Early treatment is imperative, because valve damage, heart failure, and emboli may limit the chances of recovery even if there is bacteriologic cure.

TREATMENT

The treatment is the use of appropriate antibiotics for a sufficiently long period to produce a bacteriologic cure. Accordingly the identification of the offending organism and its sensitivity to antibiotics is mandatory for optimal treatment. The treatment of endocarditis due to gram-positive cocci is outlined in Table 9.6; the duration of treatment varies according to the isolated organism. When the organism is not known, the following antibiotics are recommended for a two-week period:

For acute infection: nafcillin 2.0 g IV every 4 h
plus
ampicillin 2.0 g IV every 4 h
plus
gentamicin 1.5 mg/kg IV every 8 hr
For chronic infection: ampicillin 2.0 g IV every 4 h
plus
gentamicin 1.5 mg/kg IV every 8 h.
(*The Heart,* 6th ed, p 1149)

The use of anticoagulants should be avoided, if possible. Heart failure, emboli, renal failure, and mycotic aneurysms are treated in the usual manner.

FIG. 9.8 *Cross-sectional echocardiogram in the parasternal long-axis view of a patient with endocarditis shows a vegetation on the prosthetic (Hancock) mitral valve. (Courtesy of Steve Clements, MD, and Mr. John Perkins, Atlanta, Georgia).*

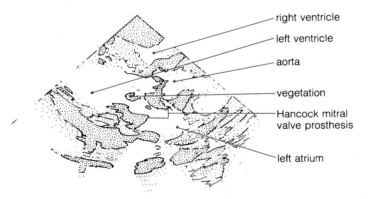

right ventricle
left ventricle
aorta
vegetation
Hancock mitral valve prosthesis
left atrium

Table 9.6 Treatment Regimens for Infective Endocarditis Caused by Gram-Positive Cocci

ORGANISM	REGIMEN	DURATION (WEEKS)	COMMENTS
Alpha-hemolytic (viridans) streptococci; *Strep. bovis*	Penicillin G 2 million units IV every 6 h *plus* streptomycin 7.5 mg/kg every 12 h IM,* *or*	2	Standard regimen, for patients less than 65 years old without renal failure, eighth-nerve defects, or serious complications
	Penicillin G 4 million units IV every 6 h *plus* streptomycin 7.5 mg/kg every 12 h IM (for first 2 weeks only),* *or*	4	For patients with complicated disease, e.g., CNS involvement, shock, moderately penicillin-resistant streptococci, failed previous treatment
	Penicillin G 4 million units every 6 h IV, *or*	4	For patients more than 65 years old, with renal failure or eighth-nerve defects
	Cefazolin 2 g IV every 8 h, *or*	4	For patients allergic to penicillins
	Vancomycin 15 mg/kg IV every 12 h	4	For patients allergic to penicillins and cephalosporins
Group A streptococci, *Strep. pneumoniae*	Penicillin G 2 million units IV every 6 h, *or*	2–4	These organisms are usually highly sensitive to penicillin; 2 weeks should be adequate for many patients
	Cefazolin 1 g IV every 8 h	2–4	
Strep. faecalis (streptomycin-sensitive) and other penicillin-resistant streptococci	Penicillin G 3 million units IV every 4 h *plus* streptomycin 7.5 mg/kg every 12 h IM* *or*	4–6	4 weeks should be adequate for most cases with symptoms present for less than 3 months
	Vancomycin 15 mg/kg IV every 12 h *plus* gentamicin 1.0 mg/kg IV every 12 h	4–6	For patients allergic to penicillin; 4 weeks should be adequate for most cases
Strep. faecalis (streptomycin-resistant) and other penicillin-resistant streptococci	Ampicillin 2 g IV every 4 h *plus* gentamicin 1.0 mg/kg IV every 8 h, *or*	4–6	4 weeks should be adequate for most cases with symptoms present for less than 3 months
	Vancomycin 15 mg/kg IV every 12 h IV *plus* gentamicin 1.0 mg/kg IV every 12 h	4–6	For patients allergic to penicillin; 4 weeks should be adequate for most cases
Staph. aureus	Nafcillin 2 g IV every 4 h, *or*	4 or longer	Standard regimen
	Nafcillin as above, *plus* gentamicin 1.5 mg/kg IV every 8 h for the first 3–5 days only, *or*	4 or longer	For patients with severe disseminated staphylococcal disease, synergy may be advantageous during early stages of treatment
	Cefazolin 2 g IV every 8 hr, *or*	4 or longer	For patients allergic to penicillins
	Vancomycin 15 mg/kg IV every 12 h	4 or longer	For patients allergic to penicillins and cephalosporins; for methicillin-resistant strains

(Table 56-7, *The Heart*, 6th ed, p 1149. Adapted; reproduced with permission of the author and publisher; see Figure Credits)
*Gentamicin 1.0 mg/kg intravenously every 12 h for 2 weeks may be substituted for streptomycin, if desired, to avoid intramuscular injections. The dose of streptomycin should not exceed 500 mg per dose in any regimen employing streptomycin.

CARDIAC SURGERY

Operative intervention may be required during the active phase of endocarditis. Such intervention has been shown repeatedly to be life-saving in spite of the risk of operating in a contaminated field. Because of this, surgery has assumed a major role in the management of patients with infective endocarditis. The need for operative intervention de-pends on the clinical presentation (Wilcox, 1985) (Fig. 9.9).

When operation is required, valve replacement is almost always necessary. Very rarely, when there is evidence of healing and/or only limited damage, a valve may be repaired rather than replaced (Fig. 9.10); however, this is the exception to the usual condition (Fig. 9.11). Most patients require extensive reconstructive surgery (Frantz et al,

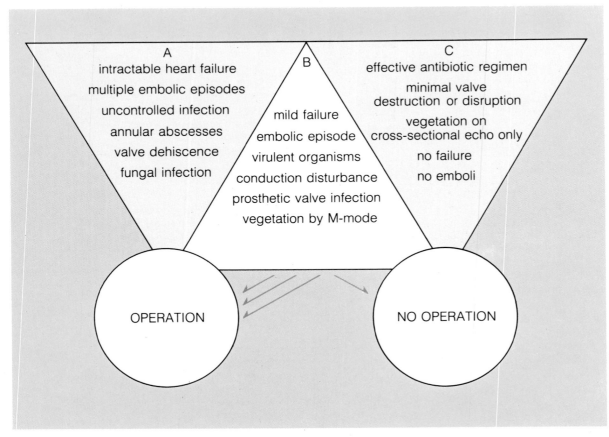

FIG. 9.9 *This schema outlines the management of patients with infective endocarditis. When one or more of the conditions listed under (**A**) are present, early surgical intervention is indicated. Early intervention is also indicated when two or three of the conditions listed under (**B**) are present. However, when only one of the latter conditions is present or when any of the circumstances listed under (**C**) exists, early operation is probably not necessary. (Redrawn; reproduced with permission of the author and publisher; see Figure Credits)*

A
intractable heart failure
multiple embolic episodes
uncontrolled infection
annular abscesses
valve dehiscence
fungal infection

B
mild failure
embolic episode
virulent organisms
conduction disturbance
prosthetic valve infection
vegetation by M-mode

C
effective antibiotic regimen
minimal valve destruction or disruption
vegetation on cross-sectional echo only
no failure
no emboli

OPERATION

NO OPERATION

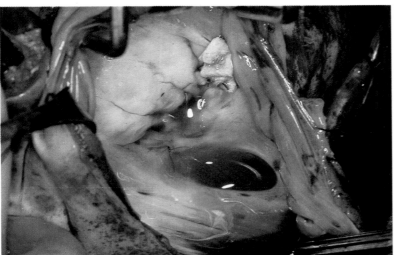

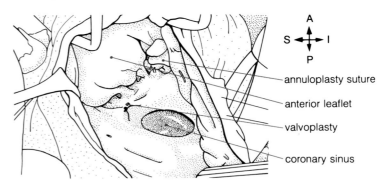

FIG. 9.10 *This operative view of a heart with tricuspid valve endocarditis in an intravenous drug abuser shows limited damage to the valve, which allowed repair using valvoplasty and annuloplasty techniques without valve replacement.*

annuloplasty suture
anterior leaflet
valvoplasty
coronary sinus

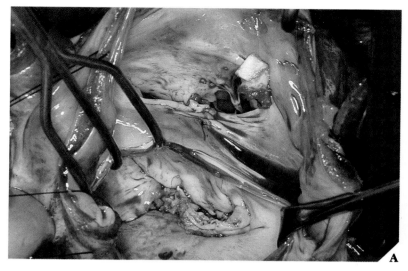

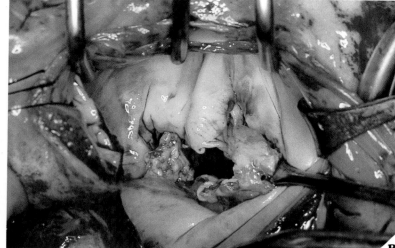

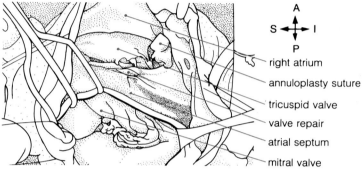

right atrium

annuloplasty suture

tricuspid valve

valve repair

atrial septum

mitral valve

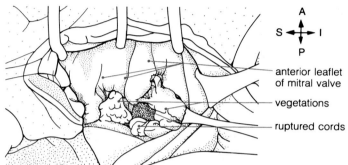

anterior leaflet
of mitral valve

vegetations

ruptured cords

FIG. 9.11 (A–C) *Operative views of the same patient seen in Figure 9.10 demonstrate the repaired tricuspid valve and the badly damaged mitral valve. Mitral valve replacement was necessary.*

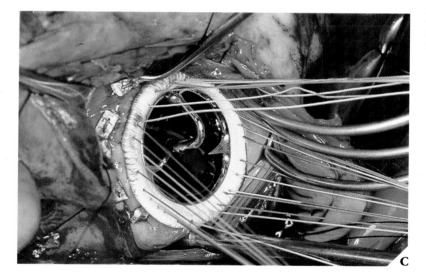

1980) in addition to valve replacement (Fig. 9.12). Complications of surgery are acceptable under these circumstances.

Operation may also be required for the treatment of a mycotic aneurysm (Fig. 9.13). Small aneurysms may not rupture after the bac-teria have been eradicated. Aneurysms that are larger than 1–2 cm in diameter may become larger and rupture even if the organisms have been eradicated. Intracranial aneurysms may be difficult to treat sur-gically because of inaccessibility and multiplicity.

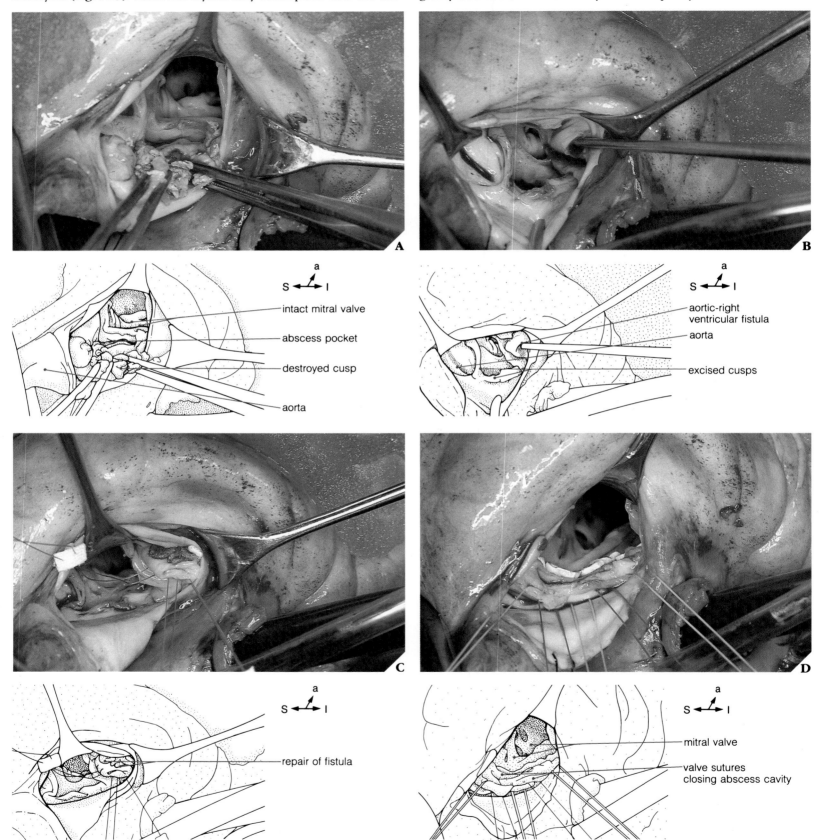

FIG. 9.12 *Considerable reconstruction is necessary in this patient with an extensively damaged aortic valve.* (**A**) *A large abscess formation separates the aorta from the myocardial mass.* (**B**) *Sinus of Valsalva–right ventricu-lar fistula also causes left-to-right shunting.* (**C**) *Direct repair of the sinus of Valsalva fistula is effected.* (**D**) *Repair of the detached aorta is incorporated in pledgeted sutures used for fixation of the prosthetic valve.*

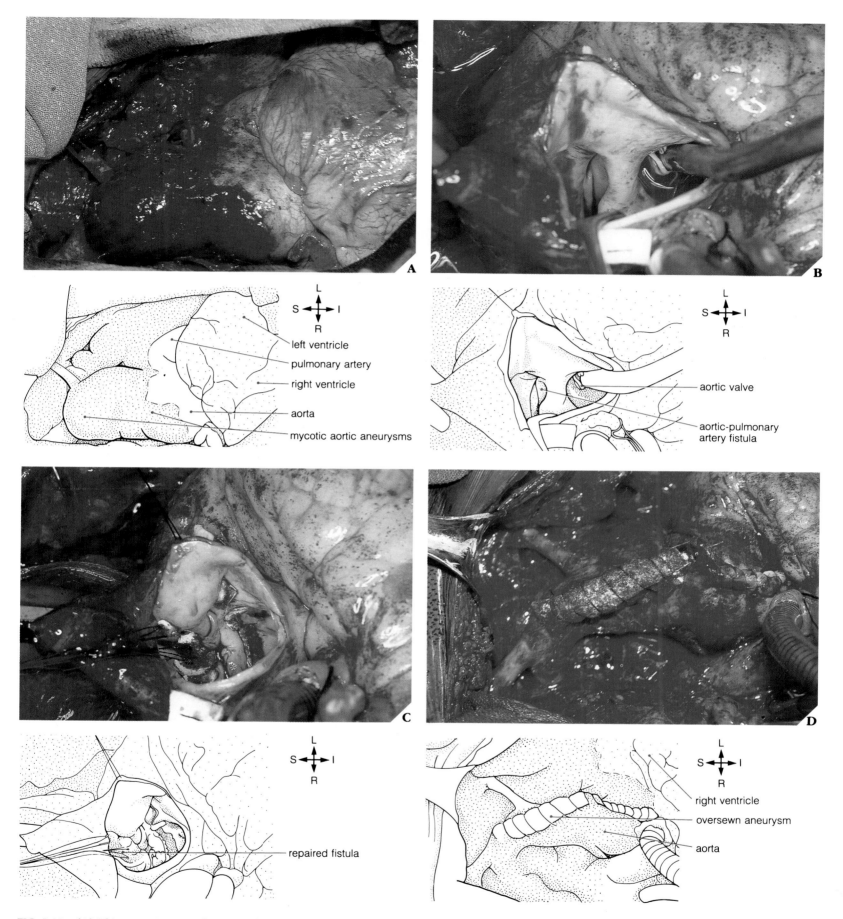

FIG. 9.13 (**A**) *This operative view shows two large mycotic aneurysms of the ascending aorta. One is located at the base of the brachiocephalic artery, and the other extends posteriorly, resulting in fistula formation into the pulmonary trunk.* (**B**) *The ascending aorta is opened, demonstrating* the large posterior fistula. (**C**) *The fistula is closed by multiple interrupted mattress sutures reinforced with Dacron pledgets.* (**D**) *The smaller aneurysm is simply excised and oversewn using continuous and interrupted sutures reinforced with Teflon felt.*

PROPHYLAXIS

There have been no definitive clinical trials to determine whether prevention of endocarditis is effective. It is customary, however, to use antibiotics prophylactically prior to and following dental work, surgical procedures when bacteremia is likely, and certain infections (Table 9.7). A committee of the American Heart Association periodically addresses the problem of prophylaxis, and publishes its recommendations in a pamphlet.*

---

*The pamphlet can be obtained by writing the American Heart Association, 7320 Greenville Avenue, Dallas, TX 75231.

REFERENCES

Carey RB, Gross KC, Roberts RB (1975) Vitamin B6-dependent *Streptococcus mitior* (*mitis*) isolated from patients with systemic infections. *J Infect Dis* 131:722.

Ellner JJ, Rosenthal MS, Lerner PI, McHenry MC (1979) Infective endocarditis caused by slow-growing, fastidious, Gram-negative bacteria. *Medicine* 58:145.

Frantz PT, Murray GF, Wilcox BR (1980) Surgical management of left ventricular–aortic discontinuity complicating bacterial endocarditis. *Ann Thorac Surg* 29:1.

Gerry JL, Greenough WB (1976) Diphtheroid endocarditis: Report of nine cases and review of the literature. *Johns Hopkins Med J* 139:61.

Katsu M (1978) Spectrum of endocarditis in Japan and current treatment. Proceedings of the 8th World Congress of Cardiology. Tokyo, p 536.

Keys TF, Hewitt WL (1973) Endocarditis due to micrococci and *Staphylococcus epidermidis. Arch Intern Med* 132:216

Richardson JV, Karp RB, Kirklin JW, et al (1978) Treatment of infective endocarditis: A 10-year comparative analysis. *Circulation* 58:589.

Stewart JA, Silimperi D, Harris P, et al (1980) Echocardiographic documentation of vegetative lesions in infective endocarditis: Clinical implications. *Circulation* 61:374.

Stinson EB (1979) Surgical treatment of infective endocarditis. *Prog Cardiovasc Dis* 22:145.

Washington JA II (1982) The role of the microbiology laboratory in the diagnosis and antimicrobial treatment of infective endocarditis. *Mayo Clin Proc* 57:22.

Wilcox BR, (1985) The role of surgery in the management of infective endocarditis, Roberts A (ed): *Difficult Problems in Adult Cardiac Surgery.* Chicago, Year Book Medical Publishers, p 199.

Wilcox BR, Murray GF, Starek PJK (1977) The long-term outlook for valve replacement in active endocarditis. *J Thorac Cardiovasc Surg* 74:860.

Wilson WR, Danielson GK, Giuliani ER, et al (1979) Cardiac valve replacement in congestive heart failure due to infective endocarditis. *Mayo Clinic Proc* 54:223.

FIGURE CREDITS

TABLE 9.6 Adapted with slight modification from Durack DT: Infectious endocarditis, in Wyngaarden JB, Smith LH (eds): *Cecil Textbook of Medicine,* 17th ed. Philadelphia, WB Saunders, 1985, p 1540.

FIG. 9.9 Redrawn from Wilcox BR: The role of surgery in the management of infective endocarditis, in Roberts A (ed): *Difficult Problems in Adult Cardiac Surgery.* Chicago, Year Book Medical Publishers, 1985, pp 199–218.

TABLE 9.7 Adapted from Durack DT: Nine controversies in the management of infective endocarditis, in Petersdorf RG et al (eds): *Update V: Harrison's Principles of Internal Medicine.* New York, McGraw-Hill, 1984, p 35.

Table 9.7 Suggested Regimens for Prophylaxis of Infective Endocarditis*

STANDARD REGIMEN

For dental procedures and oral or upper respiratory tract surgery	Penicillin V 2.0 g orally 1 h before, then 1.0 g 6 h later†

SPECIAL REGIMENS

Parenteral regimen for high-risk patients; also for gastrointestinal (GI) or genitourinary (GU) tract procedures	Ampicillin 2.0 g IM or IV *plus* gentamicin 1.5 mg/kg IM or IV, 0.5 h before†
Parenteral regimen for penicillin-allergic patients	Vancomycin 1.0 g IV *slowly* over 1 h, starting 1 h before; *add* gentamicin 1.5 mg/kg IM or IV if GI or GU tract involved†
Oral regimen for penicillin-allergic patients (oral and respiratory tract only)	Erythromycin 1.0 g orally 1 h before, then 0.5 g 6 h later†
Oral regimen for minor GI or GU tract procedures	Amoxicillin 3.0 g orally 1 h before, then 1.5 g 6 h later†
Parenteral regimen for cardiac surgery including valve replacement	Cefazolin 2.0 g IV on induction of anesthesia, repeated 8 and 16 h later‡ *or* Vancomycin 1.0 g IV *slowly* over 1 h starting on induction of anesthesia, then 0.5 g IV 8 and 16 h later‡

(Table 56-9, *The Heart,* 6th ed, p 1153. Adapted; reproduced with permission of the author and publisher; see Figure Credits)

*Note that (1) these regimens are empirical suggestions; no regimen has been proved effective for prevention of endocarditis, and prevention failures may occur with any regimen; (2) these regimens are not intended to cover all clinical situations; the practitioner should use his or her own judgment on safety and cost-benefit issues in each individual case; (3) one or two additional doses may be given if the period of risk for bacteremia is prolonged.

†Pediatric dosages: ampicillin 50 mg/kg; erythromycin 20 mg/kg for first dose, then 10 mg/kg; gentamicin 2 mg/kg; penicillin V and amoxicillin; for children who weigh more than 60 lb, use same as for adults; for children less than 60 lb, use one-half the adult dose; vancomycin 20 mg/kg.

‡Vancomycin is preferred if *Staph. epidermidis* is an important cause of postoperative infection in that hospital. Gentamicin 1.5 mg/kg IV or IM may be added to each dose, only if postoperative gram-negative infections have occurred with significant frequency.

10
TRAUMATIC DISEASE OF THE CARDIOVASCULAR SYSTEM

J. Willis Hurst, MD
Panagiotis N. Symbas, MD
Anton E. Becker, MD
Benson R. Wilcox, MD

Abstracted with permission of the authors and publisher frm Symbas PN, Arensberg D: Traumatic heart disease, Chapter 60, pp 1276–1283, in Hurst JW (ed): *The Heart,* 6th ed. New York, McGraw-Hill, 1986. Figures and tables reproduced in this chapter from the above chapter or other sources are also reprinted with permission of the authors and publishers. For the full bibliographic citations of the sources of figures and tables other than the above chapter, see Figure Credits at the end of this chapter.

Table 10.1 Penetrating Wounds of the Heart

Pericardial damage
    Laceration or perforation
    Hemopericardium with or without cardiac tamponade
    Serofibrinous or suppurative pericarditis
    Pneumopericardium
    Constrictive pericarditis
Myocardial damage
    Laceration
    Penetration or perforation
    Retained foreign body
    Structural defects
        Aneurysm formation
        Septal defects
        Aortocardiac fistula
Valvar injury
    Leaflet injury
    Papillary muscle or tendinous cords laceration
Coronary artery injury
    Laceration or thrombosis with or without myocardial
      infarction
    Arteriovenous fistula
    Aneurysm
Embolism
    Foreign body
    Thrombus (septic or sterile)
Infective endocarditis
Rhythm or conduction disturbances

(Table 60-1, *The Heart,* 6th ed, p 1277. We wish to thank Loren F. Parmley, MD, and Thomas W Mattingly, MD, for permission to modify Table 52-1, *The Heart,* 1st ed, 1966)

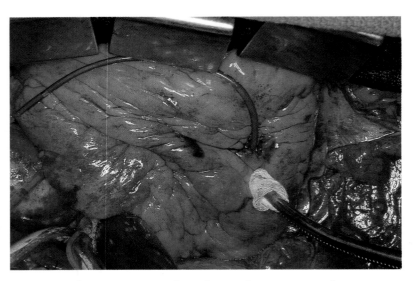

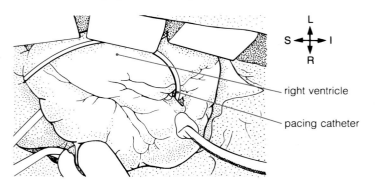

FIG. 10.1 *This operative view through a median sternotomy for coronary artery bypass surgery shows a pacing catheter inserted in the coronary care unit. The catheter perforated the right ventricular wall.*

Table 10.2 Nonpenetrating Trauma of the Heart

Pericardial injury
    Hemopericardium
    Rupture or laceration
    Serofibrinous pericarditis
    Constrictive pericarditis
Myocardial injury
    Contusion
    Rupture of free cardiac wall, early or delayed
    Rupture of septum
    Aneurysm
    Laceration
Disturbances of rhythm or conduction
Valve injury
    Rupture of valve leaflets, cusp, or tendinous cords
    Contusion of papillary muscle
Coronary artery injury
    Thrombosis with or without myocardial infarction
    Arteriovenous fistula
    Laceration with or without myocardial infarction
Great-vessel injury
    Rupture
    Aneurysm formation
    Aortocardiac chamber fistula
    Thrombotic occlusion

(Table 60-2, *The Heart,* 6th ed, p 1278. We wish to thank Loren F. Parmley, MD, and Thomas W. Mattingly, MD, for permission to modify Table 52-2, *The Heart,* 1st ed, 1966)

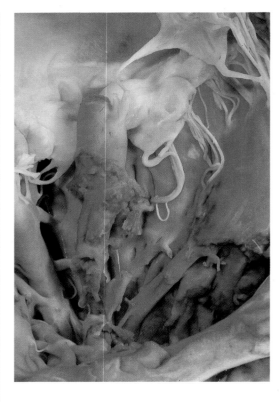

FIG. 10.2 *Laceration of the anterior papillary muscle of the tricuspid valve with complete rupture resulted from blunt chest trauma.*

The incidence of traumatic disease of the cardiovascular system has increased in recent years because of the increasing number of automobile accidents and handgun injuries. The physician must consider injury to the heart and vessels whenever trauma has occurred. Traumatic heart disease may be overlooked when other more conspicuous injuries attract the physician's immediate attention, or when diagnostic clues are not immediately apparent.

PENETRATING TRAUMA

Almost any area of the heart and great vessels may be damaged by penetrating trauma (Table 10.1). Although wounds are usually considered inflicted from without, it is useful to remember that the heart wall can also be traversed from inside outward (Fig. 10.1). This danger is perhaps becoming more prevalent with the increasing number and range of procedures that are performed in the catheter laboratory and the intensive care setting. The treatment is determined by the type and the clinical manifestations of the injury; surgical intervention is often needed.

NONPENETRATING TRAUMA

Nonpenetrating trauma may also damage the heart and vessels (Table 10.2). Myocardial laceration (Fig. 10.2), injury to valve leaflets (Fig. 10.3), and coronary artery laceration (Fig. 10.4) are among the most common complications. Rupture of the aorta may also occur (Fig. 10.5).

Significant nonpenetrating or blunt trauma of the heart may result in damage to the myocardium or to the valves themselves. When valvar damage occurs, the tension apparatus of the atrioventricular valves, more frequently the tricuspid valve, is usually affected. Myocardial

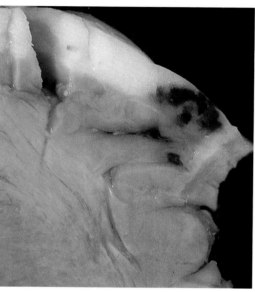

FIG. 10.4 *A laceration of the anterior descending coronary artery followed nonpenetrating trauma to the heart.*

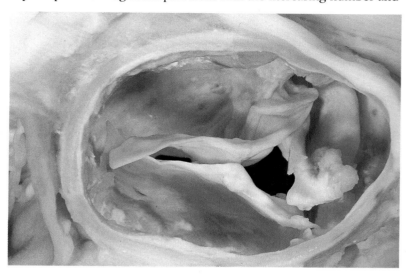

FIG. 10.3 *This torn aortic cusp resulted from blunt chest trauma.*

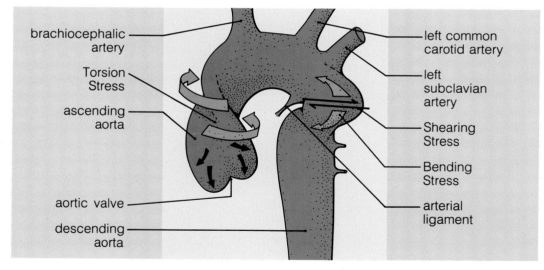

brachiocephalic artery

Torsion Stress

ascending aorta

aortic valve

descending aorta

left common carotid artery

left subclavian artery

Shearing Stress

Bending Stress

arterial ligament

FIG. 10.5 *This diagram illustrates the forces acting upon the aortic wall during rupture of the aorta from blunt trauma. (Redrawn; reproduced with permission of the author and publisher; see Figure Credits. Also, Fig. 60-1,* The Heart, *6th ed, p 1280)*

damage manifests itself either as a cardiac contusion, cardiac rupture, or a ventricular septal rupture. Ventricular aneurysm or pseudoaneurysm may be the result of such injury. This lesion is well illustrated by the case (Fig. 10.6) of a nine-year-old child who, four weeks prior to surgery, had received multiple injuries in an automobile accident. On admission to the hospital he was noted to have right bundle branch block on the electrocardiogram; cardiac enzyme analysis indicated myocardial damage. The electrocardiographic pattern evolved to show an inferior myocardial infarction; cross-sectional echocardiography demonstrated an apparent pseudoaneurysm of the right ventricle. Cardiac catheterization showed a true aneurysm of the left ventricle encroaching on the right ventricle. There was no evidence of left-to-right

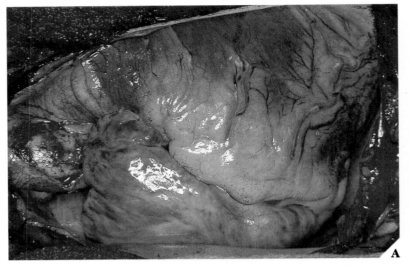

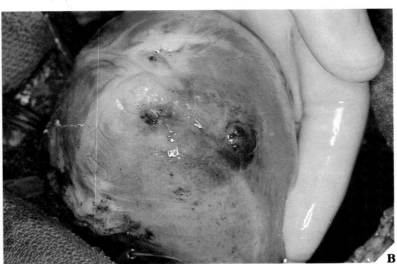

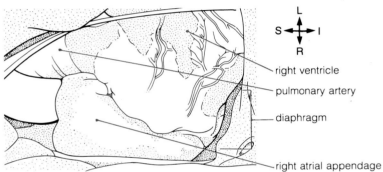

right ventricle
pulmonary artery
diaphragm
right atrial appendage

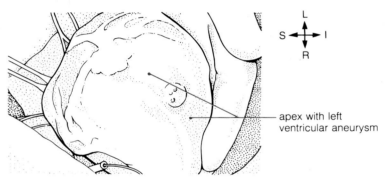

apex with left ventricular aneurysm

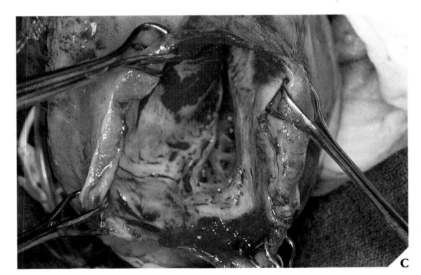

FIG. 10.6 (A) Operative view of the heart in repair of a true ventricular aneurysm caused by blunt trauma shows that the right ventricle is intact. (B) On cardiopulmonary bypass the apex is tilted out of the pericardium, and the apical aneurysm is identified. (C) The opened aneurysm shows a smooth, thin-walled, saccular deformity extending from the apex to the base of the heart (continued).

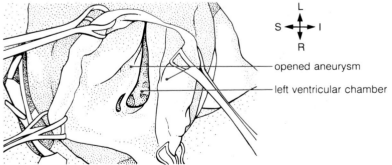

opened aneurysm
left ventricular chamber

shunting, and the cardiac valves were not damaged. Coronary angiography was not performed, but an aortic root injection demonstrated a dominant right coronary system.

At the time of operation the patient was found to have an aneurysm of the left ventricular apex that extended along the diaphragmatic surface to the base of the heart. There was no evidence of ventricular septal rupture. The apical portion of the aneurysm was excised, and the resultant defect was repaired.

FIGURE CREDITS

FIG. 10.5 Redrawn from Symbas PN: *Traumatic Injuries of the Heart and Great Vessels.* Springfield, IL, Charles C Thomas, 1971, p 153.

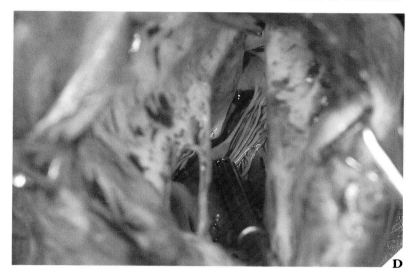

D

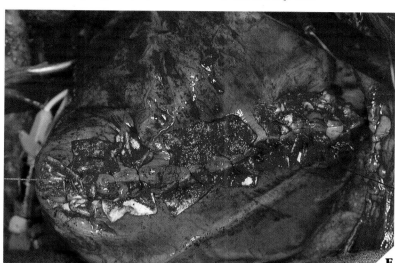

E

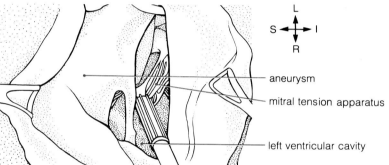

aneurysm

mitral tension apparatus

left ventricular cavity

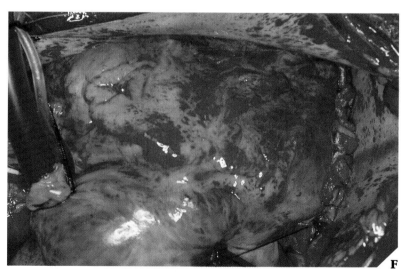

F

FIG. 10.6 (continued) (**D**) *The mitral valve tension apparatus is seen to be intact.* (**E**) *Repair of the aneurysm was effected using multiple interrupted mattress sutures over Teflon pledgets.* (**F**) *A view of the heart after completion of the repair demonstrates the extensive nature of the aneurysm.*

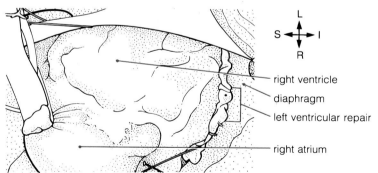

right ventricle

diaphragm

left ventricular repair

right atrium

11
SURGICAL TREATMENT OF CARDIAC ARRHYTHMIAS

J. Willis Hurst, MD
Edward L.C. Pritchett, MD
Andrew G. Wallace, MD
Anton E. Becker, MD
Benson R. Wilcox, MD

Abstracted with permission of the authors and publisher from Pritchett ELC, Wallace AG: Treatment of tachycardia by cardiac surgery, Chapter 127, pp 2013–2015, in Hurst JW (ed): *The Heart,* 6th ed. New York, McGraw-Hill, 1986. Figures reprinted in this chapter from the above chapter are also reproduced with permission of the authors and publisher.

The treatment of cardiac arrhythmias has improved considerably during the last decade, although it is not always successful. New drugs have been developed, cardiac pacemakers have been refined, the internal ventricular defibrillator has been created, and catheter ablation of the atrioventricular node can be accomplished by electrical means.

There is a small percentage of patients with serious recurrent arrhythmias that threaten life and well-being who may be treated surgically. The pathology may vary according to the underlying disease. Fibrosis amid viable myocardial cells consequent to ischemic heart disease many create micro-reentry circuits (Fig. 11.1). Macro-reentry circuits may be caused by abnormalities that involve the atrioventricular node and bundle, or more commonly by accessory atrioventricular connections (Fig. 11.2). The surgical management of these arrhythmias consists of the division of accessory conduction pathways, the operative treatment of ventricular tachycardia, or the division of the atrioventricular node from the penetrating atrioventricular bundle (of His).

DIVISION OF ACCESSORY CONDUCTION PATHWAY

Patients with the Wolff-Parkinson-White syndrome who have repeated episodes of reentrant tachycardia despite proper medical management or who have atrial fibrillation with a rapid ventricular response may

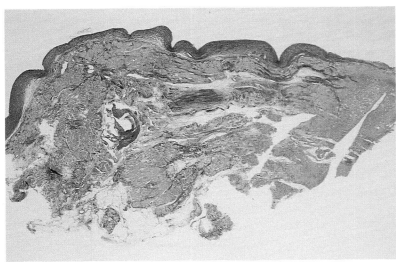

FIG. 11.1 *Histologic section of surgically excised endomyocardial tissue reveals extensive fibrosis separating viable myocardial cells, which creates the setting for a micro-reentry circuit. The resected zone was detected by intraoperative mapping (elastic tissue stain).*

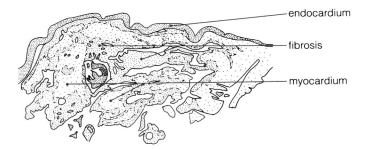

endocardium

fibrosis

myocardium

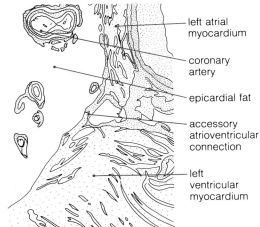

FIG. 11.2 *Accessory atrioventricular connection is composed of a strand of myocardial cells bridging the atrioventricular fibrous annulus in a patient with the Wolff-Parkinson-White syndrome (elastic tissue stain).*

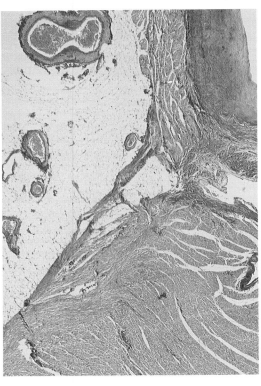

left atrial myocardium

coronary artery

epicardial fat

accessory atrioventricular connection

left ventricular myocardium

require surgical division of the accessory conduction pathway. The pathways cross the atrioventricular junction at some point outside the area of the atrioventricular node. Anatomically they can be considered in terms of left-sided, septal, and right-sided pathways. Left-sided pathways extend through the epicardial fat pad but run very close to the annulus of the mitral valve. Septal pathways may run at any point through the overlapping tissues of the muscular atrioventricular septum; these are the most difficult to divide. Right-sided pathways may pass through the fat pad close to the attachment of the tricuspid valve, or they may be more parietal. Right-sided pathways may originate in remnants of specialized conduction tissue, resulting in distinct electrophysiologic properties.

The location of the site for the incision can be identified by electrophysiologic studies on the exposed heart (Fig. 11.3). The left-sided pathways are the easiest to interrupt, using an internal incision and dissecting the fat pad via the left atrium, or approaching externally through the atrioventricular groove. Similar approaches may be used for right-sided pathways. It is most difficult surgically to divide accessory pathways in the septum because of their proximity to the atrioventricular node. Those experienced in the technique, however, have found it possible to dissect the space between the overlapping layers of the muscular atrioventricular septum, dividing pathways in this fashion. The operation is 95% successful; the operative mortality is under 1% when performed by skilled surgeons.

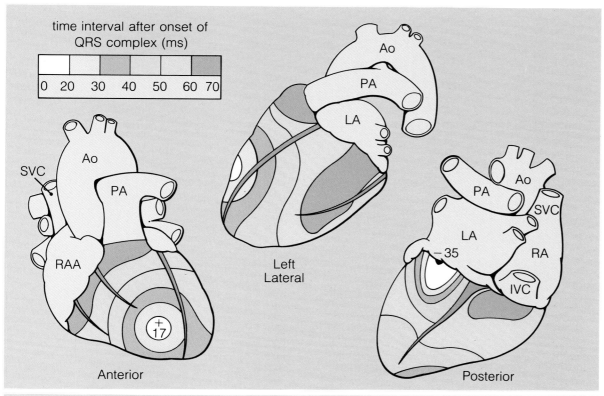

FIG. 11.3 *Epicardial map of ventricular activation during sinus rhythm was recorded in a patient with Wolff-Parkinson-White syndrome. The numbers indicated by shading are the time intervals after the onset of the QRS complex. The earliest epicardial activation was recorded at the base of the left ventricle 35 ms before the onset of the QRS complex. Epicardial activation initiated by the normal conduction system began on the surface of the right ventricle 17 ms after the onset of the QRS complex. (Redrawn; Fig. 127-1,* The Heart, *6th ed, p 2014)*

time interval after onset of QRS complex (ms)

| 0 | 20 | 30 | 40 | 50 | 60 | 70 |

Ao, aorta

PA, pulmonary artery

RAA, right atrial appendage

SVC, superior caval vein

LA, left atrium

RA, right atrium

IVC, inferior caval vein

OPERATIVE TREATMENT OF VENTRICULAR TACHYCARDIA

This operative procedure is used when recurrent ventricular tachycardia is associated with a left ventricular aneurysm due to myocardial infarction (Fig. 11.4). An incision is made in the aneurysm, and the endocardium is mapped during tachycardia. The abnormal endocardium is removed, the aneurysm is excised, and coronary bypass surgery is performed if indicated. This type of treatment has been highly successful.

Right ventricular dysplasia, a rare congenital abnormality of the right ventricle, may be responsible for uncontrolled ventricular arrhyth-mias. This condition may also be amenable to the type of surgical intervention described above.

DIVISION OF ATRIOVENTRICULAR NODE AND BUNDLE OF HIS

This technique is not often used now that the catheter ablation technique has been developed. (Catheter ablation treatment of arrhythmias is still in the developmental stage, and new modifications of the technique are now being considered.) Surgical division of the atrioventricular node and bundle of His has been used in patients who have

FIG. 11.4 (**A**) *Operative view in surgical treatment of ventricular tachycardia shows a large apical anterior ventricular aneurysm.* (**B**) *The aneurysm is opened to reveal the thin-walled, scarred myocardium with whitish, thickened endocardium.* (**C**) *The area of arrhythmogenesis is identified and excised along with the aneurysmal sac.*

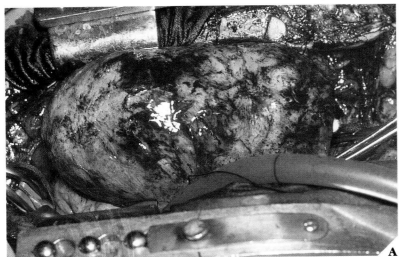

A

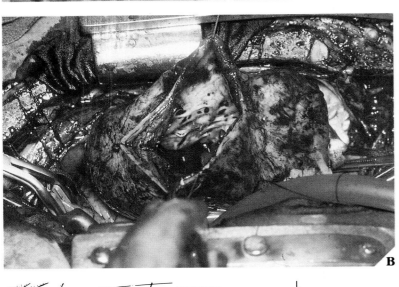

B

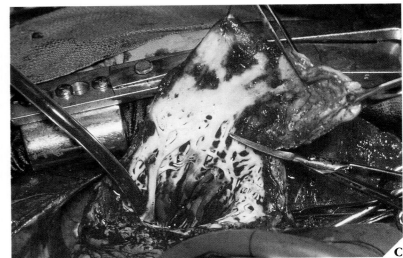

C

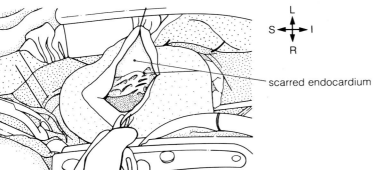

scarred endocardium

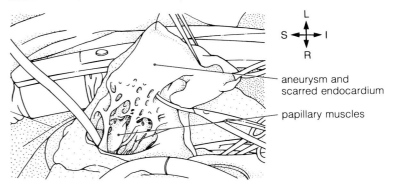

aneurysm and scarred endocardium

papillary muscles

an uncontrolled rapid ventricular rate due to atrial arrhythmia, or in patients with reentrant atrioventricular tachycardia. It is more desirable, however, to interrupt the accessory pathway in patients with reentrant tachycardia than to sever the usual connection between the atria and the ventricles by surgical means. Accordingly the surgical technique for interrupting the specialized atrioventricular conduction axis is performed less frequently now than it was a decade ago.

REFERENCES

Fontaine G, Guiraudon G, Frank R, et al (1977) Stimulation studies and epicardial mapping in ventricular tachycardia: Study of mechanism and selection for surgery, in Kulbertus HE (ed): *Reentrant Arrhythmias*. Lancaster, England, MTP Press, p 334.

Gallagher JJ, Kasell J, Sealy WC, Pritchett ELC, Wallace AG (1978) Epicardial mapping in the Wolff-Parkinson-White syndrome. *Circulation* 57:854.

Gallagher JJ, Svenson RH, Kasell J, et al (1982) Catheter technique for closed chest ablation of the atrioventricular conduction system in man: A therapeutic alternative for the treatment of refractory supraventricular tachycardia. *N Engl J Med* 306:194.

Horowitz LN, Harken AH, Kastor JA, Josephson ME (1980) Ventricular resection guided by epicardial and endocardial mapping for treatment of recurrent ventricular tachycardia. *N Engl J Med* 302:589.

Sealy WC, Gallagher JJ, Pritchett ELC (1978) The surgical anatomy of Kent bundles based on electrophysiological mapping and surgical exploration. *J Thorac Cardiovasc Surg* 76:804.

Sealy WC, Hackel DB, Seaber AV (1977) A study of methods for surgical interruption of the His bundle. *J Thorac Cardiovasc Surg* 73:424.

III

THE HEART AND OTHER CONDITIONS

12
HYPERTENSION

SYSTEMIC HYPERTENSION

J. Willis Hurst, MD
Harriet P. Dustan, MD

DIAGNOSTIC EVALUATION OF HYPERTENSION

J. Willis Hurst, MD
W. Dallas Hall, MD
Gary L. Wollam, MD
Elbert P. Tuttle, Jr, MD
Anton E. Becker, MD

TREATMENT OF HYPERTENSION

J. Willis Hurst, MD
Gary L. Wollam, MD
W. Dallas Hall, MD

Abstracted with permission of the authors and publisher from Dustan HP: Pathophysiology of hypertension, Chapter 49, pp 1038–1048; Hall WD, Wollam GL, Tuttle EP Jr: Diagnostic evaluation of the patient with hypertension, Chapter 50, pp 1048–1070; and Wollam GL, Hall WD: Treatment of systemic hypertension, Chapter 51, pp 1071–1090; all in Hurst JW (ed): *The Heart,* 6th ed. New York, McGraw-Hill, 1986. Figures and tables reproduced in this chapter from the above chapters or other sources are also reprinted with permission of the authors and publishers. For the full bibliographic citations of the sources of figures other than the above chapters, see Figure Credits at the end of this chapter.

SYSTEMIC HYPERTENSION

Systemic hypertension is a complex disorder; only the rudiments of the condition are discussed here. (The reader is referred to Chapters 49, 50, and 51 in *The Heart,* 6th ed, for further details on this subject.)

The 1984 report of the Third Joint National Committee on the Detection, Evaluation and Treatment of Hypertension (JNCIII) provides the following definitions:

Diastolic pressure: less than 85 mmHg—normal
85–89 mmHg—high normal
90–104 mmHg—mild hypertension
105–114 mmHg—moderate hypertension
115 mmHg or greater—severe hypertension.

Labile hypertension is said to be present when the pressure is intermittently elevated.

It is uncommon for the diastolic blood pressure to be elevated as an isolated abnormality unaccompanied by systolic hypertension. Isolated systolic hypertension, however, may occur with normal diastolic blood pressure. The JNCIII report defines systolic hypertension (when the diastolic pressure is less than 90 mmHg) as follows:

Systolic pressure: less than 140 mmHg—normal
140–159 mmHg—borderline isolated systolic hypertension
160 mmHg or over—isolated systolic hypertension.

PATHOPHYSIOLOGY

The maintenance of blood pressure within normal limits depends on a properly working regulatory system. The elements of the control system are carefully integrated so that the system immediately corrects a rise or a fall in systemic blood pressure. Page (1960) first proposed the idea that hypertension was a "disease of regulation." The elements of the regulating system are hemodynamic, neural, and volume factors, and the renin–angiotensin–aldosterone system.

The abnormalities vary according to the cause of the elevated blood pressure. The numerically significant types of hypertension are essential hypertension, renovascular hypertension, renal parenchymal disease, primary aldosteronism, pheochromocytoma, and coarctation of the thoracic aorta. The underlying hemodynamic fault, except in the case of coarctation of the aorta, is the failure to control peripheral resistance.

The consequences of hypertension are arterial disease, stroke, renal failure, left ventricular hypertrophy, heart failure, and coronary atherosclerosis with heart failure.

(The reader is referred to Chapter 49 in *The Heart,* 6th ed, for further discussion on the pathophysiology of hypertension.)

DIAGNOSTIC EVALUATION
BASIC DIAGNOSTIC EVALUATION

MILD OR MODERATE HYPERTENSION. The diagnostic approach to the patient with mild or moderate hypertension is outlined in Tables 12.1 and 12.2. Clues to a secondary cause for hypertension, such as renovascular disease, renal parenchymal disease, primary aldosteronism, pheochromocytoma, coarctation of the aorta, acromegaly, hyper-

Table 12.1 Key Items in the History of Patients with Mild or Moderate Hypertension

SYMPTOMS	DIET AND DRUG HISTORY	PAST DISEASE HISTORY	FAMILY HISTORY
Blurred vision	Alcohol	Angina	Coronary heart disease
Bronchospasm	Analgesics	Asthma	Diabetes
Chest pain	Blood pressure	Diabetes	Hereditary nephritis
Claudication	medications	Glomerulonephritis	Hyperlipemia
Depression	Cigarettes	Gout	Hyperparathyroidism
Dizziness	Cold remedies	Hepatitis	Hypertension
Dyspnea	Chewing tobacco	Hypertension	Pheochromocytoma
Fatigue	Licorice	Lupus erythematosus	Polycystic kidney disease
Flushing	Nasal sprays	Myocardial infarction	Renal hypoplasia
Headaches	Nonsteroidal anti-	Peptic ulcer	Thyroid disorders
Hematuria	inflammatory agents	Pyelonephritis	
Impotence	Oral contraceptives	Toxemia	
Joint pains	Potassium (dietary)	Transient ischemic	
Muscle cramps	Salt (dietary or tablets)	attacks	
Nocturia	Tricyclic antidepressants		
Palpitations			
Polyuria			
Skin rash			
Sweating			
Tingling/cold extremities			
Unsteadiness			
Weakness			
Weight loss or gain			

(Table 50-1, *The Heart,* 6th ed, p 1050)

thyroidism, hypothyroidism, and Cushing's disease, may be identified. Target organ damage may be discovered.

SEVERE, ACCELERATED, OR MALIGNANT HYPERTENSION Malignant hypertension is said to be present when the diastolic pressure is 125 mmHg or greater, and there is evidence of target organ damage and altered physiology. Target organ damage is characterized by retinal hemorrhages and exudates, papilledema, heart failure, encephalopathy, and renal failure. Physiologic abnormalities include diminished renal arteriolar perfusion with endarteritis, elevated plasma renin and aldosterone levels, increased sympathetic tone, and failure of physiologic negative feedback mechanisms.

The total examination of the patient should include the items listed in Tables 12.1 and 12.2. Diagnostic studies may also include clinical or laboratory procedures to identify renal arterial stenosis, which is much more common in whites with malignant hypertension than it is in blacks. Pheochromocytoma can usually be detected by testing the urine for catecholamines or their metabolites.

LABILE HYPERTENSION. The total examination is the same as for patients with nonlabile hypertension (Tables 12.1, 12.2).

ISOLATED SYSTOLIC HYPERTENSION. The patient should be examined for aortic regurgitation, arteriovenous fistula, coarctation of the aorta, and Paget's disease. The cause of systolic hypertension in most elderly patients is large-vessel arteriosclerosis; these patients also

Table 12.2 Key Items in the Physical and Laboratory Examinations of Patients with Mild or Moderate Hypertension

PHYSICAL EXAMINATION

GENERAL	HEENT	CHEST	ABDOMEN	EXTREMITIES	NEUROLOGIC
Appearance Blood pressure (supine or sitting; standing; both arms; one leg) Heart rate (supine or sitting; standing)	Carotid bruit Fundi Neck veins Ocular bruits Temporal arteries	Breast Diastolic murmur Rales S_3 S_4 Systolic murmur Wheezes	Bruit Femoral pulses Palpable kidneys	Edema Peripheral pulses Peripheral bruits	Focal signs Proximal muscle strength

LABORATORY EXAMINATION

GENERAL	KIDNEY	METABOLIC	MISCELLANEOUS
Hemoglobin Hematocrit White blood cell count	Blood urea nitrogen Creatinine Urine dipstix Urine sediment	Calcium Cholesterol Glucose (fasting) HDL cholesterol Potassium Uric acid	Chest radiograph Electrocardiogram

(Table 50-2, *The Heart,* 6th ed, p 1051)

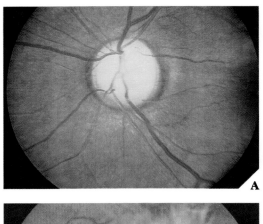

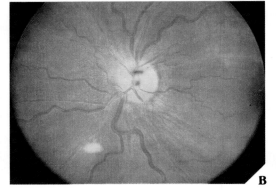

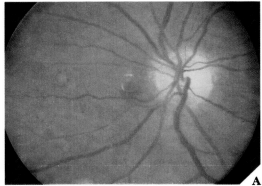

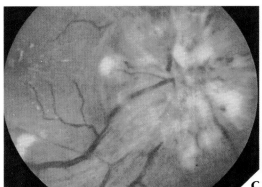

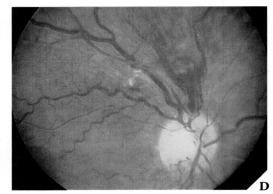

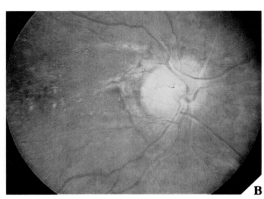

FIG. 12.1 *Retinal changes associated with systemic hypertension.* (**A**) *The retina of a 49-year-old black woman with asymptomatic essential hypertension of at least 10 years' duration displays arteriolar narrowing and straightening, increased light reflex, irregular caliber, loss of small arteriolar branches, and early arteriovenous crossing changes.* (**B**) *A 42-year-old black woman with essential hypertension and blood pressure levels averaging 260/130 was asymptomatic except for headaches. Retinal examination reveals severe vascular sclerosis, seen as marked irregularity of arteriolar caliber, "sheathing," and nearly complete loss of the arterioles. A "cotton wool" exudate is seen at seven o'clock. The nasal disk margin is blurred, which may occur normally.* (**C**) *A 38-year-old black man with malignant hypertension, bilateral papilledema, and azotemia had no visual*

disturbance. Retinal examination reveals massive edema, hemorrhages, and exudates completely obscuring the disk and burying the blood vessels. The veins are congested, and the arterioles show diffuse thickening ("copper wire"). There are hard exudates (edema residues) forming in the nerve bundle grooves in the macular region at ten o'clock. (**D**) *The retina of a 50-year-old black woman with severe hypertension of 25 years' duration shows evidence of arteriosclerosis: marked narrowing, irregular caliber, increased light reflex, and arteriovenous crossing changes. Atherosclerosis is also suggested by the large fan-shaped superficial hemorrhage, due to occlusion of a branch of the superior temporal vein as it enters the disk region.* (**A–D**: *Courtesy of Joseph A. Wilber, MD, Atlanta, Georgia. Also,* Color Plate 5, The Heart, *6th ed, between pp 318, 319*)

FIG. 12.2 *Retinal changes associated with systemic hypertension.* (**A**) *The retina of a 68-year-old white man with hypertension and mild diabetes mellitus shows very small red dots, or capillary aneurysms, scattered between the disk and the macular region. There is also a faint "cotton wool" exudate at seven o'clock.* (**B**) *A 36-year-old white woman with pseudoxanthoma elasticum presented with severe hypertension, marked visual disturbance, and renal insufficiency. Retinal examination reveals characteristic brownish angioid streaks around the disk, extending toward the macula. Also seen are marked retinal arteriosclerotic changes, sheathing, irregular caliber, occluded vessels, and hard exudates with a "smudge" hemorrhage at seven o'clock.* (**A,B**: *Courtesy of Joseph A. Wilber, MD, Atlanta, Georgia. Also,* Plate 6B,D, The Heart, *6th ed, between pp 318, 319*)

FIG. 12.3 *Globose heart* (**A**) *is opened* (**B**) *to reveal left ventricular wall hypertrophy, an adaptive phenomenon to long-standing systemic hypertension.*

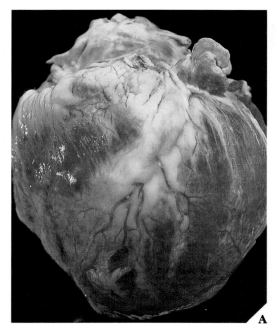

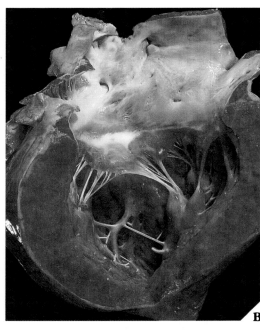

have increased risk of stroke. In years past systolic hypertension was not treated, but with the availability of better drugs today the condition is often treated, pending the results of ongoing clinical trials.

DIAGNOSIS OF TARGET ORGAN DAMAGE

HYPERTENSIVE RETINOPATHY. Figures 12.1 and 12.2 present several cases with retinal changes due to hypertension.

HYPERTENSIVE CARDIOVASCULAR DISEASE. Hypertension is one of the risk factors for the development of coronary atherosclerotic heart disease (see Chapter 6). Hypertension produces a large globoid heart due to left ventricular wall hypertrophy (Fig. 12.3); heart failure may occur. Left ventricular hypertrophy is detected on physical examination by the discovery of an apex impulse that is larger and more sustained than normal. The chest radiograph may reveal left ventricular enlargement. The electrocardiogram (ECG) (Fig. 12.4) and the echocardiogram may show left ventricular hypertrophy.

HYPERTENSIVE CEREBROVASCULAR DISEASE. *Strokes.* Micro-hemorrhages or occlusion of the small vessels in the brain may pro-

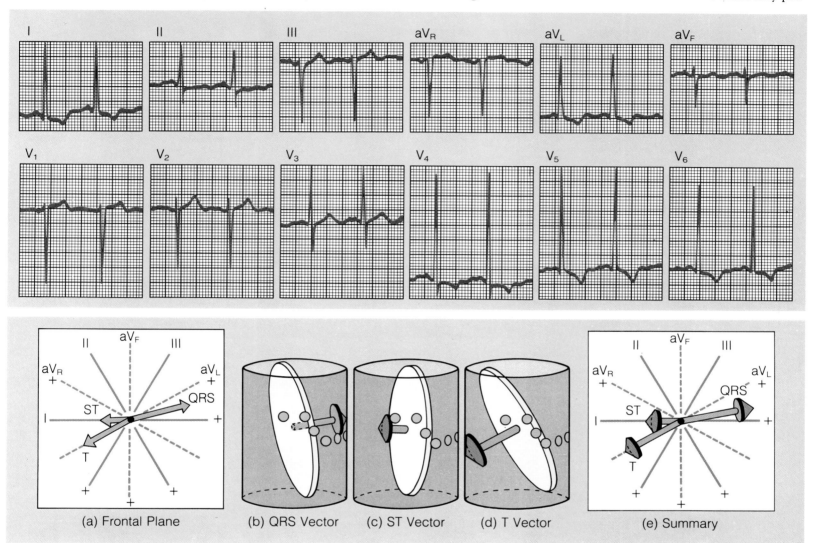

FIG. 12.4 *This ECG from a 61-year-old patient with essential hypertension illustrates left ventricular hypertrophy.* (**a**) *The QRS complex is large and positive in lead I, resultantly positive in lead II, and resultantly negative in lead aV$_F$. The mean QRS vector is therefore directed relatively parallel to the positive limb of lead I, but it must be directed slightly cephalad in order to project a slightly negative quantity on lead aV$_F$. The T wave is large and negative in lead I and flat in lead II. The mean T vector is therefore directed perpendicular to lead II. The ST-segment displacement is greatest in lead I and least in lead aV$_F$. Accordingly the mean ST vector is directed parallel to the negative limb of lead I.* (**b–d**) *The spatial orientation of the mean QRS, ST, and T vectors is illustrated. The mean QRS vector is directed 20° posteriorly, because the transitional pathway passes between V$_2$ and V$_3$. The mean ST vector is directed 30° anteriorly, because the transitional pathway passes between V$_3$ and V$_4$. The mean spatial ST vector is relatively parallel to the mean spatial T vector.* (**e**) *Final summary figure shows the spatial arrangement of the vectors. The mean QRS vector is directed to the left and posteriorly, and the mean T vector is directed to the right and anteriorly. The QRS voltage is increased, and the spatial QRS-T angle is 175°. The mean ST vector is relatively parallel to the mean T vector and represents forces of repolarization. (Redrawn; reproduced with permission of the authors and publisher; see Figure Credits)*

duce lacunar infarcts (Fig. 12.5). The neurologic deficits usually clear in days to weeks, but multiple lacunar infarcts may result in pseudo-bulbar palsy and multi-infarct dementia.

Cerebral hemorrhage (Fig. 12.6) or infarction may produce major neurologic deficits. Computed tomography (CT) is useful in separating the two etiologies.

Transient ischemic attacks are usually due to emboli originating in atheromatous lesions in the carotid arteries or the aortic arch. This condition is not directly related to hypertension, but it must be differentiated from the lacunar infarcts due to hypertension. A carotid bruit may be heard. Noninvasive techniques, such as ultrasonography and Doppler recording, may reveal evidence of obstructive atherosclerotic disease of the carotid arteries.

Hypertensive encephalopathy usually occurs in patients with accelerated-malignant hypertension; it does not usually produce focal neurologic signs. The patient may complain of a severe headache and may become confused or lethargic. He or she may be nauseated, and complain of scotoma and transient amaurosis. The condition of the patient may worsen; seizures, mental obtundation, and blindness can develop. Papilledema, retinal hemorrhages, and exudates are often

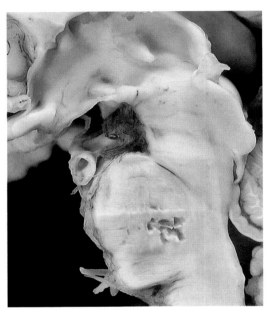

FIG. 12.5 *Median section through the pons reveals a clustering of multiple lacunar infarcts due to hypertension.*

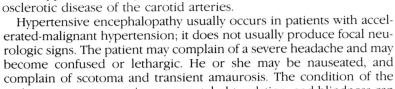

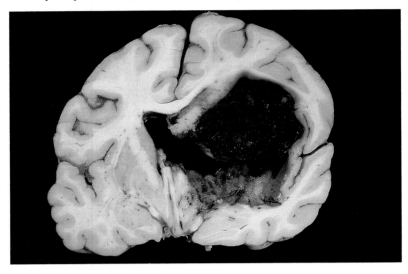

FIG. 12.6 *A massive intracerebral hemorrhage ruptured into the ventricular system.*

FIG. 12.7 *Rupture of a berry aneurysm is visible close to the site of the medial cerebral and internal carotid arteries.*

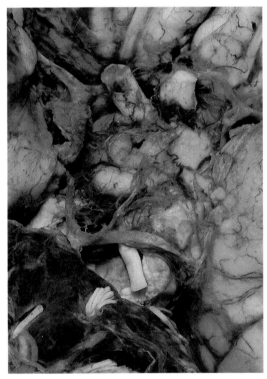

- medial cerebral artery
- optic chiasm
- internal carotid artery
- floor of third ventricle
- aneurysm
- basilar artery
- hemorrhage

seen on examination of the eyes. CT scan may be used to identify focal areas of intracerebral hemorrhage or infarction. The condition must be separated from uremic encephalopathy. Hypertensive encephalopathy is usually reversed by lowering the blood pressure.

Berry aneurysms of the cerebral arteries are more likely to rupture in patients with hypertension (Fig. 12.7).

NEPHROSCLEROSIS. When the urinalysis, blood urea nitrogen, and creatinine are normal in a patient with hypertension, it is safe to assume that the condition is not due to renal parenchymal disease.

Benign Nephrosclerosis. The diagnosis of benign nephrosclerosis can be made when a patient with long-standing hypertension exhibits proteinuria (less than 1 g/day) and granular casts, a decrease in creatinine clearance, and small kidneys (as noted on ultrasound or abdominal radiography). The pyelogram may show poor excretion of contrast material with no evidence of anatomic distortion. Other tests are usually not indicated.

Selective renal arteriography, although not usually indicated, shows "corkscrewing" of the renal arteries, with a normal ratio of parenchymal to vascular tissue. Kidney biopsy is not indicated unless there is some suggestion of collagen vascular disease or hematuria, red blood cell casts, or considerable proteinuria.

Malignant Nephrosclerosis. The characteristic pathologic change in malignant nephrosclerosis is fibrinoid necrosis of the walls of arterioles and small arteries (Fig. 12.8). Patients with malignant nephrosclerosis usually have evidence of retinopathy, encephalopathy, and congestive heart failure. Urinalysis may be negative in patients whose problem is confined to the arterioles, but it may reveal severe proteinuria, hematuria, and red blood cell or pigmented casts in the urine in patients with associated glomerulitis or interstitial bleeding. Although usually not necessary clinically, the diagnosis can be made by renal arteriography using only 10 mL of contrast medium injected into the renal artery. Aortography, which requires a larger amount of contrast material, should be avoided. The "pruning" of the vascular tree with relatively large, poorly perfused kidneys indicates malignant nephrosclerosis (Fig. 12.9). Renal biopsy carries an increased risk in these patients and should be avoided when possible. To reemphasize, aortography and renal biopsy are usually not needed.

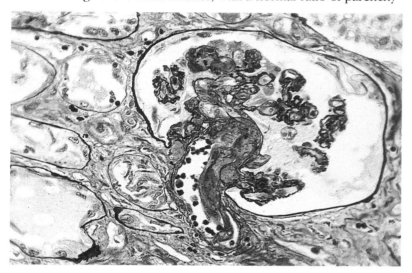

FIG. 12.8 *Fibrinoid necrosis of a glomerular afferent arteriole and the capillary tufts is evident in a patient with the malignant phase of hypertension.*

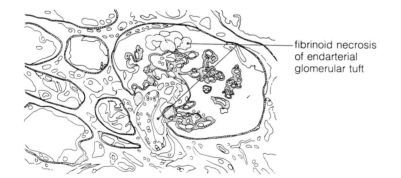

fibrinoid necrosis of endarterial glomerular tuft

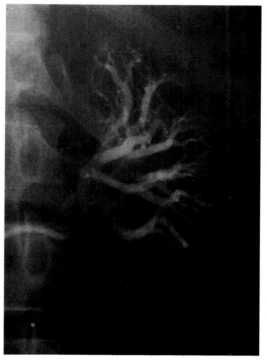

FIG. 12.9 *In this cortical nephrogram of a patient with malignant nephrosclerosis distended main branches show "pruning" of small arteries and minimal opacification despite preservation of the renal mass. (Fig. 50-3, The Heart, 6th ed, p 1057)*

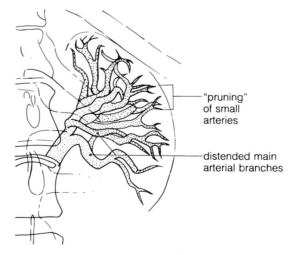

"pruning" of small arteries

distended main arterial branches

SECONDARY HYPERTENSION

The prevalence of causes of secondary hypertension in adults is shown in Table 12.3.

RENOVASCULAR HYPERTENSION

Renovascular hypertension should be considered when hypertension develops prior to age 30 or after the age of 50, when elevated blood pressure was previously controlled but becomes abruptly difficult to control, when an abdominal bruit is heard, and when advanced retinopathy is present.

Renovascular hypertension is most commonly due to atherosclerosis of the renal arteries, particularly at the site of origin from the abdominal aorta (Fig. 12.10). In younger patients fibromuscular dysplasia may be the underlying cause. There are various forms of renovascular hypertension; all share an abnormal structure of the arterial wall, most frequently characterized by thickened fibromuscular ridges alternating with aneurysmal-like pouches (Fig. 12.11).

Renal arterial stenosis can be detected by a number of noninvasive tests. Selective renal arteriography, when performed safely, provides the most reliable information (Fig. 12.12). When renal arterial stenosis is identified, it is then necessary to determine if the stenosis is the cause of the hypertension. This is accomplished by determining the renal vein renin ratio (ie, the ratio of plasma renin activity in blood samples obtained from the venous effluent of each kidney) after the administration of 40 mg of oral furosemide two or three times daily for 24–48 hours in conjunction with a low-sodium diet. A renal vein renin ratio of 1.5 or greater suggests that the stenotic side is responsible for the hypertension. A single dose of captopril may be useful prior to the determination of the level of renal vein renin in patients who would be at risk by discontinuing their antihypertensive therapy

Table 12.3 Secondary Hypertension in Adults: Results of Five Major Studies

REFERENCE	GIFFORD (1969)	KENNEDY (1965)	FERGUSON (1975)	BECH (1975)	BERGLUND (1976)
PATIENT POPULATION NUMBER (%)	PARTLY REFERRED 4939	PARTLY REFERRED 750	PARTLY REFERRED 246	PARTLY REFERRED 482	RANDOMLY SELECTED* 689
Essential hypertension	89	73	89	79	94
Chronic renal disease	5	17	2	13	4
Renovascular disease	4	6	3	5	0.6
Primary aldosteronism	0.4	0.3	0.4	0.4	0.1
Coarctation	0.6	—	—	0	0.1
Cushing's syndrome	0.2	—	—	—	—
Pheochromocytoma	0.2	0.1	—	0.2	—
Miscellaneous†	—	4	4	3	1

(Table 50-4, *The Heart*, 6th ed, p 1057)
*Randomly selected men between the ages of 47 and 54 years with blood pressure > 175/115.
†Includes oral contraceptive hypertension as well as patients not thoroughly investigated for secondary causes.

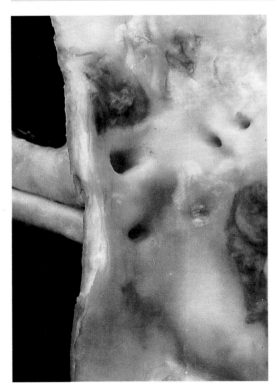

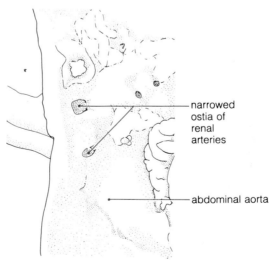

FIG. 12.10 *Abdominal atherosclerosis leads to narrowing of the orifices of the renal arteries; in this case there are two separate arteries for the right kidney. This condition may underlie renovascular hypertension.*

prior to the procedure. However, acute worsening of renal function may be precipitated with this method in patients with severe bilateral renal arterial stenosis or with renal arterial stenosis in a solitary or transplanted kidney.

PARENCHYMAL RENAL DISEASE

In contrast to patients with essential hypertension, urinalysis is usually abnormal in patients with parenchymal renal disease.

ACUTE PARENCHYMAL RENAL DISEASE

Acute diffuse glomerulonephritis may be diagnosed when there is hematuria, red blood cell or hematin-pigmented casts, proteinuria, edema, and elevation of the blood urea nitrogen (BUN)-to-creatinine ratio to 15:1 or greater. The plasma renin level is usually normal or slightly low. An abdominal radiograph or ultrasound usually reveals normal-sized or enlarged kidneys. The retrograde pyelogram shows large kidneys; intracapsular swelling produces compression of the collecting system. Other positive test results include bacteriologic and serologic signs of streptococcal infection, antinuclear antibodies, and depressed serum complement. If considerable proteinuria is present, 24-hour urine protein and creatinine clearance should be determined in order to diagnose a nephrotic type of protein wastage.

A renal biopsy is indicated in patients with acute glomerulonephritis when the nephrotic syndrome is diagnosed, or when renal function remains severely impaired after two weeks of antibiotic, antihypertensive, and diuretic treatment. The immunologic and ultrastructural classification of the condition can be used to determine prognosis and treatment.

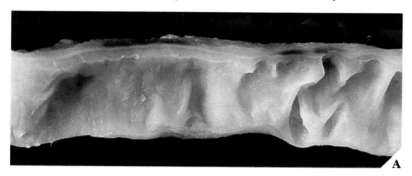

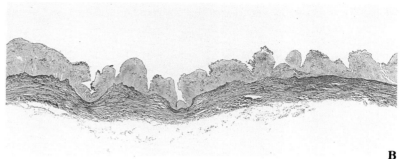

FIG. 12.11 (A) *Fibromuscular dysplasia of the renal artery, as seen in this specimen, is characterized by transverse, thickened, muscular ridges and localized saccular pouches with a thin wall.* (B) *Longitudinal section* through such an artery shows the distinct structural abnormality of the media. Fibromuscular dysplasia may be a cause of renovascular hypertension, particularly in young adults.

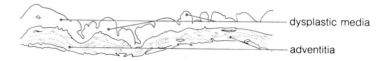

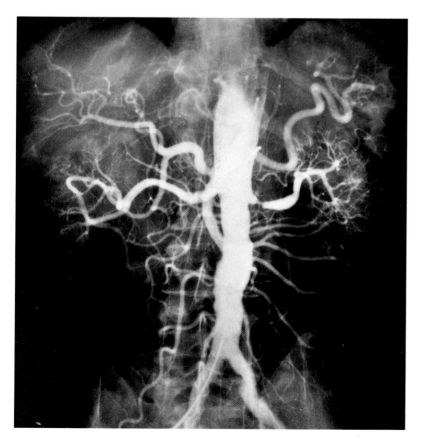

FIG. 12.12 *Renal arteriogram in a 68-year-old male with hypertension shows a small kidney on the left and extreme narrowing of the renal artery due to atherosclerosis. (Courtesy of Louis G. Martin, MD, Atlanta, Georgia)*

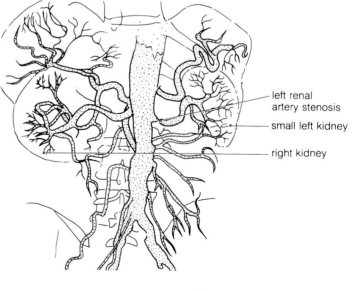

The hypertension of acute glomerulonephritis is usually managed successfully with diuretics and antisympathetic drugs.

CHRONIC PARENCHYMAL RENAL DISEASE

The loss of nephrons due to chronic renal disease of several types produces hypertension. The creatinine and urea clearances are reduced, and the BUN-to-creatinine ratio is normal (10:1). Examination of the urine reveals red blood cells and granular casts in the setting of glomerulonephritis, and white blood cells, white blood cell casts, and bacteria when there is pyelonephritis. Pyuria may also be present in patients who have analgesic renal disease. Moderate proteinuria (0.5–2 g/day) is found in patients with chronic parenchymal renal disease.

Abdominal ultrasonography reveals smaller than normal kidneys. The kidneys are smooth and of equal size in chronic glomerulonephritis, pyelonephritis lenta, or intercapillary nephrosclerosis due to diabetes; however, they may be irregular in patients with focal pyelonephritis.

Renal arteriograms reveal small kidneys and a profuse number of arterioles that reach almost to the capsule, since there is little cortical tissue (Fig. 12.13).

The renal disease of diabetes may be due to intercapillary glomerulosclerosis, large- or medium-vessel atherosclerosis, or interstitial fibrosis (Fig. 12.14). Renal artery obstruction due to atherosclerosis must always be considered.

Patients with end-stage renal disease are often treated with hemodialysis. The hypertension is usually volume-dependent, but it may be renin-dependent.

PRIMARY ALDOSTERONISM

This rare cause of hypertension should not be overlooked; most cases are identified in patients who are 30–50 years of age. The hypertension is usually not severe; there may be no other clinical clues to separate this condition from essential hypertension. Hypokalemia with its associated muscle weakness, nocturia, polyuria, polydipsia, intermittent paralysis, rhabdomyolysis, hypomagnesemia, and paresthesias may occur. The hypokalemia may be induced by diuretics, or it may occur in the untreated patient. When the serum potassium is less than 2.8–3.0 mEq/L in a hypertensive patient who is receiving a thiazide-type or loop diuretic, it is proper to consider primary aldosteronism or some other variety of mineralocorticoid hypertension (Table 12.4). Diuretics alone do not commonly produce such a severe reduction of serum potassium. A normal serum potassium, moreover, does not exclude primary aldosteronism.

Primary aldosteronism is diagnosed by demonstrating excess autonomous production of aldosterone, usually in conjunction with low plasma renin activity (see Table 12.4). (Methods used to diagnose and to distinguish between an adrenal adenoma and bilateral hyperplasia of the adrenal glands are discussed in Chapter 50, *The Heart*, 6th ed, pp 1063–1064.)

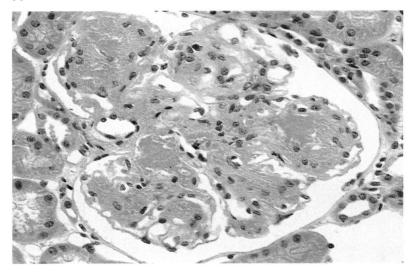

FIG. 12.14 *A histologic section of a glomerulus shows nodular sclerotic changes of the glomerular tufts characteristic of diabetic glomerulopathy (classic Kimmelstiel-Wilson syndrome).*

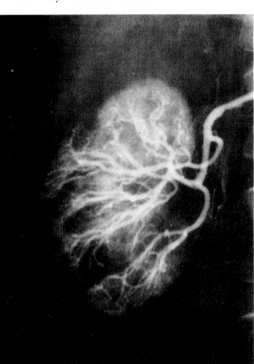

FIG. 12.13 *Renal arteriogram demonstrates disproportionately profuse small-caliber vasculature extending to the capsule of the small kidney with an atrophic cortex in chronic parenchymatous nephritis due to various causes. (Fig. 50-4,* The Heart, *6th ed, p 1061)*

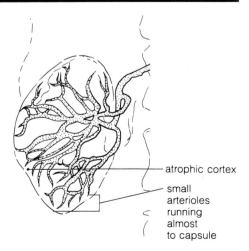

atrophic cortex

small arterioles running almost to capsule

Table 12.4 Mineralocorticoid Hypertension*

DIAGNOSIS	AGE OF ONSET	CLINICAL FEATURES	LABORATORY ABNORMALITIES
PRIMARY ALDOSTERONISM			
Aldosteronoma	More common between 30 and 50, but can occur at any age	Usually asymptomatic; may present with muscle weakness or periodic paralysis. More common in females.	↑ Plasma and urinary aldosterone; ↓ PRA; normal urinary 17-OHCS and 17-KS
Hyperplasia	As above, but tend to be 5 to 10 years older	As above, except male-to-female ratio is approximately 1:1.	As above
Glucocorticoid-suppressible primary aldosteronism	Usually childhood or adolescence	Often familial; clinical and laboratory abnormalities are reversed with dexamethasone.	As above
Indeterminate hyperaldosteronism		Usually associated with mild hypertension; serum potassium frequently normal.	As above; ↑ plasma and urinary aldosterone reported to be suppressed by DOC administration (Biglieri et al, 1972)
CUSHING'S SYNDROME			
	Any age	Cushingoid appearance with or without excessive pigmentation	↑ Plasma cortisol; ↑ urinary 17-OHCS, usually not suppressed by low-dose dexamethasone
CONGENITAL ADRENAL HYPERPLASIA			
11-β-hydroxylase deficiency	Usually childhood; occasionally adolescence or early adulthood	Virilization with or without pseudohermaphroditism in females. Precocious puberty in males. Hypokalemia is occasionally observed.	↑ Plasma DOC and 11-deoxycortisol, ↑ urinary 17-OHCS and 17-KS (usually suppressed by dexamethasone), ↓ plasma and urinary aldosterone and cortisol, ↓ PRA
17-α-hydroxylase deficiency	Adolescence	Primary amerorrhea and absence of secondary sex characteristics in females. Pseudohermaphroditism in males.	↑ Plasma DOC and corticosterone, ↓ urinary 17-OHCS and 17-KS, ↓ plasma and urinary aldosterone and cortisol, ↓ PRA
EXOGENOUS MINERALOCORTICOIDS			
Licorice,† carbenoxolone,‡ fluorocortisone, or 9α-fluoroprednisolone	Any age	Excessive licorice ingestion, antacid therapy with carbenoxolone (in use in Great Britain and Canada) or the use of nasal sprays containing 9α-fluoroprednisolone (in use in Europe, Africa, and Central and South America) (Mantero et al, 1981) Fluid retention may occur with all compounds.	↓ Plasma and urinary aldosterone, ↓ PRA

(Table 50-6, *The Heart,* 6th ed, p 1063)
17-OHCS, 17-hydroxycorticosteroids; 17-KS, 17-ketosteroids; DOC, 11-deoxycorticosterone; PRA, plasma renin activity.
*All can cause hypertension, hypokalemia, and inappropriate kaliuresis.
†Active ingredient is glycyrrhizinic acid.
‡A derivative of glycyrrhizinic acid.

PHEOCHROMOCYTOMA

Pheochromocytoma (Fig. 12.15) should be suspected whenever a patient has initial-onset hypertension and complains of severe headache, sweating, and palpitations. It is also a possible diagnosis when chronic hypertension becomes difficult to control, when the hypertensive patient has sinus tachycardia or orthostatic hypotension, when the patient has a severe hypertensive response to anesthesia and surgery (especially cholecystectomy), when there is a pressor response to beta-blocking drugs, when the family history is positive for pheochromocytoma or hypertension with either thyroid carcinoma or hyperparathyroidism, and when there is evidence of neurofibromatosis, café-au-lait spots, von Hipple–Lindau disease, Sturge–Weber disease, or tuberous sclerosis.

Patients with any of the above clues should have special tests performed to determine the urinary excretion of total catecholamines, vanillylmandelic acid, and metanephrine (Table 12.5). The excretion of metanephrine is the best indication of pheochromocytoma, but false-positive tests may occur in patients with increased intracranial pressure as well as leaking intracranial aneurysms. False-negative tests may occur within 24 hours of the use of contrast medium for angiography. The clonidine suppression test is useful to separate the patient with essential hypertension and elevated plasma catecholamines from the patient with pheochromocytoma.

CT scan localizes intra-abdominal pheochromocytoma in 90% of patients. Scintigraphic imaging with [131]meta-iodobenzylguanidine may also demonstrate the tumor when CT scan is negative.

COARCTATION OF THE AORTA

The reader is referred to pages 3.37–3.45 in Chapter 3, Congenital Heart Disease, for a discussion of secondary hypertension in relation to coarctation of the aorta.

TREATMENT OF HYPERTENSION

Discussion of the treatment of hypertension is beyond the scope of this *Atlas*. The reader is referred to Chapter 51 in *The Heart,* 6th ed. In brief the treatment of essential hypertension with modern drugs has become increasingly successful over the last 20 years. The treatment of renovascular disease due to renal arterial stenosis with angioplasty and surgery has become commonplace (Fig. 12.16). The surgical removal of aldosterone tumors, pheochromocytoma, and coarctation (see Chapter 3) can be accomplished. The management of patients on hemodialysis and those who have renal transplantation has further developed during the last several years.

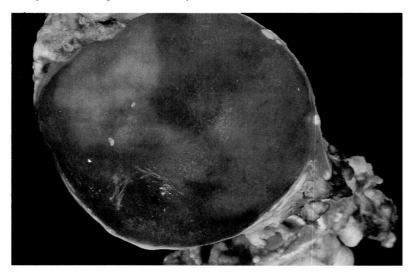

FIG. 12.15 *Cut surface of a pheochromocytoma that was surgically excised from a patient with hypertensive crises.*

Table 12.5 Frequency of Positive Urinary Tests in Patients with Pheochromocytoma

	TOTAL CATECHOLAMINES	VANILLYLMANDELIC ACID	METANEPHRINES
Mayo Clinic (Remine et al, 1974)	47/60 (79%)	37/52 (71%)	50/52 (96%)
Cleveland Clinic (DeOreo et al, 1974)	18/27 (67%)	27/33 (82%)	25/25 (100%)
NIH (Sjoerdsma et al, 1966)	60/62 (97%)	59/62 (95%)	60/62 (97%)

(Table 50-8, *The Heart,* 6th ed, p 1065)

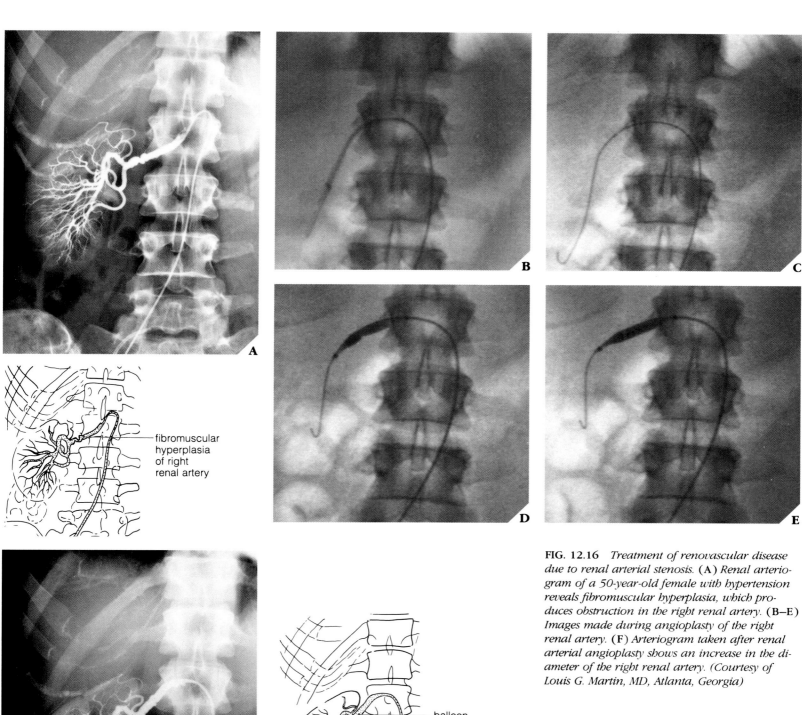

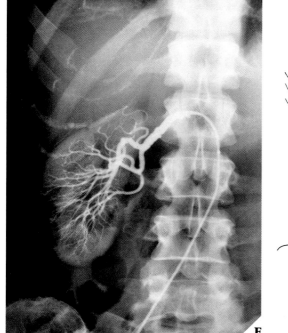

fibromuscular hyperplasia of right renal artery

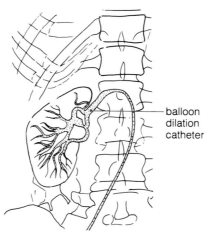

balloon dilation catheter

FIG. 12.16 *Treatment of renovascular disease due to renal arterial stenosis.* (**A**) *Renal arteriogram of a 50-year-old female with hypertension reveals fibromuscular hyperplasia, which produces obstruction in the right renal artery.* (**B–E**) *Images made during angioplasty of the right renal artery.* (**F**) *Arteriogram taken after renal arterial angioplasty shows an increase in the diameter of the right renal artery. (Courtesy of Louis G. Martin, MD, Atlanta, Georgia)*

REFERENCES

Bech K, Hilden T (1975) The frequency of secondary hypertension. *Acta Medica Scand* 197:65.

Berglund G, Andersson O, Wilhelmsen L (1976) Prevalence of primary and secondary hypertension: Studies in a random population sample. *Br Med J* 2:554.

Biglieri EG, Stockigt JR, Schambelan M (1972) Adrenal mineralocorticoids causing hypertension. *Am J Med* 52:623.

Bravo EL, Tarazi RC, Fouad FM, et al (1981) Clonidine-suppression test. A useful aid in the diagnosis of pheochromocytoma. *N Engl J Med* 305:623.

Conn JW, Cohen EL, Rovner DR, Nesbit RM (1965) Normokalemic primary aldosteronism. A detectable cause of curable "essential" hypertension. *JAMA* 193:100.

Conn JW, Knopf RF, Nesbit RM (1964) Clinical characteristics of primary aldosteronism from an analysis of 145 cases. *Am J Surg* 107:159.

DeOreo GA Jr, Stewart BH, Tarazi RC, Gifford RW Jr (1974) Preoperative blood transfusion in the safe surgical management of pheochromocytoma: A review of 46 cases. *J Urol* 111:715.

Ferguson RK (1975) Cost and yield of the hypertensive evaluation: Experience of a community-based referral clinic. *Ann Intern Med* 82:761.

Gifford RW Jr (1969) Evaluation of the hypertensive patient with emphasis on detecting curable causes. *Milbank Memorial Fund Quarterly* 47:170.

Gitlow SE, Mendlowitz M, Bertani LM (1970) The biochemical techniques for detecting and establishing the presence of a pheochromocytoma: A review of ten years' experience. *Am J Cardiol* 26:270.

Kennedy AC, Luke RG, Briggs JD, Stirling WB (1965) Detection of renovascular hypertension. *Lancet* 2:963.

Mantero F, Armanini D, Opocher G, et al (1981) Mineralocorticoid hypertension due to a nasal spray containing 9-fluoroprednisolone. *Am J Med* 71:352.

Miller R, Stark DCC, Gitlow SE (1976) Paroxysmal hyperadrenergic state. A case during surgery for intracranial aneurysm. *Anesthesiology* 31:743.

Page IH (1960) The mosaic theory of hypertension, in Bock KD, Cottier PT (eds): *Essential Hypertension*. New York, Springer–Verlag, p 1.

Remine WH, Chong GC, van Heerden JA, Sheps SG, Harrison EG Jr (1974) Current management of pheochromocytoma. *Ann Surg* 179:740.

Report of the Third Joint National Committee on the Detection, Evaluation and Treatment of High Blood Pressure 1984 *Arch Intern Med* 144, May 1984.

Sheps S, van Heerden J, Sheedy P II (1981) Current approach to the diagnosis of pheochromocytoma, in Blaufox MD, Bianchi C (eds): *Secondary Forms of Hypertension. Current Diagnosis and Management.* New York, Grune & Stratton, p 11.

Sisson JC, Frager MS, Valk TW, et al (1981) Scintigraphic localization of pheochromocytoma. *N Engl J Med* 305:12.

Sjoerdsma A, Engelman K, Waldmann TA, Cooperman LH, Hammond WG (1966) Pheochromocytoma: Current concepts of diagnosis and treatment. *Ann Intern Med* 65:1302.

Stewart BH, Bravo EL, Haaga J, et al (1978) Localization of pheochromocytoma by computed tomography. *N Engl J Med* 299:460.

FIGURE CREDITS

FIG. 12.4 Redrawn from Hurst JW, Woodson GC: *Atlas of Spatial Vector Electrocardiography.* New York, The Blakiston Company, 1952, pp 92, 93.

13
NEOPLASTIC DISEASE OF THE HEART

J. Willis Hurst, MD
Robert J. Hall, MD
Anton E. Becker, MD
Benson R. Wilcox, MD

Abstracted with permission of the authors and publisher from Hall RJ, Cooley DA: Neoplastic heart disease, Chapter 61, pp 1284–1305, in Hurst JW (ed): *The Heart,* 6th ed. New York, McGraw-Hill, 1986. Figures and tables reproduced in this chapter from the above chapter or other sources are also reproduced with permission of the authors and publishers. For the full bibliographic citations of the sources of figures other than the above chapter, see Figure Credits at the end of this chapter.

The heart may be the site of primary neoplastic disease, secondary involvement by neoplastic processes adjacent to the heart, or metastasis from distant locations. The clinical manifestations of neoplastic heart disease include pericarditis, myocardial disease, heart failure, obstructive disease simulating valve disease, cardiac arrhythmias, peripheral emboli, and fever (Table 13.1). Therefore neoplasms must always be included in the consideration of the etiology of these clinical syndromes.

Primary tumors of the heart, benign or malignant, are found in 0.001%–0.28% of all autopsies. The type and frequency of primary tumors and cysts of the heart as reported by McAllister and Fenoglio (1978) are shown in Table 13.2. Some of the more common primary neoplasms are discussed below.

BENIGN PRIMARY TUMORS
CARDIAC MYXOMAS

Myxomas comprise 50% of the benign primary tumors of the heart. Seventy-five percent of these are located in the left atrium, 18% in the right atrium, 4% in the right ventricle, and 4% in the left ventricle.

Cardiac myxoma usually presents as a pedunculated mass. Large-sized left atrial myxomas may obstruct the mitral orifice (Fig. 13.1) or the pulmonary venous orifices. Histologically they are composed of polygonal myxoma cells embedded within a mucoid ground substance (Fig. 13.2).

CLINICAL MANIFESTATIONS

Patients with cardiac myxomas may be asymptomatic. When symptoms occur, they are systemic, embolic, or obstructive.

SYSTEMIC MANIFESTATIONS. Most patients with cardiac myxomas have systemic symptoms, including fever, weight loss, fatigue, anemia (including hemolytic), elevated sedimentation rate, elevated immunoglobulin levels, leukocytosis, thrombocytopenia, clubbing, Raynaud's phenomenon, breast fibroadenomas, and erythrocytosis. When certain of these symptoms occur simultaneously, the physician may mistakenly diagnose a collagen vascular disease. The neoplasm itself may produce fever, emboli, and cardiac murmurs, mimicking endo-

---

Table 13.1 General Manifestations of Neoplastic Heart Disease

Pericardial Involvement
  Pericarditis, pain
  Pericardial effusion
  Radiographic evidence of enlargement
  Arrhythmia, predominantly atrial
  Tamponade
  Constriction
Myocardial Involvement
  Arrhythmias, ventricular and atrial
  Electrocardiographic changes
  Radiographic evidence of enlargement
    Generalized
    Localized
  Conduction disturbances and heart block
  Congestive heart failure
  Coronary involvement
    Angina, infarction
Intracavitary Tumor
  Cavity obliteration
  Valve obstruction and valve damage
  Embolic phenomena: systemic, neurologic, coronary
  Constitutional manifestations

(Table 61-1, *The Heart,* 6th ed, p 1285)

Table 13.2 Tumors and Cysts of the Heart and Pericardium

TYPE	NUMBER	PERCENT
Benign		
Myxoma	130	24.4
Lipoma	45	8.4
Papillary fibroelastoma	42	7.9
Rhabdomyoma	36	6.8
Fibroma	17	3.2
Hemangioma	15	2.8
Teratoma	14	2.6
Mesothelioma of atrioventricular node	12	2.3
Granular cell tumor	3	
Neurofibroma	3	
Lymphangioma	2	
Subtotal	319	59.8
Pericardial cyst	82	15.4
Bronchogenic cyst	7	1.3
Subtotal	89	16.7
Malignant		
Angiosarcoma	39	7.3
Rhabdomyosarcoma	26	4.9
Mesothelioma	19	3.6
Fibrosarcoma	14	2.6
Malignant lymphoma	7	1.3
Extraskeletal osteosarcoma	5	
Neurogenic sarcoma	4	
Malignant teratoma	4	
Thymoma	4	
Leiomyosarcoma	1	
Liposarcoma	1	
Synovial sarcoma	1	
Subtotal	125	23.5
Total	533	100.0

(Reproduced; see Figure Credits. Also, Table 61-2, *The Heart,* 6th ed, p 1285)

carditis. The tumor may become infected with a variety of organisms, resulting in positive blood cultures; this clinical picture simulates endocarditis even more closely.

EMBOLIC MANIFESTATIONS. Systemic emboli are common when the myxoma is located in the left atrium. A myxoma may be initially suspected when a skin biopsy of a necrotic area or a systemic embolus removed at surgery is examined microscopically. Emboli may lodge in the skin, brain, retinae, coronary arteries, kidneys, extremities, or the aortic bifurcation.

OBSTRUCTIVE SYMPTOMS AND SIGNS. *Left Atrial Myxomas.* These neoplasms may obstruct the mitral valve orifice or the pul-

monary veins, producing pulmonary venous hypertension, secondary pulmonary arterial hypertension, pulmonary congestion, dyspnea on effort, pulmonary edema, cough, hemoptysis, fatigue, syncope, or sudden death. The symptoms may occasionally be provoked or relieved by changing the body position; for example, assuming the recumbent position may relieve the symptoms in some patients.

The physical examination is suggestive of mitral stenosis. The first heart sound may be loud, a diastolic rumble is heard at the apex, and a systolic murmur may be detected. A tumor "plop" simulating the opening snap of the mitral valve may be heard, and the pulmonary valve closure sound may be loud. The tumor, which is often mobile in the left atrium, may damage the mitral valve, producing severe mitral regurgitation; this is known as the "wrecking ball" effect.

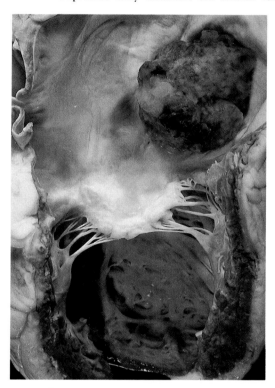

FIG. 13.1 *This large left atrial myxoma caused obstruction of the mitral orifice.*

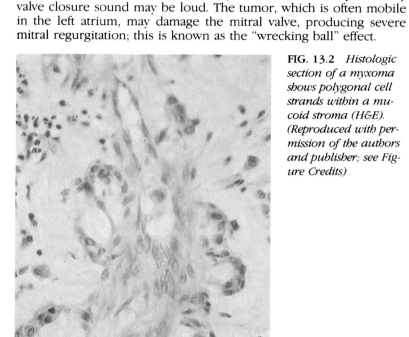

FIG. 13.2 *Histologic section of a myxoma shows polygonal cell strands within a mucoid stroma (H&E). (Reproduced with permission of the authors and publisher; see Figure Credits)*

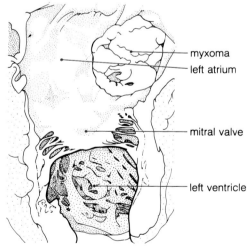

- myxoma
- left atrium

- mitral valve

- left ventricle

Abnormalities on chest radiography may suggest mitral stenosis; calcification within the tumor may be seen. The M-mode echocardiogram may simulate the abnormalities associated with mitral stenosis (Fig. 13.3). Cross-sectional echocardiography enhances visualization of the tumor (Fig. 13.4) and usually precludes the need for cardiac catheterization and angiography (see Fig. 4.60). Computed tomography (CT) and magnetic resonance imaging (MRI) may also reveal the tumor.

Cardiac catheterization reveals pulmonary hypertension, a notch on the ascending limb of the left ventricular pressure curve, a rapid y descent in the left atrial or the wedge pressure curve, and a large V wave in the wedge pressure curve. The angiogram reveals the myxoma (see Fig. 4.60). Coronary arteriography may reveal a tumor blush from small arteries that supply the myxoma. However, because echocardiography is so reliable in identifying myxomas, a coronary arteriogram is usually performed before surgery for myxoma only to identify coronary atherosclerosis.

Left atrial myxomas simulate mitral valve disease, endocarditis, and collagen vascular disease. The incidence is about 1% in patients requiring mitral valve surgery.

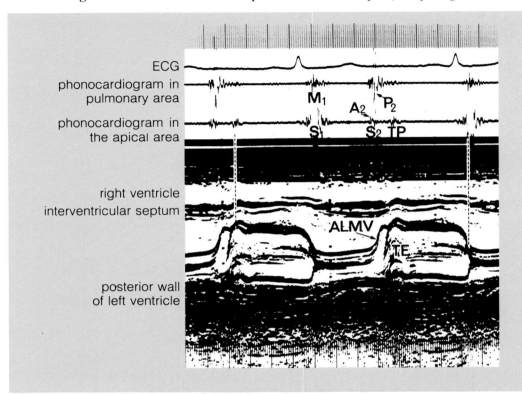

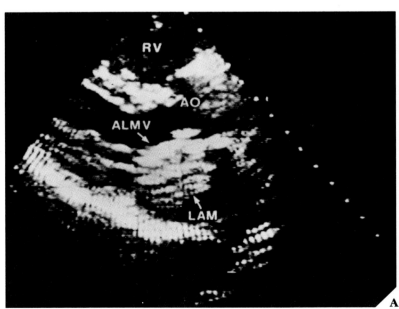

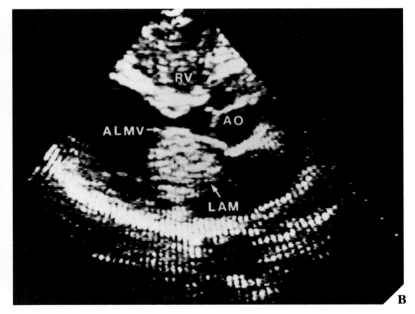

FIG. 13.3 *Recordings from a patient with a cystic left atrial myxoma include an ECG, phonocardiograms from the pulmonary and apical areas at medium frequency, and an M-mode echocardiogram at the level of the mitral valve. Time lines indicate 0.01-s intervals. The right ventricle, the interventricular septum, and the posterior wall of the left ventricle are identified. The loud component of the first sound (M$_1$) is delayed (Q–M$_1$ = 0.09 s). The pulmonary second sound (P$_2$) is accentuated. Multiple linear tumor echoes (TE) are seen behind the anterior leaflet of the mitral valve (ALMV), first appearing at the mitral level 0.04 s after the onset of mitral opening. The forward movement is completed 0.09 s after the onset of mitral opening, at which point the tumor plop (TP) is recorded. The A$_2$–TP interval measures 0.10 s. (Fig. 61-2, The Heart, 6th ed, p 1287)*

FIG. 13.4 *Cross-sectional echocardiograms in the long-axis parasternal view were recorded during systole (**A**) and diastole (**B**) in a 56-year-old woman. A large left atrial myxoma (LAM) is seen in the left atrium behind the anterior leaflet of the mitral valve (ALMV). The myxoma prolapses and fills the mitral orifice during diastole. This tumor was attached to the posterior leaflet of the mitral valve and the adjacent posterior wall of the left atrium (RV, right ventricle; Ao, aorta). (Fig. 61-3, The Heart, 6th ed, p 1289)*

Right Atrial Myxomas. Systemic symptoms are less common than in patients with left atrial myxoma. Polycythemia and cyanosis may occur because of a right-to-left shunt through the oval foramen. Erythrocytosis may also be the result of erythropoietin produced by the myxoma.

The patient may exhibit a large **a** wave in the deep jugular venous pulse, ascites, edema, enlarged liver, cyanosis, syncope, and episodes of dyspnea. The "wrecking ball" action of the mobile tumor may damage the tricuspid valve, producing tricuspid regurgitation. Pulmonary emboli may occur, and myxomatous material may infiltrate the pulmonary arteries, producing aneurysms. Paradoxical embolism may occur.

A loud sound may be heard in systole after the first sound, and it may be preceded by a murmur. These auscultatory abnormalities are due to the rapid movement of the tumor from the right ventricle into the right atrium. There is a diastolic rumble heard best at the lower sternal border and a loud systolic murmur due to tricuspid regurgitation caused by a damaged tricuspid valve. A tumor plop is sometimes heard. These sounds may be altered by the position of the patient.

The electrocardiogram (ECG) may be normal, or it may reveal a right atrial abnormality, a right axis deviation of the mean QRS vector, and right bundle branch block. The chest radiograph may show right atrial enlargement, right ventricular enlargement, and calcification of the tumor (Fig. 13.5). M-mode echocardiography reveals the presence of the tumor (Fig. 13.6).

Cardiac catheterization reveals a prominent **a** wave in the right atrium and a pressure gradient across the tricuspid valve. There may be a conspicuous notch on the upstroke of the right ventricular pressure curve. A rapid **y** descent can be seen. The right atrial myxoma can be visualized with angiography.

This condition must be differentiated from rheumatic tricuspid stenosis, Ebstein's anomaly, pulmonary emboli, and carcinoid syndrome.

Left Ventricular Myxomas. These neoplasms are rare (Wilcox and Carter, 1971); they occur more commonly in young women than young men. Emboli occur frequently, and systemic symptoms are rare. Syncope is common. The symptoms and the physical abnormalities are suggestive of aortic valve stenosis or subaortic obstruction. The echocardiogram shows the tumor moving during systole into the open aortic valve area. A pedunculated left ventricular thrombus may simulate a left ventricular myxoma, but usually the thrombus is located in the left ventricular apex. Angiography is usually diagnostic.

Right Ventricular Myxomas. These neoplasms produce right-sided heart failure, syncope, fever, and a murmur suggesting pulmonary valve stenosis. Pulmonary emboli may occur. A tumor plop may be heard in diastole, an ejection sound may be detected, and the pul-

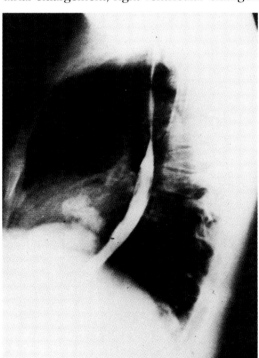

FIG. 13.5 *Lateral chest radiograph reveals the dense calcification of a right atrial myxoma. (Fig. 61-5, The Heart, 6th ed, p 1291)*

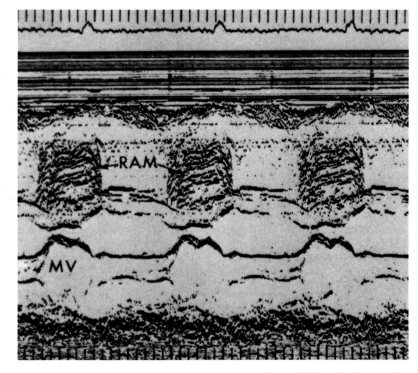

FIG. 13.6 *This M-mode echocardiogram was obtained through the ventricular chambers; it demonstrates a mass of echoes filling the tricuspid funnel* (RAM, arrows). *At surgery this patient had a large right atrial myxoma* (MV, mitral valve). *(ECG at top of tracing is for reference.) (Reproduced with permission of the authors and publisher; see Figure Credits)*

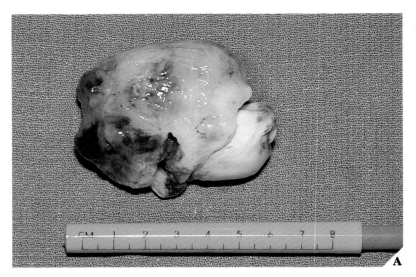

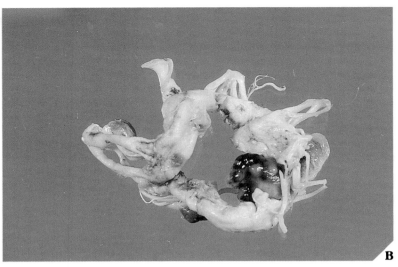

FIG. 13.7 **(A)** *This resected specimen of a left ventricular myxoma was found at surgery to arise from the posterior papillary muscle. It resulted in* *mitral stenosis and insufficiency, and necessitated a resection of the mitral valve* **(B)**.

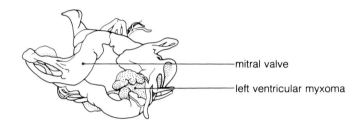

mitral valve

left ventricular myxoma

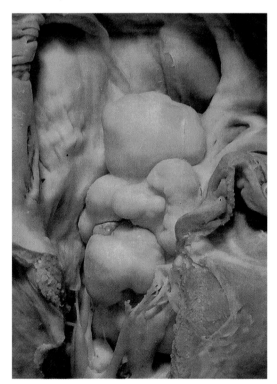

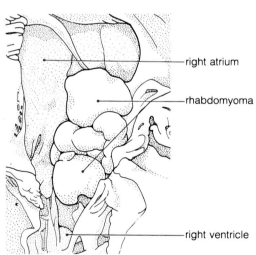

right atrium

rhabdomyoma

right ventricle

FIG. 13.8 *This specimen of rhabdomyoma of the heart demonstrates intracavitary extension through the tricuspid orifice. (Reproduced with permission of the authors and publisher; see Figure Credits)*

FIG. 13.9 *Histologic section of rhabdomyoma shows bizarrely vacuolated cells with centrally placed nuclei suspended by thin cytoplasmic strands (H&E). (Reproduced with permission of the authors and publisher; see Figure Credits)*

monary valve closure sound may be delayed. A calcified myxoma may be seen on the chest radiograph. An echocardiogram usually reveals the tumor, and angiography is diagnostic.

TREATMENT OF MYXOMAS

The treatment of myxomas of the heart is surgical removal of the tumor (Fig. 13.7).

RHABDOMYOMA

Rhabdomyomas are the most common tumors in infants and children. Their clinical significance is largely determined by their size and location within the myocardium. Intracavitary extension is particularly frequent in patients with functional impairment (Fig. 13.8). The demonstration of an intracardiac mass in a symptomatic child under five years of age is strongly suggestive of this diagnosis. Histologically the tumor is composed of grotesquely swollen myocytes with an almost empty cytoplasm traversed by strands of cellular matrix (Fig. 13.9). The tumor usually presents with obstructive symptoms, such as syncope and hypoxic spells, that result from occlusion of the pulmonary valve, the aortic valve, or the mitral valve. Cardiac arrhythmias including atrioventricular block, pericardial effusion, and sudden death are common. The tumor can be identified by echocardiographic exami-

nation, radionuclear angiography, cardiac angiography, and cardiac catheterization.

TREATMENT. The treatment of rhabdomyoma of the heart is surgical removal of the tumor.

FIBROMA

Cardiac fibromas are often circumscribed, slow-growing, and potentially aggressive lesions with a distinct tendency to occur in the ventricular septum (Fig. 13.10). Histologically the lesion is composed of interweaving bundles of collagen fibers, elastin fibers, and smooth muscle cells (Fig. 13.11). These benign cardiac tumors occur most often in infants and children. They may produce sudden death, cardiac arrhythmias, and ventricular outflow tract obstruction. These tumors are usually identified by echocardiography and angiography.

TREATMENT. The treatment of fibroma of the heart is surgical excision of the tumor. Cardiac transplantation may be possible when the tumor cannot be removed surgically.

PAPILLARY FIBROELASTOMA

These benign tumors arise from the cardiac valves or the endocardium

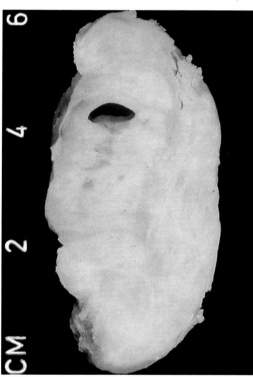

FIG. 13.10 *The cut surface of a surgically excised cardiac fibroma demonstrates the typical appearance of a fibromatous lesion. (Reproduced with permission of the authors and publisher; see Figure Credits)*

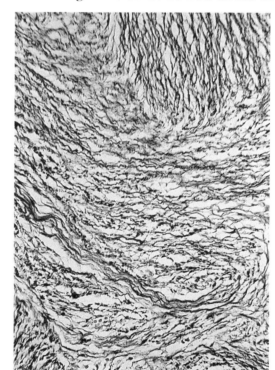

FIG. 13.11 *Histologic section of the tumor shown in Figure 13.10 shows a bundled arrangement of collagen and elastin fibers sparsely intermingled with smooth muscle cells.*

(Fig. 13.12). The villous growth may also arise from the aortic valve and obstruct the coronary ostia, producing angina pectoris and sudden death. Tumors of the tricuspid valve may obstruct the outflow tract of the right ventricle. Fibroelastomas may be recognized by echocardiographic examination and angiography.

TREATMENT. The treatment of a papillary fibroelastoma of the heart is surgical removal of the tumor.

LIPOMA

Lipomas are small or large benign tumors that may occur in the pericardium, the atrial septum, or the ventricular myocardium. They may produce no symptoms, pericardial effusion, cardiac arrhythmias, or sudden death. The tumor may be identified by echocardiography and angiography.

TREATMENT. The treatment of a lipoma of the heart or pericardium is surgical resection of the tumor.

MESOTHELIOMA OF THE ATRIOVENTRICULAR NODE

These unusual benign tumors involve the atrioventricular node, producing complete heart block and Stokes–Adams attacks. Even a small tumor in this region can produce sudden death. The tumors, which occur predominately in females, are recognized at autopsy, but they should be suspected in any child or young adult who dies suddenly.

TREATMENT. Management consists of treating complete heart block and Stokes–Adams attacks in a patient for whom the etiologic diagnosis is unknown.

HEMANGIOMAS

These rare, benign tumors may be suspected when coronary angiography reveals a tumor blush. Hemangiomas are usually discovered at autopsy (Fig. 13.13).

TREATMENT. To date there is little reported experience with the removal of these tumors.

MALIGNANT PRIMARY TUMORS
ANGIOSARCOMA

This malignant tumor is more common in males than females; it usually arises from the right atrium or the pericardium (Fig. 13.14). A continuous murmur may be heard because of the enormous vascularity of the tumor. A pericardial tumor may produce hemorrhagic pericardial effusion and cardiac tamponade. Intracavitary tumors may produce valvar obstruction and heart failure. The diagnosis may be suggested by echocardiography or angiography. Coronary arteriography may reveal abnormal vessels over the tumor area. This malignant tumor may metastasize to many areas.

TREATMENT. Surgical removal is usually impossible, and radiation therapy and chemotherapy have limited value.

RHABDOMYOSARCOMA

This malignant tumor, more commonly found in males, may involve multiple sites in the heart; valvar obstruction is present in one half of patients. Echocardiography and cardiac angiography may aid in identifying the location of the neoplasm.

TREATMENT. The prognosis is poor despite surgery, radiation therapy, and chemotherapy.

OTHER MALIGNANT NEOPLASMS

Fibrosarcoma, liposarcoma, primary malignant lymphoma, and sarcomas of other varieties comprise the remaining malignant tumors of the heart. These tumors may fill the cardiac chambers, obstructing the cardiac valves.

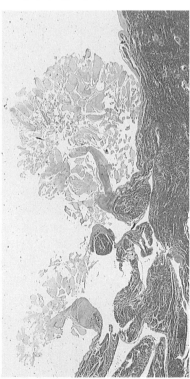

FIG. 13.12 *A fibroelastoma on this histologic section is seen to arise from the mural endocardium (H&E). (Reproduced with permission of the authors and publisher; see Figure Credits)*

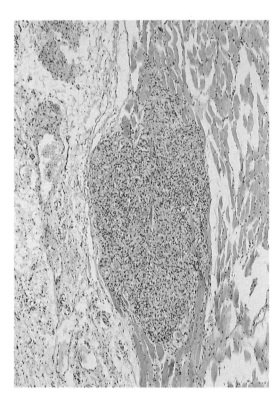

FIG. 13.13 *Histologic section reveals a capillary hemangioma of the heart (H&E).*

TREATMENT. Surgical removal of the tumors, radiation therapy, and chemotherapy may produce palliation.

TUMORS OF THE PERICARDIUM
PERICARDIAL CYST

This benign tumor, as noted on chest radiography, is usually located in the right costophrenic angle. The cyst rarely connects with the pericardial space. The tumor is usually asymptomatic, but it may produce chest pain, dyspnea, cough, or paroxysmal rapid heart action. Cross-sectional echocardiography and CT scan assist in making the diagnosis.

TREATMENT. Surgical excision is curative.

TERATOMA OF THE PERICARDIUM

This tumor, which is rarely malignant, occurs most commonly in female infants. It arises and receives its blood supply from the root of the aorta or the pulmonary artery. Most of these tumors are extracardiac and lie within the pericardial space; rarely intracardiac tumors are identified. Intrapericardial teratoma should be considered in a child who has recurrent nonhemorrhagic effusion. Cardiac function can be compromised when the tumor attains a large size. Echocardiography and computed tomography assist in the identification of tumors.

TREATMENT. Surgical removal of the neoplasm is usually curative.

MESOTHELIOMA OF THE PERICARDIUM

This malignant neoplasm involves the pericardium and myocardium (Fig. 13.15). It occurs more commonly in males than females. The patient experiences pericarditis, constrictive pericardial disease, or obstruction of the superior caval vein. The pericardial fluid is bloody, and malignant cells may be found in the fluid.

TREATMENT. Surgical intervention, radiation treatment, and chemotherapy produce only transient benefits.

INTRAPERICARDIAL PHEOCHROMOCYTOMA

Pheochromocytoma may, on rare occasion, be found within the pericardium.

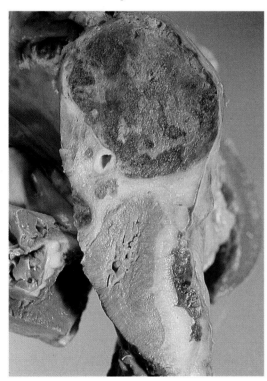

FIG. 13.14 *This angiosarcoma of the heart is localized in the atrioventricular groove.*

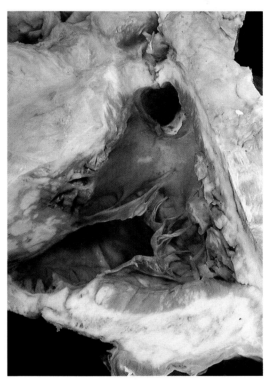

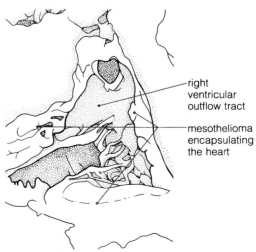

right ventricular outflow tract

mesothelioma encapsulating the heart

FIG. 13.15 *The right side of the heart is opened to reveal a primary mesothelioma of the pericardium. The tumor presents as a thick pericardial layer covering the heart, with local invasion into the myocardium.*

SECONDARY TUMORS OF THE HEART

Neoplasms originating in many organs may metastasize to the heart. The secondary tumors of the heart and the pericardium are 20–40 times as common as primary tumors of the heart. Cardiac involvement may be the result of contiguous growth from a nearby structure (Fig. 13.16), hematogenous or lymphatic spread (Fig. 13.17), or direct growth into the pulmonary veins or caval vein.

DeLoach and Haynes (1953) reported the results of 2547 consecutive autopsies performed at Walter Reed Army Hospital. They found malignant disease of the heart in 980 cases; 13.9% of these cases had metastatic disease of the heart or pericardium. Cancer of the lung involved the heart and pericardium more often than any other process

(21% of 105 cases). Lymphatic leukemia also invaded the heart and pericardium in about the same number of cases.

Metastatic involvement of the heart may be discovered at autopsy. Clinical manifestations may be related to invasion of the pericardium, myocardial involvement, coronary artery involvement, and intracavitary tumor growth.

PERICARDIAL INVOLVEMENT

The patient with metastatic disease of the pericardium may have the signs and symptoms of pericarditis, cardiac tamponade, and cardiac arrhythmias. The echocardiogram (Fig. 13.18) and CT scan (Fig. 13.19) may reveal the fluid and the mass. The pericardial fluid is usually, but

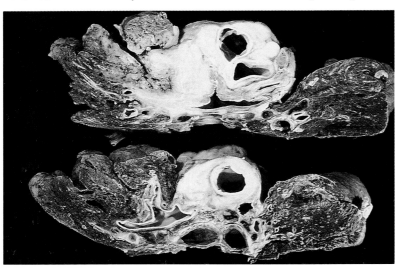

FIG. 13.16 *Cross-sections through the heart and the lungs in a patient with a central bronchial carcinoma reveals direct spread of the tumor into the heart.*

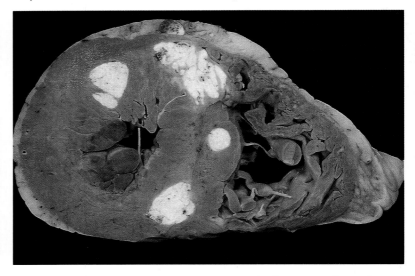

FIG. 13.17 *Hematogenous metastases appear in the myocardium of a patient with primary renal carcinoma*

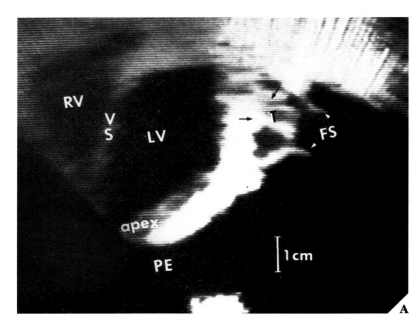

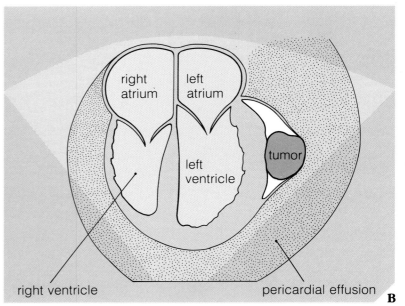

FIG. 13.18 **(A)** *A still frame, modified four-chamber view of a cross-sectional echocardiogram was obtained in a patient with a large pericardial effusion. A large tumor mass within the pericardial space is attached to the epicardium* (T, arrows) *and fibrinous strands* (FS) *extend from the tumor. This patient had had a mastectomy several years previously for adenocarci-*

noma; diagnosis was a metastatic tumor to the pericardium (RV, right ventricle; VS, ventricular septum; LV, left ventricle; PE, pericardial effusion). **(B)** *This schematic representation demonstrates the position of the tumor, as well as the view obtained on echocardiography. (Partially redrawn; reproduced with permission of the authors and publisher; see Figure Credits)* not always, bloody. Constrictive pericarditis may be the result of radiation treatment for carcinoma of the lung or the breast, or for lymphoma.

TREATMENT. Management consists of pericardial aspiration and, at times, surgical removal of the pericardium.

MYOCARDIAL INVOLVEMENT

Atrial fibrillation and flutter may occur when there is neoplastic involvement of the atria. Serious ventricular arrhythmias or heart failure may occur when the ventricles are invaded by metastatic growth. The ECG may show nonspecific ST-T wave change; on occasion it may show persistent ST-segment elevation, suggesting myocardial infarction.

TREATMENT. The treatment of the arrhythmias is usually unsatisfactory. Heart failure due to neoplastic involvement of the myocardium and chemotherapy is usually resistant to treatment.

CORONARY ARTERY INVOLVEMENT

Coronary disease manifested as angina or infarction in patients with malignant neoplasm may be due to coronary atherosclerosis unrelated to neoplasia, tumor emboli to a coronary artery, and compression or occlusion of the coronary arteries (Fig. 13.20). In addition there is evidence to support the concept that radiation of the mediastinum produces fibrosis and acceleration of atherosclerosis of the coronary arteries. Any of these conditions, as well as neoplastic invasion of the myocardium, may produce electrocardiographic signs of myocardial infarction.

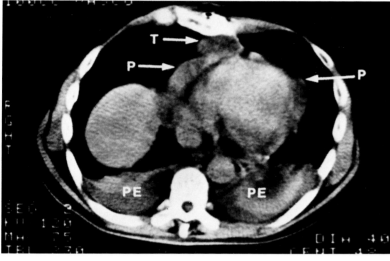

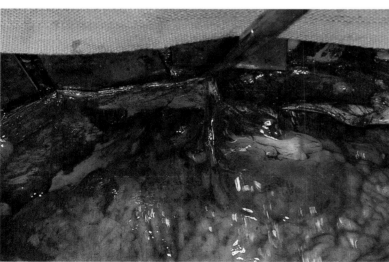

FIG. 13.19 *CT section of the chest at the cardiac level in a patient with renal cell carcinoma reveals metastases to the anterior mediastinum* (T) *and the pericardium. Extensive pericardial involvement* (P) *by the tumor and bilateral pleural effusions* (PE) *are evident. (Courtesy of F. Parker Gregg, MD, Houston, Texas. Also, Fig. 61-7,* The Heart, *6th ed, p 1297)*

FIG. 13.20 *Operative view through a median sternotomy reveals the extension of an intracavitary (right ventricle) metastatic tumor (squamous cell carcinoma) growing into the pericardium. Coronary angiography demonstrated complete obstruction of the left anterior descending coronary artery.*

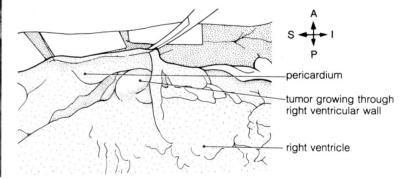

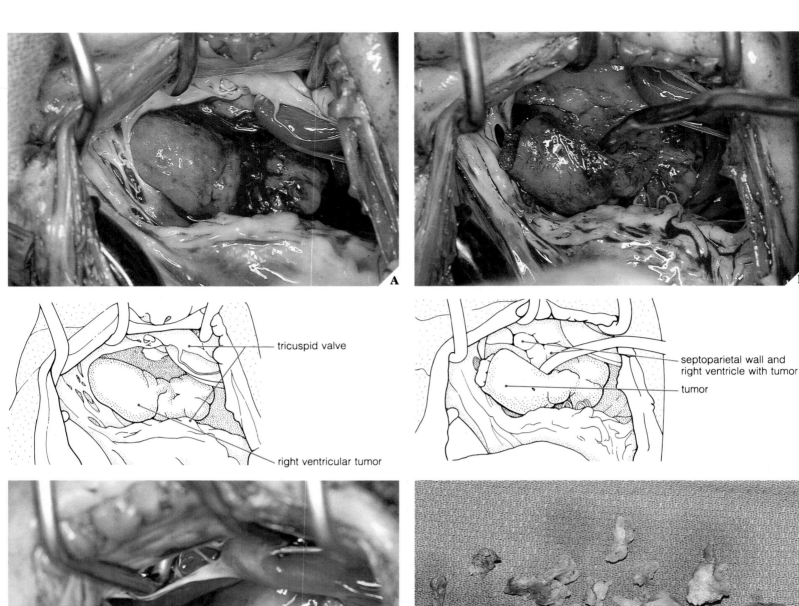

tricuspid valve

right ventricular tumor

septoparietal wall and
right ventricle with tumor

tumor

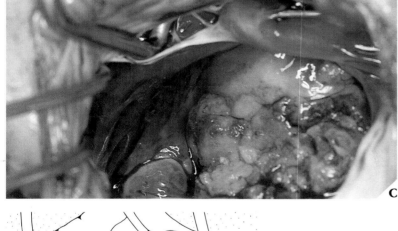

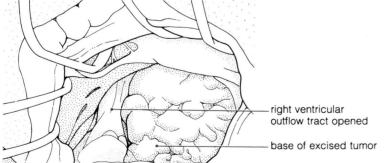

right ventricular
outflow tract opened

base of excised tumor

FIG. 13.21 *In surgical removal of a metastatic squamous cell carcinoma
of the right ventricular outflow tract in a 56-year-old man a large pedunculated metastatic tumor mass (A) is seen through the tricuspid valve.
(B) The septoparietal attachments are divided. (C) The bulk of the mass has
been removed, although tumor remains in the wall of the heart extending
into the pericardium (see Fig. 13.20). (D) Excised fragments of the tumor.
Eighteen months following incomplete removal of the tumor the patient remained symptom free with regard to his heart, although he required radiation therapy for bony metastases.*

TREATMENT.   Treatment is usually unsatisfactory and is limited to medical treatment of myocardial ischemia.

INTRACAVITARY TUMOR GROWTH

The cardiac chambers may become occluded by tumor when myocardial masses increase in size or when certain neoplasms extend into the right atrium. The latter occurs when renal cell carcinoma, hepatic carcinoma, or uterine leiomyosarcoma extend into the caval veins and the right atrial cavity. The clinical syndromes produced by intracavitary tumors simulate obstructive disease of the valves and constrictive pericarditis. Echocardiography, CT scan, and cardiac angiography assist in the diagnosis.

TREATMENT.   In situations in which the tumor causes major obstructive symptoms or threatens to embolize, excision may be beneficial (Fig. 13.21).

SPECIAL CONSIDERATIONS
LEUKEMIA

At autopsy the heart is found to be involved in about 69% of patients with leukemia. The pericardium is also involved in most of these patients.

The condition is usually not recognized prior to autopsy. Myocardial infiltration may be caused by chronic lymphatic leukemia. The mitral valve may be involved, and heart failure may occur. Rupture of the heart due to acute myeloblastic leukemia has been reported. Acute cardiac tamponade may occur in patients with chronic myelogenous leukemia due to hemorrhagic pericardial effusion. Infective endocarditis may occur in patients with acute leukemia; the invading organism is often a fungus.

TREATMENT.   Because patients with leukemia have a more favorable survival rate today than in the past, it is proper to relieve the cardiac tamponade with aspiration or surgery, to treat endocarditis, and, on rare occasion, to replace a heart valve damaged by infection.

CARCINOID HEART DISEASE

Carcinoid heart disease is produced by substances released by a distant carcinoid tumor. Serotonin is involved along with other substances, including bradykinin. (For a recent review on this subject, see Hurst et al, 1985.)

Carcinoid tumors originate in the gastrointestinal tract, including the small intestine, stomach, appendix, and rectum. The tumors also occur in the bronchus, biliary tract, pancreas, ovary, testes, and thyroid. Carcinoid tumors of the appendix rarely produce the carcinoid syndrome. A carcinoid tumor of the ileum must metastasize to the liver in order to produce the syndrome.

For the most part these tumors contain 5-hydroxytryptamine (5-HT) that is excreted in the urine as 5-hydroxyindoleacetic acid (5-HIAA). Carcinoid tumors of the bronchus, pancreas, and stomach produce different substances, differ morphologically, and metastasize more widely than carcinoid of the ileum. They also produce 5-HT and excrete 5-HIAA in the urine, but the clinical syndrome may be different from that of ileal carcinoid. Carcinoid tumors of the rectum do not produce 5-HT. The carcinoid tumors of the bronchus, pancreas, and thyroid produce substances that may produce the carcinoid syndrome.

The liver usually deactivates the substances produced by carcinoid of the ileum, but metastatic lesions produce the substances that are delivered into the hepatic and the caval veins, which damage the heart and produce the full syndrome. Ovarian carcinoid tumors and tumors arising in other extraportal vein structures can deliver the damaging substances into the ovarian vein and inferior caval vein without metastasis to the liver. The carcinoid tumors produce numerous substances; some of these damage the heart, and others (vasoactive amines) produce flushing of the skin, bronchospasm, hypermobility of the intestine, and edema.

CARDIAC LESIONS

The right side of the heart is usually involved with lesions produced by ileal carcinoid (see Fig. 4.106). Lesions known as carcinoid plaques occur on the pulmonary valve, the tricuspid valve, and the endocardium. These lesions may be present on the left side in patients who have extensive right-sided involvement or have an interatrial communication. Bronchial carcinoids tend to produce lesions, especially of the mitral valve, on the left side of the heart.

The clinical manifestations are most unusual in that the patient has episodes of flushing and cardiac lesions. There may be evidence of severe right-sided heart disease with heart failure, evidence of pulmonary valve stenosis or regurgitation, and evidence of tricuspid regurgitation. Mitral stenosis and regurgitation may occur rarely.

CLINICAL MANIFESTATIONS.   The diagnosis is usually suspected clinically because the syndrome is unique and unforgettable. The unusual flushing of the skin plus evidence of pulmonary and tricuspid valve disease should always alert the physician to consider the carcinoid syndrome. Pellagra may occasionally be present, because tryptophan is diverted into the metabolic pathway that leads to the production of 5-HIAA, which is excreted in the urine.

Echocardiography (Fig. 13.22) and cardiac catheterization reveal clues to pulmonary and tricuspid valve abnormalities. CT scan usually reveals the metastatic lesions in the liver and carcinoid tumors of the ovary.

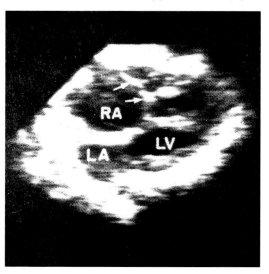

FIG. 13.22   *Subcostal cross-sectional long-axis echocardiogram of the tricuspid valve was recorded in a patient with the carcinoid syndrome. The valve leaflets* (arrows) *and cords are thickened. In this diastolic frame there is no evidence of valve opening. In real time the valve appeared completely fixed and stenotic, with no observable motion from diastole to systole. The right atrium* (RA) *is dilated* (LV, *left ventricle;* LA, *left atrium*). *(Reproduced with permission of the authors and publisher; see Figure Credits)*

TREATMENT. Although many drugs, such as alpha-adrenergic blockers and serotonin antagonists, have been used to block the substances that produce the flushing, none are entirely satisfactory. After liver metastasis has occurred, the ileal tumor is not surgically removed unless it is large and produces ileal obstruction. Removal of metastatic lesions on the liver is only temporarily beneficial. The removal of carcinoid of the ovary or a carcinoid located in some other extraportal vein area may be curative. Replacement of the diseased heart valves with prosthetic valves is beneficial. While carcinoid plaque may extend into the tissue valves, bioprostheses have been successful.

REFERENCES

Applefeld MM, Milner SD, Vigorito RD, Shamsuddin AKM (1980) Congestive heart failure and endocardial fibroelastosis caused by chronic lymphocytic leukemia. *Cancer* 46:1479.

Bjorkholm M, Ost A, Biberfeld P (1982) Myocardial rupture with cardiac tamponade as a lethal early manifestation of acute myeloblastic leukemia. *Cancer* 50:1967.

Bradham RR, Gregorie HB Jr, Howell JS Jr, Ribers CF Jr, Barnwell WH (1982) Aortic obstruction from embolizing cardiac myxoma. *J S C Med Assoc* 75:7.

Cassis N Jr, Porterfield J (1982) Massive hemopericardium as the initial manifestation of chronic myelogenous leukemia. *Arch Intern Med* 142:2193.

DeLoach JF, Haynes JW (1953) Secondary tumors of heart and pericardium: Review of the subject and report of one hundred thirty-seven cases. *Arch Intern Med* 91:224.

Hurst JW, Whitworth HB, O'Donoghue S, et al (1985) Heart disease due to ovarian carcinoid: Successful replacement of the pulmonary and tricuspid valves with porcine heterografts and removal of the tumor, in Hurst JW (ed): *Clinical Essays on the Heart,* vol 5, p 177. New York, McGraw-Hill.

Jamieson SW, Gaudiani VA, Reitz BA, et al (1981) Operative treatment of unresectable tumor of the left ventricle. *J Thorac Cardiovasc Surg* 81:797.

Kaminsky ME, Ehlers K, Engle ME, et al (1979) Atrial myxoma mimicking a collagen disorder. *Chest* 75:93.

Kopelson G, Herwig KJ (1978) The etiologies of coronary artery disease in cancer patients. *Int J Rad Oncol Biol Phys* 4:895.

Liu HY, Panidis I, Soffer J, Dreifus LS (1984) Echocardiographic diagnosis of intracardiac myxomas. *Chest* 84:63.

McAllister HA Jr (1979) Primary tumors and cysts of the heart and pericardium, in Harvey WP (ed): *Current Problems in Cardiology,* vol IV, no 2. Chicago, Year Book Medical Publishers.

McAllister HA Jr, Fenoglio JJ Jr (1978) *Tumors of the Cardiovascular System.* Armed Forces Institute of Pathology, Washington, D.C.

Meltzer V, Korompai FL, Mathur VS, Guinn GA (1975) Surgical treatment of leukemic involvement of the mitral valve. *Chest* 67:119.

Peters MN, Hall RJ, Cooley DA, et al (1974) The clinical syndrome of atrial myxoma. *JAMA* 230:694.

Roberts WC, Bodey GC, Wertlake PT (1968) The heart in acute leukemia: A study of 420 autopsy cases. *Am J Cardiol* 21: 388.

Wilcox BR, Carter JM (1971) Left ventricular myxoma: case report of successful removal. *Ann Surg* 173:131.

FIGURE CREDITS

TABLE 13.2 From McAllister HA Jr, Fenoglio JJ Jr: *Tumors of the Cardiovascular System.* Washington, DC, Armed Forces Institute of Pathology, 1978.

FIG. 13.2 From Becker AE, Anderson RH: *Cardiac Pathology.* New York, Raven Press, 1983, p 8.4.

FIG. 13.6 From Brandenburg RO: Office cardiology, in Brest AN (ed): *Cardiovascular Clinics.* Philadelphia, FA Davis, 1980, p 112.

FIG. 13.8 From Becker AE, Anderson RH: *Cardiac Pathology.* New York, Raven Press, 1983, p 8.5.

FIG. 13.9 From Becker AE, Anderson RH: *Cardiac Pathology.* New York, Raven Press, 1983, p 8.5.

FIG. 13.10 From Becker AE, Anderson RH: *Cardiac Pathology.* New York, Raven Press, 1983, p 8.6.

FIG. 13.12 From Becker AE, Anderson RH: *Cardiac Pathology.* New York, Raven Press, 1983, p 8.5.

FIG. 13.18 From Nasser FN, Giuliani, ER: *Clinical Two-Dimensional Echocardiography.* Chicago, Year Book Medical Publishers, 1983, p 185.

FIG. 13.22 From Weyman AE: *Cross-Sectional Echocardiography.* Philadelphia, Lea & Febiger, 1982, p 354.

14
THE HEART AND COLLAGEN VASCULAR DISEASE

J. Willis Hurst, MD
Bernadine P. Healy, MD
J. O'Neal Humphries, MD
Anton E. Becker, MD

Abstracted with permission of the authors and publisher from Bulkley BH, Humphries JO: The heart and collagen vascular disease, Chapter 73, pp 1435–1445, in Hurst JW (ed): *The Heart*, 6th ed. New York, McGraw-Hill, 1986. The table reprinted in this chapter from the above chapter is also reproduced with permission of the authors and publisher.

The collagen vascular diseases may affect the heart; the primary cardiac manifestations are listed in Table 14.1. Also called connective tissue disorders, they include systemic lupus erythematosus, progressive systemic sclerosis (scleroderma), polyarteritis nodosa, ankylosing spondylitis, and rheumatoid arthritis. Although the etiology of these conditions is not known, most seem to be the result of an immunologic disorder.

SYSTEMIC LUPUS ERYTHEMATOSUS
CLINICAL MANIFESTATIONS

Systemic lupus erythematosus (SLE) occurs most often in women between the ages of 20–40 years. The symptoms and signs depend on the organ that is initially or predominately involved. Accordingly the patient may have epilepsy, fever, arthritis, a characteristic skin rash (Fig. 14.1), pleurisy, pericarditis (frequently asymptomatic), myocarditis, or cardiac valve disease.

Pericarditis is a common manifestation of SLE; it is often the presenting clinical problem. Cardiac tamponade and constrictive pericarditis occur rarely. Immunosuppressed patients are at greater risk of purulent pericarditis.

Endocarditis associated with SLE was described by Libman and Sacks (1924) before its relationship to lupus was appreciated. These sterile vegetations may be located on both sides of any of the four valve leaflets, but they are more commonly located on the undersurface of the mitral valve. While these sterile lesions are similar to marantic endocarditis, focal necrosis of the valve leaflets and mononuclear infiltrates may occur (Fig. 14.2.). This type of endocarditis is more commonly observed at autopsy than it is diagnosed clinically. Healed stages of the lesions may lead to aortic or mitral regurgitation (Fig. 14.3). The sterile lesions are subject to infection in the immunosuppressed patient.

Myocarditis may occur rarely in patients with SLE. Heart failure, ventricular arrhythmias, and atrioventricular block occur rarely.

The small coronary arteries may be involved in SLE. Fibrinoid necrosis with thromboembolism may occur, but myocardial necrosis and

Table 14.1 Primary Cardiac Manifestations of the Collagen Vascular Diseases*

DISEASE	PERICARDIUM	MYOCARDIUM	ENDOCARDIUM (VALVES)	CORONARY ARTERIES
Systemic lupus erythematosus	+ +	+	+ +	+/−
Progressive systemic sclerosis	+	+ +	0	+ +
Polyarteritis nodosa	+/−	+	0	+ +
Ankylosing spondylitis	0	+/−	+ +	0
Rheumatoid arthritis	+ +	+	+	0

(Table 73-1, *The Heart*, 6th ed, p 1436)
*+ +, major site of involvement; +, may be involved, but less frequently; +/−, rarely involved; 0, not involved.

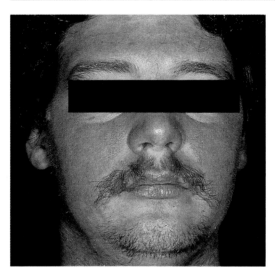

FIG. 14.1   *In this photograph of the face of a young man with SLE the intense erythema of the cheeks and the forehead following exposure to the sun is evident. This type of rash is often seen with the subacute variant of lupus erythematosus but was part of the clinical picture of this patient who had SLE. (Courtesy of Mark Holzberg, MD, Atlanta, Georgia)*

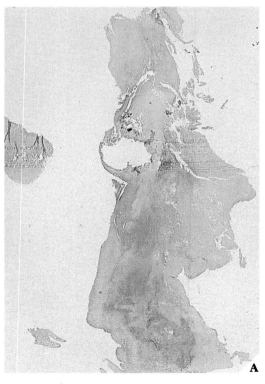

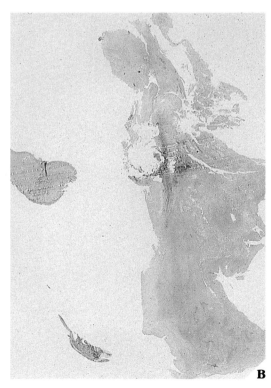

A

B

FIG. 14.2   (A, B) *These histologic sections of an aortic valve resected from a patient with SLE show evidence of necrosis of the valve tissue with a cellular infiltrate. Infective endocarditis is not present (A: elastic tissue stain; B: H&E stain).*

fibrosis are uncommon. James and colleagues (1965) reported arteritis of the sinus node artery with scarring of the sinus and the atrioventricular nodes. These abnormalities may be responsible for the arrhythmias and the conduction disturbances that are seen on rare occasion in patients with SLE.

Hypertension is a common occurrence in patients with renal lupus; it may cause left ventricular hypertrophy and heart failure. Pericarditis related to uremia may develop.

LABORATORY ABNORMALITIES

Patients with lupus erythematosus exhibit LE cells, antinuclear antibodies, anticytoplasmic antibodies, and rheumatoid factor in their blood. Serum complement is decreased. Biopsy of the kidney may reveal the different stages of a membranoproliferative (mesangiocapillary) glomerulonephritis (Fig. 14.4); a skin biopsy may show a dense linear deposition of immunoglobulins along the epidermal–dermal junction (Fig. 14.5).

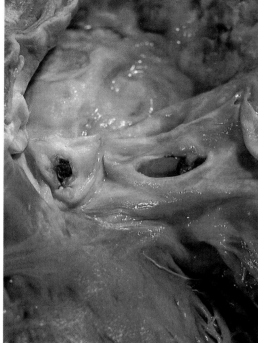

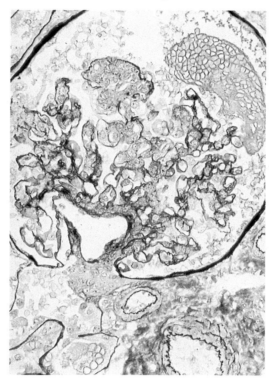

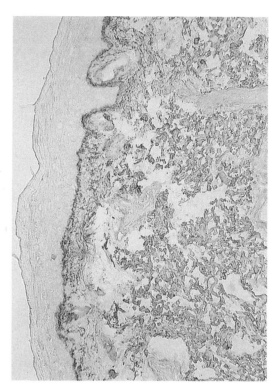

FIG. 14.3 *In the healed stage of Libman–Sacks endocarditis of the aortic valve punched-out holes remain in the semilunar cusps. The patient was known to have SLE. There were no positive signs for infective endocarditis, and the patient had not been treated with antibiotics.*

FIG. 14.4 *The histology of the glomerulus in the acute stage of SLE reveals extravasation of erythrocytes and early signs of a membranoproliferative (mesangiocapillary) glomerulonephritis (trichrome stain).*

FIG. 14.5 *Histologic section of a skin biopsy reveals a dense line of immunoglobulin deposits along the epidermal junction with an immunoperoxidase technique (C1q). The so-called lupus line suggests the diagnosis of SLE.*

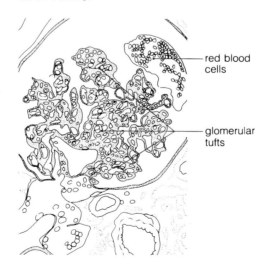

red blood cells

glomerular tufts

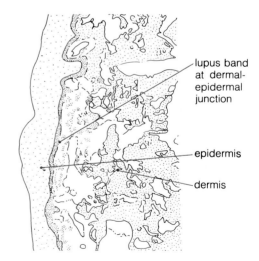

lupus band at dermal-epidermal junction

epidermis

dermis

TREATMENT

The usual treatment of SLE is cortisone; at times azathioprine and cyclophosphamide may be added. Pericardiocentesis may be needed for cardiac tamponade on rare occasion. Valve replacement may be necessary, although this too is uncommon.

PROGRESSIVE SYSTEMIC SCLEROSIS (SCLERODERMA)

CLINICAL MANIFESTATIONS

The vascular lesions of progressive systemic sclerosis produce fibrotic thickening of the skin, lesions of the fingertips and the fingers (Fig. 14.6), lesions of the esophagus, small bowel, large bowel, kidney, lung, and heart, and, usually, Raynaud's phenomenon. The CREST variant of scleroderma consists of calcinosis, Raynaud's phenomenon, esophageal abnormality, sclerodactyly, and telangiectasia.

In scleroderma the myocardium may show extensive fibrosis (Fig. 14.7); moreover, myofibrillar degeneration and contraction band changes may occur. These lesions suggest that temporary occlusion of the smaller coronary arteries has been followed by reperfusion. This has been referred to by Bulkley as Raynaud's phenomenon of the heart (*The Heart*, 6th ed, p 1442). The smaller arteries and arterioles throughout the body appear to undergo spasm for unknown reasons; this may be responsible for target organ damage in the heart as well as in other tissues. Patients with myocardial involvement have congestive heart failure, and are included in the group of patients with dilated cardiomyopathy. Patients may have angina pectoris, myocardial infarction, and sudden death; they are often misdiagnosed as having coronary atherosclerosis. Patients may have cardiac arrhythmias and conduction disturbances.

While pericarditis is often related to renal failure, primary pericarditis due to progressive systemic sclerosis does occur. Constrictive pericarditis may occur on rare occasion. Endocardial and valvar lesions almost never occur in these patients.

Patients with renal disease due to progressive systemic sclerosis develop hypertension, left ventricular hypertrophy, and heart failure.

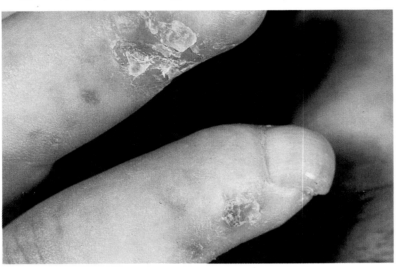

FIG. 14.6 *Photograph of the fingers of a patient with the CREST variant of progressive systemic sclerosis (scleroderma) demonstrates sclerodactyly and distal digital scars. (Courtesy of Mark Holzberg, MD, Atlanta, Georgia)*

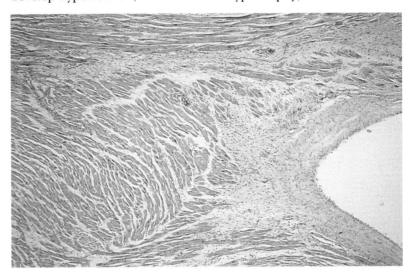

FIG. 14.7 *This histologic section demonstrates the nonspecific changes of diffuse myocardial fibrosis in scleroderma.*

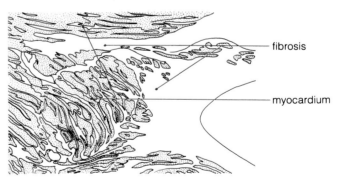

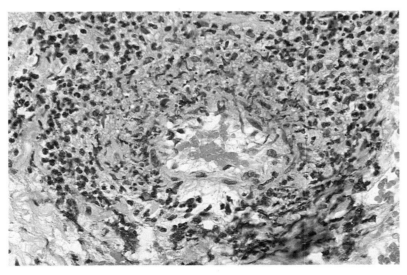

FIG. 14.8 *Histologic section of a skin biopsy from a patient with polyarteritis nodosa demonstrates a necrotizing arteritis (H&E stain).*

Pericarditis may be due to uremia. Patients with pulmonary disease due to progressive systemic sclerosis may develop cor pulmonale, right ventricular hypertrophy, and heart failure. Pulmonary arteriolar lesions may occur in the absence of pulmonary parenchymal disease. Lesions in the pulmonary arterioles may lead to a clinical syndrome that is similar to primary pulmonary hypertension. This is a serious form of the disease, and sudden death may occur.

LABORATORY ABNORMALITIES

Although the results of radiographic studies of the esophagus and the bowel may show abnormalities, biopsy of the skin and the kidney provides the most precise diagnosis.

TREATMENT

In general, treatment of scleroderma is unsatisfactory. Corticosteroids are of no value. The calcium channel blocker nifedipine may be useful for Raynaud's phenomenon that affects the fingers and the organs. Rhythm disturbances and heart failure are treated in the usual fashion.

(The reader is referred to Chapters 21 and 27 in *The Heart,* 6th ed, for further discussion of the management of heart failure, arrhythmias, and conduction abnormalities.)

POLYARTERITIS NODOSA
CLINICAL MANIFESTATIONS

Polyarteritis nodosa is a necrotizing arteritis of the small and the medium-sized arteries that leads to occlusion of vessels and, hence, may produce infarcts in multiple organs. Accordingly the skin (Fig. 14.8), gastrointestinal tract, kidneys (Figs. 14.9, 14.10), brain, spleen, lymph nodes, musculoskeletal system, and heart may be involved.

The epicardial and the subepicardial coronary arteries may also be involved in polyarteritis nodosa (Fig. 14.11). The inflammatory process extends through all arterial layers, leading to necrosis; inflammation is accompanied by thrombosis in the acute stage of the disease. Aneurysms of the coronary artery with thrombosis may appear in the healed stage. Myocardial infarction may occur. Since the disease has a ten-

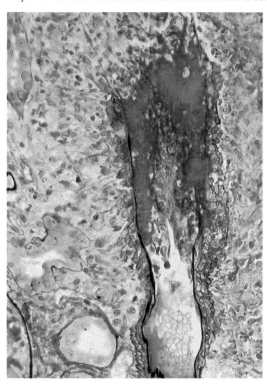

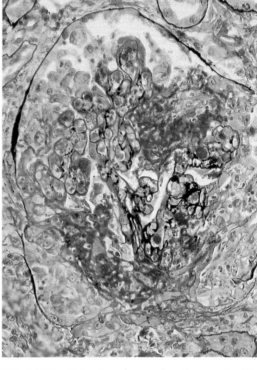

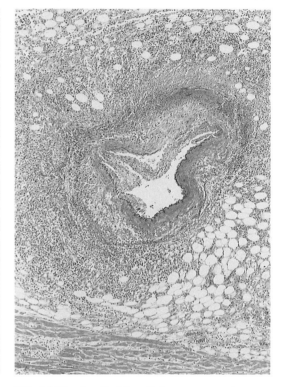

FIG. 14.9 *Histologic section shows fibrinoid necrosis of a small artery in the kidney in a patient with polyarteritis nodosa (trichrome stain).*

FIG. 14.10 *Extensive glomerular changes in this histologic section of polyarteritis nodosa are characterized by an extracapillary proliferation with vasculitis of the tufts (trichrome stain).*

FIG. 14.11 *Small epicardial coronary artery shows massive inflammatory disease with destruction of all wall layers in a patient with polyarteritis nodosa (elastic tissue stain).*

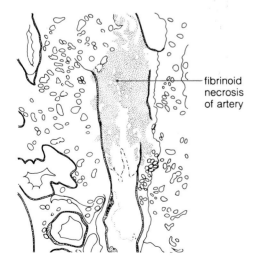

fibrinoid
necrosis
of artery

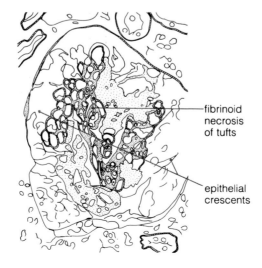

fibrinoid
necrosis
of tufts

epithelial
crescents

dency to affect multiple smaller-sized coronary arteries, the ischemic myocardial changes may be focal in nature.

Atrial arrhythmias and atrioventricular conduction defects occur when the arteries to the sinoatrial node and the atrioventricular node are involved.

Renal involvement with polyarteritis nodosa may result in hypertension, left ventricular hypertrophy, and heart failure. Kidney failure may produce uremia and pericarditis.

LABORATORY ABNORMALITIES

The sedimentation rate and the serum gamma globulin may be increased. Antinuclear antibodies and rheumatoid factor may be detected. The diagnosis is usually based on the clinical picture and biopsy.

TREATMENT

Treatment of polyarteritis nodosa is unsatisfactory. Corticosteroids are used; heart failure, myocardial infarction, and renal failure are treated in the usual fashion.

ANKYLOSING SPONDYLITIS

CLINICAL MANIFESTATIONS

Ankylosing spondylitis is due to inflammatory lesions of the spine, leading to chronic back pain, dorsal kyphosis, and fusion of the costovertebral and sacroiliac joints. An inflammatory lesion may involve the aortic root, extending into the region below the aortic valve and the basal portion of the mitral valve. This process may cause aortic or mitral regurgitation and atrioventricular block (Fig. 14.12). The longer the duration of ankylosing spondylitis, the more likely that aortic regurgitation will develop.

Almost all patients with ankylosing spondylitis have HLA-B27 histocompatibility antigen. This suggests a genetic linkage; it also indicates a relationship to Reiter's syndrome and juvenile arthritis.

TREATMENT

Corticosteroids are not indicated unless iritis occurs. Drugs such as indomethacin and phenylbutazone may provide symptomatic relief. Aortic regurgitation may become sufficiently severe to require aortic valve surgery, and a pacemaker may be needed for high-grade atrioventricular block.

RHEUMATOID ARTHRITIS

CLINICAL MANIFESTATIONS

This common collagen vascular disease, characterized by synovial inflammation that destroys the joints, is more common in women; it may be familial. The patient has pain and deformity of the joints of the hands, wrists, and upper and lower extremities (Fig. 14.13). The mandibulotemporal and the sternoclavicular joints may also be involved. Patients may have fever, weight loss, rheumatoid nodules, iritis,

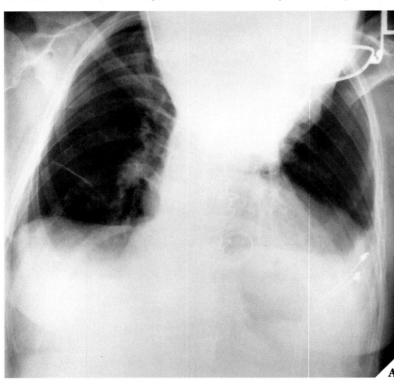

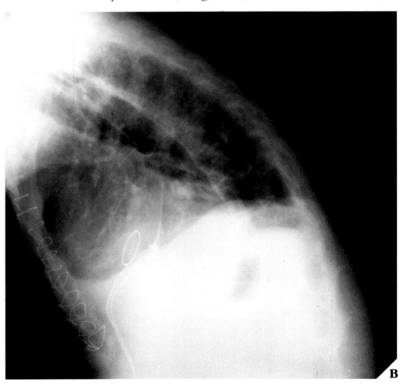

FIG. 14.12 (A) *Posteroanterior chest film of a 70-year-old man with severe ankylosing spondylitis, aortic regurgitation and complete heart block shows cardiac enlargement, the annular ring of the Hancock valve inserted in the aortic valve, and the electrodes of a cardiac pacemaker. The large dense area at the upper portion of the film is the patient's head. (B) Left lateral view shows cardiac enlargement, the annular ring in the aortic valve position, and the electrodes of a cardiac pacemaker. (Courtesy of William J. Casarella, MD, Atlanta, Georgia).*

rheumatoid lung disease, lymphadenopathy, pericarditis, pleurisy, heart disease, and arteritis.

Pericarditis and pericardial effusion may occur; cardiac tamponade and constrictive pericarditis are infrequent complications. Rheumatoid lung disease may occur, and rheumatic arteritis may produce disease of the gastrointestinal tract.

On rare occasion rheumatoid nodules may occur within the myocardium and heart valves (Figs. 14.14, 14.15). These lesions may produce sufficient myocardial damage and valvar insufficiency to produce heart failure, cardiac arrhythmias, and conduction defects. Amyloid involvement of the heart may also occur. The rheumatoid factor is usually present in the blood.

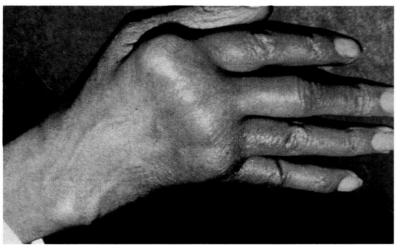

FIG. 14.13 *The hand of a patient with advanced rheumatoid arthritis demonstrates the typical appearance of the deformity associated with this condition. (Courtesy of William P. Maier, MD, Atlanta, Georgia)*

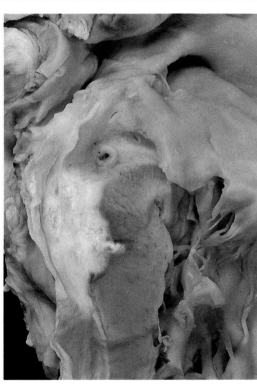

FIG. 14.14 *A rheumatoid nodule is located in the back of the heart, partially within the epicardium and partially within the mural myocardial wall.*

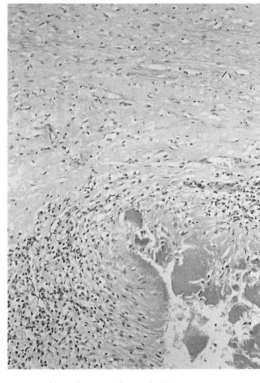

FIG. 14.15 *Histologic section of a rheumatoid nodule in the heart shows fibrinoid necrosis with a histiocytoid cellular reaction and peripheral fibrosis (H&E stain).*

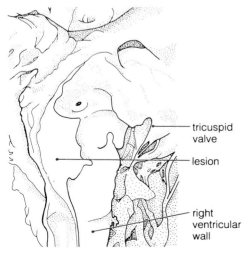

tricuspid valve

lesion

right ventricular wall

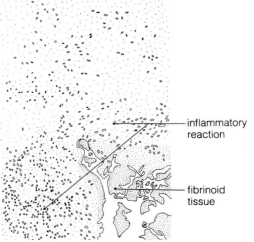

inflammatory reaction

fibrinoid tissue

TREATMENT

Numerous drugs including salicylates, indomethacin, corticosteroids, and others are used to treat this disease. Pericardiocentesis may be needed for cardiac tamponade, and constrictive pericarditis may require surgical intervention. Heart failure, cardiac arrhythmias, and conduction disturbances are treated in the conventional manner.

REFERENCES

James TN, Birk RE (1966) Pathology of the cardiac conduction system in polyarteritis nodosa. *Arch Intern Med* 117:561.

James TN, Rupe CE, Monto RW (1965) Pathology of the cardiac conduction system in systemic lupus erythematosus. *Ann Intern Med* 63:402.

Libman E, Sacks B (1924) A hitherto undescribed form of valvular and mural endocarditis. *Arch Intern Med* 33:701.

Liss JP, Bachmann WT (1970) Rheumatoid constrictive pericarditis treated by pericardiectomy: Report of a case and review of the literature. *Arthritis and Rheumatism* 13:869.

Paget SA, Bulkley BH, Grauer LE, Seningen R (1975) Mitral valve disease of systemic lupus erythematosus: A cause of severe congestive heart failure reversed by valve replacement. *Am J Med* 59:134.

15
THE HEART IN ATHLETES

J. Willis Hurst, MD
Andrew G. Wallace, MD
Anton E. Becker, MD

Abstracted with permission of the author and publisher from Wallace AG: The heart in athletes, Chapter 70, pp 1398–1403, in Hurst JW (ed): *The Heart*, 6th ed. New York, McGraw-Hill, 1986. Figures and extracts of text reprinted in this chapter from the above chapter are also reproduced with permission of the authors and publishers. For the full bibliographic citations of the sources of figures other than the above chapter, see Figure Credits at the end of this chapter.

EFFECT OF ACUTE DYNAMIC EXERCISE ON THE HEART AND CIRCULATION

The effect of dynamic exercise on the cardiac output and organ blood flow is depicted schematically in Fig. 15.1. One of the earliest consequences is a decreased resistance in the arterioles of skeletal muscles, which is due to a fall in Po_2 and to the release of vasodilator substances, such as potassium, lactic acid, CO_2, and adenosine.

There is a linear relationship between cardiac output and oxygen uptake (Fig. 15.2). Although the increase in cardiac output resulting from dynamic exercise is largely due to the increase in heart rate, other forces are operative, including the inotropic effect of increased sympathetic activity and the use of Frank–Starling forces. An increase in sympathetic activity produces arteriolar vasoconstriction in all areas except in the arterioles that supply the working muscles. The tone of the veins is also increased, which allows the venous system to enhance the venous return as the need is dictated by the right atrial pressure. Dynamic exercise also produces an increase in systolic arterial blood pressure and a decrease in diastolic pressure, resulting in a slight increase in the mean pressure.

The heat generated by working muscles is dissipated by the skin. Accordingly when dynamic exercise is intense and prolonged, dilation of the arterioles in the skin must occur in order for body heat to be controlled within safe limits. This is associated with an increase in heart rate and a drop in blood pressure, venous pressure, and stroke volume.

EFFECT OF TRAINING

Wallace discussed the physiological adaptation of the heart to endurance training as follows:

> The ability to enhance performance through training is well known. In recent years the scientific basis for this fact has been elucidated and the interest of the cardiologist has been addressed to the phenomenon.
>
> In the broadest sense, training involves enhancement of skill, strength, and endurance. It is the last of these that concerns us here. An earlier section of this chapter dealt with the changes in peripheral muscle and cardiovascular function when an individual makes the transition from rest to either submaximal or maximal sustained effort.
>
> Endurance training increases maximal aerobic capacity, i.e., maximal oxygen uptake. Since maximal oxygen uptake defines the functional capacity of the cardiovascular system and reflects the product of cardiac output and arteriovenous oxygen difference, it follows that a change in Vo_{2max} must reflect a corresponding change in maximal cardiac output

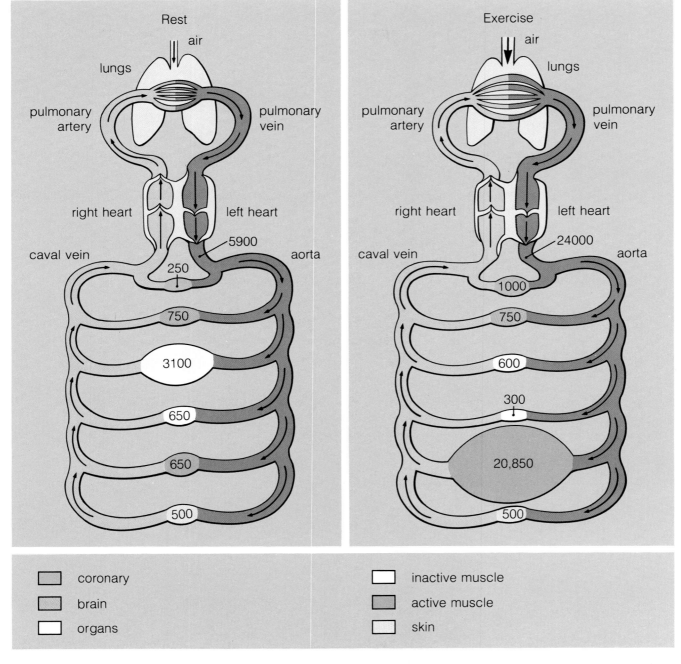

FIG. 15.1 *This schematic representation shows the cardiopulmonary system of a human in the resting state (left) and during peak upright exercise (right). Blood flow in milliliters per minute to each organ observed at rest and during maximal exercise is noted. (Redrawn; reproduced with permission of the authors and publisher; see Figure Credits. Also, Fig. 70-1, The Heart, 6th ed, p 1398)*

coronary

brain

organs

inactive muscle

active muscle

skin

or maximal extraction of oxygen by the periphery or both. The amount that Vo₂max increases with training is inversely proportional to the pre-conditioning Vo₂ and to age. For any given increase in Vo₂max due to conditioning, about half of the effect is attributable to a peripheral component, i.e., increased capacity to extract oxygen from arterial blood, and about half of the effect is due to increased perfusion. The peripheral component of this effect involves changes in skeletal muscle structure and metabolism. Numerous studies have shown that training increases the size and number of mitochondria per gram of muscle; the level of mitochondrial enzyme activity per gram of mitochondrial protein; the capacity of muscle to oxidize fat, carbohydrate, and ketones; myoglobin levels; and the capacity to generate ATP [Gollnick et al, 1971; Holloszy, 1976; Havel, 1971].

The central component of the training effect is characterized by a reduction in heart rate and blood pressure and an increase in stroke volume at any given submaximal workload [Clausen, 1977]. With maximal effort peak heart rate is unaltered by training, stroke volume is enhanced, and maximal arteriovenous oxygen difference is enhanced. The increased oxygen uptake is attributable almost equally to a widened arteriovenous oxygen difference and an increase in cardiac output. In world-class athletes maximal oxygen uptake is 65 to 85 ml/kg, and maximal cardiac output averages about 30 to 33 liters/min.

The hemodynamic and metabolic effects of training are accompanied by changes in cardiac dimensions and ultrastructure [Gilbert et al, 1975, 1977; Ehsani et al, 1978]. Cardiac size increases with training whether estimated by x-ray, by echocardiogram, or by angiography. Cardiac volume and mass increase. These are changes that can also be induced in experimental animals subjected to a training program. In one series the estimated left ventricular volume of distance runners was 60 percent greater than that of sedentary normal individuals. The left ventricular volume of distance runners was 60 percent greater than that of sedentary normal individuals. The left ventricular volume of distance swimmers was 80 percent greater than that of the control subjects. In experimental animals the ultrastructural changes that accompany hypertrophy induced by exercise have been analyzed carefully. The dimensions and volume of the myocyte appear to increase, and there is a proportional increase in myofibrils and mitochondria per cell. In summary, the structural changes appear to be physiological and are best represented as an extension of normal growth. (*The Heart*, 6th ed, p 1400)

THE ATHLETE'S HEART

The heart rate of a trained athlete is usually 40–60 beats per minute. There is often an increase in the respiratory variation of the heart rate,

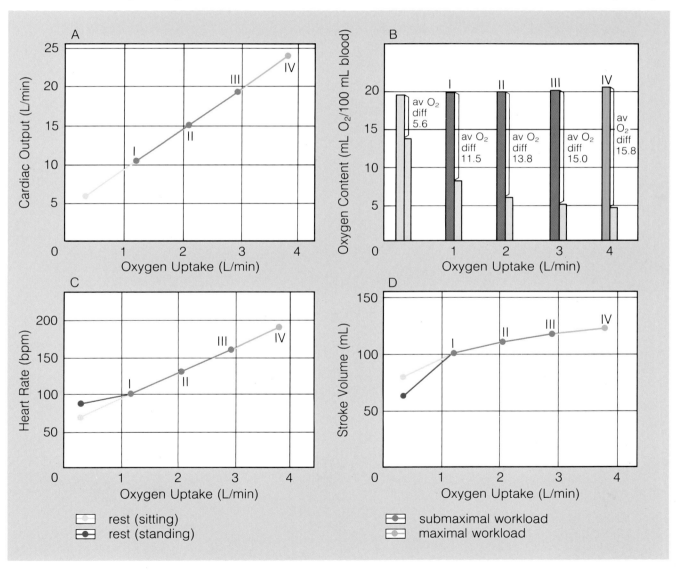

FIG. 15.2 *In these graphs of hemodynamic responses to upright exercise workload is shown as oxygen uptake on the horizontal axes; Roman numerals I to IV represent work states on the treadmill. (**A**) Changes in cardiac output. (**B**) Changes in arteriovenous oxygen difference (av O₂ diff). (**C**) Changes in heart rate. (**D**) Changes in stroke volume. (Redrawn; reproduced with permission of the authors and publisher; see Figure Credits. Also, Fig. 70-2, The Heart, 6th ed, p 1399)*

while the blood pressure and venous pressure are normal. The heart is slightly enlarged; this may be detected only on chest radiography or by echocardiography.

A ventricular gallop sound is often heard. A systolic ejection murmur is usually heard in the aortic and the pulmonary areas. Changes in the electrocardiogram may include sinus bradycardia, wandering atrial pacemaker, junctional or ventricular escape beats, increase in P-R interval, Wenckebach phenomenon, right or left atrial abnormalities, increased QRS amplitude suggesting ventricular hypertrophy, ST-segment change due to early repolarization, and an inverted T wave in leads V_1–V_3.

It is not always easy to separate idiopathic cardiac hypertrophy in an athlete from cardiac hypertrophy due to training.

SUDDEN DEATH IN ATHLETES

Sudden death of normal persons during exercise is rare. Hypertrophic cardiomyopathy appears to be a common cause of sudden death in athletes under the age of 30; over that age the cause is atherosclerotic coronary heart disease. A pathologic example of the heart of an endurance athlete who died during endurance exercise is shown in Figure 2.13.

REFERENCES

Clausen JP (1977) Effects of physical training on cardiovascular adjustments to exercise in man. *Physiol Rev* 57:779.

Ehsani AA, Hagbery JM, Hickson RC (1978) Rapid changes in left ventricular dimensions and mass in response to physical conditioning and deconditioning. *Am J Cardiol* 42:52.

Gilbert CA, Nutter DO, Felner JM (1977) Echocardiographic study of cardiac dimensions and function in the endurance trained athlete. *Am J Cardiol* 40:528.

Gilbert CA, Nutter S, Meymsfield S, Perkins J, Schlant R (1975) The endurance athlete: Cardiac structure and function. *Circulation* 51(suppl 2):115.

Gollnick PD, Ianuzzo CD, King DW (1971) Ultrastructure and enzyme changes in muscle with exercise, in *Advances in Experimental Medicine and Biology,* vol II, p 69. New York, Plenum Press.

Havel RJ (1971) Influence of intensity and duration of exercise on supply and use of fuels, in *Advances in Experimental Medicine and Biology,* vol II, p 315. New York, Plenum Press.

Holloszy JO (1976) Adaptations to muscular tissue training. *Prog Cardiovasc Dis* 18:445.

Kennedy HL, Whitlock JA, Buckingham TA (1984) Cardiovascular sudden death in young persons. *J Am Coll Cardiol* 3:485.

Spirito P, Maron BJ, Bonow RO, Epstein SE (1983) Prevalence of and significance of abnormal ST segment responses to exercise in a young athletic population. *Am J Cardiol* 51:166.

Thompson PD, Stern MP, Williams P, Duncan K, Haskell WL, Wood PD (1979) Death during jogging or running. *JAMA* 242:1265.

Waller BF, Newhouse P, Pless J, Foster L, Wills E (1984) Exercise related sudden death in 27 conditioned subjects aged less than 30 and greater than 30 years: Coronary abnormalities are the culprit. *J Am Coll Cardiol* 3:621.

FIGURE CREDITS

FIG. 15.1 Redrawn from Mitchell JH, Blomqvist G: Maximal oxygen uptake. *N Engl J Med* 284:1018, 1971.

FIG. 15.2 Redrawn from Mitchell JH, Blomqvist G: Maximal oxygen uptake. *N Engl J Med* 284:1018, 1971.

16
AGING OF THE CARDIOVASCULAR SYSTEM

J. Willis Hurst, MD
Myron L. Weisfeldt, MD
Gary Gerstenblith, MD

Abstracted with permission of the authors and publisher from Weisfeldt ML, Gerstenblith G: Cardiovascular aging and adaptation to disease, Chapter 71, pp 1403–1411, in Hurst JW (ed): *The Heart,* 6th ed. New York, McGraw-Hill, 1986. Figures and tables reprinted in this chapter from the above chapter are also reproduced with permission of the authors and publisher.

NORMAL CARDIOVASCULAR AGING

Although it is difficult to separate the effect of disease on the heart of the elderly patient from the aging process itself, there is increasing evidence that the old heart does not function as well as the young heart. Much of the data to support this view result from animal experimentation, as well as from human investigation. The following brief discussion highlights some information on the subject.

In an aging rat the rate of rise in tension and the maximum tension in the isolated cardiac muscle does not change with age (Fig. 16.1). However, the duration of ventricular contraction is prolonged because of delayed and slowed relaxation.

These findings parallel the results of studies in aging humans utilizing radionuclear scintigraphy and echocardiography, which indicate that indices of left ventricular function are maintained, but cardiac muscle relaxation is prolonged. Even this does not alter cardiac function to a significant degree unless there is underlying heart disease. Then prolonged relaxation may decrease the amount of blood flow to the subendocardial area (see Chapter 2); this is especially likely in the clinical setting of hypertension or tachycardia.

Hearts from senescent experimental animals exhibit a decrease in the inotropic response to digitalis and catecholamines. The chronotropic response to catecholamines is also diminished in hearts from aged animals compared to young. However, the shortening of the duration of contraction induced by catecholamines is unaffected by aging (Fig. 16.2).

There is decreased compliance of the arterial walls in the peripheral circulation of elderly people. Because this causes increased pulse wave velocity, it is a major factor in the production of systolic hypertension in the aged.

The factors that contribute to increased cardiac output during exercise are listed in Table 16.1. There is an increase in the dependence on the Frank–Starling mechanism to maintain cardiac output in the elderly. Healthy elderly people do not increase their ejection fractions with exercise to the same extent that young people do. Accordingly one must not assume that an elderly patient who cannot increase his or her ejection fraction with exercise has coronary disease.

The clinician should remember that although the aging heart may function well in the absence of heart disease, it may not be able to adapt to disease as well as the young heart can.

HEART DISEASE IN THE ELDERLY

Systolic hypertension is common in the elderly. The systolic pressure may rise to even higher levels with exercise; this may be responsible for the mild left ventricular hypertrophy that commonly occurs in aged individuals. Increasingly it is believed that systolic hypertension

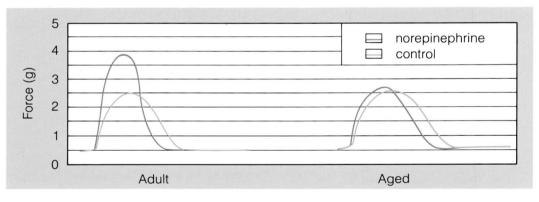

FIG. 16.1 *In this graph a typical isometric twitch of an isolated cardiac muscle from a young adult rat is compared with that of an aged rat. The rate of rise in tension and maximum tension achieved do not differ with age, but the duration of contraction is prolonged, primarily due to slowed and delayed relaxation. (Redrawn; Fig. 71-1,* The Heart, *6th ed, p 1404)*

FIG. 16.2 *Typical isometric twitches in isolated cardiac muscles from a young adult rat and in an aged rat are compared before and after exposure to norepinephrine. There are no significant increases in maximum tension or rate of tension development in the aged muscle, although the enhanced relaxation effect due to catecholamines is relatively unaffected by age. (Redrawn; Fig. 71-2,* The Heart, *6th ed, p 1406)*

Table 16.1 Factors Contributing to Increased Cardiac Output	
YOUNG HEART DURING EXERCISE	AGED HEART AT SAME WORKLOAD
Increased heart rate	Lower heart rate
Decreased afterload	Larger end-systolic volume
Increased inotropy	
Use of Frank-Starling mechanism	Larger end-diastolic and stroke volumes

(Modified; Fig. 71-3, *The Heart,* 6th ed, p 1408)

in the elderly should be treated with drugs whose primary effect is vasodilatory. The response to treatment, however, is not always pleasant and safe. Accordingly the treatment of an elderly patient must be individualized by the responsible physician.

While coronary atherosclerosis is not solely due to the aging process, this disease is more severe in the aged, and coronary events have a worse prognosis. Whereas there may be more collateral coronary circulation in the elderly than in the young, this does not fully protect the patient, and it should be considered a sign of extensive coronary disease. The clinician must remember that the diagnosis of angina is more difficult in the elderly than in the middle-aged because of inactivity and occasionally poor memory of the former.

Valvar heart disease of the elderly is predominately aortic stenosis, although mitral stenosis occurs rarely. Aortic stenosis under the age of 60–70 years is usually due to a congenital bicuspid aortic valve; after age 70 it is usually due to degenerative disease of the valve. Calcification plays an important role regardless of the etiology. Aggressive or rapidly accelerating aortic stenosis may occur. Increasingly there are reports of aortic stenosis with a left ventricular–aortic gradient of 50 mmHg that advances in one year or less to 80 mmHg. The clinician must also remember that idiopathic hypertrophic subaortic stenosis may occur in the elderly. The treatment of aortic stenosis in the elderly is discussed above (Chapter 4). Surgical replacement of the valve is undertaken for the usual indications, including heart failure, syncope, and angina. When coronary bypass surgery is performed, it is usually wise to replace the aortic valve when the left ventricular–aortic gradient is 40–60 mmHg; this may prevent the need for later reoperation for accelerated aortic stenosis. The elderly patient may also be a candidate for balloon dilation of the aortic valve (Cribier et al, 1986). Percutaneous catheter commissurotomy of the mitral valve is currently under investigation (Lock et al, 1985).

REFERENCES

Cribier A, Souudi N, Berland J, et al (1986) Percutaneous transluminal valvuloplasty of acquired aortic stenosis in elderly patients: An alternative to valve replacement? *Lancet* 1:63.

Lock JE, Khalilullah M, Shrivastava S, et al (1985) Percutaneous catheter commissurotomy in rheumatic mitral stenosis. *N Engl J Med* 313:1515.

McKay RG, Safian RD, Lock JE, et al (1986) Balloon dilatation of calcific aortic stenosis in elderly patients: Postmortem, intraoperative, and percutaneous valvuloplasty studies. *Circulation* 74:119.

Rodeheffer RJ, Gerstenblith G, Becker LC, et al (1984) Exercise cardiac output is maintained with advancing age in healthy human subjects: Cardiac dilatation and increased stroke volume compensate for a diminished heart rate. *Circulation* 69:203.

Weisfeldt ML, Loeven WA, Shock NW (1971) Resting and active mechanical properties of trabeculae carneae from aged male rats. *Am J Physiol* 220:1921.

17
THE HEART AND OBESITY

J. Willis Hurst, MD
James K. Alexander, MD
Anton E. Becker, MD

Abstracted with permission of the author and publisher from Alexander JK: The heart and obesity, Chapter 75, pp 1452–1458, in Hurst JW (ed): *The Heart,* 6th ed. New York, McGraw-Hill, 1986.

Obesity is either responsible for or aggravates several serious conditions. Even the lay public recognizes the harmful effect of obesity on diabetes mellitus. The purpose of this brief chapter is to emphasize the relationship of obesity to hypertension, coronary disease, and cardiomyopathy.

HYPERTENSION AND OBESITY

A good estimate of blood pressure can be obtained in obese patients if a 42-cm wide blood pressure cuff is used. There appears to be a type of hypertension that occurs in the obese that differs from essential or renovascular hypertension, since blood volume and renin levels in obese patients do not correlate with the presence or absence of hypertension. Furthermore systemic vascular resistance is lower in fat people than in lean people. Blood pressure may be lowered by weight reduction in about 50% of obese patients with hypertension.

CORONARY DISEASE AND OBESITY

The obese patient with angina pectoris due to coronary atherosclerosis is likely to have less angina when extra weight is significantly diminished. In addition, diabetes mellitus following weight reduction is more easily controlled with less insulin.

An argument still exists as to whether obesity is an independent risk factor for coronary atherosclerotic heart disease. Hubert and colleagues (1983) have presented evidence that it is; Alexander (1985), on the other hand, has reviewed the evidence accrued from other epidemiologic studies, as well as angiographic and pathologic studies, and has concluded that obesity is not an independent risk factor. Barrett-Connor (1985) reached the same conclusion. Until the issue is settled, one can state that while obesity is not consistently predictive of ischemic heart disease, persons with higher relative weight and body mass indices are more likely to have an unfavorable risk factor status for heart disease.

CARDIOMYOPATHY OF OBESITY

Obese patients have left ventricular hypertrophy and, at times, right ventricular hypertrophy. Heart failure is often seen in extremely obese patients. Fatty infiltration of the heart muscle, including the conduction system, may be seen, but this abnormality rarely causes any difficulty (Fig. 17.1).

Patients who are extremely obese have altered hemodynamics. Notably there is an increase in circulating blood volume, a normal or slightly increased hematocrit, increased cardiac output, an increase in

stroke volume, and a slight increase in the arteriovenous oxygen difference, as compared to subjects of normal weight. Cerebral blood flow is normal; renal blood flow may be slightly less than it is in normal subjects. The splanchnic blood flow, in contrast, may be increased as compared with subjects who are not obese.

The majority of extremely obese patients have pulmonary hypertension and systemic hypertension with high cardiac output. The left ventricular end-diastolic pressure is elevated both at rest and during exercise. Recent studies indicate that the heart failure seen in extremely obese patients may be due to one of two mechanisms. Some patients develop "diastolic" heart failure because of volume overload in the setting of decreased ventricular compliance. Other patients develop heart failure associated with myocardial systolic dysfunction. The prognosis appears to be better in those patients with diastolic dysfunction of the myocardium. The two types of heart failure can be distinguished by echocardiography, nuclear scanning, or angiography.

These patients may have recurrent bouts of worsening heart failure or sudden death, the latter perhaps as a consequence of atrial arrhythmias and conduction defects. (The reader is referred to *The Heart,* 6th ed, pp 1453–1454, for further discussion of the cardiomyopathy of obesity.)

SLEEP APNEA

About half of patients with sleep apnea are obese. The condition occurs more often in middle-aged men than women. The systemic and pulmonary blood pressures rise during apnea; at the same time the P_{O_2} decreases and the P_{CO_2} rises. Cardiac arrhythmias, such as sinus arrest, asystole, high-grade atrioventricular block, and ventricular tachycardia, also occur, possibly precipitating sudden death.

OBESITY HYPOVENTILATION SYNDROME

A small percent of obese patients have hypoventilation, hypoxemia, hypercarbia, respiratory acidosis, and erythrocytosis. This chronic syndrome often begins with sleep apnea, which dulls the hypoxic drive for ventilation. There is also decreased chest wall compliance, an increase in the work of breathing, and a decrease in the ventilatory response to CO_2. Chronic hypoxemia induces pulmonary arteriolar constriction, which, when added to the hemodynamic effects of obesity, imposes an increase in pulmonary and arterial venous pressures. This all leads to biventricular hypertrophy and failure; rarely these are associated with predominant right ventricular dysfunction. Treatment consists of weight reduction, which may result in regression of left ventricular hypertrophy.

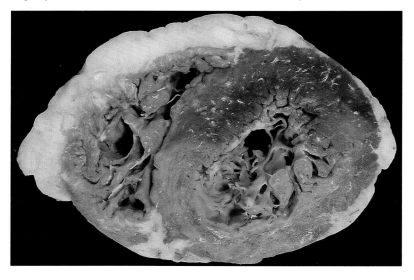

FIG. 17.1 *The heart of an obese patient displays excessive epicardial fat deposition with infiltration of myocardium. With the macro-enzyme staining technique viable myocardium stains purple.*

REFERENCES

Alexander JK (1985) Obesity and coronary heart disease, in Connor WE, Bristow JD (eds): *Coronary Heart Disease, Prevention, Complications and Treatment.* Philadelphia, Lippincott.

Alexander JK, Peterson KL (1972) Cardiovascular effects of weight reduction. *Circulation* 45:310.

Alexander JK, Pettigrove JR (1967) Obesity and congestive heart failure. *Geriatrics* 22:101.

Alexander JK, Woodard CB, Quinones MA, Gaasch WH (1978) Heart failure from obesity, in Mancini M, Lewis B, Cantaldo F (eds): *Medical Complications of Obesity.* London, Academic Press.

Balsaver AM, Morales AR, Whitehouse FW (1967) Fat infiltration of myocardium as a cause of cardiac conduction defect. *Am J Cardiol* 19:216.

Barrett-Connor EL (1985) Obesity, atherosclerosis and coronary artery disease. *Ann Intern Med* 101:1010.

Hubert HB, Feinleib M, McNamara PM, Castelli WP (1983) Obesity as an independent risk factor for cardiovascular disease: A 26-year follow-up of participants in the Framingham Heart Study. *Circulation* 67:968.

Kryger M, Quesney LP, Holder D, et al (1974) The sleep deprivation syndrome of the obese patient. *Am J Med* 56:531.

Schroeder JS, Motta J, Guilleminault C (1978) Hemodynamic studies in sleep apnea, in Guilleminault C, Dement WC (eds): *Sleep Syndromes.* New York, Alan R. Liss.

Tilkian A, Motta J, Guilleminault C (1978) Cardiac arrhythmias, in Guilleminault C, Dement WC (eds): *Sleep Syndromes.* New York, Alan R. Liss.

18
THE HEART AND ALCOHOL

J. Willis Hurst, MD
Timothy J. Regan, MD
Anton E. Becker, MD

Abstracted with permission of the author and publisher from Regan TJ: The heart, alcoholism, and nutritional disease, Chapter 74, pp 1446–1451, in Hurst JW (ed): *The Heart,* 6th ed. New York, McGraw-Hill, 1986.

Paul White (1951) was among the first to call attention to the relationship of alcohol and cardiac dysfunction, arrhythmias, and angina. The advent of modern technology has permitted the identification of certain cardiac abnormalities that may be related to overconsumption of alcohol of any type.

ALCOHOLIC CARDIOMYOPATHY
ETIOLOGY AND PATHOLOGY
The patient with alcoholic cardiomyopathy has ingested alcohol for many years. It is not possible to state that all patients who have cardiomyopathy and drink alcohol have alcoholic cardiomyopathy, because such patients often have hypertension or they may have had unrecognized viral myocarditis. There is, however, an increasing body of circumstantial evidence indicating that alcohol is harmful to the myocardium in certain susceptible patients. The biochemical derangement produced by alcohol within the myocardial cell is discussed by Sarma and colleagues (1976).

Prior to the development of heart failure the asymptomatic alcoholic patient exhibits reduced cardiac contractility (Regan et al, 1969). Early in the course of the illness the echocardiogram reveals a normal internal diameter of the left ventricle and increased ventricular wall thickness. Later in the illness there is evidence of an increase in the internal diameter of the heart with a normal ventricular wall thickness (Matthews et al, 1981).

The gross and microscopic pathology of the cardiomyopathy associated with alcohol abuse is nonspecific. In advanced stages the heart usually exhibits features of dilated cardiomyopathy (Fig. 18.1).

CLINICAL MANIFESTATIONS
The clinical features are those of dilated cardiomyopathy (see Chapter 5). The heart is enlarged with no diagnostic murmurs; atrial and ventricular gallop sounds may be heard. The chest radiograph shows a large heart with or without pulmonary congestion. The electrocardiogram (ECG) may show atrial fibrillation, other arrhythmias, or bundle branch block, while the echocardiogram displays a decrease in cardiac contractility. Heart failure ensues, gradually worsening over a period of months and years. Sudden death is common.

TREATMENT
The outcome of the treatment of alcoholic cardiomyopathy is poor. Patients may improve if abstinence from alcohol can be achieved and if the heart damage is not too advanced. Digitalis is not very useful, unless there is atrial fibrillation. Drugs to reduce afterload, diuretics, and drugs to control arrhythmias are useful. A few patients who abstain from alcohol may be candidates for cardiac transplantation. However, alcoholic patients often have damage to other organs, and there are no assurances that abstinence will be permanent.

CARDIAC ARRHYTHMIAS RELATED TO ALCOHOL
CLINICAL MANIFESTATIONS AND TREATMENT
A cardiac arrhythmia may be the first sign of alcoholic heart disease, although it is not usually appreciated as such at the time. Patients with the "holiday heart" syndrome may not have clinical signs of cardiomyopathy (Ettinger et al, 1978). These patients are often chronic users of alcohol who have cardiac arrhythmias in association with an acute binge. Supraventricular arrhythmias predominate, most commonly atrial fibrillation. Other arrhythmias and sudden death may occur. The exact chemical derangement that is responsible for the arrhythmias is not known.

The treatment of arrhythmias consists of correcting electrolyte abnormalities, including potassium and magnesium deficiencies. Propranolol may be useful, but it may decrease myocardial contractility (Zilm et al, 1980).

REFERENCES
Ettinger PO, Wu CF, de La Cruz C Jr, et al (1978) Arrhythmias and the "holiday heart": Alcohol-associated cardiac rhythm disorders. *Am Heart J* 95:555.

Matthews EC Jr, Gardin JM, Henry WL, et al (1981) Echocardiographic abnormalities in chronic alcoholics with and without overt congestive heart failure. *Am J Cardiol* 47:570.

Regan TJ, Levinson GE, Oldewurtel HA, et al (1969) Ventricular function in noncardiacs with alcoholic fatty liver: Role of ethanol in the production of cardiomyopathy. *J Clin Invest* 48:397.

Sarma JSM, Shigeaki I, Fischer R, et al (1976) Biochemical and contractile properties of heart muscle after prolonged alcohol administration. *J Mol Cell Cardiol* 8:951.

White P (1951) *Heart Disease.* New York, Macmillan, p 597.

Zilm DH, Jacob MS, Macleod SM, et al (1980) Propranolol and chlordiazepoxide effects on cardiac arrhythmias during alcohol withdrawal. *Alcoholism: Clin Exp Res* 4:400.

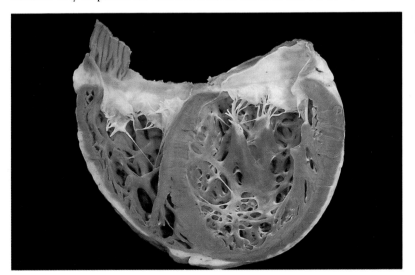

FIG. 18.1 *Cross-section of the heart of a patient with chronic alcohol abuse shows dilation of both ventricular chambers, which is also seen in other types of dilated cardiomyopathy.*

INDEX